ENDOCRINOLOGY

ENDOCRINOLOGY

Basic and Clinical Principles

SECOND EDITION

Edited by

SHLOMO MELMED, MD

*Cedars Sinai Medical Center
and UCLA School of Medicine*

P. MICHAEL CONN, PhD

*Oregon Health & Science University
Beaverton, OR*

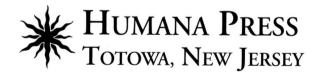

HUMANA PRESS
TOTOWA, NEW JERSEY

Cover design by Patricia F. Cleary.

This publication is printed on acid-free paper. ∞
ANSI Z39.48-1984 (American National Standards Institute) Permanence of Paper for Printed Library Materials.

Photocopy Authorization Policy:
Authorization to photocopy items for internal or personal use, or the internal or personal use of specific clients, is granted by Humana Press Inc., provided that the base fee of US $30 is paid directly to the Copyright Clearance Center at 222 Rosewood Drive, Danvers, MA 01923. For those organizations that have been granted a photocopy license from the CCC, a separate system of payment has been arranged and is acceptable to Humana Press Inc. The fee code for users of the Transactional Reporting Service is: [1-58829-427-7/05 $30].

Printed in the United States of America. 10 9 8 7 6 5 4 3 2 1

Library of Congress Cataloging-in-Publication Data
Endocrinology : basic and clinical principles / edited by Shlomo Melmed, P. Michael Conn.— 2nd ed.
    p. cm.
  Includes bibliographical references and index.
  ISBN 1-58829-427-7 (alk. paper) eISBN 1-59259-829-3
  1. Endocrinology. 2. Hormones. 3. Endocrine glands—Diseases. I. Melmed, Shlomo. II. Conn, P. Michael.
  QP187.E555 2005
  612.4—dc22   2004018638

PREFACE

Endocrinology: Basic and Clinical Principles, Second Edition aims to provide a comprehensive knowledge base for the applied and clinical science of endocrinology. The challenge in its presentation was to produce a volume that was timely, provided integration of basic science with physiologic and clinical principles, and yet was limited to 500 pages. This length makes the volume suitable as a text; and the timeliness we have striven for allows the book to serve as an off-the-shelf reference. Our goal was achieved largely through the selection of authors who are both expert writers and teachers. Tables and illustrative matter were used optimally to present information in a concise and comparative format.

Endocrinology: Basic and Clinical Principles, Second Edition will be useful to physicians and scientists as well as to students who wish to have a high-quality, current reference to the general field of endocrinology. The use of an outline system and a comprehensive index will allow readers to locate promptly topics of particular interest. Key references are provided throughout for individuals requiring more in-depth information. The volume covers the comprehensive spectrum of current knowledge of hormone production and action, even including nonmammalian systems and plants, coverage rarely included in similar volumes.

The editors wish to express appreciation to our distinguished chapter authors for their efforts, as well as diligently meeting publication deadlines and to the staff at Humana Press for their cooperation and useful suggestions.

Shlomo Melmed
P. Michael Conn

CONTENTS

Part IV.   Hypothalamic–Pituitary

CONTRIBUTORS

RICARDO AZZIZ, MD, MPH, MBA • *Department of Obstetrics and Gynecology, Cedars-Sinai Medical Center, UCLA School of Medicine, Los Angeles, CA*

RACHEL L. BATTERHAM, MBBS, PhD • *University College London, London, UK*

DANIEL G. BICHET, MD • *Clinical Research Unit and Nephrology Service, Hospital du Sacre-Coeur de Montreal, Montreal, Canada*

GLENN D. BRAUNSTEIN, MD • *Department of Medicine, Cedars-Sinai Medical Center, UCLA School of Medicine, Los Angeles, CA*

GREGORY A. BRENT, MD • *Departments of Medicine and Physiology, UCLA School of Medicine, Los Angeles, CA*

GEORGE P. CHROUSOS, PhD • *National Institute of Child Health & Human Development, National Institutes of Health, Bethesda, MD*

P. MICHAEL CONN, PhD • *Oregon National Primate Research Center, Oregon Health and Science University, Beaverton, OR*

MICHAEL A. COWLEY, PhD • *Oregon National Primate Research Center, Oregon Health and Science University, Beaverton, OR*

LAWRENCE I. GILBERT, PhD • *Department of Biology, University of North Carolina, Chapel Hill, NC*

MICHAEL S. HARBUZ, PhD • *Department of Medicine, Henry Wellcome Laboratories for Integrated Neuroscience and Endocrinology, University of Bristol, Bristol, UK*

ANTHONY P. HEANEY, MD, PhD • *Division of Endocrinology and Metabolism, Cedars-Sinai Medical Center, UCLA School of Medicine, Los Angeles, CA*

GEOFFREY N. HENDY, PhD • *Department of Medicine, Royal Victoria Hospital, McGill University, Montreal, Canada*

DEREK V. HENLEY, PhD • *Laboratory of Reproductive and Developmental Toxicology, National Institute of Environmental Health Sciences, National Institutes of Health, Research Triangle Park, NC*

AMIYA SINHA HIKIM, PhD • *Division of Endocrinology, Department of Medicine, Harbor-UCLA Medical Center and Education and Research Institute, UCLA School of Medicine, Torrance, CA*

HONGXIANG HUI, MD, PhD • *Division of Endocrinology, Cedars-Sinai Medical Center, UCLA School of Medicine, Los Angeles, CA*

TAKAHIKO KOGAI, MD, PhD • *Division of Endocrinology and Diabetes, VA Greater Los Angeles Healthcare System, UCLA School of Medicine, Los Angeles, CA*

KENNETH S. KORACH, PhD • *Laboratory of Reproductive and Developmental Toxicology, National Institute of Environmental Health Sciences, National Institutes of Health, Research Triangle Park, NC*

ASHIM KUMAR, MD • *Department of Obstetrics and Gynecology, Cedars-Sinai Medical Center, UCLA School of Medicine, Los Angeles, CA*

STEVEN W. J. LAMBERTS, MD, PhD • *Department of Medicine, Erasmus Medical Center, Rotterdam, The Netherlands*

DEREK LEROITH, MD, PhD • *Diabetes Branch, National Institutes of Health, Bethesda, MA*

STAFFORD L. LIGHTMAN, PhD • *Department of Medicine, Henry Wellcome Laboratories for Integrated Neuroscience and Endocrinology, University of Bristol, Bristol, UK*

JONATHAN LINDZEY, PhD • *Department of Natural Sciences, Clayton College and State University, Morrow, GA*

WILLIAM L. LOWE JR., MD • *Department of Medicine, Northwestern University Medical School, Chicago, IL*

DENIS MAGOFFIN, PhD • *Department of Obstetrics and Gynecology, Cedars-Sinai Medical Center, UCLA School of Medicine, Los Angeles, CA*

KELLY E. MAYO, PhD • *Department of Biochemistry, Molecular Biology, and Cell Biology, Center for Reproductive Science, Northwestern University, Evanston, IL*

JOHN A. MCCRACKEN, PhD • *University of Connecticut, Storrs, CT*

SHLOMO MELMED, MD • *Division of Endocrinology and Metabolism, Cedars-Sinai Medical Center, UCLA School of Medicine, Los Angeles, CA*

MASASHI MUKOYAMA, MD, PhD • *Department of Medicine and Clinical Science, Kyoto University Graduate School of Medicine, Kyoto, Japan*

KAZUWA NAKAO, MD, PhD • *Department of Medicine and Clinical Science, Kyoto University Graduate School of Medicine, Kyoto, Japan*

KLAUS PALME, PhD • *Institute for Biology, Albert-Ludwigs-Universität Freiburg, Freiburg, Germany*

IVAN PAPONOV, PhD • *Institute for Biology, Albert-Ludwigs-Universität Freiburg, Freiburg, Germany*

RICHARD J. PIETRAS, MD, PhD • *Department of Medicine, Division of Hematology-Oncology, Jonsson Comprehensive Cancer Center, UCLA School of Medicine, Los Angeles, CA*

WILLIAM J. RAUM, MD, PhD • *Departments of Medicine and Surgery, Louisiana State University Medical Center, New Orleans, LA*

WILLIS K. SAMSON, PhD • *Department of Pharmacologic and Physiologic Science, St. Louis University School of Medicine, St. Louis, MO*

NEENA B. SCHWARTZ, PhD • *Department of Neurobiology and Physiology, Northwestern University, Evanston, IL*

ILAN SHIMON, MD • *Institute of Endocrinology, Sheba Medical Center, Tel-Hashomer, Israel*

ELIOT R. SPINDEL, MD, PhD • *Oregon National Primate Research Center, Oregon Health and Science University, Beaverton, OR*

FREDRICK STORMSHAK, PhD • *Departments of Biochemistry/Biophysics and Animal Sciences, Oregon State University, Corvalis, OR*

CONSTANTINE A. STRATAKIS, PhD, DSC • *National Institutes of Health, Bethesda, MD*

RONALD S. SWERDLOFF, MD • *Division of Endocrinology, Department of Medicine, Harbor-UCLA Medical Center and Education and Research Institute, UCLA School of Medicine, Torrance, CA*

CLARA M. SZEGO, PhD • *Department of Molecular, Cellular, and Developmental Biology, Molecular Biology Institute, University of California, Los Angeles, CA*

MEGHAN M. TAYLOR, PhD • *Department of Pharmacologic and Physiologic Science, St. Louis University School of Medicine, St. Louis, MO*

WILLIAM TEALE, PhD • *Institute for Biology, Albert-Ludwigs-Universität Freiburg, Freiburg, Germany*

OLAF TIETZ, PhD • *Institute for Biology, Albert-Ludwigs-Universität Freiburg, Freiburg, Germany*

CHRISTINA WANG, MD • *Division of Endocrinology, Department of Medicine, General Clinical Research Center, Harbor-UCLA Medical Center and Education and Research Institute, UCLA School of Medicine, Torrance, CA*

RICHARD J. WURTMAN, MD • *Department of Brain and Cognitive Sciences, Clinical Research Center, Massachusetts Institute of Technology, Cambridge, MA*

BULENT YILDIZ, MD • *Interdepartmental Clinical Pharma-cology Center, UCLA School of Medicine, Los Angeles, CA*

RUN YU, MD, PhD • *Division of Endocrinology, Cedars-Sinai Medical Center, UCLA School of Medicine, Los Angeles, CA*

IRINA V. ZHDANOVA, MD, PhD • *Department of Anatomy and Neurobiology, Boston University School of Medicine, Boston, MA*

Value-Added eBook/PDA on CD-ROM

This book is accompanied by a value-added CD-ROM that contains an eBook version of the volume you have just purchased. This eBook can be viewed on your computer, and you can synchronize it to your PDA for viewing on your handheld device. The eBook enables you to view this volume on only one computer and PDA. Once the eBook is installed on your computer, you cannot download, install, or e-mail it to another computer; it resides solely with the computer to which it is installed. The license provided is for only one computer. The eBook can only be read using Adobe® Reader® 6.0 software, which is available free from Adobe Systems Incorporated at www.Adobe.com. You may also view the eBook on your PDA using the Adobe® PDA Reader® software that is also available free from Adobe.com.

You must follow a simple procedure when you install the eBook/PDA that will require you to connect to the Humana Press website in order to receive your license. Please read and follow the instructions below:

1. Download and install Adobe® Reader® 6.0 software.
   You can obtain a free copy of the Adobe® Reader® 6.0 software at www.adobe.com
   *Note: If you already have the Adobe® Reader® 6.0 software installed, you do not need to reinstall it.

2. Launch Adobe® Reader® 6.0 software

3. Install eBook: Insert your eBook CD into your CD-ROM drive
   PC: Click on the "Start" button, then click on "Run"
             At the prompt, type "d:\ebookinstall.pdf" and click "OK"
             *Note: If your CD-ROM drive letter is something other than d: change the above command
                    accordingly.
   MAC: Double click on the "eBook CD" that you will see mounted on your desktop.
             Double click "ebookinstall.pdf"

4. Adobe® Reader® 6.0 software will open and you will receive the message
   "This document is protected by Adobe DRM" Click "OK"
   *Note: If you have not already activated the Adobe® Reader® 6.0 software, you will be prompted
             to do so. Simply follow the directions to activate and continue installation.

Your web browser will open and you will be taken to the Humana Press eBook registration page. Follow the instructions on that page to complete installation. You will need the serial number located on the sticker sealing the envelope containing the CD-ROM.

If you require assistance during the installation, or you would like more information regarding your eBook and PDA installation, please refer to the eBookManual.pdf located on your cd. If you need further assistance, contact Humana Press eBook Support by e-mail at ebooksupport@humanapr.com or by phone at 973-256-1699.

*Adobe and Reader are either registered trademarks or trademarks of Adobe Systems Incorporated in the United States and/or other countries.

PART
I

INTRODUCTION

1 Introduction to Endocrinology

P. Michael Conn, PhD

1. INTRODUCTION

The earliest bacterial fossils date back about 3 billion years. That was a simpler time! Communications between cells were more modest than those required to maintain a multicellular organism and were probably focused on the ability to signal the presence of beneficial substances (food) or deleterious substances (toxins) in the local environment.

2. DEFINITIONS

Substances that provide the chemical basis for communication between cells are called *hormones*. This word, coined by Bayliss and Starling, was originally used to describe the products of ductless glands released into the general circulation in order to respond to changes in homeostasis. *Hormone* has taken on a broader usage in recent years. Sometimes hormones are released into portal (closed) circulatory systems and have local actions. The word *paracrine* is used to describe the release of locally acting substances. This word also describes local hormone action as the diffusion of gastric juice acts on neighboring cells. Hormonal substances released by an animal that influence

From: *Endocrinology: Basic and Clinical Principles, Second Edition*
(S. Melmed and P. M. Conn, eds.) © Humana Press Inc., Totowa, NJ

responses in another animal are referred to as *pheromones*.

Sometimes the word hormone is used as a reference to substances in plants (phytohormones) or in invertebrates that have open "circulatory" systems very different from those found in vertebrates. On other occasions, growth factors are (appropriately) called hormones, because they mediate signaling between cells. In recent years, the word has become a catchall to describe substances released by one cell that provoke a response in another cell even when the messenger substance does not enter the general circulation. The science of endocrinology has broad coverage indeed.

3. HORMONES CONVEY INFORMATION THAT REGULATES CELL PROCESSES

Characteristically, hormones transmit information about the status of one organ to another, regulating corrective actions to maintain homeostasis. For example, elevated glucose in the blood signals the pancreas to release insulin. Insulin travels through the circulation, signaling target cells in liver and fat cells to increase their permeability to glucose; conversely, processed sugar is stored in cells as blood levels drop.

To be effective, hormones should not be degraded too quickly (i.e., before arrival at the target site). If degradation is too slow, on the other hand, the information conveyed will be obsolete and may evoke an inappropriate response. Accordingly, it is not surprising that different hormones have varying half-lives in the circulation, depending, in part, on the distance that the signal must travel and the nature of the information to be conveyed.

Concentrations of hormones are sensed by receptors, usually proteins, located on the surface (i.e., plasma membrane) or inside target cells. Receptors bind their respective hormone ligands with high affinity and specificity. For example, although estrogen and testosterone are chemically similar, receptors must distinguish between them because they mediate very different cellular responses indeed. When hormone receptors are situated on the surface of target cells and the response involves intracellular changes (e.g., evoking secretione), transduction of the hormonal message must occur. Such transduction molecules are termed *second messengers of hormone action.*

It is a general truth that the chemical structures of hormones do not change markedly during evolution; instead, nature identifies and conserves molecules that already have information value and develops systems that preserve and utilize that information. Steroids, thyroid hormones, and peptides are present in some species that do not utilize them for the same endocrine purpose as do mammals.

4. IDENTIFYING HORMONES

The effects of ablation of endocrine organs have been documented back to the time of Aristotle (384–322 BC), who described changes in secondary sex characteristics and loss of reproductive capacity associated with castration in men. Much insight into the role of endocrine substances has come from disease states, surgical errors, and animal experimentation in which damage to endocrine organs is correlated with particular phenotypic changes in the organism.

Ancient medical procedures prevalent in many cultures were based on the premise that administration of extracts from healthy organs aids in the recovery of diseased organs. This practice may be viewed as a predecessor to hormone replacement therapy. Restoration of function by supplements derived from healthy endocrine organs administered to animals with endocrine ablations has formed the basis of discovering active principles of the endocrine system.

In the mid-1800s, Berthold showed that the effects of castration in avians could be reversed by placing a testis in the body cavity. Since the transplant was ectopic and not innervated, he concluded that the testes released a substance that controlled secondary sex characteristics.

A few years later, Claude Bernard, providing evidence to support a model of homeostasis, showed that the liver could release sugar to the blood. From the mid-1850s to the twentieth century, endocrinology grew at a dramatic pace. Assays became more sensitive and specific; biosynthetic and genetic engineering techniques now allow synthesis of biologically active and highly purified hormones.

5. HORMONE-DERIVED DRUGS

The identification of new hormonal activities often follows a similar pattern. The observation is made that damage to a particular gland is associated with loss of a certain function. Efforts are then focused on isolating the active principle from the gland. The active principle is then administered to restore the function to the animal patient who has ablated glandular function. The development of drugs is usually directed toward preparing purified fractions that can be used in replacement therapy. The hormone itself and, ultimately, chemical analogs can now readily be synthesized. Analogs can be designed to possess desirable properties, such as prolonged circulation half-lives, chemical stability, or specific receptor or tissue targeting. The availability of purified fractions or synthetic hormone preparations often spawns studies designed to understand the cellular and molecular basis of hormone action. This information is then used to design even more useful drugs that recognize the target cell receptor with higher specificity and affinity; antagonists can also be prepared that block the receptor or its signaling. The science of endocrinology is poised to take advantage of our understanding of intricate second-messenger systems, sensitive and precise assay systems (radioimmunoassays, bioassays, radioligand assays), and advances in structural and functional molecular biology. As the tools of endocrinology have become more precise, we have discovered that even the brain, heart, and lung possess substantial endocrine functions.

6. ENDOCRINOLOGY AS A LEAD SCIENCE

Endocrinology continues to be a lead science. Many Nobel Prizes have recognized the contributions of endocrinologists. The first cloned gene products to reach the clinical pharmaceutical market were endocrine substances. Many advances in our understanding of cellular transduction systems, receptor binding, and physiologic regulation are derivatives of the studies conducted in endocrine laboratories. Why is this so? A likely answer is found by understanding that endocrinologists study the actions of specific chemicals that cause cells to undergo specific and (usually) easily quantifiable and regulated responses. These are very simple, basic, and well-defined processes. Accordingly, clear and interpretable experiments can be designed at a complexity ranging from molecular to physiologic. This is part of the general appeal and high level of achievement of this science—and much of the reason that those who call themselves endocrinologists have made a major contribution to our understanding of regulatory biologic processes.

PART II

HORMONE SECRETION AND ACTION

2 Receptors

Molecular Mediators of Hormone Action

Kelly E. Mayo, PhD

1. INTRODUCTION

The appropriate proliferation and differentiation of cells during development and the maintenance of cellular homeostasis in the adult require a continuous flow of information to the cell. This is provided either by diffusible signaling molecules or by direct cell–cell and cell–matrix interactions. All cells utilize a wide variety of signaling molecules and signal transduction systems to communicate with one another, but within the vertebrate endocrine system, it is the secreted hormones that are classically associated with cellular signaling. Hormones are chemical messengers produced from the endocrine glands that act either locally or at a distance to regulate the activity of a target cell. As discussed in detail elsewhere within this volume, prominent groups of hormonal agents include peptide hormones; steroid, retinoid, and thyroid hormones; growth factors; cytokines; pheromones; and neurotransmitters or neuromodulators.

Endocrine signaling molecules exert their effects by interacting with specific receptor proteins that are generally coupled to one or more intracellular effector systems. The presence of an appropriate receptor therefore defines the population of target cells for a given hormone and provides a molecular mechanism by which the hormone elicits its biologic actions. These hormone receptor proteins are the focus of this chapter. Section 2 considers general concepts of receptor action, including receptor structure, interaction with the hormone ligand, activation of cellular effector systems, and receptor regulation. Sections 3 and 4 then examine the major families of hormone receptors, grouped with respect to their structures and signaling properties, in greater detail, using specific examples that illustrate the general features of each family. Finally, Section 5 discusses some of the endocrinopathies that result from known alterations in hormone receptor structure or function.

2. GENERAL ASPECTS OF RECEPTOR ACTION

2.1. Receptors as Mediators of Endocrine Signals

The concept that hormone action is mediated by receptors is most often attributed to the work of Langley on the actions of nicotine and curare on the neuromus-

From: *Endocrinology: Basic and Clinical Principles, Second Edition*
(S. Melmed and P. M. Conn, eds.) © Humana Press Inc., Totowa, NJ

cular junction (Langley, 1906). Langley referred to the target for these compounds as the "receptive substance," and postulated that "it receives the stimulus, and by transmitting it, causes contraction," a clear description of the role of receptors in mediating the actions of signaling molecules. Of course, Langley could not know the nature of these receptive substances, suggesting only that they were "radicals of the protoplasmic molecule." Indeed, despite a wealth of physiologic evidence in support of the receptor concept, firm biochemical evidence for the existence of specific receptors was not forthcoming until radiolabeled hormones became available. For hormones unable to traverse the cellular membrane, such as the polypeptide hormones, specific binding sites could be demonstrated, but their membrane association and low abundance precluded their characterization for many years. Only with the advent of molecular cloning techniques was it possible to establish firmly the structures of the hormone receptors, and to show that these proteins could, in effect, convert a nontarget cell into a target cell by conferring to the cell the ability to bind and, in some cases, appropriately respond to the corresponding hormone.

A second key event in the development of the receptor concept was the demonstration by Sutherland (1972) that cyclic adenosine monophosphate (cAMP) could mediate the intracellular effects of many different hormones, establishing the notion of "second messengers" and providing a cogent molecular explanation of how hormones and hormone receptors might elicit their widespread effects on cellular activity. The notion that many different signaling molecules, working through distinct receptors, could stimulate a common intracellular signaling pathway, together with the subsequent discovery of additional effector enzymes and intracellular second messengers, provided a rational explanation for the tremendous diversity in cellular responses to hormones.

At about the time that second-messenger systems were being discovered, different concepts were evolving on the mechanism of action of the small lipophilic steroid hormones. Radiolabeled steroids, such as estrogen, were synthesized by Jensen and others and were found to accumulate preferentially in known target organs for the hormone (Jensen and Jacobson, 1962). Specific steroid-binding proteins were subsequently identified, and the important finding that binding of agonists and antagonists to these receptors correlated with their biologic activity provided evidence that they were direct mediators of steroid action. These steroid receptors were shown to be soluble intracellular proteins, differentiating them from the membrane-associated receptors for the polypeptide hormones, and

facilitating their early purification, beginning with the identification of the estrogen receptor by Toft and Gorski (1966). The findings that the steroid receptors associated with chromatin in the cell nucleus and that steroid hormones affected RNA and protein synthesis provided the basis for models of direct genomic actions of the hormone-receptor complex that we now know to be correct.

2.2. Membrane-Associated vs Intracellular Receptors

Substances that act as signaling molecules have extremely diverse structures and chemical properties. They include complex multisubunit proteins such as follicle-stimulating hormone (FSH), small peptides such as somatostatin, steroids such as estrogen, amino acid derivatives such as thyroid hormone or the catecholamines, vitamin derivatives such as the retinoids or calcitrol, fatty acid derivatives such as prostaglandins, and simple compounds such as nitric oxide (NO), to provide but a few examples. Despite this structural complexity, most hormones act on target cells through one of two basic mechanisms. Small lipophilic molecules such as the steroids, retinoids, calcitrol, and thyroid hormone are able to enter cells directly by diffusion across the lipid bilayer, where they bind to intracellular receptors that mediate their subsequent action by directly regulating gene expression. By contrast, hydrophilic molecules such as the protein and peptide hormones must bind to their receptor at the cell surface, and the receptors are therefore typically integral membrane proteins that activate intracellular signal transduction cascades. Thus, it is common to differentiate between membrane-bound and intracellular receptors when considering mechanisms of hormone action.

The consequence of hormone-receptor interaction is the activation of pathways that lead to an appropriate biologic response in the target cell, an area referred to as a signal transduction, which is discussed in depth in Chapter 3. Briefly, most intracellular receptors, such as the steroid hormone receptors, are ligand-activated transcription factors that directly regulate the transcriptional activity of target genes. By contrast, cell-surface receptors transduce a signal to the cell interior, directly or indirectly altering the activity of proteins within the cell. This action often involves the enzymatic generation of a second messenger, and the activation of protein phosphorylation or dephosphorylation cascades. More important, the eventual consequence of the activation of enzymatic signaling pathways by cell-surface receptors is often a change in gene transcription; conversely, changes in enzymatic

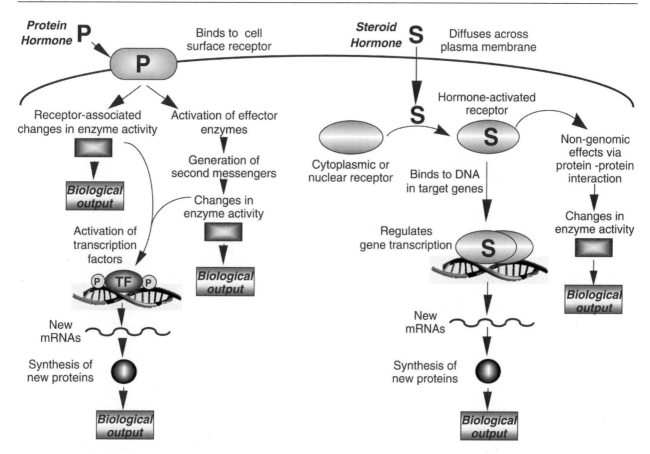

Fig 1. Hormonal signaling by cell-surface and intracellular receptors. Protein hormones (P) bind to cell-surface receptors that activate intracellular effector enzymes, often leading to the production of second messengers or the initiation of protein phosphorylation cascades. A longer-term effect is gene transcription and new protein synthesis. By contrast, steroid hormones (S), or other lipophilic ligands, bind to intracellular receptors that are ligand-activated transcription factors (TF) that directly mediate gene transcription, leading to new protein synthesis.

activities often follow as a consequence of altered gene activity when intracellular receptors are activated. Furthermore, there are many emerging examples of "cross talk" between cell-signaling pathways (Dumont et al., 2001). Finally, as our understanding of the complexity of receptor signaling increases, exceptions to these general modes of action of membrane-bound vs intracellular receptors are being identified. Thus, many of the historical mechanistic boundaries between cell-surface and intracellular receptors are breaking down. Nonetheless, these categories provide a useful way of organizing thinking about receptor action and are therefore used to classify the receptors in this chapter. Figure 1 illustrates some of the similarities and differences in hormone signaling through intracellular vs cell-surface receptors.

The membrane-associated receptors are an extremely diverse group of signaling molecules. Their common feature is the presence of one or more hydrophobic domains that span the cell membrane and anchor the receptor at the cell surface. Extracellular regions of the protein often participate in hormone binding, and intracellular sequences generally either have direct enzymatic function or associate with intermediary proteins or effector enzymes. The functional cell-surface hormone receptor is often composed of multiple protein subunits that may play a role in hormone binding, signaling, or both activities. It is clear that the receptors for structurally and functionally diverse hormones can be closely related to one another, most commonly within their intracellular domains. Thus, a limited number of basic signaling strategies are used repetitively by a very large number of receptor proteins, defining distinct receptor families, which are considered in Section 3.

The intracellular receptors for the steroid hormones were the first to be biochemically purified. Following the molecular cloning of the receptors for all of the classic steroid hormones (Evans, 1988) it became clear that

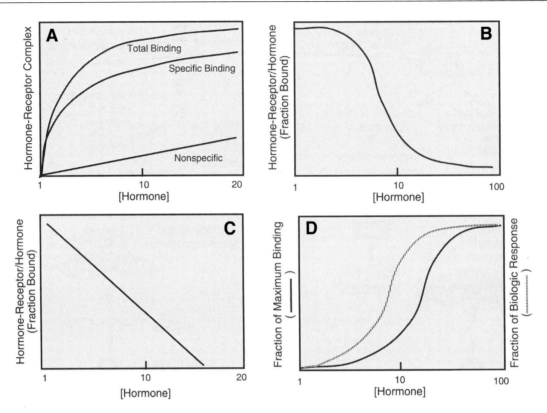

Fig. 2. Measurement of hormone-receptor interactions by binding analysis: (**A**) saturable binding to a target cell preparation as concentration of radiolabeled hormone is increased; (**B**) competition or displacement experiment in which binding of a radiolabeled tracer to the receptor is competed as excess unlabeled hormone is added; (**C**) Scatchard linear transformation of binding data, from which receptor number and affinity for hormone can be determined; (**D**) consequence of spare receptors. The biologic response is fully activated when only a fraction of the receptors is occupied by hormone. See text for details.

these receptors comprise a family of highly related proteins consisting of distinct structural domains. The highly conserved central DNA-binding domain (DBD) is generally flanked by a carboxyl-terminal region that is necessary for hormone binding by one or more additional domains that are important for activation of target gene transcription. The subsequent identification of the thyroid hormone, retinoic acid, and vitamin D receptors placed them in this nuclear receptor superfamily, along with an expanding number of "orphan receptors" that act in a ligand-independent fashion or for which appropriate ligands have not yet been identified (Willson and Moore, 2002). Not all intracellular receptors are structurally related to the steroid hormone receptors, some examples being the NO and arylhydrocarbon receptors.

2.3. Measurement of Receptor-Ligand Interaction

Hormone receptors are most commonly detected and measured using direct binding assays. This requires a labeled ligand, usually a radiolabeled hormone such as a tritiated steroid or an iodinated peptide; a source of the receptor being analyzed, typically tissue extracts, cells, or cell membranes; and a physical means of separating the bound hormone from that which is unbound, commonly centrifugation or filtration techniques. As shown in Fig. 2A, when increasing amounts of a labeled polypeptide hormone are added to a constant amount of a cell preparation, the fraction of hormone bound to the cell surface increases and eventually approaches a maximum. In addition to specific binding to its cell surface receptor, the hormone can bind nonspecifically to other cellular constituents or to the reaction vessel, and this component is commonly measured by performing the binding reaction in the presence of a large excess of unlabeled hormone, to ensure complete displacement of the labeled hormone from specific sites. Specific binding is then established by subtracting the nonspecific binding from the total binding.

In a useful variation of this assay, a competition binding experiment, a constant, small amount of the labeled hormone is mixed with cells or cell membranes in the presence of increasing concentrations of unlabeled hormone. A typical competition or displacement curve resulting from this type of experiment is shown in Fig. 2B. The binding that remains at high hormone concentrations represents the nonspecific binding, and the hormone concentration at which 50% of the radiolabeled tracer is displaced approximates the affinity constant of the receptor for its ligand, as described next.

The interaction of the hormone and its receptor can be described by the equation $H + R \rightarrow [HR]$, in which H is the free hormone, R is the free receptor, and HR is the hormone-receptor complex. Binding is assumed to be reversible, and the steady-state dissociation constant $K_d = [H][R]/[HR]$ provides a measure of the affinity of the receptor for its ligand. The total amount of receptor can be described as that which is free plus that which is liganded ($[R_T] = [R] + [HR]$), and the two equations together can be written in the form $[HR] = [R_T][H]/[H] + K_d$. When $[HR]$ is plotted as a function of $[H]$, the hyperbolic plot shown in Fig. 2A is obtained. The previous equation can be rearranged to the form $[HR]/[H] = [R_T]/[H] + K_d$, and when $[HR]/[H]$ is plotted as a function of $\log[H]$, the sigmoidal curve shown in Fig. 2B is obtained. Scatchard (1949) described a commonly used linear rearrangement of this relationship, $[HR]/[H] = -1/K_d[HR] + RT/K_d$, and as shown in Fig. 2C, the plot of $[HR]/[H]$ as a function of $[HR]$ provides the total receptor number, R_T as the intercept with the abscissa, and the affinity constant, K_d, is derived from the slope, which is $-1/K_d$. The linear relationship shown in Fig. 2C becomes curvilinear when multiple binding sites with differing affinities are present or when cooperative binding interactions occur.

Most commonly, the K_d values for hormone receptors are near the physiologic concentration of the relevant hormone, meaning that fluctuations in the hormone level can elicit both positive and negative responses with respect to receptor activation. However, in many cases it has been shown experimentally that occupancy of only a small fraction of the cell-surface receptors is needed to elicit a maximal biologic response. The term spare receptors has evolved to describe this phenomenon, which is illustrated in terms of binding and activation curves in Fig. 2D. The ability of a small fraction of occupied receptors to stimulate fully a biologic response points to the tremendous amplification potential of the enzyme effectors that act downstream of the hormone receptors. Spare receptors may allow a response to be kinetically favorable even at very low hormone concentrations.

2.4. Cellular Signal Transduction Themes

Hormones, particularly those that act on cell-surface receptors, most commonly initiate a cascade of signaling events in their target cell, ultimately leading to an appropriate biologic response. These cascades are referred to as signal transduction pathways, and although they are extremely diverse with respect to the specific molecules involved, they do have several common features. It is becoming clear that in many systems, homo- or heterodimerization of receptor proteins in response to binding of the hormone ligand is a key event in initiating cell signaling. This can lead to direct activation of a receptor's enzymatic function, or to the direct or indirect recruitment of additional effector proteins with enzymatic function. Through the actions of soluble second-messenger molecules, or through the direct enzymatic functions of the receptor or its associated proteins, protein kinases, protein phosphatases, or proteases are often activated and act to initiate cascades of protein modification that can be extraordinarily complex. Some of the modified target proteins play direct and rapid roles in the cellular response (e.g., an ion channel) whereas other modified target proteins play indirect or delayed roles in the cellular response (e.g., a transcription factor). Another common feature is the presence of regulatory mechanisms that attenuate the response to hormone and reset the signaling system. Chapter 3 provides a comprehensive treatment of signal transduction, and, therefore, only a few key points necessary for the subsequent discussion of hormone receptors and their actions are introduced in this section.

One can consider three broad classes of signal transduction themes downstream of cell-surface receptors: activation of second-messenger signaling pathways by G protein–coupled receptors (GPCRs), activation of tyrosine kinase or serine/threonine kinase receptors or receptor-associated proteins by growth factor and cytokine receptors, and activation of protein proteolysis or cell localization pathways by developmentally important receptors. Each of these is very briefly reviewed here and is considered in more detail in the following sections.

GPCRs are the largest single family of receptors in vertebrates, and derive their name from their common mechanism of action, which is to activate one or more G proteins following hormone stimulation. The G proteins are a large family of guanosine 5′-triphosphate (GTP)-binding proteins that are heterotrimeric, consisting of α-, β- and γ-subunits, and serve to stimulate or repress the activity of multiple cellular effector enzymes (Gilman, 1987). Some 16 distinct G protein α-subunits define major categories of cell responses; for example, stimulatory (G_s) and inhibitory (G_i) G proteins activate or repress, respectively, the enzyme adenylyl cyclase and thereby regulate production of the second-messenger cAMP (Schramm and Selinger, 1984), and G_q and G_{11} class G proteins regulate phopholipase Cβ activity and control the production of inositol phosphate, diacylglycerol, and calcium second messengers (Berridge, 1993). Both the α and βγ G protein subunits regulate enzyme effectors, and a cycle of GTP binding and subsequent hydrolysis to guanosine 5′-diphosphate (GDP) controls the subunit association and activity of these proteins. The second messengers that are produced as a result of G protein activation serve to regulate the activity of cellular protein kinases, such as the activation of cAMP-dependent protein kinase (protein kinase A [PKA]) and PKC by cAMP and calcium/phospholipids, respectively.

A second common signaling theme involves cell-surface receptors that have intrinsic protein kinase activity or that recruit and activate protein kinases. Three subclasses of these receptors can be considered. A large and historically important group is the growth factor receptors, which have cytoplasmic domains with intrinsic protein tyrosine kinase activity. On hormone binding, the receptor rapidly forms a dimer, and the cytoplasmic kinase domains rapidly cross-phosphorylate each other on tyrosine residues, which allows for the subsequent binding of a broad repertoire of cellular proteins that are involved in transducing the signal. A more recently characterized group is the transforming growth factor-β (TGF-β) superfamily receptors, which have cytoplasmic domains with intrinsic protein serine/threonine kinase activity. Dimerization of a hormone-binding type II receptor and a signaling type I receptor leads to the phosphorylation of target proteins of the Smad family, which transduce the signal. Finally, the cytokine receptors are not themselves protein kinases, but when activated they recruit soluble protein tyrosine kinases of the Janus kinase (Jak) family that phosphorylate both the receptor and receptor-associated effector proteins of the Stat family, which transduce the signal. Also in the same broad category are receptors that are protein tyrosine phosphatases, although much less is known about these receptors and their activation.

A third broad and emerging category includes pathways downstream of a variety of developmentally important signaling molecules such as the Wnt, Hedgehog, and DSL family ligands. The details are quite specific to each pathway, but common themes include retention of a key transcription factor or coregulator required for target gene expression in the cytoplasm until ligand activates the receptor, a switch from target gene repression to activation, and involvement of irreversible proteolysis as a key regulatory step.

2.5. Mechanisms of Receptor Regulation

It is clear that mechanisms must exist to regulate the levels of, or activity of, cell-surface receptors, allowing for modulation or termination of the response to the hormone. In some cases, the biosynthesis of receptors is tightly regulated so as to generate additional receptors when they are required. For example, the low-density lipoprotein (LDL) receptor gene is activated by a protein that acts as both a sterol sensor and transcription factor, resulting in enhanced production of the receptor when sterol levels are low (Brown and Goldstein, 1999). In other cases, the degradation of receptors, and their corresponding ligands, is tightly regulated. Many hormones that act on cell-surface receptors are internalized through the process of receptor-mediated endocytosis, which is shown in Fig. 3A. The hormone-receptor complex is internalized into clathrin-coated vesicles that are acidified and lose their clathrin coat to form endosomes, where the low pH often results in hormone-receptor dissociation. The ligand is most commonly degraded in lysosomes, effectively removing the signal from the extracellular environment. The receptor typically has one of two fates: recycling to the cell surface, where it is again available to interact productively with hormone (e.g., the insulin receptor); or degradation in the lysosome (e.g., the epidermal growth factor receptor [EGFR]). In either case, internalization effectively reduces the number of cell-surface receptors, and the process is therefore a mechanism utilized to downregulate cell-surface receptors.

A second common mode of regulation targets the ability of cell-surface receptors to bind the hormone or to subsequently transduce a signal. Probably the best-studied example of this is agonist-induced desensitization of the G protein–coupled β-adrenergic receptor. In the continual presence of the agonist epinephrine, the cAMP signal is attenuated, although the receptor continues to bind epinephrine. Desensitization is a reversible process, and it is mediated by phosphorylation of the receptor on cytoplasmic serine and threonine residues. Some of this phosphorylation is catalyzed by PKA, which is activated in response to the epinephrine-induced cAMP signal and acts in a feedback manner to downregulate the signaling pathway. Because activated PKA has the ability to phosphorylate many receptors, potentially attenuating their activity, this phenomenon is referred to as heterologous desensitization. The agonist-occupied β-adrenergic receptor is also phosphorylated by a very specific cellular kinase called the β-adrenergic receptor kinase (βARK), a member of a broader family of GPCR kinases, or GRKs (Claing et al. 2002). These kinases are broadly expressed and likely to play an important role in the desensitization of many hormonal responses mediated by GPCRs. Because βARK targets only the β-adrenergic receptor, this phenomenon is referred to as homologous desensitization. The phosphorylated β-adr-

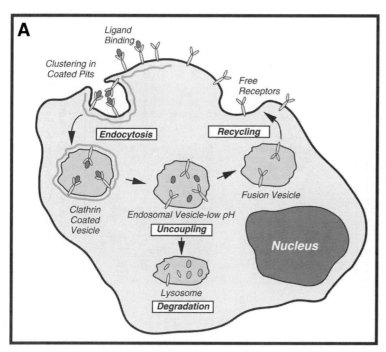

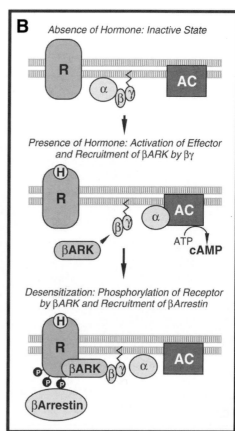

Fig. 3. Mechanisms for regulation of cell-surface receptors. (**A**) Process of receptor-mediated endocytosis. Following ligand binding, receptors rapidly move into coated pits and are internalized by endocytosis. The resulting clathrin-coated vesicles are acidified in an endosomal compartment, leading to dissociation of the ligand from the receptor. Vesicular sorting leads to a segregation of the ligand into vesicles that will fuse with primary lysosomes, resulting in degradation or utilization of the ligand. The receptor either can be degraded, as often occurs for signaling receptors, or it can be recycled to the cell surface, as often occurs for transport receptors. (**B**) Steps involved in desensitization of β-adrenergic receptor. In the continual presence of hormone, the G protein βγ-subunits recruit the β-adrenergic receptor kinase to the membrane, leading to specific phosphorylation of the receptor and an attenuation of signaling. The phosphorylated receptor is recognized by β-arrestin, further suppressing the signaling pathway. The pathway shown is homologous desensitization. As discussed in the text, heterologous desensitization involving receptor phosphorylation by PKA also occurs. ATP = adenosine triphosphate.

energic receptor is unable to couple efficiently to its G protein, resulting in the observed attenuation of the signal. In addition, many phosphorylated GPCRs, including the β-adrenergic receptor, bind proteins of the arrestin family, which serve to suppress further the signal by promoting uncoupling of the receptor and its G protein (Claing et al., 2002). Some of the regulatory processes involved in receptor desensitization are outlined in Fig. 3B. Desensitization is a major factor controlling the efficacy of action of many therapeutic agents that target GPCRs such as the β-adrenergic receptor. Although negative regulatory mechanisms for other classes of receptors have not been studied in the same depth as those for the GPCRs, they certainly exist, and several are referred to in subsequent sections.

3. CELL-SURFACE RECEPTORS

3.1. Receptors Coupled to G Proteins

The GPCRs comprise the largest known family of cell-surface hormone receptors, and it is estimated that 50% of prescription drugs target GPCRs. Hundreds of these receptors have already been cloned and characterized, many of them orphan receptors of unknown function that represent significant targets for future drug development. Their common features are seven hydrophobic potential membrane-spanning domains, and the ability to stimulate the exchange of bound GDP for GTP on associated G protein α-subunits in response to agonist binding. They are also known as the hepta-helical or serpentine receptors because of their mem-

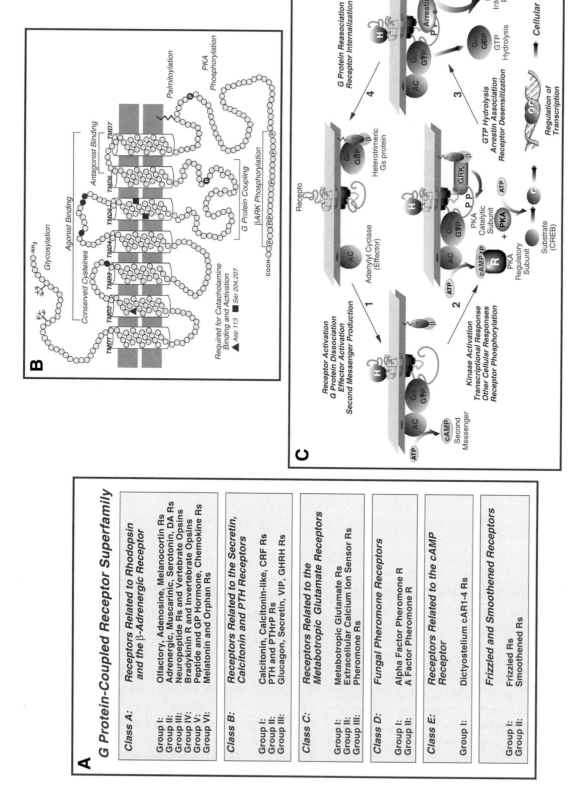

Fig. 4. Structure and signal transduction by GPCRs. **(A)** Major families and groups of GPCRs (GCPR Database; Horn et al. 2003). The mammalian receptors are largely confined to families A, B, and C. Family A is the largest and includes the diverse odorant receptors as well as prototypic GPCRs such as rhodopsin and the β-adrenergic receptor. **(B)** Schematic structure of one of the most extensively characterized GPCRs, β-adrenergic receptor. Major structural features are indicated and are expanded on in the text (After Duhlman et al., 1991). **(C)** Model for signaling through a GCPR. A receptor coupled to the cAMP pathway is illustrated, and CREB is used as an example of one substrate for PKA. This model is generic, and not all aspects will apply to all systems.

brane topology. As indicated in Fig. 4A, the GPCR superfamily can be divided into several major families that share significant sequence similarities. The three predominant mammalian families are class A (receptors related to rhodopsin and the β2-adrenergic receptor), class B (receptors related to the secretin, calcitonin, and parathyroid hormone [PTH] receptors), and class C (receptors related to the metabotropic glutamate and pheromone receptors). Further subdivisions into groups are indicated in Fig. 4, as are receptor classes D–E. Class A is by far the largest family of GPCRs, and its prototypes, rhodopsin and the β2-adrenergic receptor, are among the best-characterized receptors; therefore, much of what is known about the structure, function, and regulation of GPCRs in general comes from studies of these model proteins.

Tremendous diversity is a hallmark of the GPCR superfamily. Many of the neurotransmitter and peptide hormone receptors are encoded by multiple genes that produce related yet distinct receptors. For example, five distinct somatostatin receptors have been characterized. These are expressed with unique but overlapping tissue and cell specificity, and they are able to mediate signaling through several different G proteins. An extreme example of this is represented by the olfactory odorant receptors, a family that likely numbers in the hundreds. Other receptors are produced from a single gene, but alternative RNA processing results in the generation of multiple receptor isoforms, either produced in specific tissues or able to couple differentially to G protein–mediated signaling pathways. For example, the dopamine D2 receptor exists as two splice variants expressed in unique tissue-specific patterns, and the pituitary adenylate cyclase activating peptide receptor exists as five splice variants that differ in their ability to activate adenylate cyclase vs phospholipase Cβ (PLCβ) effectors. Further diversity may be generated by recent findings that both homo- and heterooligomerization of GPCRs is common and can impact function, potentially generating receptors with novel properties through interaction of characterized receptors with known properties (George et al., 2002).

The major structural features of a model GPCR, the β2-adrenergic receptor, are shown in Fig. 4B. The extracellular domain is relatively short, although for some class A receptors, those for the glycoprotein hormones FSH, luteinizing hormone, and thyroid-stimulating hormone, this domain is more than 300 amino acids long. There are typically several sites for asparagine-linked glycosylation within the extracellular domain. The seven membrane-spanning domains of the receptor create three extracellular loops and three cytoplasmic loops that can be quite variable in length among different

receptors. The carboxyl-terminal cytoplasmic domain is typically short and is often associated with the plasma membrane through palmitoylation of a conserved cysteine residue. As discussed above, phosphorylation plays an important role in the regulation of receptor activity, and potential sites for phosphorylation by PKA as well as the specific GRK kinases are found within the third cytoplasmic loop and the carboxyl-terminal tail of the receptor.

Mutagenesis has been extensively applied to elucidate features of the β2-adrenergic receptor important for ligand interaction and for subsequent G protein coupling. A strategy that has been particularly useful for the analysis of the GPCRs has been the generation of chimeras between two homologous receptors with distinct ligand-binding or signaling properties. Such chimeras between the β2-adrenergic and α1-adrenergic receptors have implicated the transmembrane domains and associated extracellular loops in specific agonist binding and have shown that transmembrane domain seven is particularly important in specifying antagonist binding. Similar experiments to examine signaling through the stimulation (β2-adrenergic receptor) or inhibition (α1-adrenergic receptor) of adenylate cyclase by G_s and G_i, respectively, led to the conclusion that the regions between transmembrane domains five and six, including the third cytoplasmic loop, were particularly important in determining G protein recognition. Additional mutagenesis has indicated that the carboxyl-terminal domain of the receptor, a major site of potential phosphorylation, is particularly important for desensitization, and that several conserved residues are critical for catacholamine binding and activation, including an aspartic acid residue in transmembrane domain two and two serine residues in transmembrane domain five of the β2-adrenergic receptor (Dohlman et al., 1991).

In general, much of what has been learned from model receptors such as the β2-adrenergic receptor has been applicable to additional GPCRs. The basic membrane topology of the β-adrenergic receptor, discerned through proteolysis and antibody epitope mapping studies, holds for other members of the superfamily that have been examined. There are differences in ligand-binding determinants, and, in general, receptors that interact with small molecules utilize the transmembrane domain segments more extensively for binding, and receptors that interact with larger peptides or proteins make greater use of the amino-terminal and extracellular loops. An extreme example of this is ligand recognition by the glycoprotein hormone receptors, where the large amino-terminal extracellular domain, expressed independently of the transmembrane domains, has the ability to bind the ligand with high affinity. As additional members of this family are characterized, novel modes of hormone binding and receptor activation are also being observed. For example, thrombin proteolytically cleaves its GPCR in the extracellular domain, revealing a new N-terminus that acts like a ligand to mediate activation of the receptor.

The mechanisms by which ligand binding leads to an ability of the receptor to interact productively with a G protein remain largely unknown. The first (and to date only) structure for a GPCR is that of rhodopsin (reviewed in Filipek et al., 2003), and this has provided an important foundation for modeling studies of other GPCRs. Based on a wealth of biophysical and mutagenesis data, researchers believe that activation of GPCRs involves disruption of stabilizing contacts between membrane-spanning helices, causing changes in the relative orientation of several of these helices; in particular, there is a movement of transmembrane helix 6 with respect to transmembrane helix 3, opening up the receptor in a manner that is thought to expose cytoplasmic determinants for G protein interaction. As discussed in Section 5, mutations in GPCRs that cause constitutive activity of the receptor are a common cause of disease. In addition, many GPCRs are partially active in the absence of ligand and can be further activated when overexpressed. This has been explained in terms of a two-state model in which an equili'brium exists between a signaling active and inactive state of the receptor. Agonists bind to and stabilize the active conformation, whereas inverse agonists bind selectively to the inactive conformation and stabilize it; this latter class of compounds is a potential target for drug development in regulating the activity of constitutively active mutant receptors (Strange, 2002).

As discussed earlier, the functional commonality among GPCRs is that following hormone binding they interact with the G protein so as to induce the release of GDP from the G protein α-subunit, allowing GTP to bind and facilitating dissociation of the α-subunit from the βγ complex. Several G protein structures have been solved using crystallography, and these provide substantial molecular detail into how guanine nucleotide binding impacts subunit interactions. Both the free α-subunit and the βγ complex participate in signaling, activating one or more effector enzymes. Eventually, the intrinsic guanosine 5′-triphosphatase (GTPase) activity of the α-subunit hydrolyzes GTP to GDP, promoting reassociation with the βγ complex and return to the inactive state. For some G proteins with slow intrinsic GTPase activity, this process is facilitated by GTPase-activating proteins called regulators of G protein signaling. Aspects of signaling by GPCRs are summarized in Fig. 4C, which illustrates the best-studied signaling pathway activated by this class of receptors, the G_s-stimulated cAMP pathway.

Given the diversity of the GPCRs, it is perhaps not surprising that many endocrinopathies can be attributed to mutations in specific GPCRs (Shenker, 1995). This connection first became apparent through the analysis of G proteins that these receptors interact with. It was demonstrated that mutations that constitutively activate Gsα by inactivating its intrinsic GTPase function were causative in acromegaly in association with pituitary adenoma (a late somatic mutation confined to the pituitary gland) as well as in McCune-Albright disease (an earlier somatic mutation affecting many endocrine systems). Subsequently, mutations in many GPCRs have been identified, both in human diseases and in animal models of human disease. These represent both loss-of-function and gain-of-function mutations in the targeted GPCRs. For example, inactivating mutations of the calcium-sensing receptor cause familial hypocalciuric hypercalcemia in the heterozygous state and neonatal severe hyperparathyroidism in the homozygous state, whereas an activating mutation in this same receptor causes a dominant form of hypocalcemia. In some cases, analysis of these mutations, which generally have a known phenotype, has revealed much about important structural features of these receptors. For example, more than 50 different mutations of the vasopressin V2 receptor in patients with nephrogenic diabetes insipidus have been found, providing a wealth of information on residues essential for hormone binding or activation of this receptor.

3.2. Receptors With Tyrosine Kinase Activity

The receptor protein tyrosine kinases (RTKs) are found in all multicellular organisms and mediate the actions of a broad spectrum of hormones and growth factors on cell growth, metabolism, and differentiation. They can be subdivided into several families, based largely on their structural characteristics. Examples of some of the major subfamilies, by one classification (van der Geer et al., 1994), include the platelet-derived growth factor receptor (PDGFR) subfamily, the fibroblast growth factor receptor (FGFR) subfamily, the insulin receptor subfamily, the EGFR subfamily, the nerve growth factor receptor (NGFR) subfamily, the hepatocyte growth factor receptor (HGFR) subfamily, and a series of additional receptors for which ligands have not yet been identified. Figure 5A shows examples of the major families of RTKs.

The RTKs are type I transmembrane proteins, having an external aminoterminus and a single membrane-spanning domain. The extracellular ligand-binding domains (LBDs), of these receptors are quite distinctive, but one

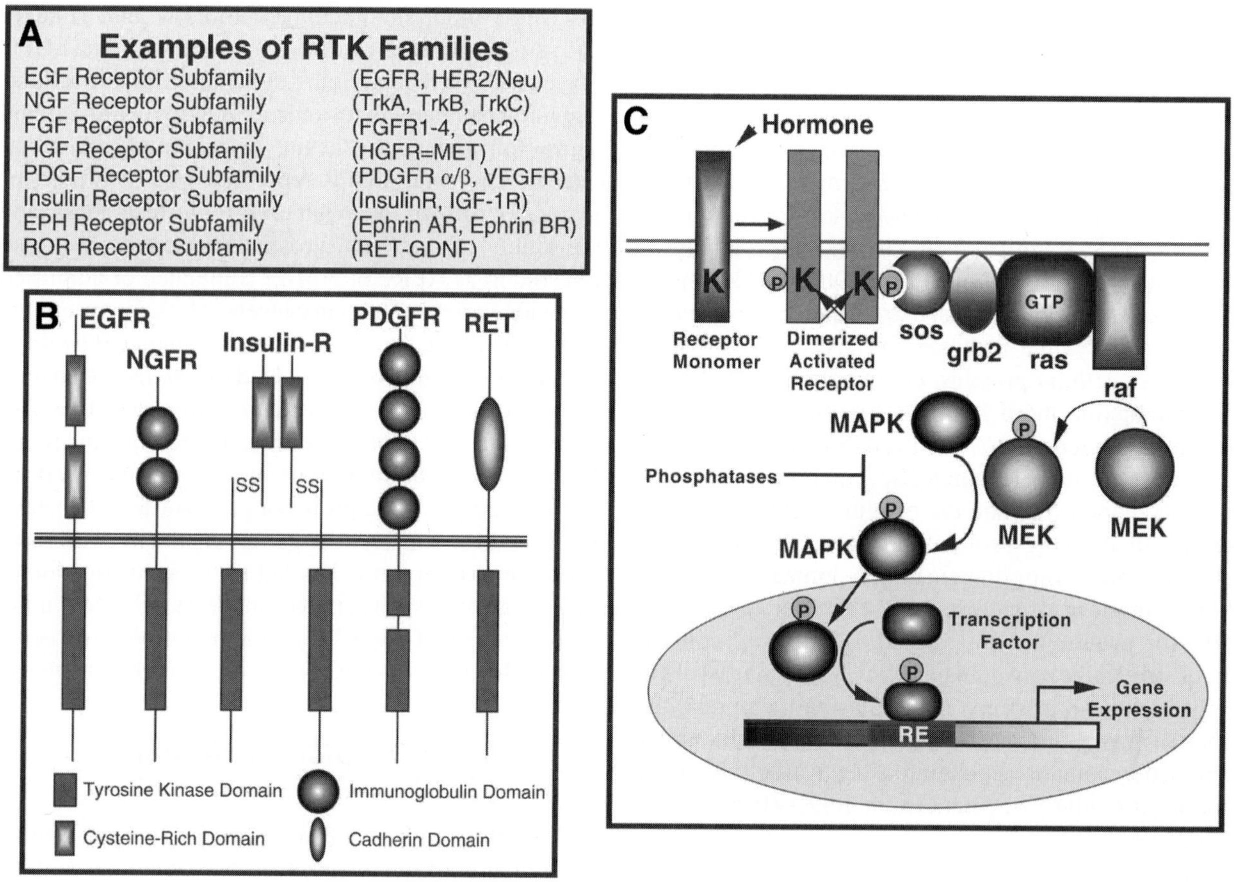

A Examples of RTK Families

EGF Receptor Subfamily	(EGFR, HER2/Neu)
NGF Receptor Subfamily	(TrkA, TrkB, TrkC)
FGF Receptor Subfamily	(FGFR1-4, Cek2)
HGF Receptor Subfamily	(HGFR=MET)
PDGF Receptor Subfamily	(PDGFR α/β, VEGFR)
Insulin Receptor Subfamily	(InsulinR, IGF-1R)
EPH Receptor Subfamily	(Ephrin AR, Ephrin BR)
ROR Receptor Subfamily	(RET-GDNF)

Fig. 5. Structure and signal transduction by RTK: (**A**) major families and specific examples of RTKs; (**B**) schematic of structures of several types of RTKs and key modular domains involved in ligand interaction; (**C**) example of generic signaling through a prototypic RTK, leading to activation of a MAPK signaling pathway as exemplified by ERK kinase.

or more of a variety of recognizable structural motifs appear in most of the LBDs. These domains include cysteine-rich regions, leucine-rich regions, immunoglobulin-related domains, fibronectin type II repeats, and EGF-like repeats, among others (Fig. 5B). For the most part, the precise roles of these extracellular domains in hormone recognition have not been well established, but structural studies are beginning to shed new light on the processes of hormone binding. The cytoplasmic catalytic domain of the RTKs is much more highly conserved, and a number of amino acid residues critical to its enzymatic function are absolutely conserved. Based on the crystallographic structures of several soluble protein kinases as well as the insulin receptor and EGFR tyrosine kinase domains, it appears that the receptor protein tyrosine kinase catalytic domains are likely to consist of two lobes, one that binds Mg^{2+}/adenosine triphosphate (ATP) utilizing a GXGXXG motif, and one that forms the actual catalytic loop. In some receptors in this family, such as the PDGFR, the tyrosine

kinase catalytic domain is interrupted by a spacer region (Fig. 5B).

The RTKs all exhibit a hormone-dependent dimerization that is crucial for subsequent signal transduction. Crystallographic studies of the extracellular domains of the EGFR and its relatives ErbB2 (Neu/HER2) and ErbB3 (HER3) demonstrate that growth factor binding to each receptor monomer promotes a structural rearrangement to expose a dimerization interface. For ErbB2, which does not have a ligand, the dimerization domain is constitutively exposed (Burgess et al., 2003). Some ligands for these receptors are themselves dimers (e.g., PDGF), whereas others are monomers (e.g., EGF), and this may affect the dimerization mechanism. The functional consequence of receptor dimerization is to bring the cytoplasmic tyrosine kinase domains into close proximity, which leads to cross-phosphorylation of the receptors and the subsequent recruitment of substrates having affinity for the tyrosine-phosphorylated receptor. These include a broad repertoire of cellular proteins that have an Src homology 2 (SH2) domain that specifically recognizes tyrosine phosphorylation sites on the receptor. Some of these SH2 domain proteins are direct substrates for phosphorylation by the receptor and can serve as effector molecules in transducing the signal. Examples of substrates include the phosphatidylinositol-3-kinase regulatory subunit, the Src family protein kinases, the protein tyrosine phosphatase Syp, and PLCγ. Other SH2 domain proteins act simply as molecular adapters; they bind to the phosphorylated receptor and also associate with additional cellular proteins, commonly through a protein interaction motif referred to as the SH3 domain. Examples include Grb2, Nck, and Crk, which bind to a variety of hormone receptors. Several proteins, including the adapter Shc and the insulin receptor substrate family of docking proteins, utilize a distinct phosphotyrosine-binding domain that recognize an Asn-Pro-x-pTyr motif in target receptors. Yet other adapter and effector proteins in this signaling pathway contain pleckstrin homology domains, which may play a role in tethering these proteins at the plasma membrane, or contain WW protein interaction motifs. Use of modular interaction domains is a common theme in cell signaling and is particularly apparent in the RTKs (Pawson and Scott, 1997).

Adapter proteins mediate a broad spectrum of cellular responses, but a common and well-characterized response leads to activation of the small GTP-binding protein Ras. Ras activation initiates a kinase cascade, the mitogen-activated protein kinase (MAPK) cascade, which eventually results in the phosphorylation and activation of nuclear transcription factors able to alter gene expression in the target cell. At many of the key regulatory steps, specific protein tyrosine phosphatases counter the actions of the kinases and, thus, exert negative control over activation, a likely component of inhibitory feedback mechanisms. A generic example of signaling of an RTK through the MAPK pathway leading to extracellular-regulated kinase (ERK) activation is shown in Fig. 5C.

The physiologic functions of many of the receptors in the tyrosine protein kinase family have been explored through gene disruption approaches in mice, or by the identification of naturally occurring mutations in these receptors in animal models or in people. It should be realized that many of the RTKs were initially discovered as transduced retroviral oncogenes that represent mutated, truncated, or inappropriately expressed versions of their cellular counterparts (Carbone and Levine, 1990). Although a complete discussion of the physiologic functions of receptor tyrosine protein kinases is beyond the scope of this chapter, a few examples related

to several important model receptors (the EGF, PDGF, and insulin receptors) are briefly considered. The EGFR played a key role in defining the relationship of cellular signaling pathways to retrovirus-induced cellular transformation and oncogenesis. A truncated and transduced form of the EGFR represents one of two oncogenes (v-erbB) of the avian erythroblastosis virus, and the highly related Neu tyrosine kinase receptor (also referred to as HER2 or erbB2) is mutated or amplified in a wide variety of human cancers. Thus, inappropriate activation of the signaling pathways mediated by these tyrosine kinase receptors can lead to cell transformation and tumorigenesis. Consistent with this, the PDGFR is involved in a number of reciprocal chromosomal translocations that lead to its constitutive activation and are associated with myeloproliferative disorders. The insulin receptor is subject to mutation in patients with insulin resistance, and this has led to the identification of many different types of mutations that affect the synthesis or function of this RTK. These mutations are associated with type A insulin resistance, leprachaunism, and lipoatrophic diabetes.

3.3. Receptors With Serine and Threonine Kinase Activity

Receptors with serine and threonine kinase activity were identified relatively recently, beginning with the expression cloning of the activin type II receptor in 1991 (Mathews, 1994). Activin is a protein hormone in the TGF-β superfamily, and this superfamily includes hormones such as Müllerian-inhibiting substance (MIS), the bone morphogenetic proteins (BMPs), and nonmammalian homologs such as *Drosophila* decapentaplegic (*dpp*) and *Xenopus* Vg-1. Receptor nomenclature has been based on early crosslinking studies with TGF-β that revealed three distinct protein bands designated type I, II, and III receptors. The type III receptor is a large proteoglycan, also known as beta glycan, which is thought to play a role as a coreceptor for TGF-β, inhibin, and possibly other family members by facilitating delivery of the hormone to the signaling receptors. Both the type I and II receptors are involved in signaling. Distinct combinations of type I and II proteins form the functional receptor for each ligand of the TGF-β superfamily, and the relative roles of the two receptor subunits vary somewhat, depending on the ligand with which they interact. Figure 6A shows several representative ligands of the TGF-β superfamily along with the type I and II receptors that mediate their actions.

Both the type I and II receptors have conserved cytoplasmic domains with protein serine or threonine kinase activity. For those ligands most closely related to TGF-β, including activin and nodal, the type II receptor is the

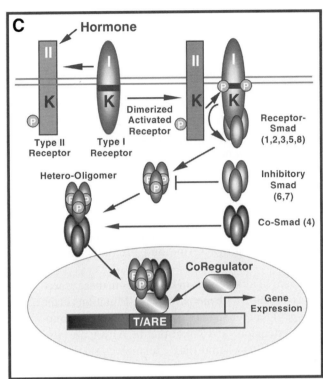

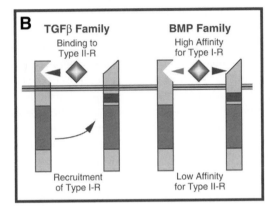

Fig. 6. Structure and signal transduction by receptor serine/threonine kinases: (**A**) representative ligands in TGF-β superfamily, their type II and I receptors, and Smad proteins they activate; (**B**) mechanisms of ligand binding to receptors for the two major subclasses of TGF-β ligands, TGF-β class and BMP class; (**C**) example of generic signaling through the Smad pathway, although this example of ligand binding illustrates initial binding to type II receptor, which is characteristic of TGF-β class.

high-affinity ligand-binding determinant. Binding of hormone allows the type II receptor to interact with the type I receptor, most likely in the form of a heterotetramer that interacts with the homodimeric ligand (Fig. 6B). The type II receptor, which has constitutive kinase activity, then phosphorylates the type II receptor in a serine-rich juxtamembrane region known as the GS box, leading to activation of the type I receptor kinase. By contrast, for ligands related to the BMPs, including the growth and differentiation factors (GDFs) and MIS, it is the type I receptor that has a higher affinity for ligand, although the type II receptor does contribute to ligand binding (Fig. 6B). Oligomerization leads to phosphorylation and activation of the type I receptor. Substantial insight into the interactions between ligand and receptor in this system has emerged from crystallographic and nuclear magnetic resonance structural studies (Shi and Massagué, 2003). There appears to be a well-conserved mechanism for binding of BMP-related ligands to the type I receptor, but there is substantial diversity in the way in which TGF-β-related ligands interact with the type II receptor.

The major transducers of signaling downstream of the serine and threonine kinase type I receptors are a family of proteins known as the Smads in vertebrates. The name derives from the related proteins in *Caenorhabditis elegans* (Sma) and *Drosophila* (Mad). There are eight known Smad proteins that play distinct roles in signaling between the cell-surface receptor and the nucleus. Smads 1, 2, 3, 5, and 8 are known as receptor-regulated Smads (R-Smads), and they are direct targets for phosphorylation within a C-terminal SSXS motif by the type I receptor. The TGF-β-related ligands lead to phosphorylation of Smads 2 and 3, and the BMP-related ligands lead to phosphorylation of Smads 1, 5, and 8. The phosphorylated Smad proteins dissociate from the receptor and form heteromeric complexes with a common cytoplasmic Smad protein, Smad4. This heteromeric complex moves to the nucleus and acts to modulate transcription of target genes. Although there is evidence for direct DNA-binding by Smads 3 and 4, the predominant actions of Smads are thought to be mediated by their interaction with nuclear DNA binding proteins and stabilization of ternary DNA-bound complexes among the R-Smads, Smad-4, and the target transcription factor (Attisano and Wrana, 2000). The *Xenopus* transcription factor FAST-1 was the first of these interacting proteins to be identified, but it is likely that the Smads target many transcriptional regulatory proteins. Smads 6 and 7 are known as inhibitory Smads, and they act to inhibit the activation of the R-Smads by binding to the type I receptor. Smads 6 and 7 are up-regulated by BMP and TGF-β pathway signaling, respectively, and are likely part of a negative feedback system. Finally, there are numerous examples of additional proteins that interact with or modify the activity of the serine and threonine kinase receptors, and signaling crosstalk is likely a very important component in generating specificity of response. Figure 6C summarizes aspects of signaling downstream of serine and threonine kinase receptors.

There are several reports of mutations in these receptors in association with human disease. Mutations in the BMP type II receptor and in ALK1 are found in pulmonary hypertension, and mutations in ALK1 are also found in hereditary hemorrhagic telangiectasia type II. Loss of expression of the TGF-β type II receptor through microsatellite instability or as a result of transcriptional repression is found in a variety of human cancers. Much more frequent are mutations in the downstream Smad proteins, indicating a role for these proteins as tumor suppressors. Smad2 mutations are found in colorectal and lung cancers, and Smad4 mutations are found in many cancers but are particularly prevalent in pancreatic carcinoma, in which Smad4 was first identified as the tumor suppressor deleted in pancreatic cancer (dpc)-4.

3.4. Receptors That Recruit Tyrosine Kinases

Many well-characterized cell-surface receptors lack apparent enzymatic functions within their cytoplasmic regions, and their activity therefore depends on the recruitment of signaling proteins to the receptor. This family includes the receptors for the interleukins (ILs), interferons (IFNs), erythropoietin (EPO), granulocyte-macrophage colony-stimulating factor (GM-CSF), leukemia inhibitory factor (LIF), growth hormone (GH) and prolactin (PRL), among others, and is known as the cytokine receptor superfamily (Fig. 7A). The functional receptors include single-chain type I transmembrane proteins (GH, PRL, EPO), those that have a ligand-specific subunit that interacts with a common shared subunit (ILs, GM-CSF, LIF) and those that have multiple unique subunits (IFNs). Some examples of cytokine family receptors of each type are shown in Fig. 7B. Although these receptors all lack tyrosine kinase activity, conserved membrane-proximal regions of their cytoplasmic domains mediate ligand-dependent interaction with one or more cytoplasmic protein tyrosine kinases, the Janus kinases, or Jaks (Ihle and Kerr, 1995). These kinases, including Jak1, Jak2, Jak3, and Tyk2, have amino-terminal homology domains of unknown function, and two carboxyl-terminal kinase domains, although the first of these lacks critical residues necessary for catalytic activity and is inactive. The Jak kinases are tyrosine phosphorylated and activated following ligand binding to the cytokine receptors, and this requires an association of the Jak kinases with two conserved membrane-proximal motifs in the receptor referred to as box 1 and box 2. It is thought that receptor dimerization brings the associated Jak kinases into close proximity and allows cross-phosphorylation and activation to occur, and, thus, two Jak kinases associate in the same manner as two cytoplasmic kinase domains of the RTKs associate. In addition to Jak kinase phosphorylation, the activation process is associated with phosphorylation of the receptor itself on specific tyrosine residues, which can lead to activation of some of the same pathways activated by the conventional RTKs, such as the MAPK pathway.

The pathway from Jak kinase activation to changes in target cell gene expression was completed through the analysis of proteins mediating the transcriptional responses to IFN, a family of proteins known as the Stat (signal transducer and activator of transcription) proteins (Darnell et al., 1994). Following cytokine receptor phosphorylation by a Jak family kinase, Stat proteins are recruited to the receptor and phosphorylated on a single tyrosine residue near the C-terminal transactivation domain of the protein. The phosphorylated and activated Stat proteins form homo- or heterodimers, translocate to the nucleus, and bind to specific DNA elements (originally called γ IFN activation sequences, or GAS elements) near target genes to regulate transcription. Stat proteins include a highly conserved SH2 domain as well as an SH3-related domain in the C-terminal regions, in addition to the conserved C-terminal tyrosine phosphorylation site, and are reported to interact with a broad spectrum of other transcription factors and coregulators. Seven Stat proteins that fall into three groups have been identified, and it appears that these serve as the major link between cytokine receptor activation and cellular transcriptional responses. There are likely several modes of negative regulation of this pathway, but a major mechanism involves Stat protein induction of the suppressor of cytokine signaling (SOCS) family of proteins, which then act through mechanisms that remain unclear to block Stat signaling, most likely at the level of the receptor or Jak kinase (Cooney, 2002).

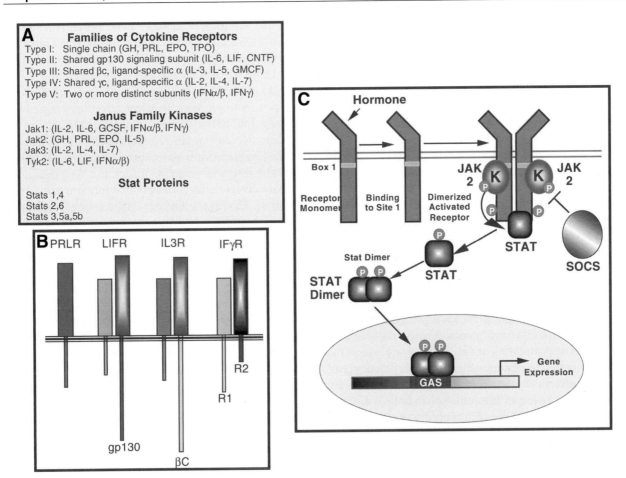

Fig. 7. Structure and signal transduction by cytokine superfamily receptors: (**A**) examples of some of the major families of receptors, along with Janus family kinases and Stat proteins they activate; (**B**) representative schematic structures demonstrating subunit composition of various types of cytokine superfamily receptors; (**C**) example of generic signaling through a type I cytokine receptor to the Jak-Stat pathway.

It is clear that different receptors in the cytokine receptor superfamily preferentially associate with one or more of the four Jak kinases and subsequently preferentially activate one or more of the seven Stat proteins, but the mechanisms of specificity are largely unknown. The various Jaks and Stats have unique tissue distributions, and this likely explains in part why particular receptors signal through particular Jak-Stat pathways. Because the cytokine receptor superfamily is large, and the receptors utilize diverse signaling mechanisms, it is informative to consider one example focused on the endocrine system in greater detail. One of the best-studied receptors in this class is the GHR. It is representative of the single-chain class of cytokine receptor and has the two pairs of conserved cysteines in the extracellular domain that are a hallmark of this family. Interestingly, two receptor chains bind to a single GH molecule at distinct sites on the hormone, and thus a single ligand molecule catalyzes receptor dimerization and subsequent signal

transduction. This has been demonstrated by determination of the crystallographic structure of the extracellular domain of the GHR complexed with GH. Site 1 on GH must be occupied prior to occupancy of site 2. At high concentrations of hormone, saturation of all receptors by binding to site 1 on GH is predicted to inhibit receptor dimerization and the subsequent biologic response. This has been experimentally demonstrated in several systems and may represent an additional mode of receptor regulation. The GHR is unique in that the extracellular domain of the receptor also functions as a soluble serum-binding protein for GH. The extracellular domain is released from the mature receptor by proteolysis in some species, and it is encoded by a distinct mRNA generated by alternative RNA processing in other species. The activated GHR associates with the Jak2 kinase, leading to the phosphorylation and activation of Stats 1, 3, and 5. In addition, the MAPK pathway is also activated by GH, presumably through the interaction of adapter proteins with the phosphorylated GHR, or with Jak2 itself. Signaling through a single-chain cytokine superfamily receptor such as the GHR is illustrated in Fig. 7C.

The GHR is also a good example of the potential involvement of receptors within this superfamily in endocrine disease. Mutations in the GHR/binding protein are responsible for the GH resistance observed in Laron-type dwarfism, in which serum GH is elevated in association with classic symptoms of GH deficiency, including reduced levels of insulin-like growth factor-1 (IGF-1) and short stature. Dozens of distinct mutations in the receptor have been found, and nearly all are in the extracellular domain and result in gross alteration in receptor structure, generally through premature termination of translation. Other cytokine family receptors involved in disease include the leptin receptor, which is mutated in a syndrome of obesity and pituitary dysfunction, and the GCSF receptor, which is truncated in severe congenital neutropenia. A particularly important example is mutation of the common γc chain of the IL receptor in severe combined immunodeficiency. Not surprisingly, the downstream Jak and Stat proteins are also likely to be targets for mutation in human disease, and Jak2 and Stat5B are both reported to act as fusion partners in chromosomal translocations is particular forms of leukemia.

3.5. Receptors That Activate Developmental Signaling Pathways

Several highly conserved signaling pathways, in addition to those already described, play important roles in the development of metazoan organisms and have common features that warrant their consideration as a single group. These include DSL ligand signaling through the Notch receptor, Wnt signaling through the Frizzled receptor, and Hedgehog signaling through the Patched and Smoothened receptors. In each of these cases, receptor activation is associated with movement of a key regulatory molecule from the cell surface or cytoplasm to the cell nucleus, regulated proteolysis is a key event in transducing the signal and genes that are otherwise repressed become activated through a corepressor/coactivator switch.

The Notch family of receptors (Mumm and Kopan, 2000) are large type I transmembrane proteins with an extracellular LBD. However, the ligands for Notch are themselves cell-surface type I transmembrane proteins of the Delta, Serrate, and Lag2 (DSL) family, so that Notch mediates direct cell-cell signaling. Another surprising feature of the Notch receptor is that the cytoplasmic domain, which has signaling function, appears to act in the nucleus to modulate transcription. In response

to ligand binding, proteases of the presenelin family cleave the Notch receptor, releasing the Notch intracellular domain. This domain has a nuclear localization signal, and it enters the nucleus to form a complex with proteins of the CBF-1, Su(H), Lag-1 family (CBL) and converts these proteins from transcriptional repressors to transcriptional activators, stimulating target gene expression. Notch signaling is illustrated in Fig. 8A.

The Frizzled family of receptors (Wodarz and Nusse, 1998) bind to a large array of secreted Wnt ligands to mediate diverse effects on cell proliferation and differentiation. The Frizzled receptors are seven-membrane-spanning domain receptors and thus can be classed with the GPCRs, but there is still no strong evidence to indicate that these receptors are in fact G protein coupled. The best, although still incompletely, characterized pathway of Wnt signaling involves the stabilization of cytoplasmic β-catenin. In the absence of Wnts, β-catenin is phosphorylated by the kinase GSK3, which triggers its ubiquitination and degradation. This occurs within a multiprotein complex, and the activity of this complex is modulated by the Dishevelled protein, which is genetically downstream of Frizzled receptor signaling. In the presence of a Wnt ligand, the activity of the complex promoting β-catenin degradation is repressed. The net effect is an increase in cytoplasmic β-catenin levels, allowing β-catenin to enter the nucleus and interact with the transcription factor TCF/LEF. This interaction promotes the recruitment of transcriptional coregulators and stimulates the expression of Wnt target genes. This pathway of Wnt signaling is illustrated in Fig. 8B. In addition, there are reports of Wnt signaling through pathways as diverse as Jun N-terminal kinase activation and calcium mobilization.

The Hedgehog family of ligands, which in vertebrates includes Sonic, Indian, and Desert Hedgehog, signals through a mechanism that is similar in many respects to the Wnt pathway. In this example, the Hedgehog binding receptor, Patched, is a 12-transmembrane domain protein that modulates the activity of a coreceptor, the 7-transmembrane domain Smoothened receptor (Ingham and McMahon, 2001). There is no strong evidence for G protein coupling of the Smoothened protein, and it does not interact directly with the ligand Hedgehog. Instead, Hedgehog binding to Patched appears to relieve Patched-mediated repression of Smoothened, allowing activation of Smoothened and transduction of the signal. Events immediately downstream of Smoothened are unknown but act on a multiprotein complex to modify the proteolytic processing of a key signal transducer, a zinc-finger protein known as Ci (in *Drosophila*) or Gli (in vertebrates). In the absence of a Hedgehog signal, Ci/Gli is processed

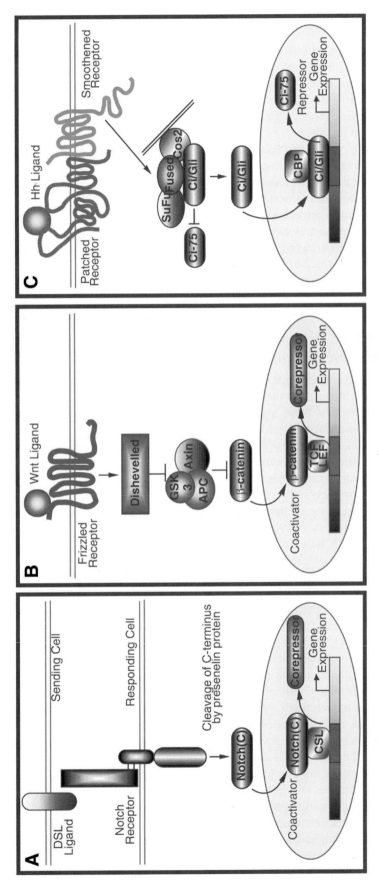

Fig. 8. Key developmental signaling pathways and their receptors. (**A**) signaling through Notch receptor in response to cell-bound DSL ligand; (**B**) Wnt signaling through Frizzled receptor; (**C**) Hedgehog signaling through Patched receptor and Smoothened coreceptor. These are generic pathways and in each case represent the best characterized of several signaling pathways that are activated by these ligands and receptors. The three pathways shown have many common features, as discussed in the text.

to a truncated form that enters the nucleus and acts to suppress Hedgehog target genes. When Smoothened is actvated, the full-length form of Ci/Gli is stabilized, and it enters the nucleus and promotes transcription of Hedgehog target genes. Signaling through the Hedgehog pathway is summarized in Fig. 8C.

Although mutational studies of these related pathways have been largely the domain of model organisms, it is becoming appreciated that these receptors and signaling pathways are of key importance to development and organogenesis in vertebrates. Mutations in the Notch ligand JAG1 are causative in arteriohepatic dysplasia. A Frizzled-4 receptor mutation has been reported in familial exudative vitreoretinopathy. Mutations in the Patched receptor and, as documented in a few reports, the Smoothened coreceptor are a major cause of basal cell carcinoma.

3.6. Receptors With Protein Tyrosine Phosphatase Activity

A large number of protein tyrosine phosphatases have been identified by molecular cloning, and their structures suggest that at least seven of these are transmembrane proteins with the potential to act as ligand-regulated phosphatases (Fischer et al., 1991). They are distinct from the serine and threonine protein phosphatases and might be expected to participate in cellular signal transduction by countering the activities of the RTKs. Despite the striking similarity of these transmembrane protein tyrosine phosphatases to receptors, distinct ligands that might activate these proteins have not been identified. Some of these proteins have extracellular domains that include regions resembling segments of fibronectin or neural cell adhesion molecule, suggesting that the transmembrane protein tyrosine phosphatases might be involved in signaling in response to direct cell-cell communication or cell-matrix interaction.

The best characterized of the potential receptor protein tyrosine phosphatases is the leukocyte common antigen CD45. It consists of an external segment that is cysteine rich and resembles a ligand-binding motif, a single transmembrane domain, and two tandem cytoplasmic protein tyrosine phosphatase domains. Multiple forms of CD45 arise through alternative RNA-processing mechanisms, and these are differentially glycosylated and expressed on distinct subsets of lymphocytes. CD45 is known to be essential for antigen-stimulated proliferation of T-lymphocytes and for thymic development, and mutations in CD45 are implicated in autoimmunity. Recent studies indicate that members of the Src family of cytoplasmic protein tyrosine kinases are likely to be the major physiologic substrates for the CD45 tyrosine phosphatase.

3.7. Receptors With Guanylyl Cyclase Activity

As their name implies, the receptors in this small family have cytoplasmic domains that possess guanylyl cyclase (GC) activity, promoting the production of a cyclic guanosine 5′-monophosphate (cGMP) second messenger. They are distinct from, but related to, the soluble GCs. They are single-chain transmembrane proteins with an extracellular LBD, a membrane proximal cytoplasmic domain that resembles a protein kinase domain but is catalytically inactive, and the carboxyl-terminal GC domain (Garbers, 1999). There are seven identified transmembrane GCs. GC-A, GC-B, and GC-C all represent receptors for natriuretic peptides or heat-stable enterotoxins. The GC-A receptor binds atrial natriuretic peptide as well as the related BNP, GC-B binds the natriuretic peptide CNP, and GC-C binds heat-stable enterotoxin and probably binds the novel peptide guanylin. GC-D is expressed in olfactory sensory neurons; GC-E and GC-F are expressed within the eye; and GC-G is expressed in lung, intestine, and skeletal muscle. These latter four remain orphan receptors with no known ligand and suggest a subfamily of GC receptors (D,E, and F) restricted to sensory tissues. Interestingly, the GC receptors appear to exist in a dimeric or tetrameric state prior to activation. Ligand binding is thought to induce a conformational change that brings the catalytic guanylyl cyclase domains into proximity to form an active dimer. Phosphorylation strongly modifies receptor activity, although the kinase responsible has not been identified.

3.8. Tumor Neurosis Factor Receptors

A large and diverse family of receptors mediate the actions of the tumor necrosis factors (TNFs). There are 18 identified TNF family ligands that promote cell proliferation, cell survival, or cell death, and, remarkably, they bind to at least 30 distinct receptor proteins (Gaur and Aggarwal, 2003). Ligands appear to be able to bind to multiple receptors, and the receptors are expressed in a tissue-specific fashion. The receptors have homologous extracellular domains and can be divided into two broad groups based on the structure of their cytoplasmic domain. At least six receptors in the TNF family have an intracellular death domain. The death domain is responsible for recruiting a broad spectrum of intracellular signaling proteins that eventually result in the activation of caspases and initiation of the apoptotic response. TNF receptors that lack the death domain can also induce apoptosis, although the signaling mechanisms involved are not clearly understood.

A second major signaling pathway activated by all TNF receptors is the nuclear factor-κB (NF-κB) pathway. This is mediated by the recruitment of TNF receptor–associated factors (TRAFs), of which at least six are activated in a ligand- and receptor-specific fashion. TRAFs in some manner lead to activation of the IκB kinase, phosphorylation and degradation of the inhibitor IκB, and release of NF-κB to enter the nucleus, where it regulates genes that suppress apoptosis and are involved in inflammatory responses. TNFs induce the NF-κB pathway in all cells, whereas they stimulate cell death in a smaller subset of cells. At least two TNF family receptors are implicated in human disease. Mutations in TNF-R1 cause a familial periodic fever syndrome, and mutations in the receptor Fas are found in malignant lymphoma and in autoimmune lymphoproliferative syndrome type I.

3.9. Transport Receptors

A significant number of cell-surface receptors may not have classic signaling functions but, rather, serve to transport substances into the cell from the plasma. These include the receptors for transferrin, LDLs, asialoglycoproteins, mannose-6-phosphate (M-6-P), and other plasma proteins. These receptors bind their ligand, cluster into coated pits, and are rapidly endocytosed into endosomal or lysosomal vesicles, where the ligand can be dissociated and utilized, and the receptor either degraded or recycled back to the cell surface, as described in Fig. 3A. Several of these receptors have proven to be important models for investigating the cell biology of cell-surface receptor trafficking. Two receptors that exemplify this family of transport receptors, the LDL receptor and the M-6-P/IGF-2 receptor, are discussed subsequently.

The LDL receptor extracellular domain consists of a cysteine-rich and negatively charged ligand-binding region, an EGF precursor homology domain, and a juxtamembrane domain rich in O-linked glycosylation sites (Brown and Goldstein, 1986). The cytoplasmic domain is short and has no obvious signaling features but is critical for clustering the receptor into coated pits for subsequent endocytosis, and eventual lysosomal hydrolysis of the cholesterol esters of LDL, to generate cellular stores of cholesterol. The importance of this receptor in the transport of LDLs is underscored by the finding of many different defects in the LDL receptor in patients with the disease familial hypercholesterolemia, in which plasma levels of cholesterol are highly elevated. These mutations affect nearly all aspects of receptor function, including synthesis, transport, binding, and internalization of the receptor.

The M-6-P/IGF-2 receptor is referred to as a multifunctional protein because it is known to bind at least two ligands utilizing distinct sites on the extracellular domain of the receptor (Kornfield, 1992). The receptor is a large protein of 275 kDa, more than 90% of which is extracellular. Fifteen conserved repeat sequences of approx 150 amino acids, each with eight conserved cysteines and 16–38% overall identity, constitute the large extracellular domain of the receptor, and the cytoplasmic domain is small and includes multiple potential phosphorylation sites. The receptor binds proteins containing M-6-P and is important for both the sorting of newly synthesized lysosomal enzymes and the endocytosis of extracellular lysosomal enzymes. A second M-6-P receptor, the cation-dependent receptor, is a 46 kDa protein that has an extracellular domain that is a single copy of the conserved repeat sequence of the larger M-6-P/IGF-2 receptor, and it is important for the sorting of newly synthesized lysosomal proteins. Although IGF-2 binds to the M-6-P/IGF-2 receptor with high affinity at a site distinct from the M-6-P-binding site, the role of this receptor in IGF-2 signaling remains uncertain, and it has been suggested that IGF-2 may instead act through the IGF-1 receptor, a member of the RTK family. An additional feature of interest regarding the M-6-P/IGF-2 receptor is that the gene encoding this receptor is subject to genomic imprinting effects, and only the maternal allele is expressed.

4. INTRACELLULAR RECEPTORS
4.1 Nuclear Receptor Superfamily

The receptors in the nuclear receptor superfamily are structurally and functionally distinct from the cell-surface receptors, in that they are located in either the cytoplasm or nucleus, where they bind hydrophobic ligands that are able to diffuse passively through the plasma membrane of the cell. In response to hormone binding, these receptors undergo a conformational change and become competent to bind to specific DNA elements that act as hormone-dependent enhancers of gene expression. The steroid hormones and their receptors are considered in greater detail in Chapter 4; the intent of this section is to contrast briefly the structure and function of the intracellular receptors with the cell-surface receptors, rather than to review this class of receptors comprehensively.

The nuclear receptor superfamily includes the receptors for the classic steroid hormones such as estrogens, progestins, androgens, and glucocorticoids; the receptors for thyroid hormones, retinoids, and vitamin D; and a large number of orphan receptors that share basic features of the superfamily but that have no known activating ligand. Many receptors initially identified as orphans are now known to have specific ligands or physiologic functions (Willson and Moore, 2002). Some of the ~50 vertebrate nuclear receptors are listed in Fig. 9A. Most

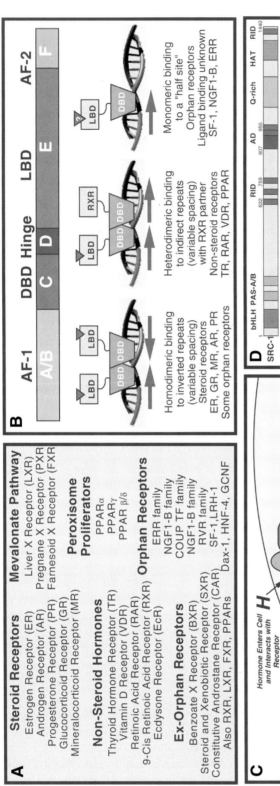

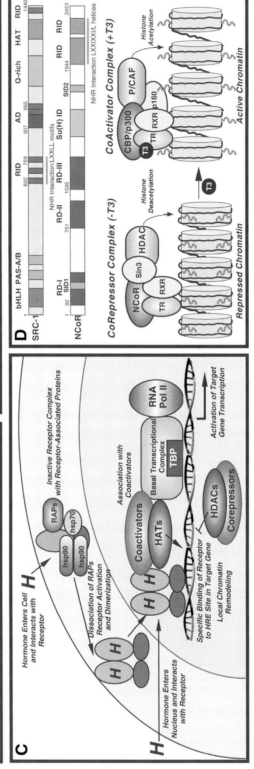

Fig. 9. Structural features and mechanism of action of nuclear receptors. (**A**) Examples of major classes of nuclear receptors, including orphan receptors. (**B**) General features of nuclear receptors. The predominant domains are the DBD, the LBD and the transactivation domains AF-1 and AF-2, as discussed in the text. Also indicated in (**B**) are three potential modes of DNA binding. Some orphan receptors bind DNA in a monomeric form; steroid receptors bind DNA as homodimers; and thyroid, retinoid, and vitamin D receptors bind DNA as heterodimers with the partner RXR. Arrows indicate the number and orientation of core motifs in the DNA-binding site. (**C**) Generic model for signal transduction by steroid hormones and related compounds. The unliganded receptor can be either cytoplasmic or nuclear and is often found in a complex with chaperone proteins. Hormone binding leads to the dissociation of these chaperones and the formation of receptor dimers competent to bind to DNA. Binding of the receptor at HREs alters target gene transcription through interactions with the basal transcriptional complex that are likely to be mediated by coactivator proteins, which also serve to remodel chromatin. (**D**) Schematic structures of a representative coactivator (SRC-1) and corepressor (NcoR) protein, illustrating the distinct nuclear hormone receptor (NHR) interaction motifs. The bottom half of the panel is a schematic of the switch between corepressors and coactivators induced by binding of some hormones to their nuclear receptors, in this example, the TR.

28

of the nuclear receptors have a distinct and common structure composed of six conserved domains (A–F), shown schematically in Fig. 9B. The defining feature of these proteins is the presence of a highly conserved DBD that includes two zinc fingers of the Cys-4 type. Sequences within this domain, particularly those near the end of the first zinc finger and the beginning of the second zinc finger, are important for determining the DNA-binding specificity of each receptor. These receptors bind to specific DNA elements near target genes termed *hormone response elements* (HREs), which are usually either direct or inverted repeats of a 6-bp core consensus sequence, separated by a variable-length spacer, the combination of which is unique for each receptor class. Sequences within the DBD and the adjacent C-terminal domain are also required for nuclear localization of the receptor, and for dimerization. The receptors bind to HREs as either monomers (some orphan receptors such as NGFI-B), homodimers (steroid receptors such as the glucocorticoid receptor [GR] and estrogen receptor [ER]), or heterodimers (the thyroid hormone receptor [TR], retinoic acid receptor [RAR], and vitamin D receptor [VDR]). In the latter class, the retinoid X receptor (RXR) serves as a common heterodimerization partner. These modes of DNA binding are illustrated in Fig. 9B. There is a region of highly variable length and sequence N-terminal to the DBD, and in many receptors this region includes a domain important for transcriptional activation termed activation function-1 (AF-1). The C-terminal region of the receptor includes the specific LBD, as well as a second transactivation domain, AF-2, and regions necessary for dimerization.

In the absence of hormone, the steroid, thyroid, and retinoid receptors appear to be localized predominantly in the nucleus. Some, particularly those that partner with RXR, may be bound to the DNA in the absence of ligand. An exception is the GR, which appears to be predominantly cytoplasmic in the absence like the GR of hormone. Unliganded steroid hormone receptors are associated with an array of chaperone proteins such as the heat-shock proteins hsp90 and hsp70, and the immunophilin FKBP52. These chaperones likely play an important role in the folding of the receptor protein during synthesis, in the maintenance of the inactive receptor in a high-affinity steroid-binding conformation, and in the transformation to the active state of the receptor following hormone binding. A model depicting the dissociation of receptor-associated chaperone proteins on hormone binding, the dimerization of the receptor, its binding to HREs in DNA, and the regulation of target gene transcription by the hormone-activated receptor is presented in Fig. 9C.

Transcriptional control of gene expression by the nuclear receptors requires their interaction with coactivators or corepressors that stimulate or repress, respectively, expression of the target gene. The first coactivator identified was steroid receptor coactivator-1 (SRC-1), and many such proteins have now been identified (McKenna and O'Malley, 2002). Coactivators do not bind directly to DNA but likely facilitate interactions between the DNA-bound nuclear receptor and the basal transcription complex. Some coactivators have intrinsic histone acetyltransferase (HAT) activity, whereas others recruit HATs to the gene promoter. Acetylation of amino-terminal lysine residues of the core histone proteins of nucleosomes loosens their association with DNA and is associated with enhanced transcriptional activity. Conversely, deacetylation of histones is associated with a compacted chromatin structure and transcriptional repression, and several corepressor proteins exert their actions by recruitment of histone deacetylases (HDACs) to the gene promoter. Major corepressor proteins involved in steroid hormone action are the nuclear receptor corepressor (NCoR) and the silencing mediator of retinoic and thyroid receptors (SMRT). These coregulatory proteins play key roles in mediating NHR signaling. Figure 9D shows schematic structures of a key coactivator (SRC-1) and corepressor (NcoR) for nuclear receptor action. In many examples, the unliganded receptor is maintained in the repressed state through the actions of corepressors and the liganded receptor becomes active through both loss of corepressor interactions and establishment of coactivator interactions. This is best described for the nonsteroid nuclear receptors such as TR and RAR. This concept as applied to thyroid hormone action is illustrated in Fig. 9D.

Many steroid hormone antagonists exert their actions by promoting a receptor conformation that favors interaction with corepressor proteins, whereas agonists promote interaction with a coactivator. The cellular composition and concentration of coregulatory proteins therefore have important influences on steroid hormone action, and this finding has been exploited in the development of selective steroid receptor modulators, drugs that act as agonists in some tissues and antagonists in others. Crystallographic structures of nuclear receptor LBDs, in the unliganded state and bound to agonists or antagonists, provide a likely explanation for these findings, in that the ligand induces structural changes, particularly in helix 12 within the AF-2 domain, that promote interaction with either a coactivator or corepressor dependent on the bound ligand.

There are mechanisms by which some of the steroid receptors, and other nuclear receptors, can be activated in a ligand-independent fashion (Weigel and Zhang, 1998). Stimulators of cellular kinase activity (such as cAMP) or inhibitors of cellular phosphatase activity (such as okadaic acid) can activate some of the nuclear receptors in the absence of any ligand. For example, the PR, ER, and VDR can all be activated by the neurotransmitter dopamine in a manner that does not involve binding to the receptor, and the ER can be activated by a variety of polypeptide growth factors. In other cases, ligand-independent activation is not observed. The pathways mediating this activation appear to involve both receptor and coactivator phosphorylation. The steroid receptors are phosphoproteins, and some receptors such as the PR are inducibly phosphorylated on ligand binding by a variety of cellular kinases. Ligand-independent activation of these receptors may provide an important mechanism of cross talk between the steroid receptor pathway and other cellular signal transduction pathways. In addition, not all of the effects of steroid hormones are mediated by the nuclear receptors, and there is ample evidence for "nongenomic" actions of these hormones.

The nuclear receptors play critical roles in endocrine communication, and it is therefore not surprising that receptor mutations are associated with a range of endocrine disorders. Resistance to thyroid hormone can involve mutation or deletion of the TR β gene, and familial glucocorticoid resistance can be caused by deletions or point mutations in the GR gene. Hypocalcemic vitamin D–resistant rickets results from mutations in the VDR that can affect hormone binding, DNA binding, or nuclear translocation of the receptor. More than 200 distinct mutations in the AR have been found in patients with androgen insensitivity syndromes. A single example of mutation of the ER gene in a man with estrogen resistance has been reported, but no mutations of the PR in humans are known. Although these latter findings might imply lethality of ER or PR mutations, disruption of these genes in mice results in animals that live to adulthood, although they have impaired reproductive function. RARα is a translocation fusion partner in acute promyelocytic leukemia. Mutations in the orphan receptor Dax-1 cause congenital adrenal hyperplasia, and mutation of the orphan receptor SF-1 results in XY sex reversal and adrenal failure.

4.2. Additional Mechanisms of Intracellular Hormone Action

Although the nuclear receptors are the largest and best studied of the intracellular receptors, several other examples that involve intracellular receptors that function as transcription factors are briefly mentioned in this section. The first of these is the arylhydrocarbon (Ah) receptor. Ahs include 2,3,7,8-tetrachlorodibenzo-*p*-dioxin and related dioxin-like environmental pollutants such as the polychlorinated biphenyls, as well as compounds such as indolo[3,2-*b*]carbazole, that are generated naturally through the digestion of plant metabolites. These toxic, carcinogenic, and highly persistent compounds act through specific binding to a soluble intracellular receptor, the Ah receptor, also known as the dioxin receptor, to modulate gene expression. It is not clear if the Ah receptor's primary function is in defense against these foreign chemicals, but there are no known endogenous ligands for this receptor, and target genes for Ah receptor regulation include enzymes that metabolize these foreign chemicals to forms that can be excreted. The Ah receptor is a ligand-activated transcription factor (Schmidt and Bradfield, 1996). Although it has a similar mode of action to the nuclear receptors described in the previous section, its structure is not consistent with it being a member of this family. The Ah receptor is instead a basic helix-loop-helix (bHLH) transcription factor that is a member of the PAS domain family (for *Per*, AhR, Ah receptor nuclear translocator [ARNT], and *Sim*). The related ARNT protein does not bind dioxins but, rather, acts as a heterodimerization partner for the Ah receptor. The unliganded Ah receptor is found in the cytoplasm and associates with hsp90, much like the steroid receptors. Following ligand binding, hsp90 dissociates, and the receptor translocates to the nucleus and binds to ARNT to form the heterodimer. The Ah receptor–ARNT complex binds to selective DNA elements known as xenobiotic response elements to regulate target gene transcription.

A somewhat similar example, although not involving a hormonal ligand, is the system for oxygen sensing in cells, with the key player being another PAS family bHLH transcription factor, hypoxia-inducible factor-α (HIF-α). Although HIF-α is not the direct receptor that senses oxygen tension, changes in oxygen tension lead to its posttranslation modification through asparagine and proline hydroxylation, stabilizing and activating the protein such that it can regulate target genes involved in the hypoxic response. Surprisingly, the ARNT protein acts as a heterodimerization partner for HIF-α much as it does for the Ah receptor (Semenza, 2002).

Sterol sensing in cells involves a membrane-bound sterol sensor called the sterol-response element binding protein (SREBP). The N-terminal domain of SREBP is a bHLH transcription factor that is proteolytically cleaved and liberated from the endoplasmic reticulum membrane, allowing it to enter the nucleus to regulate target genes necessary for sterol biosynthesis. High levels of sterols, in turn, inhibit the proteolysis and lead to the degradation of any nuclear SREBP (Brown and Goldstein, 1999).

A final example of an intracellular receptor is the soluble form of GC (Koesling, 1999). These enzymes are α-β heterodimers and serve as the target for the signaling molecule NO, leading to the formation of a cGMP second messenger. A bound heme confers sensitivity to NO in these proteins. Thus, members of the GC family have functions as both membrane-associated and intracellular receptors for diverse signaling molecules.

5. RECEPTORS, HEALTH, AND DISEASE

Given the central roles of receptors in intercellular communication, it is not surprising that many of them are targets for mutation in diseases of the endocrine system. Illustrative examples have been pointed out in each of the previous specific sections, but to summarize some of this information, Table 1 lists some of the many mutations in cell-surface or intracellular receptors that disrupt their function and lead to human disease. This partial list is stunning in the diversity of conditions, both within and outside the endocrine system, that result from mutations in receptor proteins. A few points are worth considering. First, for many of these receptors, both gain-of-function and loss-of-function mutations have been reported. Gain-of-function mutations are most common in the GPCRs and generally result in constitutive activity of the receptor. Second, the combination of identifying disease-causing mutations in these receptors with the tremendous advances that are being made in protein structure determination has resulted in a powerful ability to understand structure-function relationships that impact receptor activity. Third, Table 1 lists only human disease-causing mutations, and many more of the receptor proteins discussed in this chapter have been mutated in a targeted way in the mouse or other model organisms, providing both animal models for human disease and a wealth of new information on the physiologic functions of the receptors.

In addition to genetic disease-causing mutations, many receptors are likely to be inappropriately expressed or regulated in human disease and, thus, are significant targets for pharmaceutical intervention. Agonists and antagonists of many of these receptors have critical therapeutic value. The GPCRs alone are thought to be the target of about half of all prescription drugs, and the nuclear receptors may represent the fastest-growing targets for prescription drug design today. Of importance, both of these families include many poorly characterized orphan receptors that represent tantalizing targets for future drug discovery. The RTKs have also recently been the target of substantial drug development efforts, particularly ligand antagonists or kinase inhibitors,

Table 1
Representative Mutations in Receptor Proteins Associated With Human Disease [a]

Condition	Receptor	Type
Hirschsprung disease	Endorhelin B	GPCR
Pituitary dwarfism	HH	GPCR
Retinitis pigmentosa	Rhodopsin	GPCR
Diabetes insipidus	Vasopressin	GPCR
Glucocorticoid deficiency	ACTH	GPCR
Male precocious puberty	LH	GPCR
Hypercalcemia	Ca-sensing	GPCR
Hyperthyroidism	TSH	GPCR
Color blindness	Opsins	GPCR
Chondrodysplasia	PTH	GPCR
Gastric Carcinoma	CCK2	GPCR
Congenital bleeding	Thromboxane A_2	GPCR
Ovarian failure	FSH	GPCR
Hypogonadism	GnRH	GPCR
Resistance to TH	TRβ	NR
Glucocorticoid resistance	GR	NR
Hypocalcemic rickets	VDR	NR
Androgen insensitivity	AR	NR
Promyelocytic leukemia	RARα	NR
Adrenal hyperplasia	Dax-1	NR
XY sex reversal	SF-1	NR
Pseudohypoaldosteronism	MR	NR
Insulin resistance	PP	NR
Parkinson Disease	NR4A2	NR
S-cone syndrome	NR2E3	NR
MODY	HNF4A	NR
Insulin resistance	Insulin	RTK
Craniosynostosis	FGFR2	RTK
EN Type II	RET	RTK
Brachydactyly type B	ROR	RTK
Renal cell carcinoma	MET	RTK
Venous malformation	TIE2	RTK
Piebaldism	KIT	RTK
Hereditary	VEGFr3	RTK
CIPA	TrkA	RTK
Dwarfism	FGFR3	RTK
Pfeiffer syndrome	FGDR1	RTK
Pulmonary hypertension	BMPR2	STK
Telangiectasia type II	ALK1	STK
Colon carcinoma	TGFβR2	STK
Brachydactyly type A2	BMPR1	STK
Laron dwarfism	GH	CRS
Obesity/pit dysfunction	Leptin	CRS
Congenital neutropenia	GCSF	CRS
SCID	ILR-γc	CRS
Benign erythrocytosis	Epo	CRS
Atopy/IgE syndrome	IL-4	CRS
Periodic fever syndrome	TNFR1	TNF
ALPS	Fas	TNF
Hypercholesterolemia	LDL	TR
Hepatocellular carcinoma	IGF-2	TR
Hemochromatosis type III	Transferrin-2	TR

[a] The disease or condition is listed along with the receptor that is mutated and the classification of the receptor. GPCR = G protein–coupled receptor; NR = nuclear receptor; RTK = receptor tyrosine kinase; STK = serine and threonine kinase receptor; CRS = cytokine receptor superfamily; TNF = TNF receptor superfamily; TR = transport receptor.

given the critical roles that these receptors play in cell proliferation and in cancer.

6. SUMMARY

In assessing the structure and function of hormone receptors, several interesting issues emerge. It is clear that a fairly limited number of general strategies have been utilized repeatedly to generate the tremendous diversity of cellular responses to hormonal stimuli that are observed. Thus, superfamilies and families of receptors that have hundreds of members often represent subtle variations on a general structural or functional theme, such as tyrosine kinase activation, G protein coupling, or DNA binding. This knowledge is extremely useful for identifying novel receptors, based on conserved structural features, and for attempting to understand the mechanism of action of novel receptors once they are isolated. At a second level, aspects of receptor function such as heterodimerization with multiple partners or generation of multiple isoforms through alternative RNA processing further contribute to diversity. It is also apparent that substantial functional diversity can be generated at the level of the signal transduction cascades that receptors utilize. For example, coupling of a receptor to different G proteins, leading to the activation of distinct effectors, or interaction of a receptor with different adapter proteins, leading to the activation of distinct kinases, may occur in a tissue- or cell-specific fashion or in a developmentally regulated manner, generating dissimilar signaling responses to a single receptor.

In most of the examples considered in this chapter, our knowledge of the signaling pathways from hormone-receptor interaction to biologic response is still at best rudimentary. Despite tremendous progress in isolating receptors, in deciphering signal transduction cascades, and in unraveling the intricacies of gene transcription, there are relatively few examples for which a complete response pathway has been elucidated, and perhaps no example for which the complexities of the interaction of multiple signaling pathways in generating an appropriate cellular response is fully appreciated. It seems certain that substantial progress is needed to better characterize the signaling processes that are already known, and to uncover the novel receptor activation and signal transduction pathways that surely await discovery.

An important outcome of the quest to understand the actions of hormone receptors has been a recognition of the critical role that receptors play in cellular and organismal homeostasis and of the consequences of aberrant receptor function in endocrine diseases. The number of specific diseases or disorders associated with gain-of-function, loss-of-function, or alteration-of-function mutations in hormone receptors has increased dramatically since the first edition of this volume. This knowledge has already had immediate application in the diagnosis of endocrine disease and is likely to have eventual application in the rational design of therapeutic strategies for the prevention or treatment of these diseases. Finally, receptor biology provides a focal point for the scientific investigation of many of the critical outstanding areas of question in biology, including the control of cell proliferation, cell differentiation, and cell death; the coordinated interaction of cells during the development of a multicellular organism; and the generation of appropriate cellular responses to environmental and sensory stimuli. Further understanding of receptor-mediated signal transduction promises to contribute greatly to these fundamentally important issues.

REFERENCES

Attisano L, Wrana JL. Smads as transcription co-modulators. *Curr Opin Cell Biol* 2000;12:235.

Berridge MJ. Inositol triphosphate and calcium signaling. *Nature* 1993;361:315.

Brown MS, Goldstein JL. A proteolytic pathway that controls the cholesterol content of membranes, cells, and blood. *Proc Natl Acad Sci USA* 1999;96:11,041.

Brown MS, Goldstein JL. A receptor-mediated pathway for cholesterol homeostasis. *Science* 1986;232:34.

Burgess AW, Cho H-S, Eigenbrot C, Ferguson KM, Garrett PTJ, Leahy DJ, Lemmon MA, Sliwkowski MX, Ward CW, Yokohama S. An open and shut case? Recent insights into the activation of EGF/ErbB receptors. *Mol Cell* 2003;12:541.

Carbone M, Levine A. Oncogenes, antioncogenes, and the regulation of cell growth. *Trends Endocrinol Metab* 1990;1:248.

Claing A, Laporte SA, Caron MG, Lefkowitz RJ. Endocytosis of G protein–coupled receptors: roles of G protein–coupled receptor kinases and beta-arrestin proteins. *Prog Neurobiol* 2002;66:61.

Cooney RN. Suppressors of cytokine signaling (SOCS): inhibitors of the Jak/Stat pathway. *Shock* 2002;17:83.

Darnell JE Jr, Kerr IM, Stark GR. Jak-STAT pathways and transcriptional activation in response to INFs and other extracellular signaling proteins. *Science* 1994;265:1415.

Dohlman HG, Thorner J, Caron MG, Lefkowitz RJ. Model systems for the study of seven-transmembrane-segment receptors. *Annu Rev Biochem* 1991;60:653.

Dumont JE, Pecasse F, Maenhaut C. Crosstalk and specificity in signaling. *Cell Signaling* 2001;13:457.

Evans RM. The steroid and thyroid hormone receptor superfamily. *Science* 1988;240:889.

Filipek S, Stenkamp RE, Teller DC, Palczewski K. G protein–coupled receptor rhodopsin: a prospectus. *Annu Rev Physiol* 2003;65:851.

Fischer EH, Charbonneau H, Tonks NK. Protein tyrosine phosphatases: a diverse family of intracellular and transmembrane enzymes. *Science* 1991;253:401.

Garbers DL. The guanylyl cyclase receptors. *Methods* 1999;19:477.

Gaur U, Aggarwal BB. Regulation of proliferation, survival and apoptosis by members of the TNF superfamily. *Biochem Pharmacol* 2003;66:1404.

George SR, O'Dowd BF, Lee SP. G protein coupled receptor oligomerization and its potential for drug discovery. *Nat Rev Drug Discov* 2002;1:808.

Gilman AG. G proteins; transducers of receptor-generated signals. *Annu Rev Biochem* 1987;56:615.

Horn F, Bettler E, Oliveira L, Campaign F, Cohen FE, Vriend G. GCPRBD information system for G protein–coupled receptors. *Nucleic Acids Res* 2003;31:294.

Ihle JN, Kerr IM. Jaks and stats in signaling by the cytokine receptor superfamily. *Trends Genet* 1995;11:69.

Ingham PW, McMahon AP. Hedgehog signaling in animal development: principles and paradigms. *Genes Dev* 2001;15:3059.

Jensen EV, Jacobson JU. Basic guide to the mechanisms of estrogen action. *Recent Prog Horm Res* 1962;18:387.

Koesling D. Studying the structure and regulation of soluble guanylyl cyclase. *Methods* 1999;19:485.

Kornfield S. Structure and function of the mannose-6-phosphate/ insulin-like growth factor II receptors. *Annu Rev Biochem* 1992; 61:307.

Langley JN. On nerve endings and on special excitable substances in cells. *Proc Roy Soc Lond* 1906;78:170.

Mathews LS. Activin receptors and cellular signaling by the receptor serine kinase family. *Endocr Rev* 1994;15:310.

McKenna NJ, O'Malley BW. Combinatorial control of gene expression by nuclear receptors and coregulators. *Cell* 2002;108:465.

Mumm JS, Kopan R. Notch signaling: from the outside in. *Dev Biol* 2000;228:151.

Pawson T, Scott JD. Signaling through scaffold, anchoring, and adaptor proteins. *Science* 1997;278:2075.

Scatchard G. The attraction of proteins for small molecules and ions. *Ann NY Acad Sci* 1949;51:660.

Schmidt JV, Bradfield CA. Ah receptor signaling pathways. *Annu Rev Cell Dev Biol* 1996;12:55.

Schramm M, Selinger Z. Message transmission: receptor controlled adenylate cyclase system. *Science* 1984;25:1350.

Semenza G. Signal transduction to hypoxia-inducible factor 1. *Biochem Pharmacol* 2002;64:993.

Shenker A. G protein–coupled receptor structure and function: the impact of disease-causing mutations. *Baillières Clin Endocrinol Metab* 1995;9:427.

Shi Y, Massague J. Mechanism of TGFβ signaling from cell surface to nucleus. *Cell* 2003;113:685.

Strange PG. Mechanism of inverse antagonism at G protein coupled receptors. *Trends Pharmacol Sci* 2002;23:89.

Sutherland EW. Studies on the mechanism of hormone action. *Science* 1972;177:401.

Toft D, Gorski J. A receptor molecule for estrogens: isolation from the rat uterus and preliminary characterization. *Proc Natl Acad Sci USA* 1966;55:1574.

van der Geer P, Hunter T, Lindberg RA. Receptor protein-tyrosine kinases and their signal transduction pathways. *Annu Rev Cell Biol* 1994;10:251.

Weigel N, Zhang Y. Ligand-independent activation of steroid hormone receptors. *J Mol Med* 1998;76:469.

Willson TM, Moore JT. Genomics versus orphan nuclear receptors: a half-time report. *Mol Endocrinol* 2002;16:1135.

Wodarz A, Nusse R. Mechanisms of Wnt signaling in development. *Annu Rev Cell Dev Biol* 1998;14:59.

3 Second-Messenger Systems and Signal Transduction Mechanisms

Eliot R. Spindel, MD, PhD

1. INTRODUCTION

1.1. Signal Transduction: From Hormones to Action

Hormones are secreted, reach their target, and bind to a receptor. The interaction of the hormone with the receptor produces an initial signal that, through a series of steps, results in the final hormone action. How does the binding of a hormone to a receptor result in a cellular action? For example, in times of stress, epinephrine is secreted by the adrenal glands, is bound by receptors in skeletal muscle, and results in the hydrolysis of glycogen and the secretion of glucose. Signal transduction is the series of steps and signals that links the receptor binding of epinephrine to the hydrolysis of glycogen. Signal transduction can be simple or complex. There can be only one or two steps between receptor and effect, or multiple steps. Common themes, however, are specificity of action and control: the hormone produces just the desired action and the action can be precisely regulated. The multiple steps that are involved in signal transduction pathway allows for precise regulation, modulation, and a wide dynamic range.

There are two major mechanisms of signal transduction: transmission of signals by small molecules that diffuse through the cells and transmission of signals by phosphorylation of proteins. The diffusible small molecules that are used for signaling are known as second messengers. Examples of second messengers are cylic adenosine monophosphate (cAMP), calcium (Ca^{2+}), and inositol triphosphate (IP_3). Equally important is the transmission of hormonal signals by phosphorylation. Hormone-induced phosphorylation of proteins is a key way to activate or inactivate protein action. For example, the interaction of epidermal growth factor (EGF) with its receptor stimulates the phosphorylation of a tyrosine residue in the EGF receptor (EGFR). This in turn triggers the phosphorylation of other proteins in sequence, finally resulting in the phosphorylation of a transcription factor and increased gene expression. Enzymes that phosphorylate are called kinases. Balancing kinases are enzymes that remove phosphate groups from proteins; these are called phosphatases. In a typical signal transduction pathway, both second messengers and phosphorylation mechanisms are used. For example, cAMP transmits its message by activating a kinase (camp-dependent protein kinase A, or simply protein kinase A [PKA]).

From: *Endocrinology: Basic and Clinical Principles, Second Edition*
(S. Melmed and P. M. Conn, eds.) © Humana Press Inc., Totowa, NJ

35

Some hormones produce effects without a membrane receptor. The best examples of these are the steroid hormones that bind to a cytoplasmic receptor and the receptor then translocates to the nucleus to produce its desired effects. Even these actions, however, are modified by the actions of kinases and phosphatases. Steroid receptors are discussed in detail in Chapter 4.

Nature and evolution are parsimonious. Mechanisms that originally evolved for the regulation of yeast are also used for endocrine signaling in mammals. Similarly, mechanisms used for regulation of embryonic development are also used for endocrine signaling, and mechanisms used for neuronal signaling are also used for endocrine signaling. Thus, fundamental discoveries about the growth of yeast, early embryonic development, regulation of cancerous growth, and neurotransmission in the brain have led to fundamental discoveries of endocrine mechanisms of signal transduction. Similar receptors and signaling pathways underlie signaling by neurotransmitters and by hormones. Growth and differentiation factors trigger cell growth and development by similar mechanisms as do hormones. Thus, signal transduction is a major unifying area among endocrinology, cell biology, developmental biology, oncology, and neuroscience.

1.2. A Brief Overview of Signal Transduction Mechanisms.

One approach to classifying signal transduction mechanisms is as a function of the structure of the hormone receptor. Thus, while both thyroid stimulating hormone (TSH) and growth hormone (GH) are both pituitary hormones, the TSH receptor is a seven-transmembrane G protein–coupled receptor linked to cAMP, and the GH receptor is a single-transmembrane kinase-linked receptor. The fact that both hormones are pituitary hormones tells nothing about the signal transduction mechanism. By contrast, knowledge of the receptor structure involved provides some information as to the potential mechanisms of signal transduction and of the potential mediators involved. Complicating matters, however, hormones can have multiple receptors often with different signal transduction mechanisms. A good example of this is acetylcholine, which has more than a dozen receptors, some of which are seven-transmembrane G protein–coupled receptors and some of which are ligand-gated ion channels.

The major classes of membrane receptors are seven transmembrane, single transmembrane, and four transmembrane. Within each of these classes of receptors, there are multiple signal transduction mechanisms, but certain unifying concepts emerge. The seven-transmem-

brane receptors are G protein linked, and initial signaling is conducted by the activated G protein subunits. The single-transmembrane receptors convey initial signals via phosphorylation events (sometimes direct, sometimes induced by receptor dimerization), and the four-transmembrane receptors are usually ion channels.

As discussed in Section 2, the seven transmembrane receptors are linked to G proteins. G proteins are composed of three subunits, and binding of the ligand to the receptor G protein complex causes disassociation of the G protein. The disassociated subunit then acts to stimulate or inhibit second-messenger formation. Thus, seven-transmembrane receptors signal through second messengers such as cAMP, IP$_3$, and/or calcium. Examples of G protein–linked hormones are parathyroid hormone (PTH), thyrotropin-releasing hormone (TRH), TSH, glucagons, and somatostatin. The four-transmembrane receptors are typically ligand-gated ion channels. Binding of the ligand to the receptor opens an ion channel, allowing cellular entry of Na or Ca. Examples of the four-transmembrane receptors are the nicotinic receptors, the AMPA and kainate glutamate receptors, and the serotonin type 3 receptor. The single-transmembrane receptors form the most diverse class of hormone receptors including both single and multisubunit structures. These receptors signal through endogenous enzymatic activity or by activating an associated protein that contains endogenous enzymatic activity.

1.3. Hormone Action: The End Result of Signal Transduction

After hormone binding, there are multiple signaling steps until the hormone actions are achieved. Hormones almost always have multiple actions, so there must be branch points within the signal transduction cascade and the ability to regulate independently these multiple branches. This need for multiple, independently controlled effects is one reason that signal transduction pathways are so diverse and complicated. End effects of the signal transduction cascade fall into three general groups: enzyme activation, membrane effects, and activation of gene transcription. These individual actions are covered in more detail in the specific chapters on hormones, but it is important to understand the general concepts of how signals link to the final action.

The classic example of hormone-induced enzyme activation is epinephrine-induced glycogenolysis in which binding of epinephrine to its receptor (β_2-adrenergic receptor) stimulates formation of cAMP, which activates a kinase (cAMP-dependent protein kinase, PKA). PKA then phosphorylates the enzyme phosphorylase kinase, which, in turn, phosphorylates glycogen phosphorylase, which is the enzyme that liberates glucose from glycogen. Phosphorylation is the most common mechanism by which hormonally induced signal transduction activates enzymes.

One example of membrane action is cAMP regulation of the cystic fibrosis transmembrane conductance regulator (CFTR), which is a chloride channel that opens in response to PKA-mediated phosphorylation. Another important example of a membrane effect is insulin-induced glucose transport, in which insulin increases glucose transport by inducing a redistribution of the Glut4 glucose transporter from intracellular stores to the membrane.

Hormone-induced gene transcription is mediated by hormone activation of transcription factors or DNA-binding proteins. For steroid hormones and the thyroid hormones, the hormone receptor itself is a DNA-binding protein. How these hormones interact with nuclear receptors to stimulate gene transcription is discussed in Chapter 4. As might be predicted from the preceding paragraphs, membrane-bound receptors stimulate gene transcription through phosphorylation of nuclear binding proteins. Typically, these factors are active only when properly phosphorylated. Transcription factor phosphorylation can be mediated by hormone-activated kinases such as PKA-induced phosphorylation of the cAMP-responsive transcription factor CREB. This is discussed in Section 2.2. GH or prolactin (PRL) stimulates gene transcription by a series of steps leading to phosphorylation of the STAT transcription factors, which then bind and transactivate DNA.

2. SIGNALING THROUGH G PROTEIN–LINKED RECEPTORS

2.1. Overview of G Proteins

As described in the previous chapter, the seven-transmembrane receptors signal through G proteins. The G proteins are composed of three subunits: α, β, and γ. The α-subunit is capable of binding and hydrolyzing guanosine 5′ triphosphate (GTP) to guanosine 5′ diphosphate (GDP). As shown in Fig. 1, the trimeric G protein with one molecule of GDP bound to the α-subunit binds to the unliganded receptor. Binding of ligand to the receptor causes a conformational shift such that GDP disassociates from the α-subunit and GTP is bound in its place. The binding of GTP produces a conformational shift in the α-subunit causing its disassociation into a βγ dimer and an activated α-subunit. Signaling is achieved by the activated α-subunit binding to an effector molecule and by the free βγ dimer binding to an effector molecule. Specificity of hormonal signaling is achieved by different α-subunits

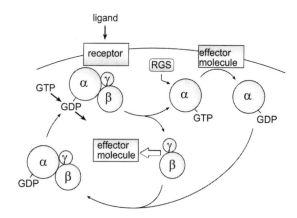

Fig. 1. The G protein cycle. The α-subunit with GDP bound binds to the βγ dimer. The αβγ trimer then binds to the receptor. Binding of ligand to the receptor causes a change in the G protein's conformation such that GDP leaves and GTP is bound. Binding of GTP causes the α-subunit to disassociate from the βγ dimer and assume its active conformation. The activated α-subunit then activates effector molecules. The intrinsic GTPase activity of the α-subunit hydrolyzes the bound GTP to GDP, allowing the α-subunit to reassociate with the βγ dimer. The α-subunit remains activated until the GTP is hydrolyzed. RGS proteins bind to the activated α-subunit to increase the rate at which GTP is hydrolyzed.

coupling to different effector molecules. The α-subunit remains activated until the bound GTP is hydrolyzed to GDP. On hydrolysis of GTP to GDP, the α-subunit reassociates with the βγ-subunit and returns to the receptor to continue the cycle. The α-subunit contains intrinsic guanosine 5′ triphosphatase (GTPase) activity (hence, the name G proteins), and how long the α-subunit stays activated is a function of the activity of the GTPase activity of the α-subunit. An important and large family of proteins, the regulators of G protein signaling (RGS) proteins bind to the free α-subunit and greatly increase the rate of GTP hydrolysis to increase the rate at which their ability to signal is terminated.

As shown in Fig. 2, the free βγ dimer can bind to and activate G protein receptor kinases (GRKs) that play a key role in desensitizing G protein–coupled receptors. The activated GRK then phosphorylates the G protein–coupled receptor, which then allows proteins known as β-arrestins to bind to the receptor. The binding of the β-arrestin to the receptor then blocks receptor function both by uncoupling the receptor from the G protein and by triggering internalization of the receptor. Besides the βγ dimers, other signaling molecules can activate GRKs to provide multiple routes to regulate G protein signal transduction.

There are multiple subtypes of the α-, β- and γ-subunits. The subtypes form different families of the G

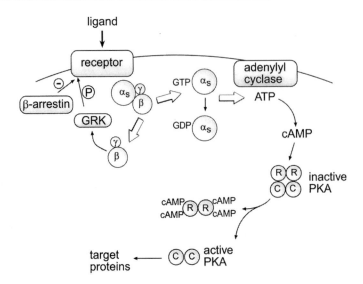

Fig. 2. Signaling by G_s. Binding of ligand to the receptor causes formation of the activated α-subunit of G_s. Activated $G\alpha_s$ then activates adenylyl cyclase. Adenylyl cyclase forms cAMP from adenosine triphosphate. Two molecules of cAMP bind to each regulatory subunit of inactive PKA and cause the regulatory subunits to disassociate from the catalytic subunits. The now-active catalytic subunits can then phosphorylate their target proteins. The free $\beta\gamma$ dimer also signals including triggering receptor desensitization by activating GRK proteins to phosphorylate the receptor, which allows the binding of β-arrestin proteins.

proteins. Most important are the subtypes of the α-subunits because they regulate the effector molecules that the G protein activates. The major families of the G proteins are G_s, G_i and G_q. Specificity of hormone action is achieved because only specific G proteins (composed of the proper subunits) will couple to specific hormone receptors and because the free $\beta\gamma$ dimer and the activated α-subunit subtypes will couple only to specific effector molecules. The G_s family couples to and increases adenylyl cyclase activity and also opens membrane K^+ channels; the G_i family couples to and inhibits adenylyl cyclase, opens membrane K^+ channels, and closes membrane Ca^{2+} channels; and the G_q family activates phospholipase Cβ (PLCβ) to increase IP_3, diacylglycerol (DAG), and intracellular Ca^{2+}. The signaling of these three families is discussed further in Sections 2.2–2.4.

In addition to the trimeric G proteins discussed above, there is also a class of small G proteins that consist of single subunits, of which Ras, Rho and Rac are important members. These proteins also hydrolyze GTP and play a role in coupling tyrosine kinase receptors to effector molecules, as discussed in Section 3.

2.2. Hormonal Signaling Mediated by G_s

Hormones that signal through G_s to activate adenylate cyclase and increase cAMP represent the first signaling pathway as described by the pioneering work of Sutherland and coworkers in the initial discovery of

cAMP. Elucidation of this pathway led to Nobel Prizes for the discovery of cAMP and for the discovery of G proteins. Examples of hormones that signal through this pathway are TSH, luteinizing hormone, follicle-stimulating hormone, adrenocorticotropic hormone, epinephrine, and glucagons, among others. Signaling in this pathway is outlined in Fig. 2. As described in Section 2.1, the binding of hormone to the receptor-G_s complex results in the active α-subunit binding to an effector molecule, in this case adenylate cyclase. Adenylate cyclase is a single-chain membrane glycoprotein with a molecular mass of 115–150 kDa. The molecule itself has two hydrophobic domains, each with six transmembrane segments. Binding of the activated α-subunit of G_s results in catalyzing the formation of cAMP from ATP. Eight different isoforms of adenylate cyclase have been described to date. These isoforms differ in their distribution and regulation by other factors such as calmodulin, $\beta\gamma$ subunits, and specificity for α-subunit subtypes. Next cAMP binds to and activates the cAMP-dependent PKA. PKA is a serine/threonine kinase that phosphorylates proteins with the recognition site Arg-Arg-X-(Ser or Thr)-X in which X is usually hydrophobic. PKA is a heterotetramer composed of two regulatory and two catalytic subunits. The regulatory subunits suppress the activity of the catalytic subunits. The binding of cAMP to the regulatory subunits causes their disassociation from the catalytic subunits, allowing PKA to phosphorylate its targets.

There are a number of PKA subtypes, but the key difference reflects the type I regulatory subunit (RI) vs the type II (RII) subunit in which the RI subunit will disassociate from PKA at a lower concentration of cAMP than will the RII subunit. Recent reports have also demonstrated that cAMP can also signal by activating other proteins besides adenylate cyclase.

PKA phosphorylates multiple targets including enzymes, channels, receptors, and transcription factors. Enzymes can be activated or inhibited by the resulting phosphorylation at Ser/Thr residues. An example of regulation of glycogen phosphorylase was discussed in Section 1.3. An example of a PKA-regulated channel is the CFTR chloride channel that requires phosphorylation by PKA for chloride movement. PKA also phosphorylates seven-transmembrane receptors as part of the mechanism of receptor desensitization similar to the function of GRKs.

A key function of cAMP is its ability to stimulate gene transcription. The basic concept is that cAMP activates PKA, which phosphorylates a transcription factor. The transcription factor then stimulates transcription of the target gene. Several classes of cAMP-activated transcription factors have been characterized. These include CREB, CREM, and ATF-1. Probably the most is known about CREB, so it is used here as an example (Fig. 3). CREB is a 341-amino-acid protein with two primary domains, a DNA-binding domain (DBD) and a transactivation domain. The DBD binds to specific DNA sequences in the target genes that are activated by cAMP. When CREB is phosphorylated, it recruits a coactivator protein, CREB-binding protein (CBP). This positions CBP next to the basal transcription complex, allowing interaction with the Pol-II transcription complex to activate transcription. CBP also stimulates gene transcription by a second mechanism by functioning as a histone acetyltransferase. The transfer of acetyl groups to lysine residues of histones is another key mechanism to activate gene transcription. As is almost always the case in signaling cascades, there is important negative regulation of the CREB pathway. A key element of the negative regulation is mediated by phosphorylated-CREB-inducing expression of Icer, a negative regulator of CREB function. Defects in CBP lead to mental retardation in a disease called Rubinstein-Taybi syndrome (RTS), one of the first diseases discovered that is caused by defects in transcription factors.

2.3. Hormonal Signaling Mediated by G_i

Hormonal signaling through seven-transmembrane receptors linked to G_i is similar to that linked to G_s except $G\alpha_i$ inhibits adenylyl cyclase rather than stimu-

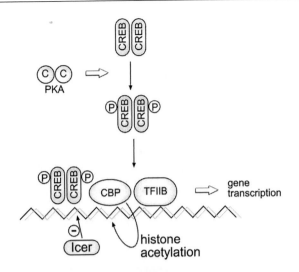

Fig. 3. Role of CREB in regulating gene transcription. PKA phosphorylates CREB on Serine 133. CREB can be phosphorylated while in the cytoplasm (as shown) or while already bound to DNA. The phosphorylation of CREB allows it to bind CBP, which then acts as a transcriptional coactivator by interacting with the pol-II transcription apparatus. CBP also increases gene transcription by acting as a histone acetyltransferase. Icer is an important negative regulator of CREB activity that is induced by CREB.

lates it, as does $G\alpha_s$. Thus, adenylyl cyclase activity represents a balance between stimulation by $G\alpha_s$ and inhibition by $G\alpha_i$. $G\alpha_i$ also couples to calcium channels (inhibitory) and potassium channels (stimulatory). Receptors that couple to G_i include somatostatin, enkephalin, and the α_2-adrenergic receptor, among others. For G_i signaling, the $\beta\gamma$ dimer also plays key signaling roles by activating potassium channels and inhibiting calcium channels on the cell membrane.

2.4. Hormonal Signaling Mediated by G_q

Hormonal signaling through seven-transmembrane receptors linked to G_q proceeds by activation of PLCβ. Examples of hormones that bind to G_q include TRH, gastrin-releasing peptide, gonadotropin-releasing hormone, angiotensin II, substance P, cholecystokinin, and PTH. Binding of hormone to its receptor leads to formation of active $G\alpha_q$ or $G\alpha_{12}$, which then activates PLC to hydrolyze phosphoinositides (Fig. 4) to form two second messengers, IP_3 and DAG. IP_3 diffuses within the cell to bind to specific receptors on the endoplasmic reticulum (ER). The IP_3 receptor is a calcium channel, and the interaction of IP_3 with its receptor opens the channel and allows calcium to flow from the ER into the cytoplasm, thus increasing free cytosolic calcium levels. The IP_3 receptor is composed of four large subunits (≈ 310 kDa) that each bind a single molecule of IP_3.

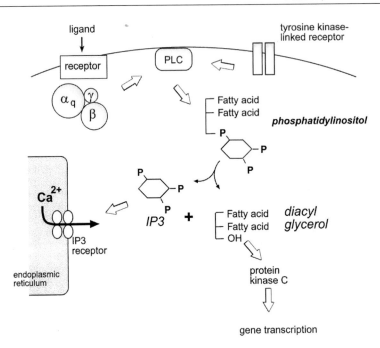

Fig. 4. Signaling by G_q. Activated $G\alpha_q$ activates PLCβ (PLC). PLCβ then hydrolyzes phosphatidylinositol to form two second messengers, DAG and IP$_3$. The binding of IP$_3$ to the IP$_3$ receptor on the ER stimulates calcium efflux from the ER to increase intracellular calcium. DAG activates PKC. PKC can then stimulate transcription by phosphorylation of transcription factors. Tyrosine kinase–linked receptors activate PLCγ to produce DAG and IP$_3$ as well.

The binding of IP$_3$ to the subunits opens the channels and also desensitizes the receptor to binding additional IP$_3$. Thus, IP$_3$ leads to increased Ca^{2+} which is the next step in signaling. Calcium is returned to the ER by ATP-dependent Ca^{2+} pumps (SERCA). Thapsigargin is a drug that blocks the SERCA, thus resulting in transient high intracellular Ca^{2+} levels, but it also depletes Ca^{2+} levels in the ER, making it a convenient tool to study IP$_3$-dependent Ca^{2+} release. In excitable cells, a similar mechanism triggers calcium release from internal stores, except here calcium directly triggers additional Ca^{2+} release from the ER via the ryanodine receptor. Depolarization opens voltage-sensitive Ca^{2+} channels on the cell membranes, allowing influx of Ca^{2+}, and this calcium then binds to the ryanodine receptor (very similar to the IP$_3$ receptor, except the ryanodine receptor is gated by Ca^{2+}) and allows Ca^{2+} efflux from the ER. The ryanodine receptor also allows Ca^{2+} efflux from the sarcoplasmic reticulum in muscle. IP$_3$, in turn, is rapidly metabolized by specific phosphatases.

Calcium is a major intracellular second messenger, and its levels are tightly regulated by calcium pumps in the ER (SERCA), calcium pumps in the membrane (PMCA), voltage-gated calcium channels, and ligand-gated calcium channels. Resting cell Ca^{2+} is 100 nM, far

lower than the 2 mM levels that occur extracellularly; thus, there is ample room to rapidly increase intracellular Ca^{2+}. Increased intracellular Ca^{2+} signals primarily by binding to proteins and causing a conformational shift that activates their function. Examples include Ca^{2+} binding to troponin in muscle cells to stimulate contraction and Ca^{2+} binding to calmodulin. The Ca^{2+}-calmodulin complex then binds to a variety of kinases. There are two general classes of Ca^{2+}-calmodulin kinases, dedicated, i.e., with only a specific substrate and multifunctional, with many substrates. Examples of dedicated CAM kinases are myosin light chain kinase and phosphorylase kinase. The multifunctional CAM kinases can phosphorylate transcription factors to effect gene transcription. For example, CAM kinase can phosphorylate CREB, which provides a mechanism for cross talk between receptors linked to G_s and G_q. CAM kinases can also phosphorylate other kinases such as mitogen-activated protein kinase (MAPK) or Akt to activate other signaling pathways. In addition, CAM kinases play a key role in mediating signaling by ligand-gated ion channels, as discussed in Section 5.

The other second messenger of the PLC pathway is DAG. The primary action of DAG is to activate PKC, a serine-threonine kinase. PKC modifies enzymatic activity by phosphorylation of target enzymes, and like PKA, PKC can modify gene transcription by regulating phosphorylation of transcription factors. PKC is activated by the class of compounds known as phorbol esters that were originally described for their ability to promote tumor growth. One phorbol ester that potently stimulates PKC activity is 12-*O*-tetradecanoylphorbol-13-acetate (TPA or PMA). It was initially shown that TPA could activate gene transcription through a DNA sequence element known as the AP-1-binding site. Isolation of the transcription factors that bound to AP-1 led to the isolation of *Jun* and *Fos*, which bind to the AP-1 site as hetero- or homodimers to regulate transcription. Thus, hormones that signal through G_q regulate gene transcription through DAG, which activates PKC, leading to phosphorylation of jun and fos. PKC, like PKA, can also regulate receptor activity by directly phosphorylating ion channels and seven-transmembrane receptors.

3. SIGNALING THROUGH RECEPTORS LINKED TO TYROSINE KINASES OR SERINE/THREONINE KINASES

The second major signaling pathway involves cascades of phosphorylation events. These pathways can be divided into those that commence with a tyrosine phosphorylation event and those that commence with a serine/threonine phosphorylation event. These pathways are similar in that they are a series of protein-binding and/or phosphorylation events. There are two primary mechanism by which the binding of hormone to its receptor causes signal propagation. In the first mechanism, hormone binding triggers receptor autophosphorylation via an intrinsic receptor kinase. Receptor phosphorylation then allows binding of additional proteins that recognize the phosphotyrosines. The EGFR uses this pathway. In the second mechanism, hormone binding triggers a receptor conformational change that stimulates binding of a second protein to the receptor. One important way in which hormone binding to the receptor triggers conformational change is by causing receptor dimerization. Examples of this are the GH and PRL receptors. These are discussed in greater detail in Section 3.2.

3.1. Signaling Through Receptors With Intrinsic Tyrosine Kinase Activity (EGF, Insulin, Insulin-like Growth Factor-1)

Hormones and growth factors that signal through receptors with intrinsic tyrosine kinase activity include the EGFR, the vascular endothelial growth factor receptor, and the insulin receptor. Binding of ligand to the receptor stimulates the receptor's intrinsic tyrosine kinase, resulting in autophosphorylation (i.e., the receptor phosphorylates itself), which then induces binding of the next signaling protein or effector protein. Within this category there are differences depending on receptor structure. Prototype signaling mechanisms are discussed below.

3.1.1. EGFR Signaling

The EGFR is a single-transmembrane receptor that binds EGF as a monomer. EGF binding causes a change in conformation that induces dimerization with a second EGF- EGFR complex. Dimerization of the EGFR complexes activates the EGFR's intrinsic tyrosine kinase, and each receptor in the dimer transphosphorylates the other receptor at multiple tyrosine residues. These phosphotyrosines then serve as docking sites for src homology 2 (SH2) domain proteins. SH2 domains are conserved regions of approx 100 amino acids that serve to target proteins to phosphotyrosines. Depending on the amino acids adjacent to the phosphotyrosine, different SH2 domain proteins will have different affinities for the phosphotyrosine residue. Thus, depending on which tyrosine residues are phosphorylated, and the sequences surrounding those tyrosines, different proteins will dock on the ligand-activated receptor. This provides specificity of effector action and the ability for multiple proteins to dock on a single receptor. The binding of the SH2 domain protein to the receptor propagates signals by a number of mechanisms including 1 bringing an effector molecule to the membrane where it is next to its target molecule, 2 binding that triggers a conformational change that can activate endogenous enzymatic activity in the SH2 proteins (e.g., kinase activity), and 3 binding that can position the SH2 protein so that it can be phosphorylated and activated. The EGFR employs these mechanisms as follows.

As shown in Fig. 5, the binding of EGF to its receptor activates the MAPK pathway, PLCγ, phosphatidylinositol 3-kinase (PI3K), and transcription factors. Many growth factors use pathways similar to EGF, so it is important to consider the multiple pathways of EGF signal transduction. As previously described, Ras is a small G protein with GTPase activity like Rho. When the EGFR is phosphorylated, the SH2 domain protein GRB-2 (growth factor receptor–binding protein-2) binds to the receptor and then binds through its SH3 domain to a guanine nucleotide exchange factor (GEF), which activates RAS by stimulating the exchange of GDP for GTP by RAS. The GEF that binds to the EGFR is known as SOS, or "son of sevenless," because of its homology to the *drosophila* protein) (Fig. 6). This brings SOS close to the membrane and in close proximity to Ras, which is anchored in the membrane. SOS then converts ras-GDP

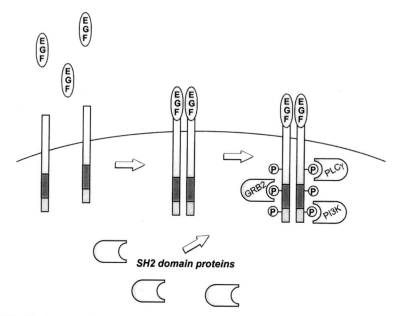

Fig. 5. Signaling by EGFR. Binding of EGF to its receptor causes dimerization of liganded receptors. Receptor dimerization causes receptor autophosphorylation by activating the receptor's intrinsic tyrosine kinase activity (shown in dark gray). SH2 domain proteins such as GRB-2, PLCγ and PI3K then bind to the phosphotyrosine residues. This results in activation of the SH2 domain proteins by either phosphorylation, localization, or both.

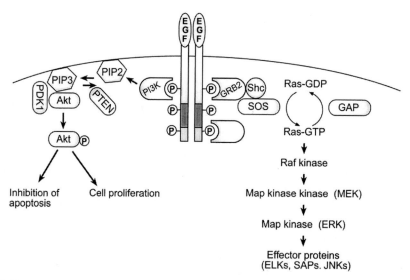

Fig. 6. The MAPK and Akt signaling cascades. Binding of EGF induces phosphorylation of the EGFR, which activates both the MAPK signaling cascade and signaling by Akt. For MAPK activation, the GRB-2-SOS complex binds to the receptor, positioning it near membrane-bound Ras-GDP, which is then activated. The activated Ras GTP activates Raf kinase, which activates MAPK kinase, which activates MAPK which then activates the final effector proteins, many of which are transcription factors. Active Ras-GTP is converted into inactive Ras-GDP by GAP. For Akt signaling, PI3K binds by the SH2 domain, is activated, and converts membrane-bound PIP_2 to PIP_3. PDK1 and Akt bind to PI3K through the Pleckstrin homology domain. This results in phosphorylation to activate Akt, which then triggers cell proliferation by both growth pathways and inhibition of apoptosis. PTEN is a key negative regulator that acts by dephosphorylating Akt.

into the active ras-GTP form. In some systems, SOS does not bind directly to GRB-2, but an intermediate adapter protein, Shc, is recruited, which then binds SOS. Ras-GTP then activates Raf kinase, which activates

MAPK kinase, which activates MAPK, which phosphorylates the final effector proteins that regulate growth or cellular metabolism. As always, there is important negative regulation, this time by GTPase-activating proteins

(GAPs) that increase the rate of hydrolysis of GTP bound to RAS to convert RAS to the inactive state. Thus, the GAPs are very similar to the RGS proteins that negatively regulate G protein signaling by increasing the rate of GTP hydrolysis by α-subunits.

There are in fact a number of parallel MAPK pathways with different MAPKs and MAPK kinases. Other MAPK pathways include MEK kinase, which is equivalent to MAPK kinase, and extracellular-regulated kinase (ERK), which is equivalent to MAPK. Transcriptional targets for ERK include the ELK and SAP transcription factors. One important MAPK subtype is Jun kinase, which activates the Jun transcription factors. Specificity of these pathways comes in part from the initial SH2 docking protein that binds to the tyrosine kinase pathways and also from multiple inputs from other proteins. MAPKs are, in turn, rapidly inactivated by phosphatases.

The second major signaling pathway of tyrosine kinase receptors such as the EGFR is through activation of PLCγ. While PLCγ is activated by Gα_q, PLCγ is an SH2 domain protein. Thus, when EGF stimulates phosphorylation of the EGFR, PLCγ, through its SH2 domains, binds to phosphotyrosines in the EGFR. This serves two purposes: first, it brings PLCγ close to the membrane adjacent to phosphatidyl inositols; and, second, it allows the EGFR to phosphorylate PLCγ. Phosphorylation activates PLCγ resulting in hydrolysis of phosphatidylinositol to IP$_3$ and DAG. Thus, tyrosine kinase–linked receptors, like G$_q$-linked receptors, also signal through IP$_3$ and DAG.

The third major pathway by which the EGFR signals is by activation of other enzymes of which PI3K is one of the most important. PI3K phosphorylates phosphoinositols such as phosphatidylinositol-4,5-bisphosphate (PIP$_2$) in the 3 position to create phosphatidylinositol-3,4,5-trisphosphate (PIP$_3$). These phosphoinositols remain membrane bound. The kinase Akt then binds to PIP$_3$ through a sequence known as the Pleckstrin homology domain. The kinase PDK1 then binds to the Akt and PIP$_3$ also through the Pleckstrin domain and activates Akt by phosphorylation. Phosphorylated Akt then stimulates cell growth both by inhibiting apoptosis through the BAD pathway and by stimulating growth. Growth stimulation proceeds in part through the phosphorylation of mTOR, leading to activation of protein translation. Negative regulation is provided by the phosphatase PTEN, which dephosphorylates PIP$_3$. PTEN, because of its ability to counter the growth stimulatory effects of Akt, is an important tumor suppressor. Finally, the EGFR can also directly activate some nuclear transcription factors by phosphorylation.

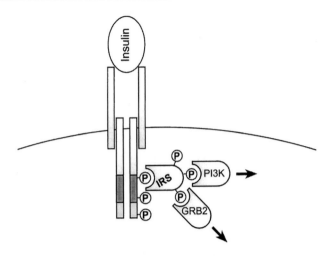

Fig. 7. Signaling by insulin receptor. Binding of insulin to its receptor causes autophosphorylation. This stimulates binding of the IRS protein, which is then phosphorylated by the insulin receptor. SH2 proteins such as GRB-2 and PI3K then bind to the IRS and signal as described for the EGFR. The binding of PI3K to the IRS plays a key role in stimulating glucose entry into cells.

The EGFR has been discussed in depth because it serves as a model for most other tyrosine kinase receptors. The key concept is that ligand binding induces autophosphorylation and SH2 proteins then bind to phosphotyrosines to activate multiple signaling mechanisms. Specificity is achieved in that different SH2 proteins recognize different phosphotyrosines.

3.1.2. Signaling by Insulin and Insulin-like Growth Factor Receptors

The signal transduction mechanism employed by the insulin receptor is a variation of that employed by the EGFR (Fig. 7). Binding of insulin to the insulin receptor (a heterotetramer composed of two α-subunits and two β-subunits), like binding of EGF to its receptor, triggers receptor autophosphorylation. However, the insulin receptor does not signal by directly binding SH2 domain proteins. Rather, ligand-induced receptor autophosphorylation stimulates binding of bridging proteins called insulin receptor substrate (IRS) proteins (IRS1–4). Four IRSs have been described to date, though IRS1 and IRS2 play the key role in insulin signaling. IRSs bind to the insulin receptor and are phosphorylated, and then multiple SH2 proteins bind in turn to the IRSs. Just as EGF-induced signaling depends on which SH2 domain proteins bind to the EGFR, insulin signaling depends on which SH2 proteins bind to the IRS. Examples of proteins that bind to IRSs include GRB-2 and PI3K. GRB-2 then activates the Ras pathway and PI3K activates Akt as discussed above. Akt and PI3K then play key roles in activating glycogen

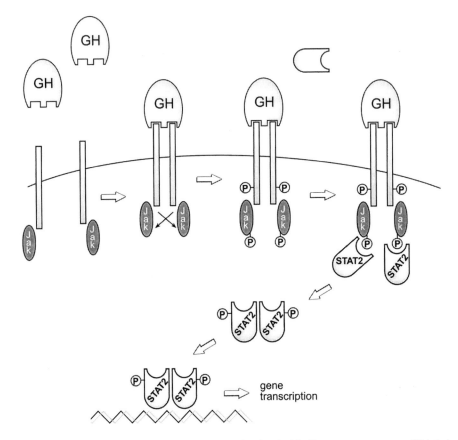

Fig. 8. Signaling by GH receptor (GHR). GH causes receptor dimerization by binding to two receptors. This brings two Jak kinases that are bound to the GHR into close apposition and allows each Jak kinase to phosphorylate the other and the reciprocal GHR (transphosphorylation). Stat proteins then bind through SH2 domains to the Jak kinases and are phosphorylated. The phosphorylated STAT proteins then form homo- or heterodimers, translocate to the nucleus, and stimulate gene transcription.

synthesis and glucose transport into the cell. IRSs do not bind to the insulin receptor via SH2 domains but, rather, appear to utilize Pleckstrin homology domains and phosphotyrosine-binding domains, though the exact details are yet to be determined.

3.2. Signaling Through Receptors That Signal Through Ligand-Induced Binding of Tyrosine Kinases (GH, PRL)

The GH and PRL receptors belong to a large superfamily of receptors that include the cytokine receptors for interleukin-2 (IL-2), IL-3, IL-4, IL-5, IL-6, IL-7, IL-9, IL-11, IL-12, erythropoietin, granulocyte macrophage colony-stimulating factor, interferon-β (IFN-β), IFN-γ, and CNTF. Many of these receptors are heterodimers consisting of an α-ligand-binding subunit and a β-signaling subunit. However, the GH and PRL receptors have single subunits that contain both the ligand-binding and signaling domains. The receptors in this family lack intrinsic tyrosine kinase

activity. Instead, these receptors associate with kinases belonging to the JAK kinase family. Ligand binding to the receptor induces receptor dimerization bringing two JAK kinases in close apposition, which results in activation of the associated JAK kinases by reciprocal phosphorylation (Fig. 8). The JAK kinases then phosphorylate target proteins and signaling commences. The name *JAK kinase* is short for Janus kinase; Janus is the ancient Roman god of gates and doorways who is depicted with two faces, one looking outward, and one looking inward (it has also been claimed that JAK stands for Just Another Kinase). There is a family of JAK kinases and different receptors associate with different kinases. At the present time, four members of the family have been described: Jak1, Jak2, Jak3, and tyk2. The different kinases phosphorylate different targets to achieve signaling specificity. For example, the PRL and GH receptors bind Jak2, the IL-2 and IL-4 receptors bind Jak 1 and Jak3, and the IFN receptors bind tyk2.

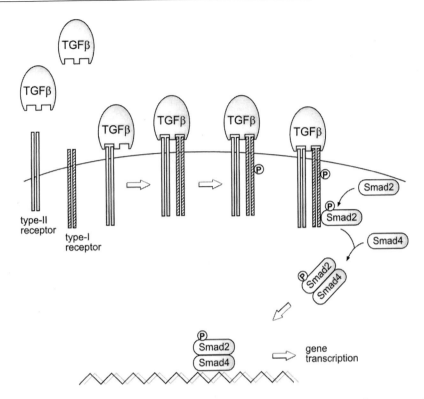

Fig. 9. Signaling by TGF-β receptor. Binding of TGF-β to the type II receptor recruits the type I receptor, which is then phosphorylated. This triggers binding of a Smad protein, which is phosphorylated, dimerizes with a second Smad, and translocates to the nucleus to stimulate transcription.

The activated JAK kinases phosphorylate the signal transduction and activation of transcription (STAT) proteins among others. Seven STAT proteins have been described to date, though there are likely more members of this important gene family. STAT proteins contain an SH2 domain and a single conserved tyrosine residue that is phosphorylated in response to ligand binding. Phosphorylation of STAT releases the STAT from the receptor, and the SH2 domains in the STAT allow them to form as homodimers or as heterodimers with other STATs or with unrelated proteins (Fig. 8). The dimerized STATs can then bind to DNA to stimulate transcription. For example, IFN-α stimulates gene transcription by activation of Stat1 and Stat2, which heterodimerize and bind to DNA. Similarly, CNTF or IL-6 results in binding of Stat1 and Stat3 heterodimers to DNA. A key question remaining to be clarified is, How is exact signal specificity achieved? There are more receptors and ligands than JAK kinases and STATs. Specificity may reside in the time course of activation (reflecting the balance between kinases and phosphatases), which STATs are activated, phosphorylation status of other proteins, and the binding of other transcriptional regulators elsewhere in the gene.

Negative regulation results both from STAT-induced transcription of negative regulators and from phosphatases (SHP-1) that dephosphorylate STATs.

3.3. Signaling Through Receptors With Intrinsic Serine/Threonine Kinase Activity (Activin, Inhibin, Transforming Growth Factor-β)

Receptors with intrinsic serine/threonine kinase activity form a large family of receptors. These receptors include the transforming growth factor-β (TGF-β), activin, inhibin, and bone morphogenic proteins. Signaling for TGF-β is best characterized and serves as a model for the signal transduction mechanism of serine/threonine kinase–linked receptors (Fig. 9). TGF-β binds to a type II receptor dimmer, which then recruits a type I receptor dimer. The type II receptor then phosphorylates the type I receptor, which results in the recruitment of Smad proteins, which are the signaling intermediates of the TGF-β receptor. First, Smad2 or Smad3 binds to the TGF-β receptor. Second, the Smad is phosphorylated, disassociates from the receptor, and dimerizes with Smad4. Third the Smad2/3-Smad4 heterodimer translocates to the nucleus and stimulates gene transcription. Negative regulation is achieved by inhibitory

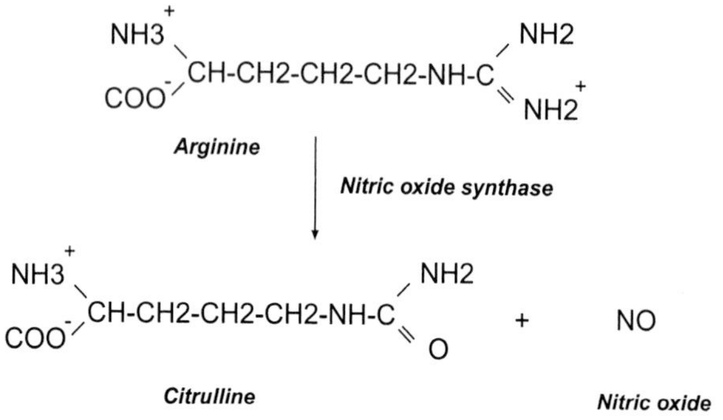

Fig. 10. Formation of NO. NOS and NADPH catalyze the oxidation of arginine to citrulline and NO.

Smads (Smad6, Smad7) which can dimerize with the Smad2 or Smad3 or bind to the TGF-β receptor to prevent signaling.

4. SIGNALING THROUGH NITRIC OXIDE AND THROUGH RECEPTORS LINKED TO GUANYLATE CYCLASE

4.1. Signaling Through Nitric Oxide and Soluble Guanylate Cyclase

Nitric oxide (NO) is one of the more recently characterized signaling molecules. Knowledge of this signaling pathway arose in part from the discovery that NO is the active metabolite of nitroglycerin and other nitrates used for vasodilation. NO is synthesized by oxidation of the amidine nitrogen of arginine through the actions of the enzyme NO synthase (NOS) (Fig. 10). Study of the role of NO has been greatly facilitated by substituted arginine analogs such as L-NAM, which act as potent NOS inhibitors. Because NO has a short half-life, is not stored, and is released immediately on synthesis, NO release reflects regulation of NOS. There are three major forms of NOS: an inducible form present in macrophage, a brain-specific form, and an endothelium-specific form. The brain and endothelial forms are activated by calcium and calcium- calmodulin complexes. The primary signaling mechanism of NO appears to be through cyclic guanosine 5′-monophosphate (cGMP). NO binds specifically to a soluble guanylate cyclase (GC) to stimulate the formation of cGMP. CGMP, in turn, activates ion channels and also activates a cGMP-activated protein kinase (PKG) that can then activate enzymes and signal similarly to PKC and PKA. The soluble GC that acts as the NO receptor is a heterodimer of $Mr = 151,000$. However, activation of GC likely does not explain all of NO's actions, and other NO signal transduction mechanisms remain to be determined. NO likely plays an important role in signaling by sensory neurotransmission mediated by neuropeptides such as substance P, vasoactive intestinal peptide, and somatostatin that increase intracellular calcium.

4.2. Hormones That Signal Through Membrane-Bound GC (Natriuretic Peptides)

The action of the atrial natriuretic peptides is mediated by a membrane-bound form of GC. There are three natriuretic peptides: ANP, BNP, and CNP. ANP and BNP bind to GC A (GC-A), and CNP binds to guanylate cyclase B (GC-B). There is a third natriuretic peptide receptor that binds all three peptides. This receptor has been thought to be primarily a clearance receptor, but recent studies suggest that it may also have independent signal transduction properties. GC-A and GC-B are single-transmembrane domain receptors with an extracellular ligand-binding domain, a transmembrane domain, and an intracellular catalytic (GC) domain. Binding of natriuretic peptide to GC-A or GC-B activates the receptors' GC activity, thus stimulating the formation of cGMP. cGMP then signals as discussed above. A third type of membrane-bound GC (GC-C) has also been described in the gastrointestinal tract and kidney. The endogenous ligand of this cyclase may be the small peptide guanylin.

5. SIGNALING THROUGH LIGAND-GATED ION CHANNELS (ACETYLCHOLINE, SEROTONIN)

Although serotonin (5-hydroxytryptamine [5-HT$_1$]) and acetylcholine (ACh) are most typically thought of as neurotransmitters, they also function as autocrine and paracrine hormones. Serotonin is secreted by pulmonary and gut neuroendocrine cells and ACh by lung airway epithelium. The nicotinic ACh receptors (nAChR) and the serotonin 5-HT$_3$ receptors are receptors that belong to the family of ligand-gated ion channels. As shown in Fig. 11, binding of the ligand allows calcium or sodium to enter the cell. Depending on the subunit composition, the selectivity for sodium or calcium can vary significantly. Primary signaling is by calcium, which signals by diverse mechanism. Changes in cell potential can open voltage-sensitive calcium channels (VSCCs) to allow more calcium entry to amplify the initial signal. The elevated calcium can then signal through CAM kinase II, which activates the MAPK, Akt pathways, and adenylyl cyclase pathways. Calcium can also activate CAM kinase kinase directly, which further activates Akt. A second important signaling route for calcium is activation of the Ras signaling pathways through mechanisms that involve the EGFR and Pyk2 kinase.

6. CROSS TALK BETWEEN SIGNALING SYSTEMS

As might be imagined, given the complexity and multiplicity of the signaling systems described in this chapter, there is considerable opportunity for cross talk between signal transduction systems. Although signaling systems in this chapter have been discussed as if isolated, it is important to realize that in the cell there is abundant cross activation. For example, multiple hormones can activate the same kinases, and the same kinase can, in turn, phosphorylate targets in more than one signaling pathway. Conversely, one hormone can activate multiple signaling pathways. Thus, signal transduction should not be considered a linear pathway but, rather, a network of activation, and signaling events represent the summation of activation. Equally important is the time course of activation as reflected by the half-life of second messengers and the balance between phosphorylation and dephosphorylation. Cross talk can be at the level of the receptor, second messenger, signaling protein, or transcription factor activation. CREB, e.g., as well as being activated by cAMP, is activated by PKC, Akt, MAPK, and CAM kinase II, making it an important integrator of multiple signaling pathways.

7. DISEASES ASSOCIATED WITH ALTERED SIGNAL TRANSDUCTION

As might be expected, given the diverse mechanisms and multiple effector molecules, there are a number of disease entities associated with signal transduction. A few examples are highlighted here, and more are described elsewhere in this book.

7.1. Oncogenes and Tumor Suppressors

Given the relation between signal transduction and growth, it is not surprising that mutations in signal transduction molecules can lead to unregulated growth and tumorigenesis. Genes that when mutated can cause transformation are called oncogenes (the normal unmutated gene is a protooncogene). Alterations in receptor structure can lead to constitutive activation and constant stimulation of the signaling cascade. An example of this includes the neu oncogene, a point mutation of the EGFR, which leads to rat neuroblastoma and the trk oncogene, a truncation of the nerve growth factor receptor, which occurs in human colon carcinomas. Mutations of the transcription factors jun and fos result in oncogenes carried by avian and murine retroviruses. Similarly, other avian retroviruses carry mutated forms of the tyrosine kinases ras and src. Loss of genes that shut off signaling pathways such as PTEN also results in tumors. This is discussed further in Chapter 19.

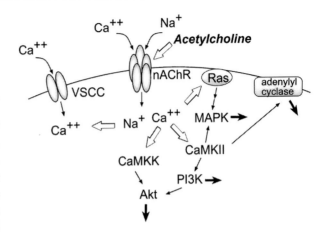

Fig. 11. Signaling by nAChR, a ligand-gated ion channel. The binding of Ach allows calcium or sodium to flow through the channel. Calcium and sodium activate VSCCs and calcium, in turn, can signal through multiple mechanisms. These include activation of CAM kinase II, CAM kinase kinase, Ras, adenylyl cyclase, PI3 kinase, Akt kinase, MAPKs, Pyk2 kinase, and the EGFR.

7.2. Alteration of G Protein Function

7.2.1. Pertussis and Cholera Toxin

Pertussis and cholera toxin are two toxins of major clinical importance that achieve their actions in part by interacting with G protein α-subunits. Cholera toxin causes adenosine 5′-diphosphate ribosylation of the α-subunit of G_s. This has the effect of inhibiting the α-subunit's GTPase activity, thus "locking" the subunit in its active GTP-bound conformation, which increases its ability to activate adenylyl cyclase and results in increased levels of cAMP. Increased levels of cAMP in the intestinal epithelial cells causes fluid secretion throughout the intestinal tract and the massive diarrhea that characterizes cholera. Pertussis toxin causes ADP ribosylation of the α-subunit of G_i. This results in uncoupling of the G protein from the receptor and leads to constitutive activation of adenylyl cyclase and increased levels of cAMP.

7.2.2. Type 1 Pseudohypoparathyroidism

Type I pseudohypoparathyroidism (PHP), also known as Albright's hereditary osteodystrophy (AHO), is a genetic disorder caused by defects in $G\alpha_s$. AHO is characterized by a distinctive phenotype of short stature, round face, obesity, shortened metacarpals, and subcutaneous ossification. In examining kindreds of type I PHP, multiple defects in $G\alpha_s$ have been described. These include point mutations, frame shifts, and splicing mutations that all produce decreased levels of $G\alpha_s$. This results in decreased responsiveness to PTH, which signals through G_s and, hence, the appearance of apparent hypoparathyroidism. As would be expected, given that G_s mediates signaling for multiple other hormones, patients with PHP exhibit multiple hormone resistance and a variety of cell types have lowered levels of adenylyl cyclase. As well as the hallmark symptoms associated with PTH resistance, patients with AHO frequently exhibit hypothyroidism and hypogonadism. PHP is discussed further in another chapter.

7.3. Alterations in cAMP-Induced Gene Transcription (RTS)

RTS is a well-defined syndrome with facial abnormalities, broad thumbs, broad big toes, and mental retardation. It has recently been discovered that RTS is caused by genetic defects in CBP. Kindreds of RTS have chromosomal break points, microdeletions, or point mutations in the CPB gene. The disease occurs in patients heterozygous for the mutation. Because CPB mediates the ability of cAMP and CREB to stimulate gene transcription, mutations in CPB will interfere with a large number of target genes. How this results in the specific syndrome remains to be determined.

7.4. Alterations in cGMP Signaling (Heat-Stable Enterotoxin)

Some strains of pathogenic bacteria produce a heat-stable enterotoxin. These toxins are a major cause of diarrhea in humans and animals and are a major cause of infant mortality in developing countries. Patients typically present with a watery diarrhea and no fever. These toxins act by binding to the membrane-bound forms of GC to increase cGMP. The increased cGMP appears to cause the diarrhea. There are two forms of heat-stable enterotoxin: STa and STb. STa binds to GC-C which is found in the intestinal mucosa. The exact mechanism by which STa activates GC remains to be determined. Some of the effects of STa may also be mediated by cGMP activation of PKA.

SELECTED READING

Cabrera-Vera TM, Vanhauwe J, Thomas TO, Medkova M, Preininger A, Mazzoni MR, Hamm HE. Insights into G protein structure, function, and regulation. *Endocr Rev* 2003;24: 765–781.

Cross MJ, Dixelius J, Matsumoto T, Claesson-Welsh L. VEGF-receptor signal transduction. *Trends Biochem Sci* 2003;28: 488–494.

Hollinger S, Hepler JR. Cellular regulation of RGS proteins: modulators and integrators of G protein signaling. *Pharmacol Rev* 2002;54:527–559.

Kohout TA, Lefkowitz RJ. Regulation of G protein–coupled receptor kinases and arrestins during receptor desensitization. *Mol Pharmacol* 2003;63:9–18.

Kopperud R, Krakstad C, Selheim F, Doskeland SO. cAMP effector mechanisms: novel twists for an 'old' signaling system. *FEBS Lett* 2003;546:121–126.

Mayr B, Montminy M. Transcriptional regulation by the phosphorylation-dependent factor CREB. *Nat Rev Mol Cell Biol* 2001;2: 599–609.

McManus KJ, Hendzel MJ. CBP, a transcriptional coactivator and acetyltransferase. *Biochem Cell Biol* 2001;79:253–266.

Petrij F, Giles RH, Dauwerse HG, Saris JJ, Hennekam RC, Masuno M, Tommerup N, van Ommen GJ, Goodman RH, Peters DJ. Rubinstein-Taybi syndrome caused by mutations in the transcriptional co-activator CBP. *Nature* 1995;376:348–351.

Proskocil BJ, Sekhon HS, Jia Y, Savchenko V, Blakely RD, Lindstrom J, Spindel ER. Acetylcholine is an autocrine or paracrine hormone synthesized and secreted by airway bronchial epithelial cells. *Endocrinology* 2004;145:2498–2506.

Spiegel AM, Weinstein LS. Inherited diseases involving g proteins and g protein-coupled receptors. *Annu Rev Med* 2004;55:27–39.

Sutherland EW. Studies on the mechanism of hormone action. *Science* 1972;177:401–408.

Ten Dijke P, Goumans MJ, Itoh F, Itoh S. Regulation of cell proliferation by Smad proteins. *J Cell Physiol* 2002;191:1–16.

West AE, Chen WG, Dalva MB, Dolmetsch RE, Kornhauser JM, Shaywitz AJ, Takasu MA, Tao X, Greenberg ME. Calcium regulation of neuronal gene expression. *Proc Natl Acad Sci USA* 2001;98:11,024–11,031.

White MF. IRS proteins and the common path to diabetes. *Am J Physiol Endocrinol Metab* 2002;283:E413–E422.

4 Steroid Hormones

Derek V. Henley, PhD, Jonathan Lindzey, PhD, and Kenneth S. Korach, PhD

CONTENTS

1. INTRODUCTION

Steroids are lipophilic molecules used as chemical messengers by organisms ranging in complexity from water mold to humans. In vertebrates, steroids act on a wide range of tissues and influence many aspects of biology including sexual differentiation, reproductive physiology, osmoregulation, and intermediate metabolism. Major sites of steroid synthesis and secretion include the ovaries, testes, adrenals, and placenta. Based on the distance of a target site from the site of synthesis and secretion, steroid hormones can be classified as either endocrine (distant target tissue), paracrine (neighboring cells), or autocrine (same cell) factors. When secreted into the environment, steroids can also act as pheromones by conveying information to other organisms.

Owing to the pervasive effects of steroids in vertebrate biology, a number of pathologic states can occur because of problems related to steroid hormone action (*see* Section 6). These disease states include cancer, steroid insensitivity, and abnormal steroid synthesis. The purpose of this chapter is to provide an overview

From: *Endocrinology: Basic and Clinical Principles, Second Edition*
(S. Melmed and P. M. Conn, eds.) © Humana Press Inc., Totowa, NJ

of steroid synthesis, steroid hormone effects in normal physiology, molecular and biochemical mechanisms of action of steroid hormones, and pathologic states related to steroid hormone action.

2. STEROID HORMONE SYNTHESIS

Steroid hormones are lipid molecules derived from a common cholesterol precursor (Cholestane, C27). There are four major classes of steroid hormones: progestins, androgens, estrogens, and corticoids, which contain 21, 19, 18, and 21 carbons, respectively. Steroid hormones are synthesized by dehydrogenases and cytochrome P450 enzymes, which catalyze hydroxylation and dehydroxylation-oxidation reactions. Eukaryotic cytochromes P450 are membrane-bound enzymes expressed in either the inner mitochondrial or endoplasmic reticulum membranes of steroid-synthesizing tissues. A common and important rate-limiting step for the synthesis of all steroid hormones is cleavage of the side chain from cholesterol (C27) to yield pregnenolone (C21), the common branch point for synthesis of progestins, corticoids, androgens, and, hence, estrogens (Fig. 1). Expression of the side-chain cleavage enzyme cytochrome P450scc (cytP450scc),

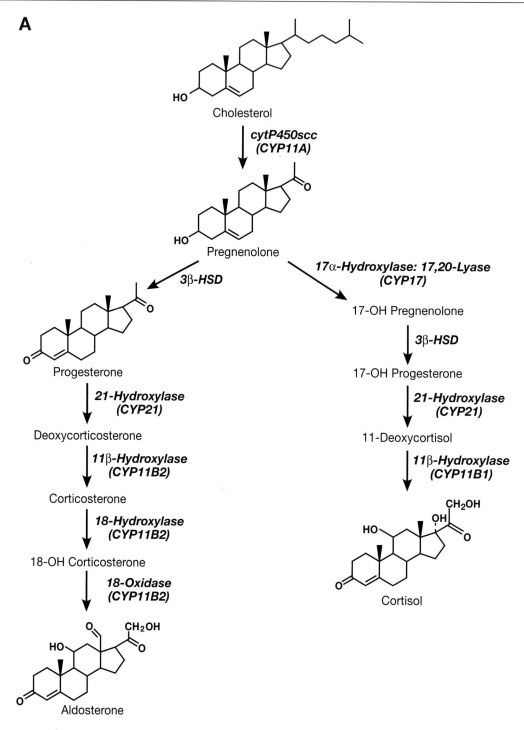

Fig. 1. (A) Synthetic pathways and structures of major progestins and corticoids found in humans. Major enzymes involved in the synthesis are in boldface.

which converts cholesterol to pregnenolone, is one of the unique features of steroidogenic cells that participate in *de novo* steroid synthesis.

In vertebrates, the synthesis and secretion of gonadal and adrenal steroid hormones are regulated by tropic hormones from the anterior pituitary such as follicle-stimulating hormone (FSH), luteinizing hormone (LH), and adrenocorticotropic hormone (ACTH). Mineralo-corticoids are also regulated by ion concentrations and circulating levels of angiotensin II. Common regulatory

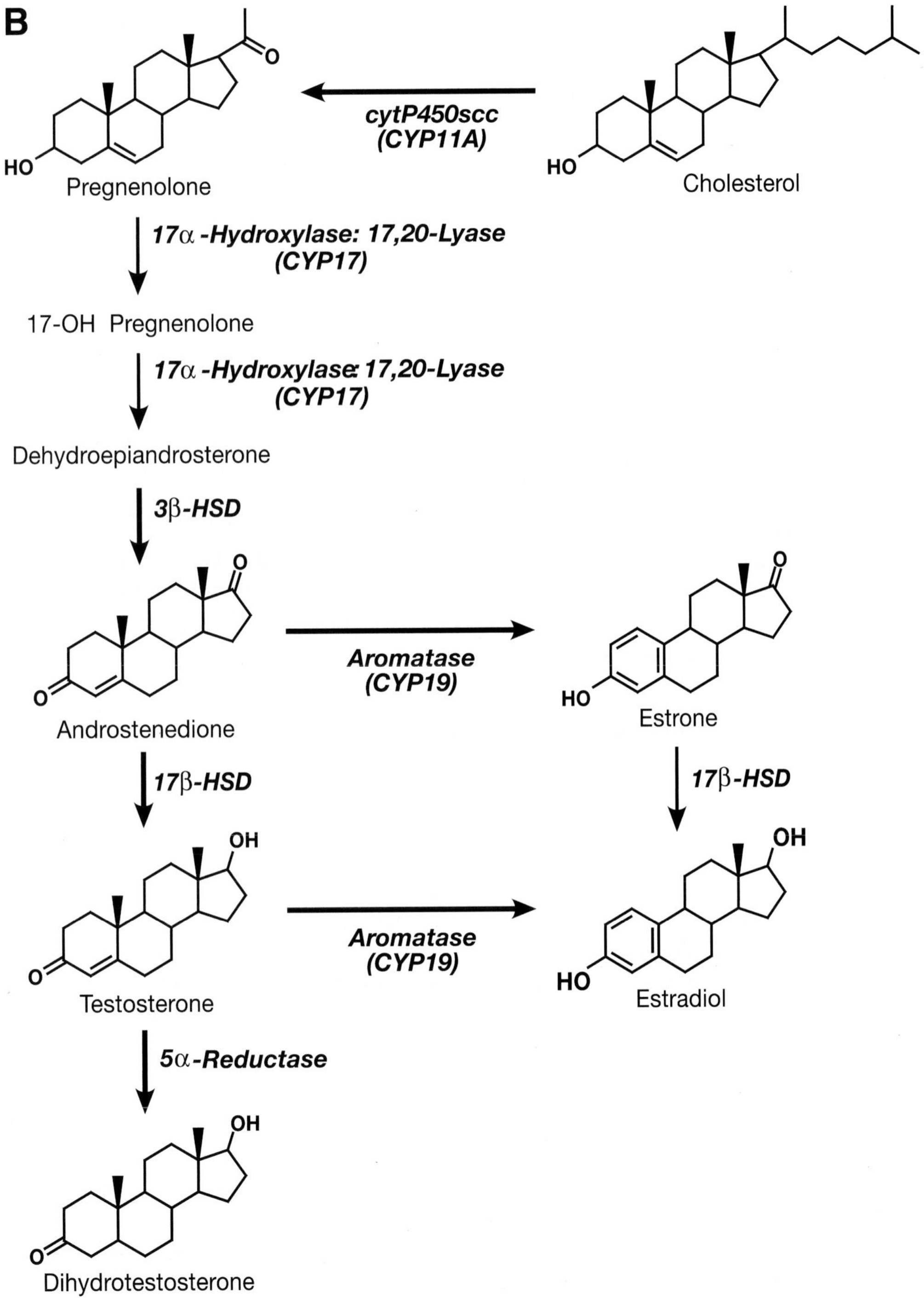

Fig. 1. (B) Synthetic pathways and structures of major androgens and estrogens found in humans. Major enzymes involved in the synthesis are in boldface.

mechanisms for steroid synthesis and release are negative feedback loops in which elevated circulating levels of steroids suppress production of tropic hormones by acting at specific sites in the brain and the anterior pituitary. The complex interplay among different components of the hypothalamic-pituitary-gonad (HPG)/adrenal (HPA) axes is an important feature of endocrine physiology and is discussed in Section 5.

2.1. Synthesis of Progesterone

Pregnenolone serves as a principal precursor to all the other steroid hormones synthesized by the ovary, testes, or adrenals. It appears that the rate-limiting step for the synthesis of progesterone is side-chain cleavage of cholesterol by P450scc. Pregnenolone is then converted into progesterone by 3β-hydroxysteroid dehydrogenase (3β-HSD). Thus, deficiencies in either P450scc or 3β-HSD have profound effects on the synthesis of all steroids.

In the ovary, progesterone is produced at all stages of follicular development as an intermediate for androgen and estrogen synthesis but becomes a primary secretory product during the peri- and postovulatory (luteal) phases. The synthesis of progesterone is under the control of FSH during the early stages of folliculogenesis and, following acquisition of LH receptors, becomes sensitive to LH later in the ovarian cycle. The synthesis of progesterone by the corpus luteum is stimulated during early pregnancy by increasing levels of chorionic gonadotropin. In addition, the placenta secretes high levels of progesterone during pregnancy, although a different isozyme of 3β-HSD is involved in the synthesis.

2.2. Synthesis of Androgen

Androgens are synthesized and secreted primarily by the Leydig cells of the testes, thecal cells of the ovary, and cells in the reticularis region of the adrenals. In most tetrapod vertebrates, testosterone is the dominant circulating androgen. Testicular synthesis and secretion of testosterone is stimulated by circulating LH, which upregulates the amount of 17α-hydroxylase:C-17,20-lyase, a rate-limiting enzyme for conversion of C21 into C19 steroids. Once taken up by target tissues, testosterone can be reduced by 5α-reductase to yield a more active androgen metabolite, 5α-dihydrotestosterone (5α-DHT). Testosterone and androstenedione can also be converted into estrogens such as 17β-estradiol (E_2) or estrone through a process termed *aromatization*. Aromatization is carried out by a cytochrome P450 aromatase enzyme that is expressed in the granulosa cells of the ovary, Leydig cells of the testes, and many other tissues including the placenta, brain, pituitary, liver, and adipose tissue. Indeed, many of the effects of circulating testosterone are owing to conversion into either 5α-DHT or E_2 within target tissues.

2.3. Synthesis of Estrogen

Estrogens and progestins are synthesized and secreted primarily by maturing follicles, corpora lutea of ovaries, and the placenta during pregnancy. The predominant estrogen secreted is E_2 and the predominant progestin is progesterone. The profile of the synthesis of estrogen changes during the course of folliculogenesis during which, under the influence of LH, the thecal cells synthesize and secrete androstenedione and testosterone, which diffuse across the basement membrane and are subsequently aromatized to estrone and E_2, respectively, by the granulosa cells. The level of aromatase and, hence, estrogens produced in the granulosa cells is under the control of FSH during midfollicular phases. Later in the cycle, the follicle/corpora lutea express greater numbers of LH receptors and LH begins to regulate E_2 production. During pregnancy, the placenta utilizes androgen precursors from the fetal adrenal gland and secretes large amounts of E_2. In addition, in male vertebrates, many target tissues such as pituitary cells and hypothalamic neurons convert circulating testosterone into E_2.

2.4. Synthesis of Corticoid

Corticoids are divided into gluco- and mineralocorticoid hormones. The predominant human glucocorticoid, cortisol, is synthesized in the zona fasciculata of the adrenal cortex. The synthesis of cortisol involves hydroxylations of progesterone at the 17α, 21 (CYP21), and 11β (CYP11B1) positions. The synthesis of cortisol is under the control of an anterior pituitary hormone, ACTH, and a negative feedback mechanism in which elevated cortisol suppresses the release of ACTH (*see* Section 5.2).

The dominant human mineralocorticoid is aldosterone, which is produced in the zona glomerulosa of the adrenal. The synthesis of aldosterone involves the synthesis of corticosterone and subsequent hydroxylation and oxidation at C18 to yield aldosterone. The synthesis of aldosterone is regulated directly by levels of potassium, and indirectly by the effects of sodium levels and blood volume on levels of angiotensin II (*see* Section 5.2).

2.5. Serum-Binding Proteins

Following synthesis, steroids are transported to their target tissues through the bloodstream. The hydrophobic nature of steroid hormones results in low water solubility; therefore, transport proteins, known as serum-binding proteins, help transport steroid hormones to their target tissues. This transport is accomplished through the binding of steroid hormones to a specific high-affinity ligand-binding domain (LBD) within the serum-binding proteins. Five serum-binding proteins have been identified: corticosteroid-binding globulin, retinol-binding protein, sex hormone–binding globulin (SHBG), thyroxine-binding globulin, and vitamin D–binding protein. As indicated by their respective names, each serum-binding protein preferentially binds a unique class of steroid hormones.

Table 1
Hormone Response Elements [a]

Type of response element	Sequence	Gene	Species
• Estrogen	GGTCAcagTGACC	vitA2	*Xenopus*
	GGTCAcggTGGCC	PS2	Human
	GG*T*CAnnnTG*A*CC	Consensus	
• Androgen	AGAACAgcaAGTGCT	PSA	Human
• Progesterone	AGTACGtgaTGTTCT	C(3)	Rat
• Glucocorticoid	AGA/*G*ACAnnnTG*T*A/CCC/T	Consensus	
• Mineralocorticoid			

[a] Sequence of some characterized response elements for ERs vs ARs, PRs, and corticoid receptors are given. Also provided are consensus sequences for an ERE and a GRE (GRE consensus sequence is identical to a PRE and an ARE). Italicized nucleotides demonstrate potential sites for mutation that can convert one class of 4 to another.

Recent studies have suggested that serum-binding proteins may serve more dynamic roles beyond steroid hormone transport. SHBG, e.g., has been shown to play a role in cell membrane–associated signal transduction through the second-messenger cyclic adenosine monophosphate (cAMP) and protein kinase A (PKA). In addition, cell-surface SHBG receptors have been identified in tissues such as the breast, testis, and prostate, further supporting a role for SHBG in cell signaling.

3. MECHANISMS OF STEROID HORMONE ACTION

The effects of steroids are typically slow in relation to the rapid time courses for the effects of second-messenger-mediated peptide hormones. This is owing both to the signal amplification inherent to second-messenger cascades and to the slower changes in gene transcription and translation exerted by steroids (genomic effects). Early experiments confirmed these paths of nuclear hormone action by utilizing protein and RNA synthesis inhibitors such as cycloheximide and actinomycin D, respectively. Though most characterized effects of nuclear hormones are mediated via nuclear receptors and genomic pathways, there are examples of very rapid, "nongenomic" effects of steroids that appear to be owing to membrane-mediated effects. In addition, alternative mechanisms of nuclear hormone receptor (NHR) activation include ligand-independent activation and genomic activation independent of a hormone-responsive element.

3.1. Genomic Mechanisms of Steroid Action

The basic genomic mechanisms of steroid action hold relatively constant across different target tissues and different classes of nuclear hormones despite the wide diversity in target tissues and the responses elicited. In the absence of hormone, estrogen receptor (ER) and progesterone receptor (PR) are principally localized in the nucleus, and glucocorticoid receptor (GR) and androgen receptor (AR) are located in the cytoplasm. Current dogma holds that steroid hormones move passively from the circulation and interstitial spaces across cell membranes and bind to and activate NHR proteins. The activated NHR-ligand complex then associates with members of a class of signal modulators termed coregulator proteins. The NHR-ligand-coregulator complex binds to specific DNA sequences termed *hormone response elements* (HREs) that are associated with promoter regions involved in regulating gene transcription. Most ligand-bound NHR complexes bind to DNA as homodimers, although some NHRs, including vitamin D and orphan receptors, can bind to DNA as heterodimers with other receptors such as the retinoid X receptor. Binding of the activated NHR-ligand complexes to an HRE is thought to position the activated NHR so that transactivation domains of the NHR interact with proteins comprising the transcriptional complex bound to a promoter and, hence, stimulate or inhibit rates of transcription.

HREs are a family of highly related DNA palindromic repeats. The estrogen, COUP factor, thyroid hormone, and retinoic acid receptors share highly homologous consensus response elements, and GR, AR, PR, and mineralocortoid receptor (MR) share very similar and, in some cases, identical elements. The high degree of homology between and within these two groups of HREs is also reflected in the high degree of homology between protein sequences of the DNA-binding domains (DBD) of the various receptors. This would seem to create a problem with specificity of hormone action but, as seen in Table 1, mutation of two nucleotides is sufficient to alter a consensus estrogen response element (ERE) into a consensus androgen response element. In addition, as other nonconsensus elements are characterized more light is shed on the nature of NHR-specific interactions with the genome.

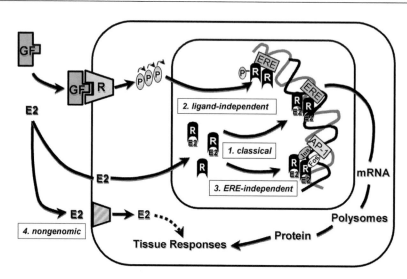

Fig. 2. Mechanisms of nuclear hormone action. E_2 and ER-mediated biologic effects occur through multiple pathways. 1. In the classic ligand-dependent pathway, E_2 diffuses across the cell membrane and binds to ER, causing dissociation of heat-shock proteins and allowing the activated ligand-ER complex to recruit transcriptional coactivators and bind to an ERE, resulting in the up- or downregulation of gene transcription. 2. Ligand-independent ER activation occurs following growth factor (GF) stimulation of kinase pathways that phosphorylate the ER. 3. E_2-ER complexes can transactivate genes in an ERE-independent manner through association with other DNA-bound transcription factors. 4. E_2 can exert rapid effects on a cell through nongenomic actions that occur at the cell surface.

The different classes of steroid hormones are all present in the circulation, and their respective levels vary with the different physiologic states of the organism. In addition, many target cells express multiple classes of NHR. This presents the organism with the problem of how to activate a specific gene by a specific steroid hormone. Specificity of steroid hormone– activated gene expression lies in (1) hormone-specific binding by the receptor, (2) DNA-specific binding exhibited by the different types of steroid receptors, and (3) control of access of steroid receptors to genes through differential organization of chromatin in the many different target cells and tissues. Many of the hormone insensitivity syndromes stem from mutations that alter steroid- or DNA-binding characteristics of the NHR.

As a whole, NHR proteins are a highly conserved group of "ligand-dependent" nuclear transcription factors (Fig. 2). NHRs are modular in nature and can be broken down into different functional domains such as transactivating domains, DBD, and LBD. Among the different classes of NHRs—AR, PR, ER, GR, and MR, the DBD is the most highly conserved region followed by the LBD and then the amino-terminal transactivating domain. The following discussion of different functional domains focuses on the ER, but many of the characteristics hold true for other NHR types.

3.2. Structure of ER Gene and Protein

Two forms of the ER have been identified, ERα and ERβ, that are coded for by separate genes located on separate chromosomes. Both ER proteins contain modular functional domain structures characteristic of the steroid hormone nuclear receptor superfamily. The ER proteins contain six functional domains that are termed *A/B, C, D, E,* and *F* domains. These domains have been found to possess the following functions: ligand-independent activation function (A/B), DNA binding (C), ligand binding (E), nuclear localization (D), and dimerization and ligand-dependent activation function (E) (Fig. 3). The ERα and ERβ proteins share a high degree of homology within their DBDs and LBDs, 97 and 60%, respectively, which results in both receptors binding to the same EREs and exhibiting a similar binding affinity for most endogenous and exogenous ER ligands. The modular nature of the different functional domains and the interdependency of these domains means that splice variants of NHR mRNAs can produce altered proteins that behave in appreciably different fashions from the full-length NHR. The importance of these variants in normal physiology is still under investigation, but splice variants may play a role in disease states such as the progression from steroid-dependent to -independent cancer (*see* Section 6.1).

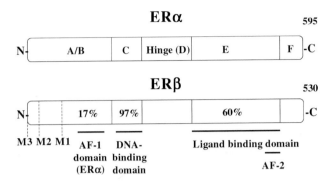

Fig. 3. Protein structure of ERs. Major functional domains of the mouse ERs and the homology between ERα and ERβ with respect to these domains is shown.

3.2.1. Ligand-Binding Domain

The LBDs (domain E) of ERα and ERβ consist of 251 and 245 amino acids, respectively, and are coded for by exons 5–9. The LBD forms a large hydrophobic pocket that exhibits specific, high-affinity binding for estradiol ($k_d \sim 0.1$ nM). Binding of estrogens to this region produces a conformational change in the ER that allows for the recruitment of transcriptional coregulators and subsequent transcriptional activation or suppression of target genes. Based on studies in which removal of the LBD results in a constitutively active or "ligand-independent" ER, it is possible that the LBD functions as a repressor of a transcription factor that would normally be constitutively active. Indeed, a constitutively active exon 5 splice variant of ERα has been detected in some human breast cancers. Finally, it appears that E_2 binding to the LBD of the ER is not always necessary for ER-mediated genomic actions. Recent evidence has shown ligand-independent ER activation of target genes owing to growth factor activation of kinase signaling pathways.

3.2.2. DNA-Binding Domain

The DBD exhibits specific binding for sequences of DNA termed EREs. This region is highly conserved and contains two "zinc finger" motifs, each of which contains cysteine residues that bind zinc. The first zinc finger dictates sequence-specific interactions with DNA, and the second appears to dictate the spacing requirements between the arms of the palindrome. These fingers are critical for DNA binding but the surrounding amino acids also influence binding. The canonical element is a palindrome inverted repeat (GGTCA nnnTGACC) although deviations from this consensus sequence are quite common (*see* Table 1). The ER binds to the DNA sequence as a dimer with one receptor

molecule contacting each 5-bp inverted repeat. Binding of the ER-ligand complex to an ERE sequence positions the ligand-activated ER and associated coactivators where they can interact with the basal transcription complexes and influence the rate of gene transcription. In addition to ERE-mediated gene expression, recent evidence indicates that the ERs are capable of transactivating genes whose promoters lack a functional ERE through protein-protein interactions with other DNA-bound transcription factors, such as Fos and Jun, at AP-1-binding sites. The result of the ER association is a tethering of the ER to DNA and an upregulation of gene expression via an ERE-independent mechanism.

3.2.3. Transcription Activation Functions

ERα contains two regions known to possess transcriptional activation functions, activation function-1 (AF-1) and AF-2, located in the A/B and E domains, respectively. Depending on the cell type and target genes, AF-1 and AF-2 can act independently or in concert. For instance, removal of AF-1 has no effect on E_2 induction of a reporter construct containing the vitellogenin ERE, whereas the same AF-1 deficient ERα has only 20% of the wild-type induction of a PS2-ERE. As mentioned earlier, removal of the LBD (containing AF-2) can lead to a constitutively active ERα. Interestingly, this constitutive activity may require phosphorylation and activation by second messengers. Studies using AF-1 and AF-2 truncated ERα have demonstrated that AF-1 responds to growth factors that act via second messengers such as cAMP or to mitogen-activated protein kinase (MAPK) signaling pathway activation, whereas AF-2 is E_2 (ligand) dependent. Thus, the ER is actually a nuclear transcription factor that responds to both steroid and second-messenger signaling pathways. In contrast to the well-characterized activation domains of ERα, the roles of the homologous regions of ERβ have not been clearly defined with respect to transcriptional activity. "Ligand-independent" or second-messenger activation of transcriptional activity has also been demonstrated for AR and PR, suggesting that this may be an important and conserved mechanism for physiologic activation of steroid receptors.

The transcriptional activation functions of AF-1 and AF-2 are mediated through transcriptional coregulators, proteins that provide the link between ligand-activated, DNA-bound receptors and the general transcriptional machinery. The conformational change induced by agonist binding to the ER allows coregulators to interact primarily with AF-2 sites on the receptor; however, interaction with AF-1 sites does occur. Many different coregulators have been identified that interact with the ligand-bound ER, including the p160 family members

SRC-1, GRIP1, and AIB1, p68 helicase, and CBP/p300. The p160 family of coregulators contains characteristic α-helical LXXLL motifs that are involved in AF recognition and binding.

3.2.4. DIMERIZATION

Most data indicate that NHRs act as homodimers, although some data suggest possible effects by NHR monomers. The region of the protein responsible for dimerization of the mouse ER overlaps with steroid-binding function and spans amino acids 501–522. These amino acids form an amphipathic, helical structure with an imperfect heptad repeat of hydrophobic amino acids reminiscent of the leucine zippers found in the JUN/FOS and CREB families of transcription factors. Mutations of amino acids in this hydrophobic stretch have proven that this area is critical for dimerization, steroid binding, and, hence, transactivation. The dimerization function is critical for the effects of NHR homodimers but may also play a role in the formation of heterodimers between NHRs and other transcription factors. Heterodimers consisting of ERα and ERβ, as well as heterodimers of ERα and SP1 proteins, have been shown to regulate expression of genes such as c-FOS and transforming growth factor-α. Thus, the dimerization function is critical for the effects of NHR homodimers but also plays a role in the formation of heterodimers between NHRs and other transcription factors with similar dimerization domains.

3.2.5. NUCLEAR LOCALIZATION SIGNAL

NHRs and many other transcription factors possess a segment of amino acids that targets the proteins to the cell nucleus. These stretches of amino acids tend to be basic and have been termed the *nuclear localization signal* (NLS). It appears that the NLS is located between amino acids 250 and 270 of the ERα, a region that shares homology with the nuclear localization domains of the glucocorticoid and progesterone receptors. The NLS for ERβ has yet to be characterized.

3.3. Nongenomic Mechanisms of Steroid Action

Although steroids typically act through the classic genomic mechanism, a process that takes several minutes to hours for effects to be seen, steroids are also capable of eliciting rapid biologic effects within seconds to minutes after administration through nongenomic mechanisms. Nongenomic steroid action results in the rapid activation of a variety of cell-signaling molecules, including MAPKs, adenylyl cyclase, and PKA and PKC. Rapid responses to estrogen have been observed in granulosa cells, endometrial cells, and oocytes, all of which exhibit increased intracellular calcium concentrations shortly, if not immediately, after E_2 exposure. Other estrogen-mediated nongenomic mechanisms have been observed in spermatozoa, breast cells, nerve cells, and vascular tissues. In addition, nongenomic mechanisms have been described for progesterone, androgens, glucocorticoids, and mineralocorticoids. Current research is under way to determine whether these nongenomic steroid mechanisms are owing to receptor-independent events at the plasma membrane, nonsteroid associated membrane receptors, or membrane-bound NHRs.

4. STEROIDS AND DEVELOPMENT

Scientists have known for years that *in utero* and neonatal exposure to steroids are critical for sexual differentiation of the brain and peripheral reproductive structures. A guiding concept for the study of developmental actions of steroidal effects is the organization-activation hypothesis. Stated simply, prenatal or neonatal exposure to steroid hormones *organizes* or alters differentiation of the phenotype such that hormonal exposure in adulthood is more likely to *activate* a particular response. A corollary of this rule is that the initial exposures must fall within certain *critical periods* of sensitivity. These critical periods typically occur during the fetal, neonatal, and pubertal stages.

Steroids affect development of organs and tissues through both induction and inhibition of growth. Inhibition occurs via active cell death, a process termed *apoptosis*. Apoptosis is an active process requiring protein synthesis and resulting in chromatin condensation, degradation of chromatin in a characteristic segmented manner that produces an observable "ladder" pattern, and development of apoptotic bodies.

4.1. Stromal-Mesenchymal Interactions

A recurring theme in development of steroid-dependent glandular tissues is the importance of stromal-mesenchymal tissue induction. In this scheme, the fate of undifferentiated epithelium is determined by the underlying mesenchyme with which it comes into contact. For instance, undifferentiated epithelium combined with prostatic or integumental mesenchyme develops a phenotype dictated by the type of mesenchyme. In the case of hormone-directed morphogenesis such as in the prostate or breast, hormonal influences on the glandular epithelium can occur either directly on epithelial cells or indirectly via inductive influences of the mesenchyme. Recent experiments demonstrate that epithelium can also influence the underlying mesenchyme, indicating a bidirectional epithelial-mesenchymal interaction.

4.2. Secondary Sex Structures

In the developing mammalian embryo, gonadal sex is determined by genotype. In turn, the embryonic gonads secrete hormones that, coupled with maternal hormones, determine the early hormonal milieu to which secondary sex structures are exposed and, hence, dictate development of male or female phenotype. Dogma holds that mammals possess a default system such that embryos develop a female phenotype in the absence of any gonadal steroid hormones. In males, as the developing testes begin to develop sex cords, the testes secrete Müllerian-inhibiting substance (MIS) and testosterone. The MIS induces ipsilateral regression of the Müllerian ducts, which prevents development of Müllerian derivatives such as the uterus and fallopian tubes. Elevated testosterone stimulates development of Wolffian derivatives such as epididymis, vas deferens, and seminal vesicles. Differentiation of external genitalia and accessory glands (such as the prostate) from the genital tubercle, scrotal folds, and urogenital sinus requires 5α-DHT. This is illustrated by 5α-reductase-deficient males who have normal Wolffian derivatives but have feminized external genitalia despite the presence of testosterone (*see* Section 6.2).

Although it is true that external genitalia and internal reproductive structures of genotypic females are grossly feminized without the influence of gonadal steroids, it is clear that steroidal effects are needed for complete and functional differentiation of some structures such as the uterus and breast. For instance, gene-targeted mice lacking functional ERα (αERKO) have uteri that possess all the normal tissue types and structures but are hypoplastic. In addition, in wild-type females, exposure to estrogens and progestins is required for differentiation of the nipple and mesenchyme surrounding the epithelium of breast tissue. Estrogen and progesterone also increase alveolar formation and branching of mammary ducts during mammary gland development.

4.3. Sexual Behavior and Sexual Dimorphisms of Brain

Sex behavior in most adult vertebrates is dependent on (1) organizational effects of hormones early in development, and (2) activational effects of circulating steroids in the adult. In many species, *in utero* and neonatal hormone exposures alter adult patterns of sexual behaviors. Historically, this observation led to the assumption that at some organizational level the brains of males and females must be morphologically or functionally distinct in order to favor female- or male-typical behaviors. In the case of the rat, sexually dimorphic nuclei have been found in the central nervous system (CNS). Male rats possess enlarged sexually dimorphic nuclei in the medial preoptic area of the hypothalamus and in the spinal cord. The development of these nuclei and subsequent function in adult males are androgen dependent; androgen ablation during early critical periods of differentiation leads to smaller, female-typical nuclei and also decreases in male-typical copulatory behavior. In rats, the effects of testicular testosterone on the sexually dimorphic nuclei of the medial preoptic area appear to be predominantly through aromatization to E_2; treatment with E_2 mimics the effect of testosterone, and the use of an aromatase inhibitor can prevent masculinization of sexually dimorphic nuclei. Similar steroid-dependent dimorphisms are found in the CNSs of gerbils, voles, songbirds, lizards, and fish. These dimorphisms may be present as differences in gross volume, cell number; cell size, dendritic arborization, and levels of expression of enzymes, neurotransmitters, neuropeptides, or receptors. Sexual dimorphisms in humans have also been reported in the anterior hypothalamus (AH), preoptic area (POA), and anterior commissure, although there are some conflicting data.

4.4. Steroids and Bone

Bone cells express ER, AR, and PR and the development and maintenance of bone structure is regulated by estrogens and androgens. Pubertal surges in estrogens and androgens initiate growth spurts including long bone growth, primarily mediated by increased insulin-like growth factor-1, and, subsequently, cessation of bone growth through epiphyseal closure. In adults, E_2 maintains bone mass and mineralization. The importance of the effects of E_2 on bone growth and development is manifest in individuals lacking in E_2 action. For instance, a human male patient lacking functional ERα exhibits continued bone growth, decreased bone density, and absence of epiphyseal closure (*see* Section 6.3). In addition, the absence of E_2 owing to either ovariectomy or menopause contributes to osteoporosis whereas exogenous E_2 helps ameliorate this condition. Excess production of cortisol results in a loss of bone mass (osteopenia).

4.5. Steroids and Liver

Liver cells express ERs and ARs which regulate production of secreted proteins and steroid-metabolizing enzymes. In humans, the liver synthesizes and secretes into the bloodstream a plasma protein termed SHBG. This protein serves to sequester and prevent steroids from being metabolized and/or cleared from the bloodstream. SHBG binds DHT with high affinity ($k_d \sim 0.5$ nM) and testosterone and E_2 with approx 5- and 15-fold lower affinity, respectively. Estrogens stimulate whereas androgens inhibit the synthesis and secretion of hepatic SHBG.

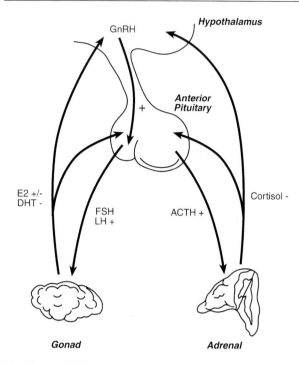

Fig. 4. HPG/HPA axes. Depicted are the pathways and major tropic hormones involved in regulating the production of gonadal and adrenal steroids.

There are distinct sex differences in the profile of steroid metabolites excreted in urine. The basis of such sex differences results from sex differences in expression of metabolic enzymes in the liver. For instance, the female liver expresses 15α-hydroxylase activity whereas the male does not express this enzyme. By contrast, males express 16α-hydroxylase, which is absent in females. In rats, these sex differences are regulated by what constitutes a hypothalamic-pituitary-hepatic axis in which neonatal androgens masculinize the growth hormone (GH) axis. In turn, the pattern of (GH) secretion imprints a male or female profile of steroid metabolism. This is evident by the fact that pulsatile surges of GH (malelike pattern) or tonic, low-level GH infusions (femalelike) into hypophysectomized rats produce a male- or female-typical pattern of enzyme expression and metabolism, respectively.

5. STEROIDS AND NORMAL PHYSIOLOGY
5.1. HPG Axes

Gonadal function is regulated by the pituitary gonadotropins (LH and FSH), which are regulated by the hypothalamic peptide, gonadotropin-releasing hormone (GnRH), steroids, and gonadal peptides (Fig. 4). GnRH is synthesized by small populations of neurons in the POA, AH, and mediobasal hypothalamus and is released

into the hypophysial portal system, which carries GnRH to the pituitary. GnRH stimulates synthesis and release of LH and FSH, which, in turn, regulate steroidogenesis and gametogenesis. Elevations in the circulating concentrations of gonadal steroids feed back on hypothalamic and pituitary sites to regulate gonadotropin synthesis and release. In addition to steroids, the gonads secrete peptide hormones (activin and inhibin) that feed back on the pituitary to regulate synthesis and release of gonadotropin.

GnRH secretion occurs as both an episodic, tonic pattern and a surge associated with ovulatory events in females. The tonic pattern of GnRH secretion occurs in a pulsatile fashion with a periodicity of approx 1 pulse/ h. Steroids feed back on the GnRH pulse generator thought to be located in the medial basal hypothalamus to regulate tonic patterns of GnRH secretion. Regulation of the ovulatory GnRH surge, however, appears to require input from the POA/AH regions. In addition, androgens and estrogens can feed back directly on pituitary gonadotropes to regulate cell growth, sensitivity to GnRH, and basal levels of gene expression of gonadotropins. A final level at which steroids feed back is on steroidogenic cells themselves. For instance, experiments indicate that androgens can downregulate LH-induced expression of steroids by Leydig cells. The feedback effects of steroids on these different levels constitute long loop (gonad-hypothalamic), short loop (gonad-pituitary), and ultrashort loop (gonad-gonad) feedback circuits (Fig. 4).

5.1.1. FEMALE REPRODUCTIVE CYCLES

Humans and most other female mammals are spontaneous ovulators, that is, the cyclical buildup of estrogen triggers a "spontaneous" pulse of gonadotropin that triggers ovulation independent of mating stimuli. However, in some species, females are reflex ovulators; that is physical mating stimuli are responsible for triggering GnRH and gonadotropin surges that provide the proximate cues for ovulation. The following discusses normal ovarian cycles in spontaneous ovulators.

As a follicle matures under the influence of basal levels of FSH, circulating levels of E_2 increase to a peak at or near ovulation. The increase in E_2 increases gonadotrope sensitivity to GnRH by upregulating GnRH receptors and, at peak levels, exerts a positive feedback effect that triggers a GnRH surge that, in turn, produces an LH surge. This LH surge induces ovulation, formation of a corpora lutea from granulosa cells of the follicle, and synthesis and secretion of progesterone and E_2. Over the course of the ovarian cycle, ovarian steroids exert control over GnRH and gonadotropins, maturation of follicles, preparation of the uterus for implantation, alterations in vaginal and cervical function, and behavior.

5.1.1.1. Feedback. Long-term ovariectomy of mice leads to a large increase in steady-state message for FSH and LH, whereas estrogen treatments reverse this effect through a negative feedback mechanism. However, this is an oversimplification of the complex effects of ovarian steroids on feedback regulation of the hypothalamus and pituitary. Estrogen appears to have biphasic effects on the synthesis and secretion of LH and FSH in which lower levels of E_2 present during postovulatory and early follicular phases can suppress gonadotropins, whereas the higher levels of E_2 found during late folliculogenesis result in (1) increased sensitivity of gonadotropes to GnRH, and/or (2) a preovulatory pulse of GnRH. Similarly, following E_2 priming, the initial exposure to progesterone results in increased sensitivity to GnRH followed by long-term inhibition. Indeed, elevated progesterone associated with formation of the corpora lutea results in suppression of estrous cycles.

5.1.1.2. Effects of Estradiol and Progesterone on Accessory Sex Structures. As E_2 levels increase during the follicular phase, the luminal epithelium of the uterus enters a proliferative phase in preparation for implantation. In mice, initial E_2 exposure rapidly induces (1–4 h) hyperemia and water imbibition followed by increases in DNA and protein synthesis, hyperplasia, and hypertrophy. An important effect of E_2 during this stage is the induction of synthesis of progesterone receptors, which allows the uterus to respond to elevated progesterone. During luteal phases, the uterus enters a proliferative phase during which elevated progesterone completes the preparation of the endometrium for implantation of the blastocyst by increasing vascularization and by thickening the mucosal layer of the epithelium. In the absence of implantation, the corpora lutea degenerate, serum progesterone levels drop, and the endometrium degenerates. The hypothalamic-pituitary-gonadal axis is then freed from progesterone suppression to resume another round of folliculogenesis.

Mammary gland function is regulated by the coordinated actions of estradiol, progesterone, and prolactin (PRL). Estradiol promotes lobuloalveolar development by acting directly on the mammary gland and by stimulating the synthesis and secretion of PRL by the anterior pituitary. Estradiol-stimulated increases in PRL also help prepare the glandular tissue for lactation. Progesterone promotes glandular development but requires (1) the presence of pituitary hormones and (2) priming with E_2, which upregulates levels of PR. While progesterone and E_2 help prepare the glandular tissue for lactation, these two hormones also suppress lactation until partu-

rition and expulsion of the placenta causes an abrupt drop in E_2 and progesterone.

5.1.1.3. Puberty. Critical stages of sex determination and sexual differentiation occur *in utero* and early in neonatal life. However, terminal differentiation of sexually dimorphic structures and the onset of reproductive fertility occur during puberty. In humans, the onset of puberty is marked by an increase in tonic, pulsatile GnRH release and increased secretion of LH and FSH. In the female, increased gonadotropin levels initiate waves of folliculogenesis and associated increases in E_2 and androgens. As levels of E_2 increase, terminal differentiation of the breasts begins and females undergo a growth spurt. As E_2 levels increase over the course of puberty, E_2 induces epiphyseal closure and cessation of the growth spurt. Exposure to increasing levels of E_2 results in an initial proliferation of the endometrium followed by the first menses (menarche) owing to a drop in E_2 at the end of a follicular wave. The initial ovulatory event takes place approx 1 yr following menarche, presumably because the mechanisms regulating a GnRH surge now respond to E_2-positive feedback. In the male, the pubertal onset of increased GnRH and gonadotropin synthesis and release is marked by testicular enlargement and initiation of spermatogenesis and steroidogenesis. As levels of circulating testosterone increase, penile enlargement, growth of pubic hair, and growth spurts commence. In addition, the glandular epithelium of secretory glands such as the seminal vesicle and prostate undergo a proliferative phase and begin to produce secretory products that become components of the semen.

5.1.1.4. Effects of E_2 and Progesterone on Sexual Behavior. In many vertebrates, E_2 and progesterone act to coordinate periods of maximum sexual receptivity with periods of maximum likelihood of fertilization. Thus, E_2 priming during follicular phases followed by a surge of progesterone associated with ovulation and luteinization results in maximum receptivity near the time of ovulation. The effects of the estrous cycle on behavior can be re-created in ovariectomized female rodents treated with E_2 followed by progesterone. The E_2 treatment has a facilitatory effect alone but is greatly augmented by subsequent progesterone treatment. Based on lesion studies and intrahypothalamic implants of E_2 and progesterone, the ventromedial hypothalamus appears to be the site of E_2 and progesterone effects on receptive and proceptive behaviors in female mammals. One effect of E_2 is to upregulate PR in the ventromedial hypothalamus. The significance of E_2 and progesterone in sexual behaviors of female humans appears less profound than in other mammals with a distinct behavioral estrus.

5.1.2. Male Reproductive Cycles

Regulation of the male HPG axis is a less dynamic process in which GnRH pulses are lower in magnitude and do not undergo surges like those associated with ovulation in females. In rodents, the male GnRH system cannot respond to exogenous E_2 with a surge, whereas in humans and monkeys injections of exogenous E_2 result in a GnRH surge. Thus, the absence of a GnRH surge in male humans is owing to the absence of the estrogen buildup associated with folliculogenesis in females.

GnRH stimulates gonadotropes to synthesize and release FSH and LH, which act on spermatogenesis and steroidogenesis, respectively. LH elevates cAMP levels, which stimulates synthesis and secretion of testosterone from the Leydig cells. Elevated testosterone assists spermatogenesis and feeds back to downregulate GnRH levels and, hence, synthesis and release of gonadotropins. It appears that testosterone may feed back both directly as an androgen and as an estrogen following aromatization. Indeed, recent studies with αERKO males demonstrated that ERα as well as AR pathway can effectively suppress serum LH at levels of both the pituitary and hypothalamus. Gonadotropes express both AR and ERα whereas GnRH neurons do not express large amounts of either AR or ERα. Thus, the hypothalamic feedback probably occurs in an indirect fashion through AR- and ERα-expressing neurons that innervate the activity of GnRH neurons from a distant site.

Sexual behavior in most adult male vertebrates is dependent on elevated circulating levels of testosterone. Testosterone acts on brain nuclei of the AH/POA to activate male-typical sexual behaviors; lesions of these brain areas or castration results in a cessation of sexual behaviors. Depending on the species, behavioral effects of androgens can be owing to both aromatization to E_2 and direct effects as testosterone or DHT. Testosterone also acts on Sertoli cells, where it can maintain spermatogenesis, even in hypophysectomized males. Another important function is stimulation of accessory sex structures such as the prostate and seminal vesicle. Circulating testosterone is converted into 5α-DHT, which causes hypertrophy of secretory epithelium, increases in RNA and protein synthesis, and increased protein secretions. As adults, the continued functioning of these androgen-dependent responses relies on exposure to circulating testosterone.

5.2. HPA Axis

Synthesis and secretion of glucocorticoids such as cortisol are stimulated by the pituitary hormone, ACTH. The release of ACTH from corticotropes is stimulated by a hypothalamic peptide, corticotropin-releasing factor (CRF), produced by the paraventricular nucleus of the hypothalamus. Increased levels of cortisol act directly at the level of the corticotroph to reduce ACTH production and at the paraventricular nucleus of the hypothalamus to suppress CRF levels (Fig. 4). Thus, hypophysectomy leads to a decrease in cortisol and adrenalectomy leads to an increase in ACTH that is reversed by cortisol treatment. Continuous ACTH secretion characteristic of chronic stress also leads to adrenal cortical hypertrophy; elevated glucocorticoid levels; and, in some cases, adrenal failure.

ACTH has a very limited tropic effect on the zona glomerulosa and aldosterone levels in mammals. Primary regulators of aldosterone synthesis include potassium (K^+), sodium (Na^+), blood volume, and angiotensin II. Elevated angiotensin II, K^+ loading, and low serum Na^+ levels, however, increase synthesis of adrenal aldosterone, which promotes Na^+ reabsorption by the kidney. Conversely, Na^+ loading produces hypertension or circulatory expansion and decreases levels of aldosterone.

Potassium appears to act directly at the level of the glomerulosa both in vivo and in vitro. Furthermore, K^+ loading appears to affect the release of renin and synergizes with angiotensin II to increase the release of aldosterone. Sodium depletion decreases blood volume, which stimulates the juxtaglomerular apparatus to secrete renin. In turn, renin cleaves angiotensinogen, producing angiotensin I and initiating a cascade that eventually leads to elevated levels of angiotensin II and subsequent elevation of aldosterone. The elevated aldosterone promotes Na^+ retention and elevates blood volume and arterial pressure, which, in turn, feeds back to decrease renin production.

5.2.1. Carbohydrate Metabolism

Adrenalectomy leads to reduced liver glycogen and low blood glucose resulting from increased oxidation of glucose and decreased gluconeogenesis from protein. Conversely, administration of cortisol leads to a rise in blood sugar and an increase in liver glycogen stores owing to decreased glucose utilization and increased gluconeogenesis. Glucagon also elevates glucose levels and promotes glycogen breakdown. Insulin, however, has the opposite effects, producing lower blood sugar (decreased gluconeogenesis) and increased glycogen synthesis and storage.

5.2.2. Stress Responses

Stress can be induced by social interactions, physical stress, and physiologic challenges. A classic stress response is increased secretion of glucocorticoids trig-

Table 2
Steroid-Based Pathologies

Defect	Phenotype
AR	X: feminization of external genitalia, androgen resistant
5α-Reductase	XY: feminization of external genitalia
ERα	XX: mammary agenesis, normal Müllerian structures, elevated androgens and gonadotropins, polycystic ovaries, infertile Human XY: tall stature, open epiphyseal plate, elevated estrogens and gonadotropins
ERβ	XX: subfertile, normal mammary gland development and lactation XY: fertile, no testicular phenotype
Aromatase	XX: mammary agenesis, ambiguous external genitalia, normal Müllerian structures, elevated androgens and gonadotropins, polycystic ovaries XY: phenotypes similar to those from ER defects but responds to estrogen therapy
PR A	XX: impaired ovulation, impaired uterine decidualization, infertility
PR B	XX: reduced mammary ductal morphogenesis and alveologenesis
P450scc	XX: asteroidogenesis, hyponatremia, altered glucose metabolism, no pubertal changes XY: same as XX, external genitalia feminized, Wolffian structures absent
3β-HSD	XX: similar to P450scc deficiency except some masculinization may be present XY: similar to P450scc deficiency
21-Hydroxylase	Inability to synthesize cortisol XX: increased androgens, ambiguous genitalia, masculinization, rapid postnatal somatic growth XY: increased androgens, rapid postnatal somatic growth

gered by increased secretions of CRH and ACTH. Hormonal responses to stress can be very fast (minutes) and dissipate quickly, or in some cases, become chronic. In stressful situations, elevated glucocorticoids stimulate an adaptive rise in glucose levels from carbohydrate energy sources. The effects of long-term elevated glucocorticoid include suppression of HPG function and suppression of the immune system.

Elevated glucocorticoids suppress production of GnRH by hypothalamic neurons and, consequently, alters gonadotropin and steroid synthesis and gametogenesis. Glucocorticoids also directly affect gonadotrope function by suppressing basal and second-messenger-induced synthesis and release of gonadotropins. At the level of the gonad, glucocorticoids also suppress gonadotropin and second-messenger-stimulated steroid synthesis. Thus, the suppressive effects of elevated glucocorticoids on reproduction are exerted at all levels of the HPG axis.

Glucocorticoids play a role in the apoptotic events leading to differentiation of the immune system and regulation of the immune system in adults. Apoptosis is an active process of programmed cell death in which a series of programmed events leads to the death of a cell. In the developing immune system, glucocorticoids induce apoptosis in autoreactive T-cells and unreacted B-cells. High levels of glucocorticoids can also lead to apoptosis of immune cells in the adult and, consequently, a compromised immune system and increased susceptibility to disease.

5.2.3. Electrolyte Balance

Salt balance is achieved primarily by mineralocorticoids and neurohypophyseal peptides such as arginine vasopressin and arginine vasotocin. Aldosterone, the principal human mineralocorticoid, reduces Na$^+$ loss by enhancing resorption by the renal tubules of the kidney. Thus, adrenalectomy or deficiencies in adrenal steroid synthesis result in rapid decreases in blood Na$^+$ and circulatory collapse unless Na$^+$ or exogenous aldosterone is provided.

6. STEROIDS AND PATHOPHYSIOLOGY

Steroid-related pathologies (Table 2) include non-heritable steroid-dependent cancers and heritable syndromes that affect the synthesis or function of steroids and their receptors, resulting in steroid insensitivity syndromes. Even though the effects of steroids on steroid-dependent cancers are environmental and non-heritable, there are clearly genetic predispositions to developing such cancers. The heritable defects in steroid action are generally autosomal recessive diseases that lead to developmental anomalies with various degrees of severity.

6.1. Cancer

A number of steroid-dependent and steroid-independent tumors occur in steroid target tissues such as the uterus, breast, and prostate. In the case of prostate cancer, a clear link with androgens is provided by the fact that castrated males never develop prostate cancer. Furthermore, many prostate cancers exhibit a period of regression and remission following castration and antiandrogen treatment. Unfortunately, many of these cancers enter a steroid-independent stage during which growth and metastases are independent of androgens or hormonal therapy.

A vital question is, Why does prostate cancer become steroid independent? Since normal proliferation and growth cycles are dependent on androgens, the question becomes, Why do these tumor cells lose their normal requirement for androgen stimulation? Two hypotheses seem viable: (1) splice variants result in a constitutively active variant AR that stimulates growth independent of androgens, and (2) key regulatory points in the cell cycle lose the requirement for androgen stimulation. These hypotheses remain to be tested in this and other steroid-independent tumors.

Breast cancer is often amenable to treatment with tissue-specific steroid antagonists, including tamoxifen and faslodex, as assessed clinically by assays for both ER and PR in mammary biopsies. The presence of receptor levels >10–15 fmol suggests that the cancer is probably steroid dependent and likely to respond to antihormone therapy. However, breast cancer can become estrogen independent and unresponsive to antiestrogens such as tamoxifen. A constitutively active ERα splice variant present in some breast tumors may provide one explanation of how cancers can progress to a steroid-independent state. Another explanation may be that the overexpression of ER coactivators, such as amplified in breast cancer-1, in breast cancer cells results in increased levels of coactivator activity that could reduce the effectiveness of ER antagonists such as tamoxifen.

6.2. Androgen-Based Developmental Defects

A number of different types of androgen-based defects have been documented. These range from a defective 5α-reductase enzyme that occurs as a rare autosomal mutation to a defective AR resulting from mutations within the X-linked AR gene. In addition, alterations in steroidogenic enzymes earlier in the synthetic pathways can also result in developmental anomalies of androgen-dependent tissues. The phenotypic manifestations of these defects range from infertility in phenotypically normal males to complete feminization of external genitalia. In cases of enzymatic deficiencies, hormone therapy can ameliorate some symptoms, whereas those symptoms related to receptor defects are resistant to hormone therapy.

6.2.1. 5α-Reductase Deficiency

5α-Reductase type 1 is expressed at low levels in peripheral tissues, and 5α-reductase type 2 is expressed at high levels in male genital structures. In males, 5α-reductase deficiencies result in varying degrees of ambiguity of the external genitalia ranging from hypospadias to complete feminization. Under the influence of elevated testosterone, Wolffian derivatives such as the epididymis and seminal vesicle develop normally whereas the external genitalia are feminized to varying degrees. In addition, Müllerian derivatives are absent owing to production of MIS by the testes. In extreme cases of feminization, this syndrome is often diagnosed at the age of puberty when a patient with female phenotype exhibits amenorrhea and/or some increased masculinization owing to the increased levels of testosterone associated with puberty. Prior to puberty, these individuals are usually raised with female gender roles, but following pubertal changes in phenotype they sometimes assume male gender roles.

6.2.2. Androgen Insensitivity Syndrome and Testicular Feminized Males

Androgen insensitivity actually presents itself as a spectrum of disorders ranging from complete external feminization to infertility in phenotypic males. A wide variety of AR gene defects have been documented ranging from point mutations that cause a premature stop codon in the testicular feminized male mouse to a complete deletion of the AR gene in a human family. Known mutations within the human AR appear to cluster primarily within the DBD and SBD of the receptor. Generally, there is a reasonable correlation between the degree of feminization and the degree to which normal function of the AR is altered, as assessed by various in vitro assays. For instance, mutations that totally abolish steroid binding lead to profound feminization, and more subtle mutations affecting thermolability and steroid dissociation rates lead to less profound effects such as infertility and hypospadia.

Fertility problems related to AR defects are resistant to therapy whereas anomalies such as mild hypospadia can be treated by surgical correction. In cases of complete feminization, inguinal and labial testes are removed owing to increased incidences of testicular cancer. Infertile completely feminized XY individuals develop female gender roles and tend to maintain these roles throughout adulthood.

6.3. Estrogen-Based Developmental Defects

Until recently, no mutations in the aromatase or ER genes had been detected. Additionally, ERα mRNA had been detected during very early embryonic stages using reverse transcriptase-polymerase chain reaction. Thus, it was suspected that estrogen is critical for development of a viable embryo and that mutations of either of the aforementioned genes would be lethal. Recent findings, however, have documented aromatase deficiency and estrogen insensitivity (ERα defects) in adult humans. In addition, gene-targeted mouse lines in which ERα(αERKO), ERβ (βERKO), or both ERα and ERβ have been disrupted (αβERKO) demonstrate that embryos can develop in the absence of functional nuclear ER. Furthermore, aromatase-deficient mice (ArKO), which lack the enzyme for converting androgens to estrogens, and therefore have no circulating estrogens, are viable. Although these data suggest that estrogens may not be critical for embryonic survival, a number of phenotypic and receptor-specific abnormalities occur owing to these gene mutations.

6.3.1. AROMATASE DEFICIENCY

Mutations in the aromatase enzyme lead to alterations in phenotypes in both males and females. A male homozygous for defective aromatase exhibited tall stature, incomplete epiphyseal closure, continued linear bone growth, and osteoporosis. Circulating androgens and gonadotropin levels were increased but gross sexual phenotype was normal. In an aromatase-deficient female, the individual presented with ambiguous genitalia at birth but normal internal Müllerian structures by subsequent laparoscopic examination. At puberty, the individual possessed the following symptoms: absence of breast development (mammary agenesis), primary amenorrhea, elevated gonadotropins, elevated androgens, and polycystic ovaries. Estrogen treatment alleviated many of these symptoms. The masculinization is owing to a lack of conversion of C19 steroids into estrogens and, hence, excess circulating androgens.

As discussed previously, ArKO mice have been generated to characterize further the phenotypes associated with aromatase and estrogen deficiency. Many of the phenotypes observed in ArKO mice are similar to those seen in aromatase-deficient humans. Male ArKO mice exhibit an osteoporotic phenotype owing to decreased bone formation, increased adipose tissue, elevated gonadotropin levels, age-dependent disruptions of spermatogenesis and fertility, and impaired sexual behavior. Female ArKO mice, like males, exhibit an osteoporotic phenotype and increased adiposity, as well as increased gonadotropin levels. Reproductive phenotypes in the female ArKO mice include underdeveloped external genitalia, uteri, and mammary glands, and infertility.

6.3.2. ESTROGEN RECEPTOR MUTATIONS

Recent work documented a normally masculinized, human male with clinical symptoms very similar to those of the aromatase-deficient male: tall stature, incomplete epiphyseal closure, osteoporosis, decreased sperm viability, and elevated testosterone and gonadotropins. Estrogen levels were also elevated and the patient exhibited no response to E_2 therapy. Molecular analysis revealed a point mutation that created a premature stop codon in the ERα gene resulting in a truncated mutant form of the receptor protein.

ERKO mice for both ERα and ERβ have been developed to elucidate the role of ER-mediated signaling in normal growth and development. The female αERKO mouse shows a number of interesting phenotypes including reduced uterine development, absent uterine responsiveness to E_2, mammary agenesis, hemorrhagic cystic ovaries, anovulation, elevated gonadotropins, and elevated testosterone and E_2. Male αERKO mice exhibit normal gross phenotype but are infertile as a result of reduced intromissions, reduced sperm counts, and decreased sperm motility. The gross sexual phenotype of the external genitalia and internal androgen-dependent structures appears normal with the exception of testicular dysmorphogenesis resulting in reduced testis size. In contrast to the complete infertility in αERKO mice, βERKO females are subfertile, have normal mammary gland development, and lactate normally, and males are fertile and have no testicular phenotype.

6.4. Progesterone-Based Developmental Defects

Defects in progesterone synthesis can arise owing to mutations in P450scc and 3β-HSD. However, because of the pivotal position of progesterone in the synthetic pathways leading to other steroids, the consequences of the absence of progesterone synthesis are clouded by the absence of other important steroids. Thus, the consequences of defects in progesterone action may be more accurately elucidated from cases involving a defective PR. To this end, a PR knockout (PRKO) mouse that was a complete knockout of both isoforms of the PR (PR-A and PR-B) was developed and characterized. The two isoforms of the PR, PR-A (81 kDa) and PR-B (116 kDa), are expressed from the same gene containing alternative translation start sites. Female PRKO mice were anovulatory, possessed underdeveloped mammary glands, and did not display lordosis behavior. However, estrogen treatments did cause uterine enlargement, hyperplasia, and edema, indicating a functional ER system. The male PRKO mouse was fertile and grossly normal except for an underdeveloped preputial gland.

To elucidate the roles of the individual PR isoforms, PR-A and PR-B knockout mice, designated PRAKO and PRBKO, respectively, were developed and characterized. Phenotypic analyses have revealed that female PRAKO mice are infertile owing to severe abnormalities in ovarian and uterine function. However, PR-A-deficient mice have normal mammary gland and thymic responses to progesterone. By contrast, PRBKO mice display normal ovarian, uterine, and thymic responses but exhibit reduced mammary ductal morphogenesis. Taken together, these observations illustrate the distinct roles for each of the PR isoforms in progesterone action.

6.5. Corticoid-Based Developmental Defects

Congenital adrenal hyperplasia is a heritable disorder in which the adrenal does not synthesize cortisol effectively. The inability to synthesize cortisol can result from defects in any of the enzymes involved in the synthesis of cortisol from cholesterol. As a consequence of these disorders, feedback inhibition of the pituitary is absent and high levels of ACTH are secreted, resulting in hypertrophy of the adrenal and, depending on the affected enzyme, high levels of precursors for cortisol synthesis. A large buildup of cortisol precursors can result in synthesis of excess androgens and subsequent masculinization of females.

Deficiency in cholesterol desmolase (P450scc) leads to a deficiency in all steroid hormones and a syndrome referred to as congenital lipoid adrenal hyperplasia. Deficiency in 3β-hydroxysteroid dehydrogenase also leads to a disorder in which synthesis of corticoids and sex steroids is deficient in adrenals and gonads. These disorders are characterized by an inability to produce cortisol and aldosterone and, hence, a reduced ability to regulate glucose metabolism, an inability to conserve salt, and severe hyponatremia. In males, the absence of sex steroids results in feminized external genitalia, and secretion of MIS by inguinal testes leads to regression of Mullerian derivatives. Females with P450scc deficiencies are normal in appearance at birth but do not undergo pubertal changes. Females with 3β-HSD deficiencies may show some masculinization of external genitalia owing to secretion of dehydroepiandrosterone, a weak androgen. Typically, treatment of these disorders involves replacement with gluco- and mineralocorticoid hormones followed by sex steroid therapy near pubertal age.

The most common form of adrenal hyperplasia is owing to deficiency in 21-hydroxylase. The resulting inability to synthesize cortisol leads to a buildup of precursors and subsequent conversion into testosterone. Clinically, females often present with ambiguous genitalia, irregular menstrual cycles, and some virilization. Both sexes undergo rapid somatic growth (postnatal), accelerated skeletal growth, and early closure of epiphyseal plates. Some patients also have defects in the ability to synthesize aldosterone, resulting in a "salt-wasting" form of the disease.

If the fetus is diagnosed prenatally via genotyping of biopsy samples, the mother can undergo treatment with dexamethasone to suppress excess production of androgens by the adrenal cortex of the fetus thus reducing masculinization of female offspring. Neonatal screening for 21-hydroxylase can be accomplished by assaying for 17-hydroxyprogesterone. This may be useful in preventing deaths related to salt-wasting forms of 21-hydroxylase deficiency.

7. CONCLUSION

Steroid hormones are synthesized and secreted by the ovary, testis, adrenal, and placenta. The majority of steroidal effects occur through binding to specific intracellular receptor proteins that regulate gene transcription in target tissues. Steroids are critical for sexual differentiation of different target organs and, in the adult, are important regulators of many aspects of normal physiology. Thus, heritable deficiencies in steroid synthesis or receptor action often lead to permanent alterations in differentiation of adult phenotype and, hence, altered function in the adult. Steroid-dependent tumors can become steroid independent by somatic mutations in receptor genes and alternate splicing of mRNAs. Recent advances in molecular endocrinology and gene targeting to generate relevant experimental animal models have allowed scientists to begin to elucidate the molecular mechanisms by which steroid hormones regulate normal physiology and pathophysiology.

SELECTED READING

Clark JH, Mani SK. Actions of ovarian steroid hormones. In: Knobil E, Neil J, eds. *The Physiology of Reproduction*, vol. 1. New York, NY: Raven, 1988:1011–1059.

Clark JH, Peck EJ, eds. *Female Sex Steroids: Receptors and Function*. New York, NY: Springer-Verlag, 1979.

Couse JF, Curtis SW, Washburn TF, et al. Analysis of transcription and estrogen insensitivity in the female mouse after targeted disruption of the estrogen receptor gene. *Mol Endocrinol* 1995;9: 1441–1454.

Couse JF, Korach KS. Estrogen receptor null mice: what have we learned and what will they tell us. *Endoc Rev* 1999;20:358–417.

Fink G. Gonadotropin secretion and its control. In: Knobil E, Neil J, eds. *The Physiology of Reproduction*, vol. 1. New York, NY: Raven, 1988:1349–1377.

George FW, Wilson JD. Sex determination and differentiation. In: Knobil E, Neil J, eds. *The Physiology of Reproduction*, vol. 1. New York, NY: Raven, 1994:3–28.

Green S, Chambon P. The oestrogen receptor: from perception to mechanism. In: Parker MG, ed. *Nuclear Hormone Receptors: Molecular Mechanisms, Cellular Functions, Clinical Abnormalities*. San Diego, CA: Academic, 1991:15–38.

Isaacs JT. Role of androgens in prostate cancer. In: Litwack G, ed. *Vitamins and Hormones*, vol. 49. San Diego, CA: Academic, 1994: 433–502.

Jordan CV, ed. *Estrogen/Antiestrogen Action and Breast Cancer Therapy*. Madison, WI: University of Wisconsin Press, 1986.

Lindzey J, Kumar MV, Grossman M, Young C, Tindall, DJ. Molecular mechanisms of androgen action. In: Litwack G, ed. *Vitamins and Hormones*, vol. 49. San Diego, CA: Academic, 1994:383–432.

Luke MC, Coffey DS. The male sex accessory tissues: structure, androgen action, and physiology. In: Knobil E, Neil J eds. *The Physiology of Reproduction*, vol. 1. New York, NY: Raven, 1994:1435–1487.

Moudgil VK, ed. *Molecular Mechanism of Steroid Hormone Action: Recent Advances*. New York, NY: Walter de Gruyter, 1985.

Parker MG, ed. *Nuclear Hormone Receptors: Molecular Mechanisms, Cellular Functions, Clinical Abnormalities*. San Diego, CA: Academic, 1991.

Sluyser M. Mutations in the estrogen receptor gene. *Hum Mutat* 1995;6:97–103.

Smith EP, Boyd J, Frank GR, Takahashi H, Cophen RM, Specker B, Williams TC, Lubahn DB, Korach KS. Estrogen resistance caused by a mutation in the estrogen-receptor gene in a man. *N Engl J Med* 1994;331:1056–1061.

White PC. Genetic diseases of steroid metabolism. In: Litwack G, ed. *Vitamins and Hormones*, vol. 49. San Diego, CA: Academic, 1994:131–195.

5 Plasma Membrane Receptors for Steroid Hormones in Cell Signaling and Nuclear Function

Richard J. Pietras, PhD, MD
and Clara M. Szego, PhD

CONTENTS

1. INTRODUCTION

Steroid hormones play an important role in coordinating rapid, as well as sustained, responses of target cells in complex organisms to changes in the internal and external environment. The broad physiologic effects of steroid hormones in the regulation of growth, development, and homeostasis have been known for decades. Often, these hormone actions culminate in altered gene expression, which is preceded many hours earlier by enhanced nutrient uptake, increased flux of critical ions, and other preparatory changes in the synthetic machinery of the cell. Because of certain homologies of molecular structure, specific receptors for steroid hormones, vitamin D, retinoids, and thyroid hormone are often considered a receptor superfamily. The actions of ligands in this superfamily are postulated to be regulated by receptors in the cell nucleus. On binding ligand, nuclear receptors associate with target genes and permit selective transcription. This

genomic mechanism is generally slow, often requiring hours or days before the consequences of hormone exposure are evident. However, steroids also elicit rapid cell responses, often within seconds (*see* Fig. 1). The time course of these acute events parallels that evoked by peptide agonists, lending support to the conclusion that they do not require precedent gene activation. Rather, many rapid effects of steroids, which have been termed nongenomic, appear to be owing to specific recognition of hormone at the cell membrane. Although the molecular identity of binding site(s) remains elusive and the signal transduction pathways require fuller delineation, there is firm evidence that primary steroid action is initiated by plasma membrane receptors.

A current challenge is to determine the precise relation of these rapid responses to intermediate and long-term effects. It appears that plasma membrane–binding sites for steroids are coupled to rapid signal transduction systems that act in concert with coactivator pro-

From: *Endocrinology: Basic and Clinical Principles, Second Edition*
(S. Melmed and P. M. Conn, eds.) © Humana Press Inc., Totowa, NJ

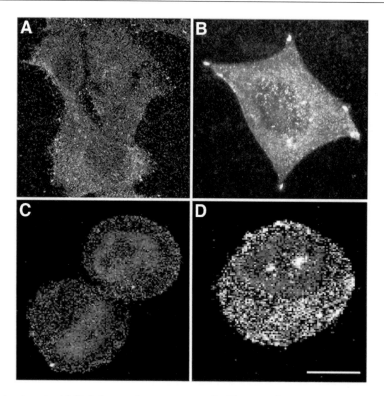

Fig. 1. Rapid response to treatment with E_2 in human breast cancer cells. Tumor cells derived from established cell lines (MCF-7), as well as those isolated from a recent tumor excision (BC), were plated on glass cover slips and grown to 60% confluency. Thereafter, cells were maintained for 24–48 h in steroid-free medium enriched with 1% dextran-coated charcoal-treated serum before the start of experiments. MCF-7 cells were treated for 2 min with control vehicle (**A**) or 2 nM E_2 (**B**), and BC cells were similarly treated for 2 min with control vehicle (**C**) or 2 nM E_2 (**D**). Cells were then immediately fixed and stained with a polycolonal antibody directed to phospho-p42/p44 mitogen-activated protein kinase (MAPK) (Thr203/Tyr204). Binding of primary antibody was detected by a fluorescent fluorescein isothiocyanate (FITC)-conjugated anti–rabbit IgG. Confocal microscope images of cells immunostained for phospho-MAPK (p-MAPK) allows *in situ* detection and subcellular resolution of fluorescent deposits. At baseline for both cell types (A,C), p-MAPK resides predominantly near the surface membrane and in the cortical cytoplasm. Treatment with estradiol (B,D) elicits rapid activation of p-MAPK, as evidenced by increased phosphorylation and enhanced translocation of the growth-promoting enzyme to the nucleus. Bar = 10 µM (H-W Chen et al., unpublished observations.)

teins and nuclear transcription factors. Hormone-receptor interactions at the surface membrane can initiate a cascade of signaling events that regulate many cellular functions, both acute and prolonged. Steroid hormones are among the most frequently prescribed drugs in the world, yet the complete mechanism of action of this important class of compounds remains to be fully elucidated. The primary purpose of this chapter is to provide an overview of emerging evidence on the nature and function of plasma membrane–associated receptors for steroid hormones in health and disease.

2. STEROID RECEPTOR SIGNALING MECHANISMS

Members of the known steroid hormone receptor family are proteins with molecular weights ranging from about 50 to 100 kDa. These "intracellular" recep-

tors share a series of common domains, usually referred to as A–F. Using the estrogen receptor (ER) as an example, there is evidence for the occurrence of four structurally distinct, functional domains in this receptor protein (Fig. 2). From the amino to the carboxy terminus of the ER molecule, these domains are the N-terminal A/B region that contributes to transcriptional activation and contains the activation function-1 (AF-1), the adjoining C-region that harbors the DNA-binding domain (DBD), the D-domain or hinge region, and the ligand-binding domain (LBD or E/F domain) at the carboxy terminus that contains the ligand-binding region as well as sites for cofactor binding and for transactivation functions (AF-2). On ligand binding, these receptors form dimers and modulate transcription by binding to their corresponding hormone response element (estrogen response element [ERE]) in the promoter region of target genes (*see* Fig. 3).

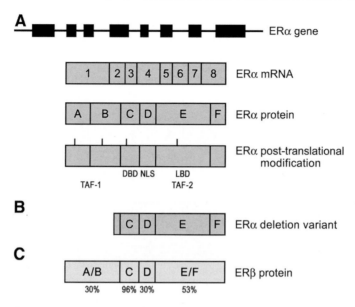

Fig. 2. Organization and functional domains of known forms of ERs compiled from the work of O'Malley, Chambon, Greene, Gustafsson, and many others. (**A**) A general diagram depicts the structure of the ERα gene; its specific transcript, ERα mRNA; and the intracellular protein product, ERα. The ERα protein has 595 amino acids, a molecular mass of 67 kDa and contains several distinct functional domains, labeled A–F. The protein product can undergo posttranslational modification, often phosphorylation of specific serine and tyrosine residues (indicated by short, vertical lines). Specific biologic activities have been localized to the different domains of the protein: transcription activation functions (TAF-1 and TAF-2), a DBD, a nuclear localization sequence (NLS), and an LBD. (**B**) Splice variant forms of ERα are known to occur. One common splice variant, a truncated 46 kDa protein with significant deletion of the A–B domains, is represented. (**C**) The ERβ protein is shown for comparison with ERα proteins. ERβ contains 530 amino acids, with the percentage of amino acid identity with that of ERα indicated in the diagram.

The first ER, termed ERα, was cloned in 1986, and the second ER, termed ERβ, the product of a gene on a different chromosome, was not discovered until 10 yr later. There is 96% amino acid identity between the two receptors in the DBD but only 53% homology in the LBD. Both ER forms bind estradiol-17β (E$_2$), and the bound complexes interact, in turn, with classic EREs with similar affinity. However, certain ligands show preferential binding to one or the other ER, and synthesis and testing of α- and β-selective ER ligands is currently in progress. The two ER subtypes have overlapping but distinct tissue distribution patterns and singular activation profiles at promoter elements of target genes, but it remains unclear how ERα and ERβ individually contribute to the physiologic effects of estrogens. In the case of ERs, several splice variants of ERα and ERβ have been described, and these variant receptors may have significant biologic activity in target cells (Fig. 2).

In general, the major target tissues of steroid hormones contain abundant levels of specific receptor proteins that bind and transduce downstream signals for modulating hormone action. Their relative distribution, whether plasma membrane, nuclear, or occurrence in additional cytoplasmic compartments, is a function of the metabolic history of the individual cell. Entry of receptor-bound ligand is extremely rapid and can deplete the surface membrane of native receptor, especially under conditions of excessive levels of steroid, and result in relatively high concentrations in other compartments including the nucleus.

In the example of ER, there are more than 20 coregulator proteins that bind to ERs and modulate their function, with each acting as either a positive (coactivator) or a negative (corepressor) transcriptional regulator. Coactivator proteins recruit other proteins of the transcriptional apparatus and also have histone acetyltransferase activity that may facilitate unwinding of tightly coiled DNA from its histone scaffold. The mechanisms by which corepressor proteins inhibit gene expression are less well understood. The relative and absolute levels of expression of coregulator proteins vary considerably among estrogen target cells, thus serving as a potential means of fine-tuning ultimate hormone action (*see* Fig. 3). Control of gene expression by steroids thus involves a series of specific molecular interactions among steroid hormones, their specific receptors, steroid receptor–associated

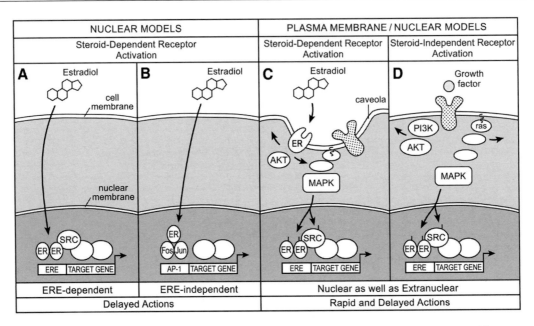

Fig. 3. Concepts of estrogen action in target cells. Nuclear, as well as plasma membrane/nuclear, models of hormone action are depicted. (**A,B**) In many prevailing models, the steroid freely enters all cells and, having crossed both plasma and nuclear membranes, is retained only in those cells in which it homes in on its receptor, localized within the nucleus. Therefore, steroid binding to ER is believed to promote alterations in receptor conformation favoring enhanced association with coactivator proteins and with specific EREs, leading, in turn, to selective gene transcription (A). However, this model fails to account for ERE-independent genomic activation. As shown in (B), the steroid may also interact with activating protein-1 (AP-1) to facilitate gene transcription via a pathway that does not require EREs. Neither nuclear model (A,B) can explain numerous, rapid cell responses to steroid treatment, such as the downstream signaling cascade. (**C**) In eliciting these acute responses, estrogens bind to a plasma membrane–associated ER to promote hormonal responses through a complementary pathway that cross-communicates, or interacts directly, with a genomic mechanism. (**D**) In addition, activation of ER may occur by steroid-*in*dependent signaling, involving mediation by growth factor receptors. Liganded membrane ER or growth factor receptor–activated ER may affect one or more of several pathways, including modulation of ion channels, leading to enhanced flux of ions, notably Ca^{2+}; interaction with peptide membrane receptors; and activation of G proteins, nucleotide cyclases, and/or MAPK, with resultant increases in their catalytic products. These membrane interactions may elicit phosphorylation of ER itself through steroid-promoted (C) or steroid-*in*dependent pathways (D). Accordingly, through these interrelated pathways, cytoplasmic and nuclear events respond in a coordinated manner to steroid hormone levels in the external environment. The intricate array of physiologic responses of cells to steroid hormones may occur as a consequence of a synergistic feed-forward circuit where steroids activate cell membrane signaling pathways that act, in turn, to enhance transcriptional activity of ER in the nucleus.

proteins, and the regulatory regions for the different target genes present in each cell.

Further complexity in the regulation of steroid hormone action is owing to the discovery of "nonclassic" modes of ligand-dependent effects, as well as ligand-*in*dependent modulation of steroid hormone–receptor function (*see* Fig. 3). Estrogens, e.g., can regulate the transcription of certain genes that lack functional EREs by modulating the activity of other transcription factors. Binding of the ER to subunits of AP-1 results in the formation of a novel transcription factor. Since most steroid hormone receptors are phosphoproteins, their function can also be altered by changes in their phosphorylation state in the absence of hormonal ligands (Fig. 3). Activators of protein kinases, such as peptide growth factors, can elicit steroid-independent activa-

tion of receptors, such as ER, by inducing phosphorylation of the receptor, usually at specific serine or tyrosine residues. Receptor tyrosine kinases and MAPKs generally modulate receptor phosphorylation in response to various extracellular signals initiated by membrane receptors (Fig. 3). Alternative pathways for activation of ER appear to be very important in vivo, and, in the case of ER, receptor activation can be induced independently of estrogens by epidermal growth factor (EGF), heregulin, transforming growth factor-α (TGF-α), insulin-like growth factor-1 (IGF-1), dopamine, and cyclic adenosine monophosphate (cAMP). The proximate and downstream signal transduction mechanisms available for promoting these initial interactions of steroid hormone receptors in hormone action (Fig. 3) are addressed more fully in the following sections.

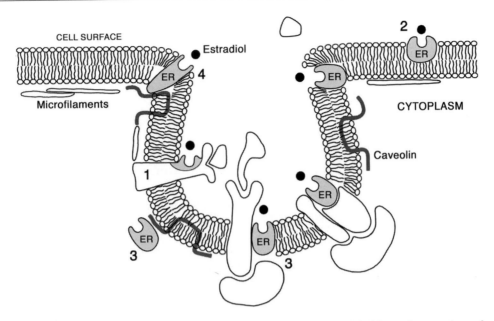

Fig. 4. Supramolecular organization of plasma membrane and occurrence of ERs. A model of the surface membrane from an estrogen-responsive cell in the region of a caveolar structure is depicted. Estradiol may interact with one of several different forms of plasma membrane–associated ERs, with examples designated as 1–4. The physical orientation and full structure of these molecules remain to be established. Of note, alternatively spliced transcripts of several steroid receptors occur, and these variant receptors give rise to proteins of different molecular mass and, possibly, modified properties (*see* Fig. 2). Membrane insertion of receptors would likely require one or more hydrophobic regions or posttranslational modification of receptor protein leading to membrane targeting. (Reprinted with permission from Szego et al., 2003.)

3. PLASMA MEMBRANE ORGANIZATION AND STEROID HORMONE RECEPTORS

As noted earlier, the "classic" mode of estrogen signaling involving nuclear interaction usually takes hours to elicit enhanced protein synthesis by activation of transcription. However, other effects of steroids cannot be fully explained by a transcriptional mechanism owing to their rapid, often instantaneous, onset. These effects can only be the result of direct steroid hormone recognition at the cell membrane.

The uptake of steroid hormones in responsive cells may occur by passive or facilitated diffusion across the plasma membrane or by one of several endocytotic mechanisms. Biophysical studies demonstrate that most steroid hormones are lipophilic molecules that partition deep within the hyrdocarbon core of lipid bilayer membranes, even those devoid of receptor proteins. However, these agonists also appear to enter target cells by a membrane-mediated process that is saturable and temperature dependent.

3.1. Membrane Models: From Fluid Mosaic to Lipid Rafts and Signaling Platforms

To understand the nature of steroid receptor association with surface membrane, it is important to consider current concepts of membrane organization (Fig. 4). The original notion of a fluid-mosaic structure of plasma membrane, wherein membrane proteins diffuse freely in a sea of lipid above a critical temperature of 15°C, is challenged by emerging evidence on the existence of macro- and microdomains that serve to concentrate key signaling molecules for more efficient coupling to specific effectors. The concept of a "signaling platform" has been advanced to characterize a supramolecular structure in which many different plasma membrane–associated receptor and effector components are assembled together in a highly coordinated hierarchical template that promotes more effective and ordered signal transduction to the cell interior.

Plasma membrane microdomains, termed *lipid rafts*, appear to arise from the phase behavior of lipid components. In the fluid bilayer of the membrane, different lipid species are asymmetrically distributed over exoplasmic and cytoplasmic leaflets of the membrane. In particular, long, saturated acyl chains of sphingolipids cluster in the presence of cholesterol to form a liquid-ordered phase relatively resistant to detergent solubilization. Saturated acyl chains of glycosylphosphatidylinositol-anchored proteins, as well as transmembrane proteins and certain tyrosine kinases, also occur within these lipid domains. Lipid raft associa-

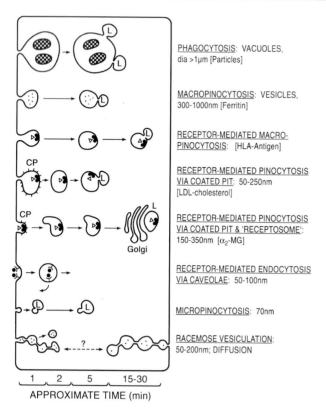

PHAGOCYTOSIS: VACUOLES, dia >1μm [Particles]

MACROPINOCYTOSIS: VESICLES, 300-1000nm [Ferritin]

RECEPTOR-MEDIATED MACRO-PINOCYTOSIS: [HLA-Antigen]

RECEPTOR-MEDIATED PINOCYTOSIS VIA COATED PIT: 50-250nm [LDL-cholesterol]

RECEPTOR-MEDIATED PINOCYTOSIS VIA COATED PIT & 'RECEPTOSOME': 150-350nm [α₂-MG]

RECEPTOR-MEDIATED ENDOCYTOSIS VIA CAVEOLAE: 50-100nm

MICROPINOCYTOSIS: 70nm

RACEMOSE VESICULATION: 50-200nm; DIFFUSION

Fig. 5. Schematic representation of pathways for internalization of extracellular agonists. Such pathways may play a role in the action of steroid hormones. For example, an especially telling analysis of the [³H]estradiol-17β translocation mechanism is available, using analytical cell fractionation at progressive time periods, beginning within 10 s of exposure. Estradiol-17β interacts specifically with membrane proteins in uterine cells and undergoes rapid internalization in nanometer-size endocytotic vesicles resulting in delivery of a portion of the steroid hormone and its associated receptor protein to the cell nucleus and nuclear protein matrix. Concomitant with a decline in plasmalemmal and presumptive endosomal fractions, a significant amount of labeled hormone occurs in Golgi and lysosomal compartments before the peak in nuclear accumulation. (Adapted and reprinted with permission from Szego and Pietras, 1984.)

tion may concentrate receptors for specific interaction with ligands and effectors on either side of the membrane, thus facilitating binding during signaling and suppressing inappropriate cross talk between conflicting signal transduction pathways.

3.2. Downstream Signaling Pathways

Caveolae (literally "little caves") are more specialized lipid raft microdomains that also concentrate and assemble components of many signal transduction pathways (Fig. 4). These membrane structures can be invaginated, flat within the plane of the membrane, detached vesicles, or fused together to form grapelike

structures and tubules (Fig. 5). As rafts, caveolae are rich in cholesterol and sphingolipids, but, unlike lipid rafts, they are lined intracellularly with clusters of the protein caveolin, a cholesterol-binding molecule that contributes to the organization of membrane lipids. The growing list of caveolae-associated molecules constitutes a virtual catalogue of cell-signaling molecules, including receptor tyrosine kinases, G protein–coupled receptors (GPCRs), protein kinase C (PKC), components of the MAPK pathway, and endothelial nitric oxide synthase (eNOS). In one such example, subpopulations of ERs are localized to caveolae in vascular endothelial cells, and, in plasma membrane caveolae isolated from these cells, estradiol directly binds to its receptors, which are coupled to eNOS in a functional signaling module to regulate the local calcium environment and blood vessel contractility.

Clathrin-coated pits are independent membrane invaginations, decorated at the inner cell membrane surface with the protein clathrin. They mediate endocytosis of nutrients and certain receptors, such as receptor-mediated uptake of low-density lipoprotein (LDL)–cholesterol complexes, and also play an important role in cell signaling. Under certain conditions, some agonists may be internalized through either clathrin-coated pits or caveolae, with one pathway apparently providing a default entry mechanism for the other.

Lipid raft–dependent signaling is often coupled with endocytotic uptake mechanisms involving both lipid rafts and caveolae. Also important in this scheme is the cytoskeletal protein actin, considered to provide constraints for the lateral mobility of lipid microdomains and to function in endocytotic trafficking. Endocytosis itself is a diverse set of processes that promote internalization of specialized regions of plasma membrane as well as small amounts of extracellular fluid (Fig. 5). Caveolae also play an important role in potocytosis, a mechanism for uptake of small molecules across plasma membrane. Finally, some cell types can internalize larger amounts of fluid by macropinocytosis or of particulates by phagocytosis (Fig. 5). In most cells, internalized materials are first delivered to early sorting endosomes, which may mature into or be transferred to late endosomes and, ultimately, to lysosomes. The potential functions of these several membrane structures and signaling domains are considered in the following sections.

3.3. Variant Forms of Steroid Hormone Receptors in Target Cell–Surface Membranes

The exact nature of the association of steroid receptors with plasma membrane remains elusive, primarily because full structural characterization of these molecules is largely incomplete. They may be known membrane components (e.g., enzymes, ion channel subunits, receptors for nonsteroid ligands) with previously unrecognized binding sites for steroids, new forms of steroid hormone receptors, "classic" receptors complexed with other membrane-associated proteins, or truly novel membrane proteins. As noted, the task of identifying these membrane-associated steroid receptors is made more challenging by the detection of multiple transcript variants of classic "intracellular" steroid receptors. In the case of ER, both ERα and ERβ are expressed in membranes, and both classes of receptor can elicit acute and late phases of cellular responses through activation of signal transduction cascades.

ER from target cell plasma membranes is a protein species with high-affinity, saturable binding specific for E_2. In addition, antibodies to nuclear ERα recognize surface sites, suggesting that membrane ER has antigenic homology with nuclear ER. Moreover, recent work reveals that membrane and nuclear ER may be derived from a single transcript. Likewise, properties of membrane glucocorticoid receptors closely resemble those of the intracellular receptor. On the other hand, properties of the aldosterone receptor, as well as those of the plasma membrane receptor for 1,25-dihydroxyvitamin D_3 (1, 25[OH]$_2$ D_3), suggest that membrane receptors for these steroids may be distinct from their "classic" intracellular counterparts. Finally, recent cloning, expression, and characterization of a membrane progestin receptor from fish ovaries showed evidence of a protein with seven transmembrane domains, a finding typical of GPCRs. Thus, a family of native steroid hormone receptors unrelated to nuclear steroid receptors may also occur in nature.

Collectively, current findings suggest that membrane receptors for steroid hormones may occur in different molecular forms. They may be duplicate or variant copies of nuclear receptors or products not related to nuclear receptor forms. Insertion of receptor proteins into plasma membrane would likely require one or more hydrophobic regions in the candidate protein. However, targeting of a receptor transcript to the membrane may also be promoted by posttranslational modification of receptor protein, including phosphorylation; glycosylation; and/or addition of lipid anchors or other modifications, such as palmitoylation or myristoylation. Thus, palmitoylation of a diminished variant form of ER occurs in vascular endothelial cells and represents an important structural modification for association of receptor with plasma membrane. ERα gene can encode the truncated ER form by alternative splicing in target cells, and the receptor then undergoes posttranslational

palmitoylation, thus promoting targeting to the cell membrane, with a C-terminus-out and N-terminus-in topology.

It remains to be determined whether surface steroid hormone receptors may also be part of a multimeric complex including a "classic" steroid receptor bound to as-yet unidentified transmembrane protein and/or coupled to membrane-associated signaling molecules. Alternatively, plasma membrane receptors for steroids may have several common structural features with, but may be distinct from, intracellular steroid hormone receptors. In the case of retinoic acid, binding to known membrane proteins, such as mannose-6-phosphate/ IGF-2 receptor (M-6-P/IGF-2R), may modulate some ligand effects. Progesterone may interact directly with oxytocin receptor, a G-linked protein, at the cell surface, with resultant inhibition of uterotonic activity of oxytocin. Progesterone congeners also bind with moderate affinity to γ-aminobutyrate type A receptors that comprise ligand-gated ion channel complexes. Similarly, acute vascular relaxation induced by pharmacologic levels of estradiol may be mediated by its binding to the regulatory subunit of Maxi-K channels in membranes, thus supporting the view that some effects of steroids, at least at high micromolar concentration, may be mediated by known membrane receptors with previously unrecognized steroid-binding sites.

In the first generation of ERα gene knockout (ERKO) mice, rapid actions of estradiol on kainate-induced currents in hippocampal neurons were noted to persist, and the effect was not inhibited by ICI 182,780, a pure antagonist of hormone binding to both ERα and ERβ. On the basis of these data, some investigators suggested that a distinct estrogen-binding site existed in neurons and appeared to be coupled to kainate receptors by a cAMP-dependent process. However, residual estrogen-binding capacity in target tissues of up to 5–10% raised doubts about whether this knockout was a true null mutation of ER. Indeed, alternatively spliced forms of ERα as well as ERβ still occur in these first-generation ERKO mice, thus complicating interpretation of such results. Nonetheless, perfection and application of this technology with the development of true, double ERα and ERβ gene knockouts should eventually prove important in deciphering the contribution of "classic" and novel receptor forms in steroid hormone action.

As with the mixed steroid hormone–binding protein systems known to occur within cells and in their extracellular fluids, it may well be that multiple forms of receptor proteins for steroids coexist in plasma membranes, thus complicating efforts to isolate and characterize *the* individual binding species in this cell compartment. Efforts to understand ligand-receptor interactions are often limited by simplistic "lock-and-key" models that may not accurately reflect the true state of complex molecular signaling cascades. Study of the molecular organization of several neurotransmitter receptor families has shown that extraordinary biologic variability occurs, with multiple "keys" and multiple "locks" sometimes involved in ligand-receptor recognition. Researchers must consider the existence of similar high-affinity, but possibly multivalent and multifunctional, receptors in the steroid hormone superfamily. Nevertheless, available evidence suggests that a finite portion of cellular steroid receptors is associated with signaling platforms in specialized microdomains of the plasma membrane.

3.4. Specific Binding of Steroid Hormones to Surface Membranes of Responsive Cells

As postulated by Paul Ehrlich more than a century ago, the outer surface of a responsive cell is equipped with specialized components that exhibit exquisite discriminatory capacity toward potential agonists when molecular conformations are mutually complementary. Indeed, in evolutionary terms, steroid recognition at the surface membrane appears to have been the primary response pathway of the primitive cell. In plant cells, no nuclear forms of steroid receptors are currently known to exist. The only recognized response pathway to plant steroids is via a membrane-associated receptor that regulates numerous functions in the intracellular economy including growth and development. Similar membrane-associated receptors for steroids have also been described in other lower organisms, such as the unicellular *Tetrahymena*.

The concept of specific membrane-associated binding sites for steroid hormones has been supported by rigorously controlled observations from many independent laboratories. Evidence is now available for the extended steroid family, which includes the retinoids, thyroid hormone, and digitalis-like steroids (Table 1). Representative examples of several approaches used to identify membrane-associated receptors for estrogen are presented in Figs. 6 and 7. Comparable observations are also available for other members of the steroid family, especially adrenocortical steroids and vitamin D metabolites. Thus, from physical, ultrastructural, immunologic, and molecular probes, as well as direct kinetic analyses of specific binding of radiolabeled steroids to the surfaces of isolated target cells or to their purified plasma membrane fractions, a large body of evidence supports this view. Such membrane proteins constitute a fraction of total receptor molecules in the target cell and have occasionally been

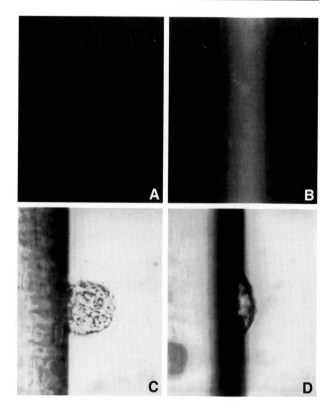

Fig. 6. Intact target cells for estrogen exhibit affinity binding to an estradiol-derivatized matrix. Estradiol was immobilized by covalent linkage to albumin-derivatized nylon fibers in order to probe for the occurrence of surface membrane–associated binding sites for estrogen. To verify the availability of steroid ligand at the fiber surface, binding of FITC-labeled antibodies to the estradiol-derivatized fiber matrix was first assessed. Experiments conducted at 22°C with (**A**) FITC-labeled nonimmune serum or (**B**) estrogen antiserum clearly demonstrated the presence of the steroid at the fiber surface, as shown in dark-field–ultraviolet fluorescence micrographs (magnification: ×100). (**C,D**) In independent experiments, estrogen target cells from liver were incubated with the estrogen-derivatized fibers in Ca^{2+}, Mg^{2+}-free Ringer solution. Washed fibers with bound cells were photographed with an immersion lens. Some cells appear fairly rounded (C), whereas others tend to flatten out at the fiber surface of the latter (D), suggesting intense interaction with immobilized estradiol (magnification: ×850). (Reprinted with permission from Pietras and Szego, 1979.)

overlooked when methods of sufficient sensitivity were not utilized. Thus, ultrastructural studies reveal extranuclear immunoreactivity for ERα associated with membrane sites along dendritic spines and axon terminals of neurons. This modern work confirms observations by Williams and Baba in 1967, at which time they reported, using electron microscopy and an excess of labeled steroids, that [3H]-aldosterone and [3H]-cortisol associated with plasma membranes of their respective target cells.

Table 1

A Brief Chronology of Selected Reports Documenting Occurrence and Activity of Plasma Membrane Receptors for Steroid Hormones in Their Cellular Targets [a]

Steroid	Year	Observation	Reference
Estradiol	1967	Elevation of uterine cAMP by estrogen within seconds	Szego and Davis
	1975	Rapid endometrial cell calcium mobilization by estrogen	Pietras and Szego
Corticosterone	1975	Binding to plasma membranes of rat liver	Suyemitsu and Terayama
Estradiol	1976	Effects on electrical activity of neurons	Dufy et al.
	1977	Specific plasma membrane binding sites for estrogen	Pietras and Szego
Cortisol	1977	Electrophysiologic effects on neurons	Kelly et al.
Progesterone	1978	Induction of oocyte maturation by steroid linked to a polymer	Godeau et al.
Estradiol	1979	Increased proliferation of cells with membrane ER	Pietras and Szego
	1980	Molecular properties of ERs in liver plasma membrane	Pietras and Szego
Vitamin D	1981	Rapid intestinal cell calcium uptake	Nemere and Szego
Progestin	1982	Specific binding to oocyte surface and role in meiotic maturation	Kostellow et al.
		Steroid receptor of 110 kDa on oocyte surface by photoaffinity labeling	Sadler and Maller
Corticosterone	1983	Binding to synaptic plasma membranes	Towle and Sze
Estradiol	1983	Increased microvilli at endometrial cell surface within seconds	Rambo and Szego
	1984	Primary internalization of ER in plasma membrane vesicles	Pietras and Szego
Thyroid hormone	1985	Characterization of plasma membrane binding sites	Alderson et al.
Estradiol	1986	High-affinity binding sites in breast cancer cell plasma membranes	Berthois et al.
		Altered cell membrane potential, density of microvilli in seconds	Pourreau-Schneider et al.
Glucocorticoid	1987	Membrane receptor associated with apoptosis in lymphoma cells	Gametchu
Vitamin D	1989	Rapid activation of PLC in rat intestine	Lieberherr et al.
		Activation of calcium channels in osteoblasts	Caffrey and Farach-Carson
Thyroid hormone	1989	Rapid induction of glucose uptake	Segal
Progesterone	1990	Stimulation of calcium influx in human sperm	Blakemore et al.
	1991	Calcium uptake mediated by sperm cell-surface binding sites	
		Action at plasma membrane of human sperm	Meizel and Turner
Corticosterone	1991	Correlation of neuron membrane receptors with behavior in newts	Orchinik et al.
Aldosterone	1991	Rapid effects on Na$^+$/H$^+$ exchange	Wehling et al.

Continued on next page

Table 1 *(Continued)*

A Brief Chronology of Selected Reports Documenting Occurrence and Activity of Plasma Membrane Receptors for Steroid Hormones in Their Cellular Targets[a]

Hormone	Year	Description	Reference(s)
Glucocorticoid	1993	Antigenic similarity between membrane and intracellular receptors	Gametchu et al.
Estradiol	1993	Binding and stimulation of HER-2 membrane receptor	Matsuda et al.
	1994	Activation of adenylate cyclase signaling pathways	Aronica et al.
Vitamin D	1994	Isolation of a plasma membrane receptor from chick intestine	Nemere et al.
Aldosterone	1994	Identification of membrane receptor in human lymphocytes	Eisen et al.
Estradiol	1995	Membrane receptor with antigenic identity to nuclear receptor	Pappas et al.
		Membrane receptor–enriched neural cells and nongenomic responses	
Androgen	1995	Rapid increase in cytosolic Ca++ in Sertoli cells	Gorczynska and Handelsman
Estradiol	1997	Membrane action and PLC regulation	LeMallay et al.
		Isolation of membrane-binding proteins from rat brain	Zheng and Ramirez
Vitamin D	1998	Hormone activation of PKC blocked by membrane receptor antibody	Nemere et al.
Estradiol	1999	Rapid Ca++ mobilization required for activation of MAPK	Improta-Brears et al.
		Rapid actions in neurons from ERα-knockout mice	Gu et al.
		Membrane ER expression reduced by antisense to nuclear ER	Norfleet et al.
		Membrane and nuclear ERα and ERβ each expressed from single transcript	Razandi et al.
		Activation of G proteins, IP$_3$, adenylate cyclase, and MAPK by membrane ER	
Androgen	1999	Rapid activation of MAPK pathway in prostate	Peterziel et al.
Progesterone	1999	Cloning, expression of binding protein from liver microsomes	Falkenstein et al.
Vitamin D	2000	Ligand-induced nuclear translocation of plasma membrane receptor	Nemere et al.
Estradiol	2000	Surface receptor in endothelial cells recognized by ERα antibody	Russell et al.
		Interaction of ER with regulatory subunit of PI3K	Simoncini et al.*
		Clustering of membrane ER in endothelial cells in caveolar domains	Chambliss et al.*
Estradiol	2001	Blockage of estrogen-induced cancer cell growth by antibody to ERα	Márquez and Pietras*
Estradiol	2003	Posttranslational palmitoylation of membrane-associated ER	Li et al.*
		Membrane ER–regulated secretion, cAMP in neurons	Navarro et al.*

[a]More than 2500 publications on membrane steroid receptors have appeared in the past 30 yr. Of these, only representative examples can be listed here. (Reprinted in expanded form with permission from Pietras et al. [2001], wherein full citations may be found, except for those references in this table followed by an asterisk, which can be found in the References at the end of this Chapter.)

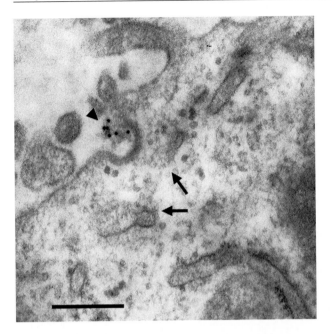

Fig. 7. Electron microscopic visualization of receptor-mediated, specific binding and internalization of 17β-estradiol-17-hemisuccinate:bovine serum albumin (BSA) that had been adsorbed to colloidal gold (E17 BSA:Au) at surfaces of human hepatoblastoma (Hep G2) cells. Note the binding of ligand to plasma membrane over a prominent invagination (arrowhead) with intracellular tubulovesicular structures beneath it (arrows). In control preparations with BSA:Au (lacking derivatization with estrogen; not shown), there is minimal internalization, despite its presence in abundant extracellular concentrations. Bar = 0.250 μm. (Reprinted with permission from Moats and Ramirez, 2000.)

Loose and reversible association of steroid hormones with transport protein in the circulation is of approximately two orders of magnitude lower than the affinity of the target cell– surface receptor for the ligand, thus permitting selective binding and accumulation by the responsive tissue. By the same token, the corollary principle of competitive displacement forms the basis for the assay of trace amounts of steroids in biologic samples.

It is also important to note that different structural conformations of a given steroid hormone may, in some instances, act as specific agonists for selected cellular response pathways. For example, $1\alpha,25(OH)_2$ vitamin D_3 produces biologic responses through two distinct receptors, one predominant in the surface membrane and the other in the cell nucleus, respectively, which are able to recognize different shapes of the conformationally flexible molecule. Accordingly, it appears that utilization of responsive mechanisms depends on the immediate steroid environment, as well as selective pathway engagement for signal transduction.

4. INTEGRATION OF MEMBRANE AND NUCLEAR SIGNALING IN STEROID HORMONE ACTION

The genomic hypothesis of steroid hormone action has generally prevailed as the exclusive mechanism since 1961, the seminal year in which the novel concepts of Jacob and Monod electrified the scientific community. In the interval to the present, extraordinary accomplishments by many molecular biologists have extended and clarified the details of these concepts for the late nuclear effects of a number of steroid hormones at their cell targets. Unfortunately, the many well-documented responses owing to primary signal transduction at the cell surface, which were being characterized independently and in parallel, were often overlooked in formulating the "classic" genomic models of steroid hormone action or misinterpreted as an alternative mechanism. Communication between events at the cell surface and the relatively remote nucleus, separated as it is from all else in the cell by a double membrane, is critical for elaborating the coordinated responses of growth and differentiation. Indeed, there is rapidly growing evidence that there is close synergism between receptor-mediated, virtually instantaneous activities at the plasma membrane and delayed effects within the nucleus.

Events initiated at the cell surface may be communicated intracellularly and, thereby, modulate transcriptional events that will eventually unfold in the nucleus. In the case of estrogen, which has received the most attention among the steroid hormones in this regard, the time course of such events encompasses several orders of magnitude, leading to its general description as a continuum (Fig. 8). A similar temporal distribution pattern also prevails for responses to other steroid hormones.

Receptor-mediated signal transduction responses have been identified for all the steroid hormones. It is significant to note that the time course of some of these cellular activities, such as nucleotide cyclase reactions, can occur within seconds or less. This is particularly well illustrated in neural responses. Acute alterations in Ca^{2+} and in Na^+/K^+ flux are likewise rapid and occur within wide differences in steroid agonist and end-organ targets. Many of these changes in the cytoplasmic microenvironment, in turn, have profound effects on enzyme reactions and on cytoskeletal structure. Indeed, there is considerable evidence that microtubules and the actin cytoskeleton of the cell play an important role in endocytotic trafficking and concomitant signal transduction. Thus, amplification of the primary hormonal signal is achieved through a limited number of receptor-mediated transduction mechanisms, linked, in part,

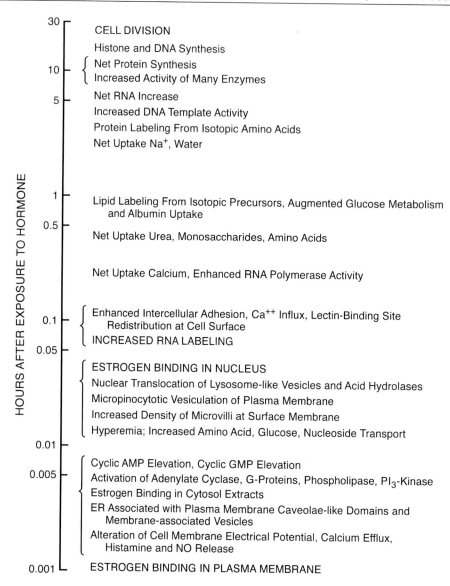

Fig. 8. Schematic representation of time course of responses of uterus to E$_2$. Times shown on the logarithmic scale refer to the onset of unequivocal change from baseline values. Thus, times indicated are dependent in part on sensitivities of the various analytic methods applied and on the somewhat arbitrary selection of initial time points for observation in the several experimental protocols. GMP = guanosine 5′-monophosphate; PI$_3$-Kinase = phosphatidylinositol 3-kinase. (Reprinted with permission from Szego and Pietras [1984], wherein additional details and sources are given.)

through heterotrimeric G proteins and other specialized signaling partners that are integral to plasma membrane.

In the case of some hormonal responses, interaction at the surface membrane may itself be sufficient to elicit an alteration in cell function. For example, estradiol can directly stimulate PKC activity in membranes isolated from chondrocytes, and the steroid also modulates calcium-dependent eNOS activity associated with its receptor in isolated plasma membranes from endothelial cells. Moreover, estrogens may enhance growth of mammary tumor cells, largely independent

of ERE-dependent transcription, by stimulating membrane-associated MAPK pathways. In ER-negative cells, transfection of transcriptionally inactive, mutant forms of ERα allows full stimulation of DNA synthesis by estradiol. Ligand-independent activation of steroid hormone receptors also occurs and may represent a more primitive response pathway, whereby cross-communication with peptide signaling systems in the cell can directly modulate the activity of steroid hormone receptors. For example, ER can be activated in the absence of estradiol through phosphorylation by

EGF-stimulated MAPK. These signaling pathways may also allow for phosphorylation of important regulatory molecules, such as the steroid receptor coactivators and corepressors that play a crucial role in steroid hormone action. As is readily appreciated, the shuttling of phosphate groups in and out of proteins critical to the signal transduction cascade is a powerful means of modifying their structure, with the immediate result of altering their folding patterns and/or relative degree of their interactions with neighboring molecules. Thus, such apparently minimal changes in composition provide a means of augmenting or attenuating their catalytic functions in a virtually instantaneous manner. It is not surprising that this efficient mechanism is so widely conserved in so many biologic contexts and across so wide an evolutionary spectrum. Any comprehensive model of steroid hormone action must account for these important cellular interactions.

Accordingly, the functions of the surface membrane–associated receptors are likely twofold. Both lead to coordination of the activities of more downstream cellular organelles. One such function is *complementary* to the more distal and time-delayed events at the genome, through communication of information from the extracellular compartment. The second function *supplements* the more deferred and metabolically expensive activities at the genome, through exclusion of the latter. Instead, the cascade of signals, transduced from binding of steroids at the cell surface, are themselves converted into immediate and more readily reversible stimuli, such as those eliciting acute ion shifts and changes in vasomotor dynamics—these being of evolutionary significance for survival. In the case of some hormone responses, such primary interactions at the plasma membrane may be sufficient to trigger a cascade of intracellular signals that lead to specifically altered cell function. Thus, within seconds of estrogen binding by surface receptors of the target cell, widespread changes are communicated to the cytoarchitecture involving striking alterations in the localized assembly and disassembly of the microtubule-microfilament scaffolding of the cell. These abrupt, but transitory, changes in the subcellular cytoskeleton may allow enhanced exchanges between membrane and nuclear compartments to promote redistribution of matériel in the pretranscriptional stage of the estrogen response cascade. Indeed, these dual capacities of membrane receptor activation underlie adaptation of the target cell to processing of information from its external environment on two independent/synergistic pathways: acute and delayed. Some selected examples of the role of membrane receptors for steroids in health and disease states are provided in the following sections.

5. MEMBRANE-ASSOCIATED STEROID RECEPTORS IN HEALTH AND DISEASE

5.1. Estrogen Receptors in Bone, Neural, Cardiovascular, and Reproductive Health and in Malignancy

As with other steroid hormones, biologic activities of estrogen in breast, uterus, and other target tissues have long been considered to be fully accounted for through activation of a specific high-affinity receptor in cell nuclei. However, it is well established that estrogen can trigger in target cells rapid surges in the levels of intracellular messengers, including calcium and cAMP, as well as activation of MAPK and phospholipase (Table 1). These data have led to a growing consensus that the conventional genomic model does not explain the rapid effects of estrogen and must be expanded to include plasma membrane receptors as essential components of cellular responsiveness to this and other steroid hormones.

The first unequivocal evidence for specific membrane binding sites for E_2 was reported about 25 yr ago. Intact uterine endometrial cells equipped with ER, but not ER-deficient, control cells became bound to an inert support with covalently linked E_2. In addition, target cells so bound could be eluted selectively by free hormone, in active form, but not by the relatively inactive estradiol-17α; and cells so selected exhibited a greater proliferative response to estrogens than cells that did not bind. Further investigations have continued to provide compelling evidence for the occurrence of a plasma membrane form of ER and support for its role in mediating hormone actions (Table 1).

Selye first demonstrated that steroids at *pharmacologic* concentrations elicit acute sedative and anesthetic actions in the brain. However, electrical responses to *physiologic* levels of E_2 with rapid onset have since been reported in nerve cells from various brain regions. Estrogen has diverse effects on brain functions, including those regulating complex activities, such as hypothalamic-pituitary circuits, cognition, and memory. Some of these estrogenic actions may be attributable to regulation of cAMP signaling by G protein–coupled plasma membrane receptors for the hormone.

New caveats from randomized controlled clinical trials on the increased risk of cardiovascular disease among healthy postmenopausal women prescribed estrogen plus progestin conflict with the long-held belief that hormone therapy might reduce a woman's risk of coronary heart disease. The results of basic research and animal models had suggested the hypothesis that estrogens were beneficial for cardiovascular health. It is likely that variations in the dose, type or timing of estrogens or the coadministration of progestogens modifies the final physiologic and clinical responses to estrogen, and these clinical variables may account for differences from the preceding laboratory and observational research studies. However, these clinical trial results also suggest that further understanding of the molecular and cellular determinants of estrogen action are required. Traditional genomic models of estrogen action in the vasculature are incomplete, but, with knowledge of the full spectrum of steroid hormone action in target cells, researchers may yet find ways to manipulate estrogenic actions that promote cardiovascular health. One starting point is to recognize that estrogen has both rapid and long-term effects on the blood vessel wall. Certain vasoprotective effects of estrogen are mediated by membrane-associated receptors. Estrogen-induced release of uterine histamine *in situ* has long been associated with rapid enhancement of the microcirculation by a process that excludes gene activation. Reinforcing these observations are data detailing the role of nitric oxide (NO) in vascular regulation by estrogen. Normal endothelium secretes NO, which relaxes vascular smooth muscle and inhibits platelet aggregation. Estrogens elicit abrupt liberation of NO by acute activation of eNOS without altering gene expression, a response that is fully inhibited by concomitant treatment with specific ER antagonists. This estrogenic effect is mediated by a receptor localized in caveolae of endothelial cell membranes. Manipulation of rapid estrogen signaling events may provide new approaches in the medical management of cardiovascular health. Direct effects of estrogen on the vasculature promote acute vasodilation and may contribute to late effects leading to inhibition of the development and progression of atherosclerosis.

Estrogen deficiency is associated with significant bone loss and is the main cause of postmenopausal osteoporosis, a disorder that affects about one-third of the postmenopausal female population. When estrogen is diminished, bone turnover increases, and bone resorption increases more than bone formation, leading to net bone loss. In randomized clinical trials, administration of estrogen plus progestin in healthy postmenopausal women increases bone mineral density and reduces the risk of fracture. However, in considering the effects of combined hormonal therapy on other important disease outcomes, such as the risk of ovarian and breast cancer, caution is recommended in the use of continuous combined hormonal therapy in the clinic. Hence, the role of membrane ER in regulating bone mass has had increasing research emphasis and could promote development of alternative treatments. Evidence for membrane-binding sites and acute effects of estrogen with an onset

within 5 s has been observed in both osteoblasts and osteoclasts. The effects of estrogens on bone homeostasis also appear to involve rapid activation of MAPK, as has been demonstrated in certain other target cells. Indeed, the "classic" genotropic effects of estrogens may be dispensable for their bone-protective effects. A novel synthetic ligand, 4-estren-3α,17β-diol, stimulates transcription-independent signaling of estrogens and increases bone mass and tensile strength in ovariectomized mice. Such therapeutic agents targeted to membrane-associated receptor forms may play a role in future treatment and prevention of osteoporosis and may offer an alternative to hormone replacement therapy for this indication. Similar considerations may apply in the case of poor patient tolerance of compounds related to etidronate and calcitonin.

Estrogen stimulates the proliferation of breast epithelial cells, and endogenous and exogenous estrogens, as well as related synthetic compounds, have been implicated in the pathogenesis of breast cancer. Human breast cancer cells exhibit specific plasma membrane reactivity with antibodies directed to the nuclear form of ERα. In addition, breast cancer cells with these membrane-associated ERs show rapid responses to estradiol, including significant increments in MAPK and phosphatidylinositol 3-kinase (PI3K)/Akt kinase, enzymic molecules that are crucial in the regulation of cell proliferation and survival. There are current indications that these membrane receptors may associate with HER-2/neu growth factor receptors in lipid raft subdomains of plasma membrane and promote tumor growth. Such signaling complexes may offer a new strategy for therapeutic intervention in patients afflicted with breast cancer.

5.2. Progestogen and Androgen Receptors in Reproduction and Malignancy

As documented for estrogens, several physiologic effects of progestogens and androgens appear to be regulated, in part, by membrane-associated receptors. Progesterone controls several components of reproductive function and behavior. Some of these activities are mediated by interaction with neurons in specific brain regions, and membrane effects appear to be important in this process. Meiosis in amphibian oocytes is initiated by gonadotropins, which stimulate follicle cells to secrete progesterone. The progesterone-induced G_2/M transition in oocytes was among the first convincing examples of a steroid effect at plasma membrane, since it could be shown that exogenous, but not intracellularly injected, progesterone elicited meiosis and that many progesterone-stimulated changes occurred even in enucleated oocytes. Moreover, this process may be related to progesterone-induced increments in intracellular Ca^{2+} and release of diacylglycerol (DAG) species that elicit a cascade of further lipid messengers.

Progesterone elicits rapid effects on the activity of second messengers and the acrosome reaction in human sperm. Assay of acute sperm responses to progesterone in subfertile patients is highly predictive of fertilization capacity. Effects of the steroid, present in the cumulus matrix surrounding the oocyte, are mediated by elevated intracellular Ca^{2+}, tyrosine phosphorylation, chloride efflux, and stimulation of phospholipases, effects attributed to activation of a membrane-initiated pathway. Indeed, two different receptors for progesterone, apparently distinct from genomic ones, have been identified at the surface of human spermatozoa; nevertheless, a monoclonal antibody against the steroid-binding domain of human *intra*cellular progesterone receptor inhibits progesterone-induced calcium influx and the acrosome reaction in sperm.

As with estrogens and progestogens, androgens promote rapid increase in cytosolic Ca^{2+} in their cellular targets. Other effects of androgens that are not attributable to genomic activation include acute stimulation of MAPK in prostate cancer cells, an action that may be important for promoting their growth. It has been demonstrated in fibroblasts that androgens can stimulate membrane-initiated signaling and the onset of DNA synthesis without activation of "classic" androgen receptor (AR)-dependent gene transcription pathways. Rather, other signaling pathways, such as those modulated by MAPK, may be operative in androgen-induced stimulation of DNA synthesis. Such observations have important implications for understanding the regulation of cell proliferation in steroid target tissues.

The androgen 5β-dihydrotestosterone induces vasodilation of aorta, which may be owing to direct action of the steroid on membranes of smooth muscle cells leading to modulation of calcium channels. In osteoblasts, membrane receptors for androgen appear to be coupled to phospholipase C (PLC) via a pertussis toxin–sensitive G protein that, after binding testosterone, mediates rapid increments in intracellular calcium and inositol triphosphate (IP_3). Testosterone also elicits Ca^{2+} mobilization in macrophages that lack a "classic" intracellular AR. These cells express an apparent G protein–coupled AR at the cell surface that undergoes agonist-induced internalization and may represent an alternative pathway of steroid hormone action.

5.3. Thyroid Hormone Receptors in Metabolic Regulation

Thyroid hormones are well known to regulate energy expenditure and development, and membrane-initiated effects may contribute to these responses. Triiodothyronine (T_3) rapidly stimulates oxygen consumption and gluconeogenesis in liver. T_3 also promotes an abrupt increase in uptake of the glucose analog 2-deoxyglucose in responsive tissues by augmenting activity of the plasma membrane transport system for glucose. In rat heart, T_3 elicits a positive inotropic effect, increasing left ventricular peak systolic pressure, as early as 15 s after hormone injection. In each tissue investigated, alterations in intracellular Ca^{2+} induced by thyroid hormone appear to modulate signal transduction to the cell interior.

Membrane-initiated effects of T_3 have been documented in bone cells by means of inositol phosphate signaling, and in brain through calcium channel activation. T_3 can also influence other cell processes, including the exocytosis of hormones and neurotransmitters, rapid effects that may be attributable to mediation by membrane receptors. Although uptake of T_3 can occur concomitantly with receptor-mediated endocytosis of LDL, and likely is accompanied by carrier proteins, direct uptake of T_3 itself is demonstrable in numerous tissues by means of a high-affinity, stereospecific, and saturable process, such as found for steroid hormones.

5.4. Glucocorticoid Receptors in Metabolic, Immune, and Neural Function

In addition to their long-established effects on mobilization of energy sources by promoting catabolism and the induction of enzymes involved in gluconeogenesis, glucocorticoids have profound effects on neuron signaling and on induction of apoptosis in lymphocytes, phenomena that appear to be membrane-initiated events. Glucocorticoids rapidly alter neuron-firing patterns. These molecular events lead to glucocorticoid modulation of specific brain functions, such as the rapid response of hypothalamic somatostatin neurons to stress. Such abrupt changes in neuron polarization are reinforced by findings of specific, saturable binding of the biologically active radioligand [^{3}H]corticosterone to neuron membranes.

Glucocorticoids play an important role in the regulation of immune function and in inflammation, especially in severe forms of hematologic, rheumatologic, and neurologic diseases. These steroids have profound anti-inflammatory and immunosuppressive actions when used at therapeutic doses. In lymphoproliferative diseases, glucocorticoids are in wide use for disease management, but the cellular mechanism leading to the therapeutic effect remains unclear. In several studies using both cell lines and freshly prepared leukemia or lymphoma cells, the presence of a membrane-associated receptor for glucocorticoids has been implicated in modulating cell lysis and death. Moreover, in lymphocytes, the membrane-binding site is antigenically related to the intracellular glucocorticoid receptor (GR) and may be a natural splice variant of this form. Some glucocorticoids have been shown to inhibit cation transport across the plasma membrane without concomitant alterations in protein synthesis through transcription. It is postulated that the steroid may thus diminish the acute immune response by interfering with immune regulatory events such as the rise in intracellular Ca^{2+}. An important pharmacologic goal is the development of a steroid compound capable of separating detrimental side effects of glucocorticoids, such as bone loss, from their beneficial antiinflammatory activity. Future approaches aimed at discrimination of the differential activities of membrane-associated and intranuclear GRs may facilitate this prospect.

5.5. Aldosterone and Digitalis-Like Steroid Receptors in Cardiovascular Health

Beyond its classic functions of promoting renal reabsorption of sodium and excretion of excess potassium, aldosterone enhances sodium absorption from the colon and urinary bladder. In each tissue, the mineralocorticoid effect is owing to enhanced activity of amiloride-sensitive sodium channels, with aldosterone rapidly augmenting Na^+/H^+ exchange. This function is Ca^{2+} and PKC–dependent but independent of nuclear receptor activation. Similarly, nontranscriptional action of aldosterone has also been reported to underlie its acute effects on cardiac function, such as increased blood pressure and reduced cardiac output, and on sodium transport in vascular smooth muscle cells.

Digitalis-like compounds are often overlooked members of the steroid superfamily. These plant-derived agents elicit inotropic and chronotropic effects on the heart but also affect many other tissues. Endogenous steroidal ligands, termed *digitalis-like* or *ouabain-like factors*, have been found in sera of humans and other animals with blood volume expansion and hypertension and may be released from the adrenal cortex. These ligands elicit inhibition of membrane-associated Na^+,K^+-adenosine triphosphatase (ATPase), likely the principal receptor for these agonists. It is notable that the steroid-binding domain of Na^+,K^+-ATPase and that of nuclear hormone receptors share significant amino acid sequence homology. In addition to membrane actions of these compounds on Na^+,K^+-ATPase, ouabain-induced hypertrophy in myocytes is accompanied by promotion of Ca^{2+} flux and initiation of protein kinase–dependent pathways leading, in turn, to specific changes in transcription and altered expression of early and late response genes. Thus, the biologic

effects of digitalis-like compounds, long considered the exception to the concept of exclusive genomic influence, may render them more closely integrated with the steroid hormone superfamily than was previously recognized.

5.6. Vitamin D Metabolite Receptors in Bone Health and Disease

Membrane-initiated effects of the secosteroid hormone $1,25(OH)_2D_3$ are well documented in bone and cartilage. In osteoblasts, interactions have been proposed between rapid effects of $1,25(OH)_2D_3$, requiring milliseconds to minutes, and longer-term effects owing to gene expression. Rapid activation of calcium channels by $1,25(OH)_2D_3$ occurs in these cells. Calcium flux, which can influence gene expression through multiple pathways, promotes key phosphorylation events in certain bone proteins. Osteoblasts exhibit rapid changes in inositol 1,4,5-triphosphate and DAG in response to vitamin D metabolites via activation of PLC. Other bone cells with rapid responses to vitamin D metabolites include osteosarcoma cells and chondrocytes. The latter system is particularly intriguing because chondrocytes elaborate matrix vesicles that appear critical in bone mineralization. Matrix vesicles, which lack nuclei, exhibit specific, saturable binding of $1,25(OH)_2D_3$, especially when derived from growth-zone chondrocytes.

Other rapid effects of vitamin D occur in a variety of cell types. Muscle cells respond within seconds to $1,25(OH)_2D_3$ via several mediators that alter cardiac output in some instances, and acute activation of calcium channels in skeletal muscle promotes contraction. Of note, in lymphoproliferative disease, $1,25(OH)_2D_3$ appears to prime monocytic leukemia cells for differentiation through acute activation or redistribution of PKC, Ca^{2+}, and MAPK. In pancreas and intestine, activation of membrane-associated signaling pathways results in vesicular exocytosis. Pancreatic β-cells respond to $1,25(OH)_2D_3$ with enhanced intracellular Ca^{2+} that is coupled to increased insulin release. In intestine, $1,25(OH)_2D_3$ stimulates exocytosis of vesicular calcium and phosphate. These cellular events may be related to vitamin D–promoted alterations in the levels of α-tubulin, thereby influencing assembly of microtubules and possibly providing a means for vectorial transport of absorbed ions. Several signal transduction pathways have been found to respond rapidly to exogenous $1,25(OH)_2D_3$, including activation of protein kinases and promotion of abrupt increments in Ca^{2+}, but integration of these signaling cascades with the physiologic response of enhanced ion absorption remains to be established.

Investigations with vitamin D congeners have recently indicated the potential hormonal nature of 24,25-dihydroxyvitamin D_3 (24,25[OH]$_2D_3$), once thought to represent merely the inactivation product of precursor 25(OH)$_2D_3$. Acute effects of 24,25(OH)$_2D_3$ have been observed in bone cells and in intestine; 24,25(OH)$_2D_3$ also inhibits rapid actions of 1,25-(OH)$_2D_3$. This may explain why abrupt effects of 1,25(OH)$_2D_3$ often fail to be observed in vivo: normal, vitamin D–replete subjects have endogenous levels of 24,25-(OH)$_2D_3$ sufficient to inhibit acute stimulation of calcium transport by 1,25(OH)$_2D_3$, thus providing a feedback regulation system.

5.7. Retinoid Receptors in Development and Malignancy

Retinoic acid exerts diverse effects in the control of cell growth during embryonic development and in oncogenesis. Effects of retinoids are widely considered to be mediated exclusively through nuclear receptors, including those for retinoic acid, as well as retinoid X receptors. However, retinoid response pathways independent of nuclear receptors appear to exist. Cellular uptake of retinol (vitamin A) may involve interaction of serum retinol-binding protein with specific surface membrane receptors followed by ligand transfer to cytoplasmic retinol-binding protein. In this regard, targeted disruption of the gene for synthesis of the major endocytotic receptor of renal proximal tubules, megalin, appears to block transepithelial transport of retinol. It is noteworthy that megalin may also be implicated in receptor-mediated endocytosis of 25-hydroxyvitamin D_3 in complex with its plasma carrier. In addition, retinoic acid binds M-6-P/IGF-2R receptor with moderate affinity and enhances its receptor function. M-6-P/IGF-2R is a membrane glycoprotein that functions in binding and trafficking of lysosomal enzymes, in activation of TGF-β, and in degradation of IGF-2, leading to suppression of cell proliferation. The concept of multiple ligands binding to and regulating the function of a single receptor is relatively novel but has important implications for modulating and integrating the activities of seemingly independent biologic pathways.

5.8. Steroidal Congeners in Regulation of Angiogenesis

Steroidal compounds are also implicated in the regulation of angiogenesis. Several steroids, including glucocorticoids, have low levels of angiostatic activity. Squalamine, a naturally occurring aminosterol, has highly potent anti-angiogenic activity. The steroidal substance does not bind to any known steroid hormone receptor, but it interacts specifically with caveolar domains at the surface membrane of vascular endothelial cells and disrupts growth factor–induced signaling for the regulation of cell proliferation. In early clinical trials, the compound showed considerable promise as a therapeutic agent to block the growth and metastatic spread of lung and ovarian cancers by interfering with tumor-associated angiogenesis. In addition, squalamine steroids may be useful for medical management of macular degeneration, a form of visual loss that is highly correlated with uncontrolled angiogenesis. At this time, there is no known cure for macular degeneration, which afflicts about 30 million people worldwide, and is the leading cause of legal blindness in adults older than 60.

6. CONCLUSION

Since the discovery of chromosomal puff induction by the insect steroid hormone ecdysone, cell regulation by steroid hormones has focused primarily on a nuclear mechanism of action. However, even ecdysone is now known to elicit rapid plasma membrane effects that may facilitate later nuclear alterations. Indeed, numerous reports of acute steroid hormone effects in diverse cell types cannot be explained by the generally prevailing theory that centers on the activity of hormone receptors located exclusively in the nucleus. Plasma membrane forms of steroid hormone receptors occur in target cells and are coupled to intracellular signaling pathways that mediate hormone action. Membrane-initiated signals appear to be the primary response of the target cell to steroid hormones and may be a prerequisite for subsequent genomic activation. Coupling of plasma membrane, cytoplasmic and nuclear responses, constitutes a progressive, ordered expansion of initial signaling events. Recent dramatic advances in this area have led to intensified efforts to delineate the nature and biologic roles of all classes of receptor molecules that function in steroid hormone–signaling pathways. Molecular details of cross-communication between steroid and peptide receptors are also beginning to emerge, and steroid receptors associated with plasma-membrane signaling platforms may be in a pivotal location to promote convergence among diverse cellular response pathways. This new synthesis has profound implications for integration of the physiology and pathophysiology of hormone action in responsive cells and may lead to development of novel approaches for the treatment of many cell proliferative, metabolic, inflammatory, reproductive, cardiovascular, and neurologic diseases.

SELECTED READING

Davis PJ, Davis FB. Nongenomic actions of thyroid hormone on the heart. *Thyroid* 2002;12:459–466.

Gruber C, Tschugguel W, Schneeberger C, Huber J. Production and actions of estrogens. *N Engl J Med* 2002;346:340–352.

Hoessli D, Llangumaran S, Soltermann A, Robinson P, Borisch B, Din N. Signaling through sphingolipid microdomians of the plasma membrane: the concept of signaling platform. *Glycoconj J* 2000;17:191–197.

Lösel R, Wehling M. Nongenomic actions of steroid hormones. *Nat Rev Mol Biol* 2003;4:46–56.

Mendelsohn ME, Karas RH. The protective effects of estrogen on the cardiovascular system. *N Engl J Med* 1999;340:1801–1811.

Migliaccio A, Castoria G, Di Domenico M, de Falco A, Bilancio A, Lombardi M, Bottero D, Varicchio L, Nanayakkara M, Rotondi A, Auricchio F. Sex steroid hormones act as growth factors. *J Steroid Biochem Mol Biol* 2003;17:1–5.

Milner TA, McEwen BS, Hayashi S, Li CJ, Reagan LP, Alves SE. Ultrastructural evidence that hippocampal α-estrogen receptors are located at extranuclear sites. *J Comp Neurol* 2001;429: 355–371.

Moss RL, Gu Q, Wong M. Estrogen: nontranscriptional signaling pathway. *Recent Prog Hormone Res* 1997;52:33–70.

Nemere I, Farach-Carson M. Membrane receptors for steroid hormones: a case for specific cell surface binding sites for vitamin D metabolites and estrogen. *Biochem Biophys Res Commun* 1998;248:443–449.

Szego CM. Cytostructural correlates of hormone action: new common ground in receptor-mediated signal propagation for steroid and peptide agonists. *Endocrine* 1994;2:1079–1093.

Szego CM, Pietras R. Membrane recognition and effector sites in steroid hormone action. In: Litwack G, ed. *Biochemical Actions of Hormones*, vol. VIII. New York, NY: Academic 1981:307–463.

Watson CS, Gametchu B. Membrane-initiated steroid actions and the proteins that mediate them. *Proc Soc Exp Biol Med* 1999; 220:93–19.

Weihua Z, Andersson S, Cheng G, Simpson E, Warner M, Gustafsson J-A. Update on estrogen signaling. *FEBS Lett* 2003; 546:17–24.

REFERENCES

Chambliss KL, Yuhanna IS, Mineo C, Liu P, German Z, Sherman TS, Mendelsohn ME, Anderson RG, Shaul PW. Estrogen receptor alpha and endothelial nitric oxide synthase are organized into a functional signaling module in caveolae. *Circ Res* 2000;87: E44–E52.

Li L, Haynes MP, Bender JR. Plasma membrane localization and function of the estrogen receptor alpha variant (ER46) in human endothelial cells. *Proc Natl Acad Sci USA* 2003;100:4807–4812.

Márquez DC, Pietras RJ. Membrane-associated binding sites for estrogen contribute to growth regulation of human breast cancer cells. *Oncogene* 2001; 20: 5420–5430.

Moats RK II, Ramirez VD. Electron microscopic visualization of membrane-mediated uptake and translocation of estrogen-BSA: colloidal gold by Hep G2 cells. *J Endocrinol* 2000;166: 631–647.

Navarro CE, Saeed SA, Murdick C, Martinez-Fuentes AJ, Arora K, Krsmanovic LZ, Catt KJ. Regulation of cyclic adenosine 3′,5′-monophosphate signaling and pulsatile neurosecretion by G-coupled plasma membrane estrogen receptors in immortalized gonadotropin-releasing hormone neurons. *Mol Endocrinol* 2003; 17:1792–1804.

Pietras RJ, Nemere I, Szego CM. Steroid hormone receptors in target cell membranes. *Endocrine* 2001;14:417–427.

Pietras RJ, Szego CM. Metabolic and proliferative responses to estrogen by hepatocytes selected for plasma membrane binding-sites specific for estradiol-17β. *J Cell Physiol* 1979;98:145–159.

Simoncini T, Hafezi-Moghadam A, Brazil DP, Ley K, Chin W, Liao JK. Interaction of oestrogen receptor with the regulatory subunit of phosphatidylinositol-3-OH kinase. *Nature* 2000;407:538–541.

Szego CM, Pietras RJ. Lysosomal functions in cellular activation: propagation of the actions of hormones and other effectors. *Int Rev Cytol* 1984;88:1–302.

Szego CM, Pietras RJ, Nemere I. Encyclopedia of Hormones. In: Henry H, Norman A, eds. *Plasma Membrane Receptors for Steroid Hormones: Initiation Site of the Cellular Response*. San Diego, CA: Academic 2003;657–671.

6 Growth Factors

Derek LeRoith, MD, PhD
and William L. Lowe Jr., MD

CONTENTS

1. INTRODUCTION

In this chapter, we discuss various aspects of classic growth factors and their relevance to endocrinology. Although "growth factors" have traditionally been considered to be represented by the family of peptide growth factors, this definition is too restricted given that nonpeptide hormones, e.g., steroid hormones such as estrogen, also stimulate cell growth. Similarly, growth factors have traditionally been considered as tissue factors, functioning locally as autocrine or paracrine factors, as compared to hormones that function in a classic endocrine fashion. We focus here on insulin-like growth factors (IGFs), which represent a paradigm that has both endocrine and autocrine/paracrine modalities. We then discuss other members of classic growth factor families, allowing the reader to compare and contrast them to the IGFs. We also briefly address the numerous cell-surface receptors and the cross talk between receptors. Because we cannot describe here all aspects of the growth factors, their receptors, and interacting proteins, we refer the reader to various other excellent reviews in the Selected Reading section.

2. INSULIN-LIKE GROWTH FACTORS

The IGF family of growth factors represents one of the best examples of the overlap of the two classic

From: *Endocrinology: Basic and Clinical Principles, Second Edition*
(S. Melmed and P. M. Conn, eds.) © Humana Press Inc., Totowa, NJ

systems: endocrine and autocrine/paracrine. The IGF family consists of three hormones (insulin, IGF-1 and IGF-2), three receptors (the insulin, IGF-1, and IGF-2 [mannose-6-phosphate, or M-6-P] receptors), and six well-characterized binding proteins (IGFBPs 1–6). The IGFs have structures that resemble insulin, hence their names, and were discovered as circulating hormones with insulin-like properties. Following the advent of molecular endocrinology, it was found that IGFs, particularly IGF-1, are produced by all tissues of the body and therefore function as both hormones and growth factors with autocrine/paracrine actions.

Insulin interacts with the insulin receptor with high affinity and with the IGF-1 receptor (IGF-1R) with much lower affinity, explaining the metabolic effects mediated by insulin at low circulating levels, whereas insulin's effect as a mitogen occurs at higher concentrations, probably via the IGF-1R. The IGFs, on the other hand, bind to and activate the IGF-1R with high affinity, whereas they stimulate metabolic effects through the insulin receptor at high concentrations owing to their low binding affinity for this receptor. The IGF-2R has no apparent signaling capacity and is not discussed further in this chapter. Both the insulin receptor and the IGF-1R belong to a subgroup of the family of cell-surface receptors with endogenous tyrosine kinase activity and are very similar in structure. They are oligomers of $\alpha\beta$–subunits that form an $\alpha2\beta2$ heterotetramer. Ligands bind to the extracellular domain of the α–subunit, which induces a conformational alteration that results in autophosphorylation on tyrosine residues in the cytoplasmic domain of the β–subunit. Tyrosine phosphorylation of the receptor results in binding of cellular substrates that mediate intracellular signaling.

It is now evident that the separation of receptors into insulin or IGF-1Rs, does not represent the full spectrum of receptor expression. Hybrid receptors may represent a significant proportion of the receptors expressed on the cell surface. These hybrids comprise an αβ–subunit from the insulin receptor and an αβ–subunit from the IGF-1R. Hybrid receptors can form in tissues that express both receptors, because their αβ–subunits are similar and are processed by identical pathways. Generally, these hybrid receptors bind IGF-1 better than insulin, which could explain how IGF-1 induces metabolic effects in certain tissues (such as muscle) even at physiologic concentrations. On the other hand, there are two isoforms of the insulin receptor, the A- and B-isoforms, each being differentially expressed by different cells and tissues. Interestingly, the A-isoform, which has an additional 11 amino acids owing to a splicing variation that includes exon 11, has greater mitogenic activity when compared to the metabolic activity of the B-isoform. IGF-2 binds the A-isoform with high affinity. Thus, the effect of the different ligands in the IGF family depends, to some extent, on the receptors expressed on the various tissues as well as the concentration and composition of the receptors. For example, liver and fat cells express mostly, if not only, insulin receptors and are primary metabolic tissues, whereas most other tissues express a mixture of receptors and may respond to these ligands either with a metabolic response or, more commonly, with mitogenic or differentiated functions.

The biologic action of the the IGFs is also dependent on the IGFBPs that bind the IGFs with high affinity but do not bind insulin. In the circulation, the IGFBPs function as classic hormone-binding proteins (e.g., the steroid hormone– binding proteins), that bind, neutralize, and protect the IGFs and form a reservoir, making the IGFs available for distribution to the tissues. Although this aspect has been well characterized, it fails to address the growing body of evidence that the IGFBPs represent a complex system of locally produced proteins that affect cellular function, thereby representing an autocrine/paracrine system in their own right. Most, if not all, cells express some complement of the six IGFBPs, which they secrete into the local environment. Cell culture experiments have shown that IGFBPs present in the local cellular milieu bind the IGFs with higher affinity than cell-surface IGF-1Rs and are capable of inhibiting their interactions with the cell. On the other hand, posttranslational modifications including phosphorylation, proteolytic cleavage, or binding of the IGFBPs to the cell surface, as opposed to the extracellular matrix, decrease their affinity for the IGFs which releases the bound ligand, thereby allowing delivery to cell-surface receptors. Finally, the IGFBPs can interact with cells and activate cellular events independent of the IGF-1R, via mechanisms presently unknown.

Both the ligands (IGF-1 and IGF-2) and the IGFBPs should therefore be viewed as endocrine and autocrine/paracrine systems that form an interesting paradigm against which to compare other growth factor families.

2.1. IGFs in Health and Disease

The IGF system plays a critical role in normal growth and development. There are examples of human disorders resulting from genetic mutations in various components of the system. An IGF-1 gene mutation was described in a severely retarded child who demonstrated growth delay, no response to growth hormone (GH) injections, but a significant response to rhIGF-1. A mutation in the IGF-1R was identified in an infant who was small for gestational age, and a mutation has recently been described in the gene encoding the acid labile-subunit (ALS) of IGFBP-3 resulting in a growth-retarded child.

The impact of loss of function of distinct genes in the IGF system has also been examined in mice with null mutations of specific genes. Mice homozygous for deletion of the IGF-1 gene show reduced birth weights with high mortality and severe postnatal growth retardation in the surviving animals. By contrast, deletion of the IGF-2 gene causes severe growth retardation from embryonic d 13 onward, although postnatal growth continues in parallel with control mice. These findings suggest that IGF-2 plays a role in prenatal growth, whereas IGF-1 plays a role prenatally and a critical role postnatally, especially during the pubertal growth spurt. Mice with deletions of the insulin receptor have relatively normal birth weights but die soon after birth secondary to ketoacidosis and severe diabetes. Mice with deletions of the IGF-1R die at birth apparently unable to breathe owing to severe muscle hypoplasia. By contrast, mice heterozygous for deletions of the IGF-1 gene exhibit an increased lifespan compared to controls. Similar findings have been observed in *Caenorhabditis elegans*, in which an insulin/IGF-1R deletion is associated with longer survival. IGF-2/M-6-P receptor deletions result in increased birth weight, suggesting that in its absence clearance of IGF-2 protein is reduced, resulting in excess growth via IGF-1R activation. Deletion of the individual genes encoding the IGFBPs has no resultant phenotype, and only double or triple crosses lead to some mild pheno-types, suggesting redundancy in the system.

Tissue-specific gene deletions have provided further insight into the endocrine and autocrine/paracrine function of the IGF system. Liver-specific deletion of the IGF-1 gene using the cre/loxP system leads to a mouse with a 75% reduction in circulating IGF-1 and a marked increase in circulating GH. The major phenotype in this model is severe insulin resistance owing primarily to the excess GH, but there is also a reduction in spleen weight and bone mineralization, suggesting that circulating IGF-1 is not redundant with tissue IGF-1. This was further emphasized when a double knockout mouse was created by crossing a mouse with liver-specific deletion of the IGF-1 gene with an ALS knockout mouse. These mice exhibited a more severe reduction in growth and bone mineralization associated with a further reduction in circulating IGF-1. Tissue-specific knockouts of the IGF-1R have been created in bone and the pancreas. In bone, deletion of the IGF-1R results in changes in the growth plate, whereas in pancreatic β-cells, absence of the IGF-1R causes a defect in glucose-stimulated insulin secretion associated with reduced expression of the GLUT-2 and glucokinase genes, two proteins critical for glucose uptake and metabolism in β-cells.

Essentially all tissues in the body express one or more components of the IGF system. Not surprisingly, every system in the body is controlled, to some degree, by the IGF system during normal growth and development. A few examples of the role of the IGFs in pathophysiology and potential therapeutic applications of IGF-1 are discussed next.

2.2. Cancer

The IGF system and its role in cancer cell growth has been the subject of intensive research during the past decade. Components of the system are expressed by virtually all cancers and have been shown to affect the growth and function of cancer cells. Most cancers express either IGF-1 or, more commonly, IGF-2, and if they fail to do so, the surrounding stromal tissue releases these ligands. In both circumstances, these ligands stimulate cell proliferation and are even more active as inhibitors of apoptosis, which supports growth of the cancer. IGF-2 is of particular interest because its gene is imprinted, and alterations in imprinting contribute to IGF-2 expression in many tumors. Interestingly, over-expression of a "big IGF-2" by some tumors leads to tumor-induced hypoglycemia, owing to the inability of IGFBP-3 and ALS to totally neutralize this unprocessed form of IGF-2 in the circulation. This leads to high cir-culating levels of unbound big IGF-2 which is then free to interact with tissue receptors (particularly the insulin receptor), resulting in hypoglycemia.

Recent epidemiologic studies have demonstrated a correlation between a relative risk of developing pros-tate, breast, colon, lung, and bladder cancer and the level of circulating IGF-1. The greatest correlation was evident in those individuals with IGF-1 levels in the upper quartile of the normal range. The relationship between these two events remains to be determined, but the results have stimulated interest in the connec-tion between the IGF system and cancer growth.

Almost all cancers overexpress the IGF-1R, which may explain their more rapid proliferation or protec-tion from apoptosis. One explanation for the overexpression has been found by studies focused on the promoter region of the IGF-1R gene, which is GC rich and normally inhibited by tumor suppressor gene products such as p53, WT1, and BRAC-1. Mutations in these proteins lead to a paradoxical increase in pro-moter activity in colon cancer cells (p53), Wilms tumor (WT1), and breast cancers (BRAC-1). IGFBPs are also expressed by the cancer cells and, in some studies, have been shown to stimulate proliferation (mostly by enhancing IGF-1 function) and, in other cases, to inhibit cell proliferation (in both an IGF-1-dependent and -independent manner).

The potential importance of the IGF system, and particularly the IGF-1R, in cancer has led to an intense effort to find blockers of IGF-1R function as potential adjuncts to chemotherapy. These include IGF-1R blocking peptides, antibodies, small molecules, as well as small molecule antagonists to the IGF-1R tyrosine kinase domain.

2.3. Diabetes

There has been considerable interest in the possible use of rhIGF-1 in cases of severe insulin resistance. Conceptually, this arose from the knowledge that the IGF-1R is similar to the insulin receptor and can enhance glucose uptake in muscle. As proof of prin-ciple, rhIGF-1 was able to overcome insulin resistance in patients with severe insulin resistance secondary to mutations in the insulin receptor. When administered to patients with type 1 or type 2 diabetes, rhIGF-1 simi-larly reduced the insulin resistance and reduced the requirements for insulin injections. More recently, it has been administered together with IGFBP-3, and, apparently, this mode of administration has fewer side effects. Outstanding questions remain regarding the long-term benefits and potential side effects of IGF-1 on the vasculature and, potentially, cancer cell growth.

OTHER GROWTH FACTORS

Table 1 lists families of growth factors. In this chap-ter, we only describe briefly some essential elements of

Table 1
Growth Factor Families

IGFs	*Insulin, IGF-1, IGF-2*
VEGFs	VEGF, VEGFB, VEGFC, VEGFD, placental growth factor
EGFs	EGF, TGF-α, heparin-binding EGF, amphiregulin, betacellulin
PDGFs	PDGF-AA, -BB, -AB
TGF-β	TGF-β1–6; inhibin A and B; activin A, B, and C; Müllerian-inhibiting substance; bone morphogenetic proteins
NGFs	NGF, neurotropins (NT-3, -4, and -5) BDNF
FGFs	22 family members

structure and function of a select few from this large and growing list of important growth factors.

3.1. Vascular Endothelial Growth Factor

Vascular endothelial growth factor (VEGF) is a potent angiogenic factor with mitogenic and chemotactic effects on endothelial cells. Mice homozygous for a null mutation of VEGF or its receptors show failure of blood vessel development during embryogenesis resulting in fetal death. Studies have demonstrated the importance of angiogenesis (and VEGF) in organ development and differentiation during embryogenesis. There are five isoforms of VEGF and three receptors, which appear to mediate different VEGF-related biologic actions. VEGF is the most potent angiogenic factor in normal tissues and tumors, being more potent than other angiogenic factors such as fibroblast growth factor (FGF), transforming growth factor-α (TGF-α), and hepatocyte growth factor (HGF). Antibodies to VEGF can inhibit tumor growth, suggesting an important role of angiogenesis (and VEGF) in tumor progression and supporting the concept that inhibitory molecules may be useful adjuncts to chemotherapy in cancer patients. A variety of studies have suggested that VEGF plays an important role in the development of diabetic retinopathy. VEGF levels are increased in the aqueous humor and vitreous of patients with diabetes and decrease following successful laser therapy. Animal models of ischemic retinal neovascularization have demonstrated increased production of VEGF in the setting of ischemia and prevention of retinal neovascularization by inhibitors of VEGF.

The VEGFs demonstrate different modes of secretion; some are retained on the cell surface, whereas others are sequestered in the matrix by heparin sulfate proteoglycans. VEGF receptors are expressed almost exclusively by vascular endothelial cells, although the recent demonstration that VEGF is able to protect neural cells from apoptosis suggests that it has effects beyond endothelial cells. As noted, three different VEGF receptors have been identified. The receptor isoform thought to mediate most of the effects of VEGF, flk1, has a split tyrosine kinase domain in the cytoplasmic portion of the molecule. The signaling pathways activated by this receptor include phospholipase C-γ (PLCγ), mitogen-activated protein kinase (MAPK), phosphatidylinositol-3′-kinase (PI3K), and ras guanosine-5′-triphosphatase (GTPase) activating proteins (Fyn and Yes).

Recently, a novel VEGF, human endocrine gland–derived VEGF (EG-VEGF) was identified during a screen for endothelial cell mitogens. Mature EG-VEGF is an 86-amino-acid peptide that is not structurally related to VEGF but exhibits homology to a snake venom protein, venom protein A, and the Xenopus head-organizer, dickkopf. EG-VEGF stimulates effects in endothelial cells similar to those of VEGF, including cell proliferation, survival, and chemotaxis. This occurs, in part, through increased activity of the MAPKs, extracellular-regulated kinase-1 (ERK-1) and ERK-2, and Akt. Interestingly, EG-VEGF is active primarily in endothelial cells of specific origin. Indeed, in humans, EG-VEGF is expressed largely in steroidogenic tissues, including adrenal, testis, ovary, and placenta, although low-level expression has been exhibited in other tissues, such as prostate. Unlike the VEGFs, the effects of EG-VEGF are mediated by a G protein-coupled receptor with seven transmembrane domains. Expression of the receptor is restricted to vascular endothelium from steroidogenic tissues, explaining the relative specificity of EG-VEGF's effects. Interestingly, like other angiogenic factors, EG-VEGF is highly expressed in neoplasms derived from its glands of origin, such as adrenal adenocarcinomas. It is highly expressed in ovaries of patients with polycystic ovary syndrome, although its possible contribution to the pathophysiology of that disorder awaits clarification.

3.2. Epidermal Growth Factor Family

Epidermal growth factor (EGF) and TGF-α and their common receptor the EGF receptor (EGFR) are the most commonly described members of the EGF family. Both growth factors are synthesized as large precursor transmembrane molecules that are then processed to release the mature 53-amino-acid molecule in the case of EGF and a 50-amino-acid molecule in the case of TGF-α. EGF family members signal through the ErbB family of receptors, which includes ErbB-1 (the EGFR), ErbB-2 (HER2 or Neu), ErbB-3, and ErbB-4. EGF family members have differing abilities to bind to various homo-

and heterodimer complexes composed of ErbB family members. Like other growth factor receptors, these receptor complexes are tyrosine kinases. The intracellular signaling pathways activated by the different receptor complexes vary, but, in general, receptor activation results in activation of the MAPK, PI3K and PLCγ pathways. The EGFR-ErbB-2 heterodimer binds EGF with higher affinity than EGFR homodimers and exhibits a decreased rate of ligand degradation. This heterodimer has been associated with enhanced tumor progression. G protein–coupled receptors (GPCRs) can modulate EGFR-mediated activation of the MAPK cascade. GPCRs activate protein kinase A (PKA) which enhances the MAPK pathway and thereby acts as the focal point for cross talk between the receptors. GPCRs also activate PLCγ, which, in turn, activates inositol triphosphate and diacylglycerol, leading to enhancement of PKC and Src tyrosine kinase activity. PKC enhances MAPK activity whereas Src activates the EGFR tyrosine kinase activity.

Both EGF and TGF-α are potent mitogens essential for normal embryonic development, EGF being important for eyelid opening, teeth eruption, lung maturation, and skin development. In adults, TGF-α has been implicated in wound healing, angiogenesis, and bone resorption. Both ligands have been implicated in tumor progression, because they and members of the ErbB family are overexpressed in different tumors. Various anti-EGFR antagonists, such as EGFR tyrosine kinase inhibitors (ZD1839 AstraZeneca), anti-EGFR antibodies (IMClone C-225), and antisense oligonucleotides, have shown promise in treating pancreatic cancers.

Another intriguing member of the EGF family is betacellulin. Betacellulin is expressed in adult and fetal pancreas, signals through the ErbB family of receptors, and stimulates the proliferation of multiple cell types, including β-cells. The potential role of betacellulin in pancreatic function and development is still being elucidated, but several lines of evidence suggest that it plays a key role in islet cell proliferation and/or differentiation. Betacellulin enhances pancreatic regeneration following 90% pancreatectomy by increasing β-cell proliferation and mass. It increases DNA synthesis in human fetal pancreatic epithelial cells and enhances β-cell development in fetal murine pancreatic explant cultures. Finally, betacellulin is expressed in islets and ducts of adult human pancreas and primitive duct cells in the fetal pancreas.

3.3. Platelet-Derived Growth Factors

Platelet-derived growth factor-A (PDGF-A) and PDGF-B are encoded by separate genes and bind as disulfide-linked homo-or heterodimers to their tyrosine kinase receptors, the PDGFα and PDGFβ receptors. PDGF receptors are expressed by vascular smooth muscle cells, fibroblasts, and glial cells but not by most hemopoietic, epithelial, or endothelial cells. PDGF-AB is the major isoform expressed by humans, especially by platelets, whereas the BB homodimer is expressed by other tissue and tumor cells. The PDGFα receptor binds all three PDGF isoforms (i.e., AA, AB, and BB), whereas the PDGFβ receptor binds only the BB isoform. Ligand binding leads to receptor dimerization, activation of the receptor tyrosine kinase, and subsequent activation of intracellular signaling pathways, including PLA$_2$, PLCγ, PI3K, and RAS-GAP.

Targeted inactivation of the growth factors or their receptors results in embryonic or perinatal lethality, indicating the importance of this family in development. PDGF is a competence factor, enabling cells to enter the G$_0$/G$_1$ phase of the cell cycle, and this allows other growth factors to induce progression through the remainder of the cell cycle. Thus, PDGF can induce proliferation of fibroblasts, osteoblasts, glial cells, and arterial smooth muscle cells. Interestingly, targeted deletion of the gene encoding PDGF in endothelial cells generates mice with decreased pericyte density in the central nervous system (CNS), including the retina. These mice develop retinal changes characteristic of diabetic retinopathy, including microaneurysms and capillary occlusion.

PDGF has been shown to be involved in wound healing. It is released by platelets, vascular cells, monocyte-macrophages, fibroblasts, and skin epithelial cells at the site of injury and acts in a paracrine fashion to induce connective-tissue cell proliferation and chemotaxis. It induces DNA synthesis and collagen synthesis by osteoblasts, thereby enabling bone formation after fractures. PDGF may also play a role in pathologic processes. PDGF receptors are expressed in the vasculature and may play an important role in atherosclerosis and restenosis following balloon angioplasty. Vascular endothelial cells and activated macrophages in the vessel express PDGF and intimal smooth muscle cells express PDGF receptors. Myelofibrosis, scleroderma, and pulmonary fibrosis are associated with increased connective-tissue cell proliferation, chemotaxis, and collagen synthesis, at least partially owing to the PDGFs and their receptors. Tumors such as gliomas, sarcomas, melanomas, mesotheliomas, and hemopoietic cell–derived tumors overexpress PDGF, whereas other tumors overexpress the receptor. Thus, PDGF may play a role in tumor progression.

Recently, two novel PDGFs have been discovered: PDGF-C and PDGF-D. PDGF-CC binds only the PDGFα receptor, whereas PDGF-DD is specific for the PDGFβ receptor. Overexpression of PDGF-C in the heart leads to cardiac hypertrophy and fibrosis, and it may be involved in physiologic and pathologic cardiac conditions. PDGF-C and PDGF-D are also expressed by numerous tumors and, therefore, may play a role in tumorigenesis. Finally, these two novel PDGFs have structural similarities with VEGF. The importance of these similarities is, as yet, not known.

3.4. Nerve Growth Factors

Nerve growth factor (NGF) is a highly conserved molecule exhibiting ~70% homology with other vertebrate NGF molecules. Other members of the family, including brain-derived neurotrophic factor (BDNF), neurotrophin-3 (NT-3), NT-4, and NT-5, also have conserved regions and similar predicted tertiary structures. The receptors responsible for mediating their effects are complexes of a low-affinity 75-kDa intrinsic membrane protein (p75) that complexes with either TRK (TRK-A) or TRK-B; TRK-A and TRK-B contain tyrosine kinase activity and when complexed with p75 form a high-affinity functional receptor. NGF binds the p75-TRK-A receptor complex, and the signaling pathways that are activated on NGF binding include PLCγ, PI-3K, RAS GTPase-activating protein, SHC, and the MAPK. TRK-B complex binds BDNF and NT-3, whereas TRK-C binds NT-3 with high affinity.

NGFs play important roles in differentiation and survival of neurons, and the specific effects are determined by the expression of the various subtypes of NGF receptors. For example, TRK-B expression is widespread throughout the CNS, suggesting that it modulates more generalized functions, whereas TRK-A is more localized in its expression.

3.5. TGF–β Family

There are five different isoforms of TGF-β (TGF-β1–5) as well as multiple other family members that include the bone morphogenetic proteins, activins, Müllerian inhibitory substance, inhibins, and other growth and differentiation factors.

TGF-β1 is a disulfide-linked dimer of two identical chains of 112 amino acids. Each of the chains is processed from a larger inactive precursor. Latent TGF-β–binding protein-1 (LTBP-1) is responsible for storage of this large inactive molecule in the matrix of costochondral chondrocytes, whereas another isoform of the binding protein, LTBP-2, is found in chondrocytes and blood vessels. Other LTBPs are more widely distributed. During secretion of TGF-β, a latency-associated peptide present in the immature form is cleaved by furin-like endoproteinases. The latency-associated peptide remains associated with mature TGF-β, however, and

activation of mature TGF-β requires dissociation of the latency-associated peptide.

The effects of the various isoforms of TGF-β and other members of the family are mediated by a complex of type I and type II receptors that possess serine/threonine kinase activity. To date, five type II and seven type I receptors have been identified. The functional receptor complex consists of two type I and two type II receptors. In the absence of ligand, the type I and type II receptors exist as homodimers in the membrane. Ligand binding induces the formation of the functional heteromeric complex. On formation of this complex, the type II receptor phosphorylates the type I receptor in a specific domain, the GS domain, which activates the kinase activity of the type I receptor. The active type I receptor phosphorylates members of the Smad family of transcription factors, which regulates the transcription of a variety of target genes. Smad-independent signaling via the MAPK pathway and the Rho family of small GTPases, including Rho, Cdc42, and Rac, also occurs. Betaglycan, an abundant membrane-anchored proteoglycan, also binds TGF-β and has been designated the type III receptor. Betaglycan is able to facilitate interaction of TGF-β with the type II receptor.

TGF–β can inhibit or stimulate cell proliferation, depending on the conditions of the cellular environment; in a mitogen-rich environment it inhibits and in a mitogen-free medium it enhances proliferation. It also enhances expression of matrix and cell adhesion receptors, thereby increasing cell-cell adhesion between mesenchymal and epithelial cells. TGF–β is expressed by macrophages at the site of wound healing or inflammation, which may explain the role of TGF–β in tissue repair and angiogenesis. Locally produced TGF–β may also enhance bone remodeling.

TGF–β has been invoked as a mediator of certain fibrotic disorders including mesangial proliferative glomerulosclerosis, lung fibrosis, cirrhosis of the liver, arterial restenosis after angioplasty, and myelofibrosis. TGF-β is also thought to play an important role in the pathogenesis of diabetic nephropathy. Increased expression of TGF-β and the type II receptor has been observed in glomeruli of diabetic animals, and increased TGF-β levels are present in the glomeruli of humans with diabetic nephropathy. Moreover, inhibition of TGF-β production or action prevents changes in the kidney characteristic of diabetic nephropathy in various animal models of diabetes. On the other hand, TGF-β has antiproliferative effects on T- and B-lymphocytes, and the potential anti-inflammatory and immunosuppressive effects of TGF–β in systemic disorders such as rheumatoid arthritis await further investigation.

3.6. Fibroblast Growth Factors

There are 22 members of the FGF family, including acidic FGF, basic FGF, and keratinocyte growth factor. FGFs bind to low-affinity, high-capacity cell-surface proteoglycans containing heparan sulfate side chains as well as to high-affinity receptors with tyrosine kinase activity. Both types of receptors (proteoglycan and tyrosine kinase) collaborate in FGF binding; the low-affinity receptor binds the FGF molecule, and allows it to dimerize, thus allowing it to bind the high-affinity receptor. Activation of tyrosine kinase leads to signaling via multiple signaling pathways, including PLCγ, one of the major substrates in the FGF receptor signaling cascade. FGFs play a critical role in the survival of neural cells and stimulate proliferation of fibroblasts, endothelial cells, and smooth muscle cells. Certain aspects of embryonic development such as mesoderm induction are dependent on FGF, and different FGF family members play a critical role in the expansion and differentiation of stem cells in vitro. Finally, one FGF family member, FGF23, is a phosphaturic hormone important in the regulation of serum phosphorus. Missense mutations in FGF23 that prevent cleavage of the mature hormone into inactive amino- and carboxy-terminal fragments cause autosomal dominant hypophosphatemic rickets.

3.7. Hepatocyte Growth Factor

HGF/scatter factor (SF) is a disulfide-linked heterodimeric molecule that is expressed primarily by mesenchymal cells and acts in an endocrine or paracrine fashion on epithelial cells that express the HGF receptor, commonly known as c-MET. HGF/SF is both a growth factor for hepatocytes and a fibroblast-derived cell motility factor (SF). Activation of MET leads to important aspects of embryonic growth and development, wound healing, tissue regeneration, angiogenesis, and morphogenic differentiation. Its role in tumorigenesis and metastasis has recently received much interest.

MET is a highly conserved member of a subfamily of heterodimeric receptor tyrosine kinases that is comprised of a highly glycosylated and entirely extracellular α-subunit as well as a β-subunit with a significant extracellular domain, a transmembrane domain, and an intracellular domain that contains a tyrosine kinase domain. The biologic effects of MET are mediated by a variety of signaling pathways. These include signaling molecules that interact with the receptor such Grb2, SHC, Gab1, and Crk/CRKL as well as various kinases and transcription factors, including PI3K, Stat3, PLCγ, Src kinase, and SHP2 phosphatase. There is significant cross talk between MET signaling pathways and those of integrins. MET, via the PI3K pathway, promotes cell adhesion on laminin, fibronectin, and vitronectin, and antibodies to multiple β integrins can inhibit MET activity on cell adhesion and invasiveness. MET also enhances expression of certain α integrins, and there is also cross talk between MET and cadherins. MET induces phosphorylation of paxillin and focal adhesion kinase, enhancing matrix adhesion and invasion by prostate cancer cells.

MET is commonly overexpressed in tumors. In many cases, this is owing to amplification of the gene. In other cases, missense mutations resulting in constitutive tyrosine kinase activity of MET have been described. In a few instances of cancer, elevated HGF/SF was detected in serum or, alternatively, overexpressed by the tumor itself. Because of the extensive evidence favoring the role of HGF/SF-MET in the pathogenesis of numerous tumors, the potential for using inhibitors of this growth factor/receptor in cancer therapy has received a significant level of interest. HGF and MET are also expressed in both osteoblasts and osteoclasts. In osteoclasts, HGF induces changes in cell shape and increases intracellular calcium and DNA replication, whereas HGF stimulates osteoblasts to enter the cell cycle. HGF together with 1,25-dihydroxyvitamin D promotes the differentiation of bone marrow stromal cells into osteogenic cells. Thus, HGF may also play a role in bone formation and metabolism.

SELECTED READING

Chang H, Brown CW, Matzuk MM. Genetic analysis of the mammalian transforming growth factor-β superfamily. *Endocr Rev* 2002; 23:787–823.

Dunbar AJ, Goddard C. Structure-function and biological role of betacellulin. *Int J Biochem Cell Biol* 2000;32:805–815.

Ferrara N, Gerber H-P, LeCouter J. The biology of VEGF and its receptors. *Nat Med* 2003;9:669–676

LeCouter J, Ferrara N. EG-VEGF and Bv8: A novel family of tissue-selective mediators of angiogenesis, endothelial phenotype, and function. *Trends Cardiovasc Med* 2003;13:276–282.

LeRoith D, Bondy C, Shoshana Yakar S, ,Liu J-L, Butler AA. The somatomedin hypothesis. *Endocr Rev* 2001;22:53–74.

LeRoith D, Werner H, Beitner-Johnson D, Roberts CT Jr. Molecular and cellular aspects of the insulin-like growth factor I receptor. *Endocr Rev* 1995;16(2):143–163.

Quarles LD. FGF23, PHEX and MEPE regulation of phosphate homeostasis and skeletal mineralization. *Am J Physiol Endocrinol Metab* 2003;285:E1–E9.

7 Prostaglandins and Leukotrienes
Locally Acting Agents

John A. McCracken, PhD

CONTENTS

1. INTRODUCTION

This chapter is not intended for the prostaglandin (PG) specialist but, rather, for those not familiar with the PG field. It provides a brief overview of the biology of the eicosanoid family and how these local mediators may function in health and disease. The term eicosanoids (from the Greek *eicosa*, which means 20) was coined to describe the broad group of compounds derived from C$_{20}$ fatty acids that, in turn, are derived from the essential dietary fatty acids. The predominant C$_{20}$ fatty acid precursor for eicosanoid biosynthesis in most mammals is arachidonic acid (AA). These eicosanoids include the PGs and thromboxanes (TXs), leukotrienes (LTs), lipoxins (LPXs), and hydroxyeicosatetraenoic acids (HETEs). Because the biologic activity of eicosanoids is diminished rapidly in both tissues and the circulation, it is likely that they act locally at the tissue and organ level, where they may regulate regional blood flow and other metabolic activities. Moreover, their formation in various inflammatory sites indicates an important mediating role for these substances in diseased states. Indeed, eicosanoid inhibition by different classes of anti-inflam-

matory drugs underlines their importance in this regard. This chapter includes a brief historical background, together with a description of nomenclature, biosynthesis, and selected local actions of PGs and LTs. For those requiring more detailed information, see the references at the end of this chapter.

2. HISTORICAL BACKGROUND

The biologic existence of PGs was established in the 1930s by the detection of smooth muscle contracting and vasodepressor activity in extracts of human and sheep seminal plasma. von Euler (1988) went on to demonstrate that these compounds were acidic lipids and the name prostaglandins was coined because it was thought, at the time, that these acidic lipids emanated from the prostate gland; however, we now know that the seminal vesicles are the main site of synthesis in the male reproductive system. It is not surprising that the biologic activity of PGs was first detected in the male system because they are present in microgram quantities in seminal plasma of many species including human, monkey, and sheep. By contrast, PGs in other tissues are present in picogram or, at best, nanogram

From: *Endocrinology: Basic and Clinical Principles, Second Edition*
(S. Melmed and P. M. Conn, eds.) © Humana Press Inc., Totowa, NJ

amounts. The function of PGs found in seminal plasma has not been fully documented, although a role has been suggested in contraction of the male accessory glands and the vas deferens. In addition, it has been proposed that they assist in sperm transport by stimulating contraction of the female genital tract, the latter also being a major source of PG synthesis and action. Indeed, the most fully established physiologic role of the PGs is that of $PGF_{2\alpha}$, a locally acting uterine luteolytic hormone in a number of mammalian species (*see* Section 6.7.).

Progress in identifying the chemical nature of the PGs was slow, partly because of World War II and partly because the technology to detect these labile and elusive compounds was not available until the 1950s and 1960s. Bergström and Sjovall (1957) isolated two different PGs in crystalline form, one of which they named PGE, found in the ether (E) fraction, and the other PGF, found in the fraction with phosphate, spelled fosfat (F) in Swedish, thus giving rise to the present nomenclature. Samuelsson and colleagues (1987) discovered a related product of AA metabolism that is a potent stimulator of platelet aggregation and named it TX. Later, Vane and colleagues discovered a potent inhibitor of platelet aggregation derived from AA and formed in endothelial cells and named it prostacyclin (PGI_2) because of its double-ring structure.

Shortly thereafter, Samuelsson described a new class of AA metabolites from leukocytes, some of which have chemotactic properties and others that increase vascular permeability. These substances were named LTs. They are produced from AA by the action of the enzyme 5-lipoxygenase (5-LO). In some of the LTs, the amino acid cysteine is incorporated into the molecule to give rise to the cysteinyl LTs (*see* below). The LTs are considered to be involved in inflammatory processes in which they most likely act synergistically with other mediators such as histamine, bradykinin, and PGs to produce the classic signs of inflammation described by Celsus: redness (rubor), heat (calor), swelling (tumor), and pain (dolor). The involvement of PGs in the inflammatory process is underlined by the effects of non steroidal anti-inflammatory drugs (NSAIDs) such as aspirin and indomethacin, which are potent inhibitors of PG biosynthesis via inhibition of cyclooxygenase (COX) activity. The NSAIDs, however, have little or no effect on the lipoxygenase pathway responsible for LT biosynthesis. Indeed, because NSAIDs so efficiently block PG synthesis, these drugs most likely amplify LT synthesis by diverting AA into the lipoxygenase pathway. Thus, in patients with asthma, in whom LTs have been identified as a major mediator of bronchoconstriction, the use of NSAIDs is contraindicated. On the other hand, corticosteroids have a potent inhibi-

tory effect on phospholipase A_2 (PLA_2) activity, thus markedly reducing the availability of AA as a substrate for both the COX and lipoxygenase pathways. As described later, corticosteroids also appear to inhibit the synthesis of the inducible form of the COX enzyme (COX-2). Corticosteroids are thus the most useful therapeutic agents for patients with asthma at present; however, drugs based on LT receptor antagonists and LT biosynthesis inhibitors have now been developed and are providing important alternatives and/or additions to long-term corticosteroid therapy (*see* Section 4.3.).

3. PG NOMENCLATURE

The major PGs of the two series are summarized as follows:

PGA_2 Dehydration product of PGE_2
PGB_2 Isomerization product of PGA_2
PGD_2 Abundant in neural tissues, sleep inducing, allergic responses
PGE_2 Vasodilator, gastric cytoprotection, pyrogenic, bone resorption
$PGF_{2\alpha}$ Vasoconstrictor, luteolysis and labor
PGG_2 Endoperoxide intermediate
PGH_2 Endoperoxide precursor for PG synthesis
PGI_2 Antiplatelet aggregation, vasodilator
PGJ_2 Dehydration product of PGD_2
TXA_2 Platelet aggregation, vasoconstrictor

3.1. Chemical Structure

As illustrated in Fig. 1, the number of double bonds in the PG molecule is designated by a subscript so that the one series of PGs has one double bond in position 13:14, e.g., $PGF_{1\alpha}$. The two series of PGs has a second double bond in position 5:6, e.g., $PGF_{2\alpha}$. The three series of PGs has a third double bond in position 17:18, e.g., $PGF_{3\alpha}$. In the case of PGF, the α designation indicates that the hydroxyl groups are in the α orientation. The principal PG precursor in most species is AA, liberated from phospholipid stores, principally by cytosolic PLA_2, which gives rise to the two series of PGs. The one series of PGs is derived from homo-γ-linolenic acid, which, in most species, is less abundant. Some species, especially when on diets rich in fish oils, produce the three series of PGs derived from eicosapentaenoic acid. It is suggested that the high consumption of fish oils by Eskimos has a protective effect on the cardiovascular system in the presence of a high-fat diet.

4. BIOSYNTHESIS
4.1. Prostaglandins

A simplified flow sheet of the major pathways of eicosanoid biosynthesis is shown in Fig. 2. Virtually all cells appear to have the capacity to synthesize PGs, the

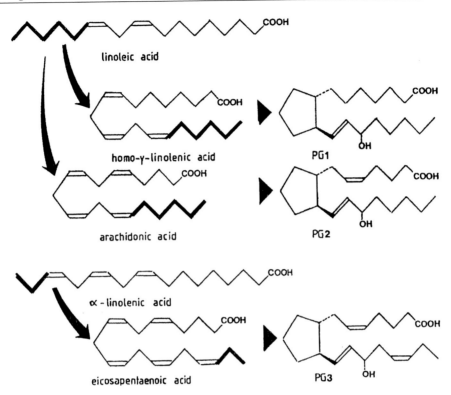

Fig. 1. Homo-γ-linolenic and arachidonic acids are converted, respectively, into prostanoids (PG) of the one series (PG$_1$), exhibiting only one double bond, and into the two series (PG$_2$) exhibiting two double bonds. These polyunsaturated acids and their precursor, linoleic acid, are members of the biologic family of ω-6 fatty acids, characterized by an end segment of 6 carbons (at the opposite end from the —COOH). Eicosapentaenoic acid, coming from the α-linolenic acid (ω-3 family), is converted into PG$_3$ (three double bonds). Thick lines represent characteristic end segments of the ω-6 and ω-3 families. (Reproduced from Deby, 1988.)

end product depending on the enzymes present that convert the endoperoxide intermediates into specific PGs. The initial step in PG biosynthesis is the formation of AA from phospholipid stores via the action of cytosolic PLA$_2$. The microsomal COX which converts AA to the endoperoxide intermediates PGG$_2$ and PGH$_2$, is now known to exist in both a constitutive form (COX-1) and an inducible form (e.g., activated by serum or endotoxin; designated COX-2). The crystal structures of COX-1 and COX-2 are almost identical except for one amino acid difference that leads to a larger side pocket in COX-2 for substrate recognition. Chandrasekaharan et al. (2002) have recently identified a variant derived from the COX-1 gene, designated COX-3, which is particularly sensitive to acetaminophen and other antipyretic drugs (*see* Section 6.4.). The NSAIDs such as aspirin or indomethacin act mainly by inhibiting the activity of the COX enzymes (also known as PGH endoperoxide synthases). Indeed, different NSAIDs have selective effects on the inducible form (COX-2) vs the constitutive form (COX-1). Corticosteroids, which act primarily by blocking the phos-

pholipase-mediated release of AA from phospholipids, also have an additional inhibitory effect by blocking the formation of the inducible form of COX (COX-2), thus contributing to the blockade of PG synthesis. Although it is well documented that PGs are an important component in acute inflammatory responses, it was observed that PGs of the E series may have certain modulating effects in some types of chronic inflammation; that is, high tissue levels of PGEs may have anti-inflammatory effects. Weissmann (1993) and, more recently, Zurier (2003), who have studied the role of PGs in inflammation for many years, suggest that the proposed anti-inflammatory action of PGE$_2$ in certain chronic inflammatory states may be mediated by its ability to generate cyclic adenosine monophosphate (cAMP). Because certain NSAIDs, such as sodium salicylate, can alleviate inflammation without inhibiting PG synthesis, it has been proposed that PGs may be modulators, rather than mediators, of inflammation (Weissmann, 1993). Moreover, PGE$_1$ has been shown to suppress adjuvant disease (induced polyarthritis) in animal models and to inhibit neutrophil-mediated tissue injury (Zurier, 2003).

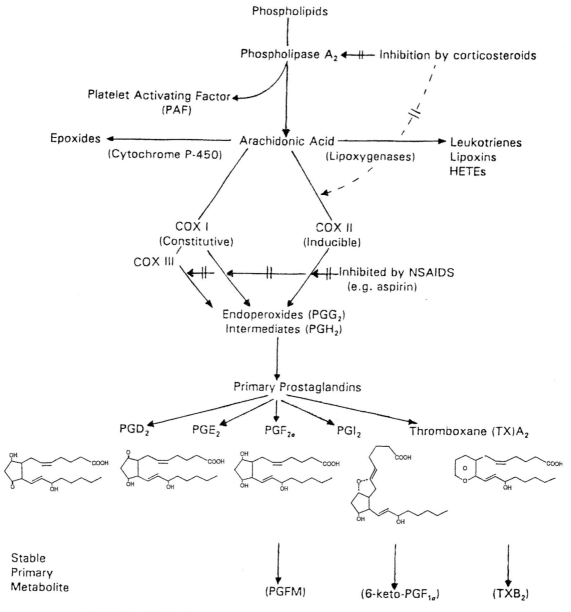

Fig. 2. Simplified pathway of eicosanoid biosynthesis. PGFM = PGF$_{2\alpha}$ metabolite.

Since the 5-LO pathway is largely unaffected by NSAIDs, LT production may be potentially enhanced by diverting AA into the lipoxygenase pathway. In some instances, generation of LTs (e.g., the production of LTB$_4$ by neutrophils), can be inhibited by PGs, suggesting that there may be a subtle balance between COX and lipoxygenase pathways. Moreover, both PGE$_2$ and PGI$_2$ have been shown to downregulate the production of tumor necrosis factor-α (TNF-α).

It has been proposed that the administration of a combination of NSAIDs and long-acting PGE analogs could act synergistically in anti-inflammatory therapy (Weiss-mann, 1993). It is likely that some of these opposing actions of PGE are related to the various PGE receptor subtypes that have now been elucidated and that can give rise to different second-messenger systems (*see* Section 5.1.).

4.2. Platelet-Activating Factor (Alkyl-acetyl-glycerophosphocholine)

Platelet-activating factor (PAF) is derived from phosphatidylcholine as a product of PLA$_2$ action, although structurally it is not an eicosanoid. However, PAF is a potent platelet-aggregating substance that can operate

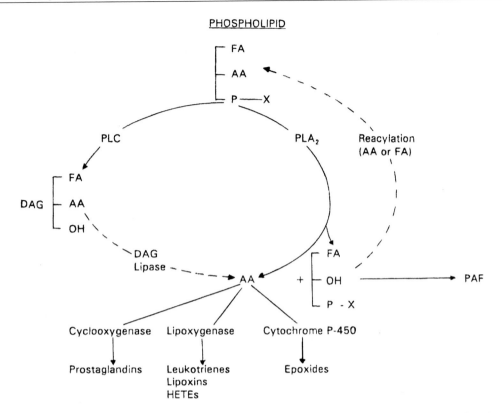

Fig. 3. Simplified diagram of pathways for biosynthesis of PAF and eicosanoid products of AA metabolism. Note that PLA_2 action forms both AA and PAF whereas the action of PLC can form lesser amounts of AA indirectly from diacylglycerol (DAG) via DAG lipase (e.g., during signal transduction). AA = arachidonic acid; FA = fatty acid.

without adenosine 5′-diphosphate or TXA_2. O'Flaherty and Wykle (2004) reviewed the biosynthesis of PAF in various tissues and concluded that PAF may act as both an intracellular and an extracellular mediator. As well as acting as an intracellular mediator, PAF appears to act in an autocrine fashion, i.e., by binding to the parent cell receptors, thus initiating other second-messenger signals. PAF appears to act in conjunction with endogenous eicosanoids with which it is often coformed during inflammatory states and allergic processes such as asthma. In addition, it has been suggested that PAF may play a local role during implantation of the embryo in the uterus, a process that also may involve PGs and other local mediators. A simplified chart showing the biosynthesis of PAF is shown in Fig. 3. In addition to the main PLA_2 pathway, the PLC pathway is illustrated to show that activation of this signal transduction mechanism may also generate AA for eicosanoid formation.

Recent studies by Cundell et al. (1995) indicate that virulent pneumococci utilize the PAF receptor to gain entry into host cells. This bacterium is a commensal in the human nasopharynx and is a major cause of sepsis, pneumonia, and meningitis. Bacterial entry into endo-

thelial cells is increased 20- to 40-fold following stimulation of PAF receptors by fibrin or TNF-α and reversed by PAF receptor antagonists. It is suggested that bacterial cell wall phosphatidylcholine is a cognate ligand for the PAF receptor and that bacterial attachment subverts the receptor (in the absence of signal transduction) to internalize the bacterium. These novel findings suggest that PAF receptor antagonists may be of therapeutic value, not only in blocking PAF action, but also by attenuating bacterial attachment, which leads to invasion of host cells.

4.3. Leukotrienes

Like the PGs, LTs are considered to be local mediators generated in the microenvironment and usually associated with inflammation. The LTs are generated from AA released from membrane phospholipids or from secretory granules of tissue cells such as neutrophils or mast cells. The main enzyme in LT synthesis, 5-LO, requires activation by Ca^{++} and translocation to a membrane-associated site. These requirements are in contrast to PG synthesis in which COX does not require specific activation but, rather, only the presence of sub-

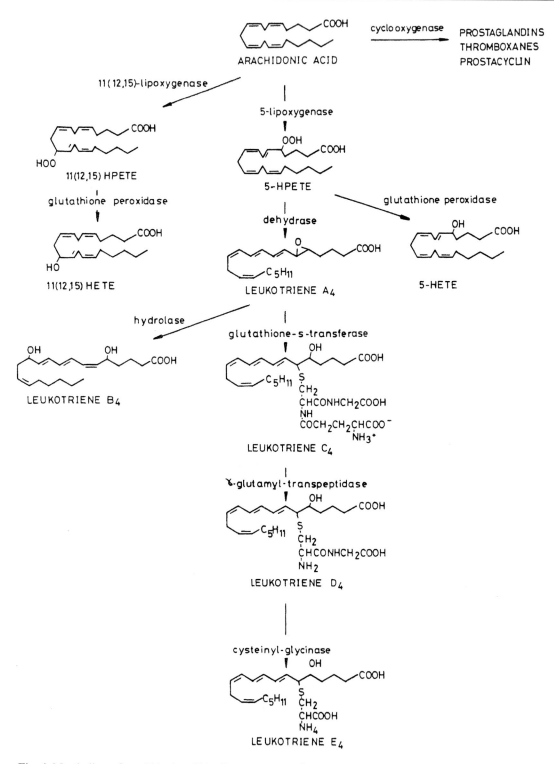

Fig. 4. Metabolism of arachidonic acid by lipoxygenase pathways. (Reproduced from Piper and Letts, 1988.)

strate (AA). An additional regulatory component in LT biosynthesis is the existence of a 5-LO activating protein (FLAP) thought to be essential for LT biosynthesis. Local synthesis of LTs is part of a cascade of events occurring during inflammation that include the release of PGs, PAF, histamine, and other cellular mediators of this process. The LT pathway from AA involves the synthesis of LTA$_4$ via the 5-LO pathway (Fig. 4).

LTA_4 is nonenzymatically converted into LTB_4 or into the cysteinyl LTs LTC_4, LTD_4, and LTE_4. Human neutrophils have the selective capacity to synthesize LTB_4 and also appear to inactivate LTB_4, thus regulating its local activity, which includes chemotaxis and neutrophil adherence to endothelial cells. Eosinophils, on the other hand, generate only LTC_4 because they possess LTC_4 synthase, whereas monocytes generate both LTB_4 and LTC_4. Cells lacking the enzymes required to produce specific eicosanoids may utilize an intermediate provided by another cell type. For example, the transfer of PG endoperoxide intermediates from platelets to endothelial cells results in the formation of PGI_2, which has antiplatelet aggregating activity. Erythrocytes lack 5-LO but can convert LTA_4 into LTB_4. These cell–cell interactions illustrate the complexity of eicosanoid synthesis likely to occur, e.g., in inflammatory processes.

The three cysteinyl LTs (LTC_4, LTD_4, and LTE_4) are now known to constitute the slow-reacting substance of anaphylaxis, and they are implicated in the pathogenesis of asthma and other pulmonary conditions. Inhalation of LTD_4 and LTC_4 by humans is 1000 times more potent than histamine in causing airflow impairment at a fixed vital capacity, whereas LTE_4 is 10 times as potent as histamine. The involvement of LTs in anaphylaxis and asthma has prompted the synthesis of a number of LT receptor antagonists including Singulair (montelukast) and Accolate (zafirlukast), which are presently in clinical use. Another approach is the development of the LT biosynthesis inhibitor Zyflo (zileuton) which has no direct effect on the 5-LO enzyme itself but binds with high affinity to FLAP, whose expression is required for LT biosynthesis. The development of these new LT-inhibiting drugs, including those binding to FLAP, will most likely help to alleviate the clinical symptoms associated with asthma and other pulmonary conditions, thus providing an alternative, or an addition, to corticosteroid therapy (Robinson et al., 2001).

Arachidonic acid can also be converted via other lipoxygenase pathways to yield a series of hydroxy-eicosatetraenoic acid derivatives (HETEs) including lipoxins (from "lipoxygenase interaction substances") and other HETEs (Fig. 2). These lipoxygenase products are considered to be associated with the immune system, as proposed by Vanderhoek (1992), where they may play a role as endogenous immunosuppressive agents. Recent studies by Klein and colleagues (2004) have indicated a potential role for 12/15 lipoxygenases in the pathogenesis of osteoporosis in a mouse model. Their findings suggest that inhibitors of the 12/15 lipoxygenase pathway, already in clinical use, may merit investigation for the prevention and/or treatment of osteoporosis. Arachidonic acid also can be metabolized to epoxides by cytochrome P-450 (Capdevila and Falck, 2001). The functional role of epoxides is only now being explored but may include control of systemic blood pressure and the pathophysiology of hypertension.

Because eicosanoids are released from tissues as soon as they are formed, they are not stored within the cell. However, in the case of the male reproductive system, PGs accumulate in large amounts in the glandular secretions found in the lumen of the seminal vesicles. Most tissues metabolize PGs very rapidly via the 15-hydroxy dehydrogenase/13:14 reductase complex, which is particularly abundant in lung tissue, thus forming the biologically inactive metabolite (e.g., PGFM from $PGF_{2\alpha}$). In many species, one passage through the lungs can inactivate >90% of the biologic activity of the primary PGs. The net effect is that, whereas returning venous blood can contain considerable amounts of PGs in the nanogram range, aortic blood contains much lower levels, probably in the low picogram range. Thus, PGs are generally regarded as *locally acting agents* because their very potent biologic activity is necessarily restricted by 15-hydroxy dehydrogenases, both at the tissue level and in the vascular system, by pulmonary metabolism and, to some extent, by metabolism in the liver and kidney.

4.4. Isoprostanes

Roberts and Morrow (1994) have identified a novel series of PG-like compounds, called F_2-isoprostanes, that are formed as products of lipid peroxidation of membrane phospholipids catalyzed by free radicals, (i.e., independent of the COX pathway). One of the isoprostanes, 8-epi-$F_{2\alpha}$, has been identified as the most potent renal vasoconstricting substance ever discovered. The marked vasoconstrictor effect of this compound has been shown to be mediated by activation of TX receptors. Current work suggests that the overproduction of isoprostanes may play a causative role in the hepatorenal syndrome, defined as unexplained renal failure in the presence of severe liver disease. Thus, in addition to being markers of lipid peroxidation, it is likely that isoprostanes may be associated with the pathophysiology of oxidant stress, suggesting that antioxidant therapy may provide a new rationale for therapeutic intervention in certain disease states.

5. EICOSANOID RECEPTORS

PGs, TXs, and LTs are considered to act locally via specific receptors located on the cell surface. However, the specificity of these receptors shows considerable overlap, so that responses to PGs within different tissues may vary or even have opposite actions. The nature

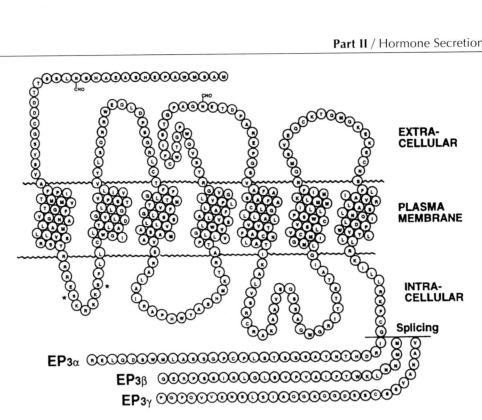

Fig. 5. Seven-transmembrane-spanning model of mouse EP3 isoforms showing alternative splicing for isoforms. CHO indicates potential sites of N-linked glycosylation. Stars indicate potential phosphorylation sites for cAMP-dependent protein kinase. (Reproduced from Negishi et al., 1995.)

and affinities of receptors for various PGs were initially studied using radiolabeled ligands. PG receptors have also been characterized pharmacologically by comparing the potencies and responses of various PGs and their analogs in a variety of bioassay systems. Based on these findings, Coleman and colleagues (1994) have described a pharmacologic classification in which each PG has its own receptor, some of which show subtypes. In the case of PGE, four subtypes have been assigned and designated EP1, EP2, EP3, and EP4. Evidence has also accumulated that TXA_2 has two receptor subtypes, designated TPα and TPβ, which regulate platelet aggregation and vascular smooth muscle contraction, respectively.

Narumiya and Fitzgerald (2001) have pioneered the cloning of the PG receptors, the first of which was TXA_2. This was accomplished by isolating and purifying it from human blood platelets followed by cloning of the cDNA. These studies indicated that the TXA_2 receptor is a G protein–coupled rhodopsin-type receptor with seven transmembrane domains. Because there is only a 10–20% homology with other rhodopsin-type receptors, it is proposed that TXA_2 and other prostanoids constitute a subfamily of the rhodopsin-type receptor superfamily. Based on this model, screening of mouse cDNA libraries revealed seven different

prostanoid receptors. Four receptor subtypes of the PGE receptor were cloned and designated EP1, EP2, EP3, and EP4, thus confirming the aforementioned pharmacologic classification. In addition to the receptors encoded by different genes, alternative splicing of the EP_3 receptor transcript has yielded three isoforms of the receptor that couple to various G proteins and induce specific signaling systems (Fig. 5). The PGD receptor exists in two forms, DP1 and DP2, with each receptor type derived from a single gene. DP1 is thought to be involved in mediating allergic asthma and DP2 is assigned a role in lymphocyte chemotaxis. Recently, two forms of the FP receptor have been cloned, designated FP_A and FP_B (Sakamoto et al., 2002). Although the role of the conventional FP receptor, FP_A, is well defined, the role of the new FP receptor, FP_B, remains to be investigated. The so-called relaxant receptors—IP, DP, EP2, and EP4—are considered to act via G protein–mediated increases in cAMP, and the so-called contractile receptors—EP1, FP, and TP—are considered to act via a G protein–mediated increase in intracellular Ca^{++}. By contrast, the EP3 receptor is thought to be the exception, because it decreases cAMP via G-protein interaction.

Although many PG receptors are located in the plasma membrane, there is also evidence that some PG receptors are located in the nuclear envelope. The finding that COX-2 is predominantly located near the perinuclear envelope thus provides a convenient interaction with the PGs so formed, with receptors in the nuclear envelope to effect increases in Ca^{++} and gene transcription. LTs also act via G protein–coupled receptors, several of which have been characterized. The LTB4 receptor (B-LT) exists in two forms, one regulating chemotaxis of leukocytes and the other regulating neutrophil secretion (Yokomizo et al., 2000). Receptors also exist for the cysteinyl LTs, LTC4 and LTD4, designated cysLT-1 and cysLT-2, respectively, and are thought to mediate the action of these LTs in the pulmonary and vascular beds. PGs and LTs may also interact with peroxisome proliferator-activated receptors, members of the nuclear superfamily that includes steroid hormone receptors. PGI_2 and PGD_2 and its metabolite PGJ_2, but not PGE_2 or $PGF_{2\alpha}$, have been shown to activate peroxisome proliferator-activated receptors.

5.1. PG Transporter

Some years ago, McCracken and colleagues showed that during luteolysis in sheep, $PGF_{2\alpha}$ diffuses from the uterine vein rather slowly through the wall of the closely adherent ovarian artery. This countercurrent mechanism allows about 1% of $PGF_{2\alpha}$ secreted by the uterus to escape metabolism by the lungs and reach the ovary directly, where it causes luteolysis (*see* Section 6.7.). In some tissues, PG transport appears to be enhanced by a carrier-mediated transporter that has been identified in epithelial cells (*see* Banu et al., 2003) as a protein with 12 transmembrane domains. Because the PG transporter appears to facilitate transport of PGs across cell membranes, it does not appear to be a receptor as such, particularly because it differs from the seven-transmembrane structure of the PG receptors. The PG transporter is thought to mediate the uptake and release of newly synthesized PGs from cells and to facilitate vectoral transport. Recently, high concentrations of the PG transporter have been identified in the bovine uterine vein/ovarian artery complex as well as other reproductive tissues (Banu et al., 2003). Such a finding may explain the mechanism underlying the countercurrent transfer of $PGF_{2\alpha}$ that occurs in the sheep and cow and several other species. Some PGs, such as PGI_2 and its metabolite, 6-keto-$PGF_{1\alpha}$, show very poor interaction with the PG transporter, which may explain the much-reduced metabolism of these compounds in the pulmonary circulation. The biologic activity of other PGs present in venous blood is rapidly reduced by metabolism in one passage through the lungs, presumably because the PG transporter very efficiently allows access to the intrac-

ellular 15-hydroxydehydrogenases present in the lung parenchyma. This explanation is consistent with the finding that, although PGI_2 is indeed a substrate for 15-hydroxydehydrogenase in cell-free systems, it probably escapes metabolism in the lungs by virtue of its very weak interaction with the PG transporter. However, it should be emphasized that PGI_2 in vivo is intrinsically unstable, being transformed nonenzymatically to its inactive metabolite, 6-keto-$PGF_{1\alpha}$, in about 20 s. Thus, it is a "local hormone" rather than a circulating one because arterial levels (about 3 pg/mL) are probably too low to have any systemic effect. LTC_4 is also known to be transported extracellularly by transporters such as multidrug resistance–associated protein, and, in this way, LTC_4 is thought to mediate the migration of dendritic cells to lymph nodes (Robbiani et al., 2000).

6. SELECTED EXAMPLES OF LOCAL ACTIONS OF EICOSANOIDS

6.1. Gastric Cytoprotection

PGE_2 appears to be an endogenous inhibitor of gastric acid secretion and to have a cytoprotective effect on the gastric mucosa. The ingestion of aspirin, indomethacin, and other NSAIDs that inhibit PG synthesis can cause severe damage to the gastric mucosa, with formation of ulcers and gastric bleeding. That inhibition of PG synthesis leads to damage to the mucosa is demonstrated by the coadministration of NSAIDs and PGE_2, or one of its various analogs, which prevents mucosal damage. Flower (2003) has recently evaluated the ability of several different NSAIDs to inhibit the two forms of COX, COX-1 (constitutive) and COX-2 (inducible) and has reviewed in detail the evolution and development of selective inhibitors for COX-2. The amino acid sequence of COX–2 shows a 60% homology with COX-1, but both enzymes have the same mol wt, about 70 kDa, and possess similar active sites for binding NSAIDs. However, the side pocket differs by one amino acid and results in a larger target for COX-2 inhibitors. Aspirin and indomethacin show greater inhibition of COX-1 (the predominant form in the gastric mucosa) than COX-2, which is consistent with the relative propensity among various NSAIDs to cause gastric ulceration. Thus, it has been possible to design NSAIDs (selective COX-2 inhibitors) that have minimal effects on gastric COX-1, but that inhibit the COX-2 induced by inflammatory mediators in other tissues. Such drugs, which include Celebrex and Vioxx (withdrawn from market 2004), permit safer oral administration for maximal systemic effects with diminished gastric side effects, which are reduced by at least 50%. However, since some of these drugs may inhibit COX-2 in endothelial cells, they could potentially skew the ratio of PGI_2 to TXA_2 and influence blood platelet aggregation. An unusual example of local action of PGs on gastric function is provided by a species of Australian frog that incubates its eggs in the stomach. Extremely high levels of gastric PGE_2 during the incubation are thought to act locally to inhibit gastric acid secretion and to promote gastric mucous secretion, thus protecting the eggs against digestion in the stomach.

The local production of LTs may also play a role in gastric function because ethanol-induced mucosal damage in the rat is accompanied by an increase in LTC_4. Moreover, nordihydroguaiaretic acid, a nonspecific lipoxygenase inhibitor, prevents ethanol-induced gastric mucosal damage and, at the same time, inhibits mucosal release of LTC_4. Thus, endogenous local production of PGE_2 has a protective effect on the stomach, although the effect is blocked by NSAIDs, whereas LTs appear to be local mediators of ethanol-induced damage to the gastric mucosa.

6.2. Local Action of PGs in Glaucoma

A biologically active substance was isolated from the iris and was found to increase during ocular inflammation. This substance, which caused a marked constriction of the pupil, was initially named irin. Subsequently, the biologic activity of irin was shown to be owing to PGs, principally $PGF_{2\alpha}$. This is consistent with previous findings that NSAIDs were effective in reducing inflammation in the eye. Paradoxically, it was found later that $PGF_{2\alpha}$ applied topically to the eye reduced intraocular pressure, suggesting a physiologic role for PGs in regulating intraocular pressure. Stjernschantz and colleagues (2000) pioneered the development of $PGF_{2\alpha}$ analogs for the treatment of glaucoma, which is characterized by a chronic increase in intraocular pressure. $PGF_{2\alpha}$ was found to reduce intraocular pressure, not by increasing outflow via the trabecular meshwork or by reducing the production of aqueous humor but, rather, by increasing the uveoscleral outflow of aqueous humor through the ciliary muscle. Some of these analogs, several of which are now in clinical use, have additional effects on the microvasculature of the eye and may increase capillary permeability. Although some modest side effects of daily topical application of $PGF_{2\alpha}$ analogs are observed, the dramatic and long-lasting reduction in intraocular pressure indicates that further development of $PGF_{2\alpha}$ analogs may provide more clinically acceptable treatments for glaucoma.

6.3. Local Effect of PGD₂ in Sleep Induction

For many years, Hayaishi and colleagues (1993) studied the role of PGD_2 production in the preoptic area (POA)

of the brain in relation to the induction of physiologic sleep. They found that microinjection or infusion of PGD_2 in femtomolar concentrations into the POA (an area considered to be the sleep center), or into the third ventricle of the rat or monkey, was effective in inducing normal sleep. They went on to show that the specific activity of the enzyme that controls PGD_2 production in the brain, PGD_2 synthase, exhibits a circadian fluctuation that parallels the sleep/wake cycle. When PGD_2 synthase activity in the POA was inhibited by the infusion of a specific inhibitor, selenium, sleep was inhibited. Such inhibition was reversed when the infusion of selenium into the POA was stopped. Hayaishi and colleagues (1993) conclude that PGD_2 is produced and acts locally in the POA of the brain as the physiologic inducer of sleep.

6.4. Mediating Role of PGE₂ in Fever

Evidence has accumulated over several years that PGE_2 is a primary mediator of fever induced by bacterial pyrogens. Skarnes and colleagues (1981) investigated the role of PGE_2 in endotoxin-induced fever in conscious sheep. They showed that PGE_2 infused into the carotid artery caused a transient increase in blood pressure (10–20%) accompanied by a sustained (3 h) increase in core body temperature that mimicked the effects seen during the first wave of fever induced by intravascular endotoxin (*see* Fig. 6). Subsequent experiments revealed that during the first phase of endotoxin-induced fever, a marked increase in both PGE_2 and $PGF_{2\alpha}$ occurred in the venous and arterial circulation. Intracarotid $PGF_{2\alpha}$ itself, however, did not exhibit the pyrogenic or pressor effects seen with intracarotid PGE_2. Further work showed that indomethacin blocked both the first and second phases of fever induced by endotoxin. More important, PGE_2 evoked both the pressor response and the first phase of fever during indomethacin blockade. It was concluded that PGE_2, formed within the vasculature, crosses the blood-brain barrier and acts on the thermoregulatory center in the hypothalamus to evoke the first phase of fever. However, since both the first and second phases of fever are blocked by indomethacin, it appeared that the presence of circulating levels of another AA metabolite might be responsible for the second phase of fever (i.e., the phase associated with leukocyte pyrogen, interleukin-1 [IL-1]). Studies by Coceani and colleagues (1989), using the cat as a model, supported the role of PGE_2 in the pathogenesis of fever induced by bacterial pyrogen. By means of a push-pull perfusion procedure, they demonstrated that iv endotoxin selectively caused an increase in PGE_2 in the anterior hypothalamic/preoptic region of the brain. The increase in PGE_2 production in these areas of the brain was consistent with the onset and progression of fever in their experimental model.

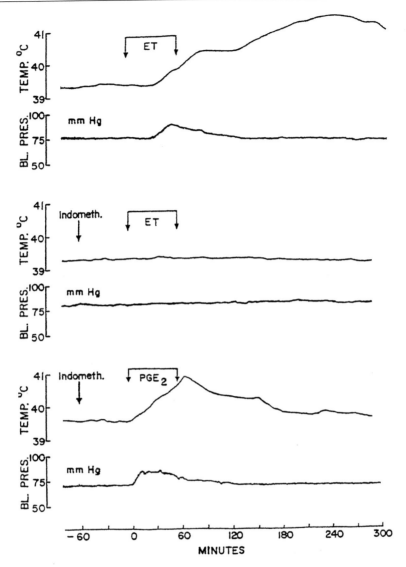

Fig. 6. Effect of indomethacin treatment (4.0 mg/kg, subcutaneously) on fever and pressor responses to an intracarotid infusion of endotoxin (ET) (10 µg/min) or PGE_2 (2.6 µg/min). Indomethacin blocked both the first and second waves of fever and the pressor response to endotoxin, but the first wave of fever and the pressor response to PGE_2 were elicited during indomethacin treatment. BL. PRES. = blood pressure. (Adapted from Skarnes et al., 1981.)

Recent work using knockout mice lacking different subtypes of the EP receptor supports and extends the key role of PGE_2 in endotoxin-induced fever. Sugimoto and colleagues (2000) showed that knockout mice deficient in the receptor subtypes EP1 and EP2 continued to exhibit a fever response after an endotoxin challenge but that no fever occurred with endotoxin in EP3 knockout mice. This same group went on to demonstrate that local synthesis of PGE_2, induced by lipopolysaccharide or a cytokine, interacts with EP3 receptors located in the neurons surrounding the organum vasculosa lamina terminalis (OVLT), considered to be the thermoregulatory center, thus inducing a fever response to endotoxin.

It now seems likely that, as demonstrated in the sheep model, the initial wave of fever and pressor responses induced by endotoxin is mediated by the rapid increase in the general circulation of PGE_2, which readily passes across the blood-brain interface to act on the themoregulatory center in the hypothalamus as well as on the vasomotor center in the medulla. The fever response to PGE_2 is very specific because, in the sheep model, intracarotid PGD_2 causes a pressor response but does not induce fever. The second and more sustained wave of fever observed in the sheep and other species may be owing to the induction of COX-2 and/or COX-3 in the OVLT by cytokines such as IL-1.

Moreover, recent studies by Engblom and colleagues (2003) provide further support for a role of centrally generated PGE_2 in the pathogenesis of fever. Using knockout mice lacking the gene for microsomal PGE synthase-1, they demonstrated that these mice did not show a febrile response to endotoxin injected intraperitoneally, whereas pyresis occurred in these same animals in response to PGE_2 injected into the cerebral ventricles. Thus, the delayed increase in the local generation of PGE_2 in the OVLT would provide an answer for the second wave of fever. Such a scenario would explain why indomethacin blocks the first wave of fever caused by peripherally generated PGE_2 as well as blocking the second wave of fever mediated by centrally generated PGE_2. The initial pressor response to intracarotid PGE_2, as well as to intracarotid endotoxin infusion, is consistent with the view that an increase in PGE_2 in the general circulation, caused either directly by PGE_2 infusion or indirectly by endotoxin, causes a central, peripherally mediated increase in arterial pressure. This most likely explains why a pressor response occurs with endotoxin only during the first wave of fever. The second wave of fever induced by endotoxin, associated with a delayed local increase in PGE_2 in the OVLT, thus does not result in a pressor response. The identification of a third form of COX, COX-3 (Chandrasekharan et al., 2002), particularly in neural tissues, together with the high sensitivity of COX-3 to inhibition by acetaminophen, supports a central role for neural COX-3 in the generation of the second sustained wave of fever.

6.5. Pheromonal and Reproductive Function of PGs in Teleost Fish

Among the more unusual actions of PGs is their recently proposed role as pheromones in male teleost fish. Sorensen and Goetz (1993) have investigated this phenomenon. $PGF_{2\alpha}$ and/or its metabolites are produced in large quantities in the ovaries of female teleost fish, where they appear to act in a paracrine fashion by stimulating follicular rupture, a phenomenon also observed during ovulation in most mammalian and nonmammalian species. In female teleost fish, $PGF_{2\alpha}$ and/or its metabolites secreted by the ovary persist in the systemic circulation (since fish do not have lungs) and act centrally in the brain to elicit female spawning behavior. Apparently the female fish releases into the water during oviposition relatively large amounts of PGF metabolites that are detectable by the highly developed chemosensory system in the male fish. The male is thus "signaled" through a sensitive olfactory system to exhibit spawning behavior.

6.6. Local Action of PGs in Uterus

Although PGs were first isolated and identified from secretions of the male reproductive tract, it was not long before they were also identified in the female reproductive system, where they serve a number of important local functions. Key findings included the discovery that human menstrual fluid was a major source of PGs, particularly PGE_2 and $PGF_{2\alpha}$, and that the administration of $PGF_{2\alpha}$ to women during the luteal phase produced menstrual-like bleeding. Moreover, Eldering and colleagues (1993) reported high production rates of several PGs (especially $PGF_{2\alpha}$) from endometrium of the rhesus monkey, primarily during the luteal phase. These findings led to extensive studies on the role of PGs in normal menstruation and in abnormal conditions such as dysmenorrhea and menorrhagia. Bygdeman and Lundstrom (1988) investigated the role of PGs in menstrual physiology. It is established that an overproduction of endometrial PGs explains the symptoms of dysmenorrhea in women. This conclusion is supported by the finding that a variety of NSAIDs alleviate the clinical symptoms of dysmenorrhea (uterine cramping) and menorrhagia (excessive blood loss). The effectiveness of different NSAIDs varies considerably, owing to the fact that in addition to blocking COX activity in the uterus and hence PG production, some of these compounds (such as the fenamates) also act as PG receptor antagonists. Intrauterine devices (IUDs) stimulate the local production of endometrial PGs, which may mediate the mechanism of action of IUDs in preventing conception. In some individuals, the presence of an IUD results in an overproduction of PGs and the occurrence of dysfunctional bleeding, which often can be controlled by NSAIDs.

6.7. Identification of PGF_{2\alpha} as a Local Uterine Luteolytic Hormone

The occurrence of PGs in human menstrual fluid and their role in menstruation provided an important lead regarding the potential role of PGs in uterine physiology in mammals. Unlike in primates, the presence of the uterus is essential for cyclic regression of the corpus luteum in many nonprimate species. McCracken and colleagues (1972) investigated the role of uterine PGs in relation to cyclic regression of the corpus luteum using sheep with autotransplanted ovaries and/or uterus. The presence of a contiguous uterine horn was found to be a requirement for luteolysis in this species. Such a requirement was subsequently explained by the local uterine production and countercurrent transfer of $PGF_{2\alpha}$ from the uterine vein to the ovarian artery, the latter vessel being highly contorted and adherent to the uter-

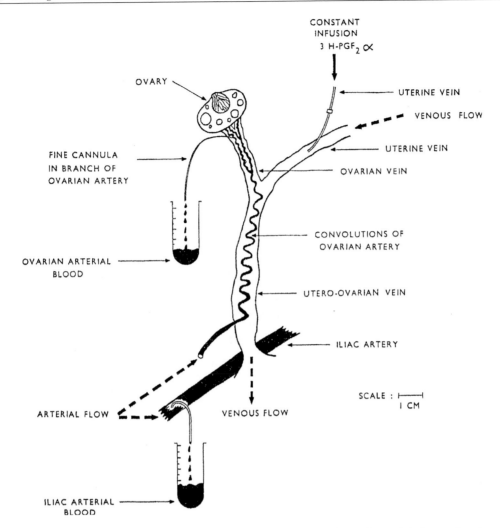

Fig. 7. Anatomic relationship of ovarian artery and uteroovarian vein in sheep and experimental design used to demonstrate countercurrent transfer of ^{3}HPGF$_{2\alpha}$ from a uteroovarian vein to its closely adherent ovarian artery. About 1% of PGF$_{2\alpha}$ secreted by the uterus reaches the ovary directly, thus bypassing metabolism in the pulmonary circulation. (Reproduced from McCracken et al., 1972.)

ine vein (*see* Fig. 7). This mechanism allows PGF$_{2\alpha}$ secreted by the uterus to avoid metabolism in the pulmonary circulation and to reach the adjacent ovary directly, hence causing luteolysis. The PG transporter, recently identified in bovine reproductive blood vessels, most likely accounts for the countercurrent transfer process. Such a bypass mechanism from vein to artery allows the transfer of about 1% of the secreted amount of uterine PGF$_{2\alpha}$ (*see* Fig. 8), which occurs as a series of episodic bursts during luteolysis. It is likely that similar countercurrent transfer mechanisms for PGs and other substances may occur where the appropriate vascular anatomy exists, such as in the testicular vascular pedicle or in the kidney vasculature. Indeed, the transfer of tritiated water, krypton, and heat is reported to occur in the testicular vasculature. In addition, ste-roids are known to be transferred within the ovarian vasculature of several species including the human. Such a transfer mechanism may permit steroids and other substances to reach the ovary, the oviduct, and perhaps the uterus itself in a concentration greater than would be supplied via the systemic circulation.

6.8. PGs and Cancer

Evidence has accumulated in recent years that the use of NSAIDs decreases the incidence of certain cancers, especially colorectal, breast, and lung cancer. Moreover, NSAIDs suppress carcinogen-induced cancers in several animal models. A number of potential targets for NSAID action in the prevention of cancer have been proposed. In a recent study, Lui and colleagues (2001) showed that overexpression on COX-2 in transgenic

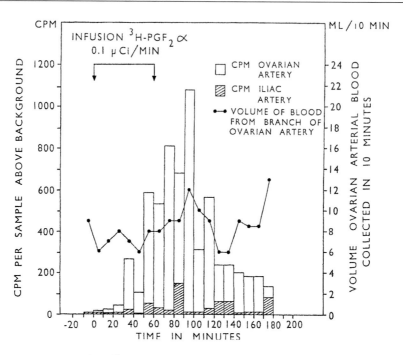

Fig. 8. Time course of countercurrent transfer of $^3HPGF_{2\alpha}$ from a uteroovarian vein to its closely adherent ovarian artery. (Reproduced from McCracken et al., 1972.)

mice is sufficient to induce tumorigenesis, suggesting that overproduction of PGs may promote cancer in certain tissues. Indeed, mammary tumors from these transgenic mice contained elevated levels of $PGF_{2\alpha}$, PGE_2, PGD_2, and 6-keto-$PGF_{1\alpha}$. Moreover, studies have indicated an involvement of the EP1 receptor subtype in precancerous lesions evoked by chemical carcinogens (Watanabe et al., 1999).

The extracellular matrix (ECM) has also been implicated in the progression of tumorigenesis, potentially via changes in gene expression, basement membrane formation, cell adhesion characteristics, and cell migration (Liotta and Kohn, 2001). Recently, $PGF_{2\alpha}$ was shown in vivo to reduce acutely protein levels of tissue inhibitors of metalloproteinases (TIMPs), primary regulators of the ECM, in luteal tissue by as much as 90% within 1 h of $PGF_{2\alpha}$ administration (*see* Fig. 9) and then to increase metalloproteinase-2 activity (Towle et al., 2002). Such a rapid reduction in TIMPs in luteal tissue may be the initial step in functional luteolysis, e.g., by altering the conformation/localization of luteinizing hormone (LH) receptors on luteal cells. The rapid effect of physiologic levels of $PGF_{2\alpha}$ on regulators of the ECM in luteal tissue in vivo suggests one possible explanation for the tumorigenic effect of PGs since the unexplained beneficial effects of NSAIDS on certain cancers may be attributed to their attenuation of PG action on the ECM. It may seem paradoxical that PGs (specifically $PGF_{2\alpha}$)

promote regression of luteal tissue, whereas there is evidence that PGs promote tumorigenesis in susceptible tissues and that NSAIDs prevent it. However, recent work has shown that, in some tissues, TIMP-2 suppresses TKR growth factor independently of metalloproteinase inhibition (Hoegy et al., 2001). Thus, acute suppression of TIMP-2 by a PG, as occurs in luteal tissue in vivo, may increase growth factor activation in certain tissues and, hence, contribute to tumorigenesis (McCracken, 2004).

6.9. NSAIDs and Alzheimer Disease

In recent years, several epidemiologic studies have indicated that the incidence of Alzheimer disease is reduced in individuals undergoing long-term NSAID therapy. Alzheimer disease is characterized by a buildup in the brain of amyloid plaques consisting of protein fibers and amyloid-β surrounded by astrocytes and microglia. The beneficial effects of NSAIDs on Alzheimer disease were considered initially to be owing to their antiinflammatory action via COX inhibition. However, a specific explanation for the protective effect of NSAIDs against Alzheimer disease has been lacking. A recent study by Weggen and colleagues (2001) has indicated that the beneficial action of NSAIDs in Alzheimer disease may be owing to the reduction of amyloid-β by a mechanism independent of COX inhibition. Using mice engineered to provide a

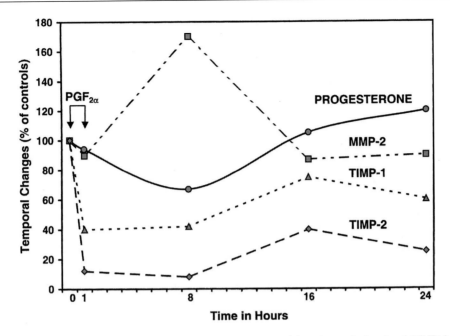

Fig. 9. In vivo temporal changes in peripheral plasma progesterone and luteal protein levels of TIMP-1, TIMP-2, and MMP-2 following administration of a 1 h luteolytic pulse of $PGF_{2\alpha}$ to sheep during midcycle; n = three sheep per time point. (Adapted from Towle et al., 2002.)

model for Alzheimer disease, as well as cultured cells, these investigators showed that ibuprofen lowered the level of amyloid-β42, which has been implicated in the pathogenesis of this disease, by as much as 80%. It seems that the beneficial effect may be limited to certain NSAIDs, since aspirin therapy, as well as selective COX-2 inhibitors, has a much less convincing effect on the incidence of Alzheimer disease. Moreover, in Weggen et al.'s (2001) study, aspirin did not block the formation of amyloid-β42 in mice. Because the action of certain NSAIDs in lowering amyloidogenic proteins is independent of anti-COX activity, the development of similar compounds lacking COX inhibition could give rise to a new generation of drugs that selectively reduce brain amyloid-β42 formation without the side effects of long-term COX inhibition, such as gastric and renal side effects. On the other hand, the anti-inflammatory action of NSAIDs may help to reduce the amyloid plaque-induced inflammatory response, that occurs in Alzheimer disease.

7. A MODEL FOR ENDOCRINE CONTROL OF PULSATILE $PGF_{2\alpha}$ SECRETION DURING LUTEOLYSIS IN SHEEP

Hormonal regulation of uterine $PGF_{2\alpha}$ secretion, which initiates luteolysis in nonprimate species, has been studied extensively in the sheep. This species offers a number of advantages as a model, such as the access to

the uterine and ovarian circulation in sheep bearing a transplanted ovary and/or uterus. Early studies indicated control of uterine $PGF_{2\alpha}$ secretion by estrogen and progesterone. However, McCracken and colleagues (1995; 1999) subsequently showed that these hormones act indirectly by regulating the formation of oxytocin receptors (OTRs) in the endometrium, the site of uterine $PGF_{2\alpha}$ synthesis in sheep. A model for the cellular control of $PGF_{2\alpha}$ synthesis in the endometrium of the sheep is shown in Fig. 10. Estradiol-17β (E_2) promotes the formation of endometrial OTRs in 6–9 h and may also increase PG synthetase and phospholipase levels. When OTRs are present on the endometrial cell membrane, oxytocin (OT) induces the immediate secretion of $PGF_{2\alpha}$. Signal transduction via the phosphatidylinositol-mediated increase in intracellular Ca^{++} is thought to activate PLA_2, resulting in liberation of AA from phospholipid stores. Some AA may also be generated from DAG via DAG lipase. Released AA is then rapidly converted into $PGF_{2\alpha}$ by PG synthetase (COX). Progesterone secreted during the luteal phase initially inhibits estrogen action and prevents the formation of endometrial OTRs. During this period of inhibition, progesterone appears to increase lipid stores in the endometrial cells (the so-called priming effect of progesterone). Finally, progesterone action diminishes toward the end of the luteal phase via catalysis of its own receptor. Such a loss of progesterone action will facilitate the return of E_2 action with the con-

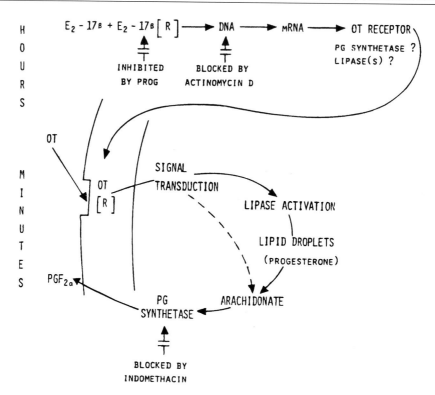

Fig. 10. Model for the endocrine control of PGF$_{2\alpha}$ synthesis in endometrial cell of sheep during luteolysis (*see* text for explanation). (Reproduced from McCracken et al., 1995.)

sequent formation of endometrial OTRs and, hence, the ability of OT to stimulate endometrial PGF$_{2\alpha}$ secretion. However, because of the effects of progesterone priming, the amount of PGF$_{2\alpha}$ secreted in response to OT is 50- to 100-fold greater than the response to OT before priming.

The model proposed in Fig. 10 explains the cellular regulation of PGF$_{2\alpha}$ synthesis via the induction of endometrial OTRs, but it does not explain the role of circulating levels of OT. In the sheep and other ruminants, the regulation of blood levels of OT is complicated by the fact that, in addition to the neurohypophysis, the corpus luteum is an ectopic site of OT synthesis. Recent work from our laboratory has confirmed that a finite store of OT exists in the ovine corpus luteum that can be released by subluteolytic levels of PGF$_{2\alpha}$. This supplemental source of OT appears to reinforce periodic signals from the central OT pulse generator to amplify the magnitude of each luteolytic pulse of PGF$_{2\alpha}$ from the uterus. A model of the endocrine control of pulsatile secretion of PGF$_{2\alpha}$ from the uterus during luteolysis in the sheep is depicted in Fig. 11 The numbers in the Fig.11 are explained as follows: (1) At the end of the cycle, loss of progesterone (P) action by catalysis of its receptor, in both the hypothalamus and the uterus, results in return-

ing E$_2$ action. (2) E$_2$ (E) increases endometrial OTRs and causes intermittent increases in the frequency of the central OT pulse generator. (3) Low-level PGF$_{2\alpha}$ is generated by the action of central OT on uterine OTR. (4) This low-level PGF$_{2\alpha}$ acts on the high-affinity PGF$_{2\alpha}$ receptor (HFPR) present on OT-containing luteal cells to stimulate OT secretion. (5) A high level of uterine PGF$_{2\alpha}$ secretion is now generated by luteal OT. (6) This high level of PGF$_{2\alpha}$ now has two effects via the low-affinity PGF$_{2\alpha}$ receptor (LFPR) in luteal cells: first, it stimulates additional luteal OT; and, second, it depresses luteal P secretion (luteolysis). The closed-loop positive feedback between the uterus (source of PGF$_{2\alpha}$) and the corpus luteum (source of OT) will continue until PGF$_{2\alpha}$ receptors in the corpus luteum are desensitized, thus terminating the release of luteal OT. Additional luteolytic pulses will follow when luteal PGF$_{2\alpha}$ receptors and/or uterine OTR recover after 6–9 h, in time to respond to the next high-frequency signal from the central OT pulse generator. However, further work will be required to determine whether a luteal contribution of OT is an absolute requirement for the luteolytic process in sheep and other ruminants. A minimum of five luteolytic pulses of PGF$_{2\alpha}$ are necessary to complete functional luteolysis.

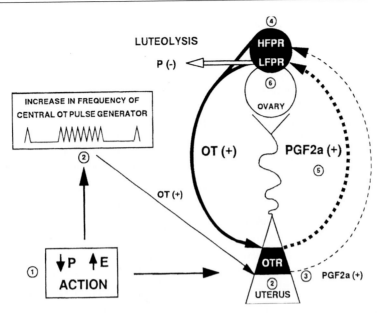

Fig. 11. Model for neuroendocrine control of pulsatile PGF$_{2\alpha}$ secretion from uterus during luteolysis in sheep (*see* text for explanation of numbers in the model). (Reproduced from McCracken et al., 1995.)

In the past few years, receptors for LH have been identified in the endometrium and other nongonadal components of the reproductive tract of several species. In the bovine species, LH receptors have been located in both the endometrium and the uterine veins, and LH stimulates the expression of COX-2 and the production of PGF$_{2\alpha}$ by these tissues (Shemesh et al., 1997). However, a potential role for uterine LH receptors in the process of luteolysis remains to be investigated.

In the sheep and other nonprimate species, in addition to the well-established interplay between ovarian steroids and the hypothalamic/anterior pituitary axis for the initiation of the ovarian cycle (via the gonadotropins), there is now good evidence for an interplay between ovarian steroids and the hypothalamic/posterior pituitary axis for the termination of the reproductive cycle (via OT). In species that do not synthesize OT in the ovary, it seems likely that OT secreted via the central OT pulse generator may alone be a sufficient stimulus for the generation of pulsatile luteolytic releases of uterine PGF$_{2\alpha}$ as in the mare and sow. Thus, in sheep and several other nonprimate species, the uterus can be regarded as a transducer that, under appropriate hormonal conditions, converts neural signals into local hormonal signals from the uterus to effect luteolysis. Although the uterus is an abundant source of PGs in primates, the presence of the uterus is not required for luteolysis because ovarian cyclicity is normal in hysterectomized subjects. However, many of the components present in the sheep uteroovarian system are present within the primate ovary itself, namely small amounts of

OT, OTRs, PGF$_{2\alpha}$, PGF$_{2\alpha}$ receptors, and different luteal cell types. Thus, a local production and action of PGF$_{2\alpha}$, or another metabolite of AA within the primate ovary itself, could account for luteolysis, but, this possibility is still under investigation.

The endocrine control for the local production of PGF$_{2\alpha}$ in the endometrium at the time of luteolysis may also occur at the end of pregnancy during the induction of labor in a number of species. Work by Fuchs and colleagues (1992) indicates an upregulation of OTRs in the endometrium and in the placental membranes in the bovine fetoplacental unit prior to the onset of labor. This upregulation of OTR is associated with the local formation of PGF$_{2\alpha}$ in these tissues. It is proposed that PGF$_{2\alpha}$, so formed, acts synergistically with low levels of OT on the myometrium to promote uterine contractions and the initiation of first-stage labor. The subsequent increase in maternal OT levels during the second or expulsive phase of labor is most likely owing to release of pituitary OT via the Ferguson Reflex (*see* Fuchs et al., 1992).

Another important local function of PGs during pregnancy is the maintenance of ductus arteriosus patency in the fetus. Momma (2004) investigated the role of PGs in ductal patency and concluded that PGE$_2$ is the prime agent in this respect. PGE$_2$ was found to be more than 1000 times more potent than PGI$_2$ in maintaining ductal patency. The levels of PGE$_2$ in the fetal circulation are 300–400 pg/mL of plasma vs 5–10 pg/mL in the adult sheep. One likely explanation for the high levels of PGE$_2$

in the fetal circulation is that the low blood flow through fetal lungs may result in diminished pulmonary metabolism of PGE_2. Thus, it appears that ductal patency is maintained by high levels of PGE_2 in the fetal circulation rather than by local mural production. Because NSAIDs and corticosteroids block PG synthesis, they can be used to effect ductal closure in the newborn and in cases of fetal prematurity. These drugs are contraindicated in women during late pregnancy because of potential harmful effects on fetal hemodynamics. It now appears that both PGE_2 and nitric oxide are involved in maintaining ductal patency, but recent work indicates that endothelin and its type A receptor are involved in the actual contraction of the ductus arteriosus at birth. Thus, corticosteroids may promote ductal closure, not only by inhibiting PGE_2 synthesis, but also by their ability to stimulate endothelin-1 synthesis.

8. CONCLUSION

The foregoing selected examples of local action of eicosanoids were described to emphasize the diversity of function of these potent biologic agents. Further examples of the diversity of action of eicosanoids may be obtained by consulting the references provided. Judging by the intense research efforts currently being extended in the eicosanoid field, it is clear that new information on the regulation and action of these biologically potent substances will continue to evolve. Moreover, their important pathophysiologic role in certain diseases gives cause for optimism that the pharmacologic control of their synthesis and action will be of considerable therapeutic value.

ACKNOWLEDGMENTS

Thanks are due to my colleagues Drs. Robert C. Skarnes and David Kupfer for critical evaluation of the text. The investigations of the author and his group that are included in this chapter were supported by National Institutes of Health grants HD-08129 and HD-20290, and US Department of Agriculture grants 98-35203-6635 and 2004-35203-14176.

REFERENCES

Banu S, Arosh JA, Chapeldaine P, Fortier MA. Molecular cloning and spatio-temporal expression of the prostaglandin transporter: a basis for the action of prostaglandins in the bovine reproductive system. *Proc Natl Acad Sci USA* 2003;100: 11,747–11,752.

Bergström S, Sjovall J. The isolation of prostaglandin. *Acta Chem Scand* 1957;11:1086–1087.

Bygdeman M, Lundstrom V. Menstruation and dysmenorrhoea. In: Curtis-Prior PB, ed. *Prostaglandins: Biology and Chemistry of Prostaglandins and Related Eicosanoids*. Edinburgh, UK: Churchill Livingstone 1988:490–495.

Capdevila JH, Falck JR. The CYP P450 arachidonic acid monoxygenases: from cell signaling to blood pressure regulation. *Biochem Biophys Res Commun* 2001;285:571–576.

Chandrasekharan NV, et al. COX-3, a cylooxygenase-1 variant inhibited by acetominophen and other analgesic/antipyretic drugs: cloning, structure and expression. *Proc Natl Acad Sci USA* 2002;99:13,926–13,931.

Coceani F, Bishai J, Lees J, Sirko S. Prostaglandin E_2 in the pathogenesis of pyrogen fever: validation of an intermediary role. *Adv Prostate Thromb Res* 1989;19:394–397.

Coleman RA, Smith WL, Narumiya S. International Union of Pharmacology Classification of Prostanoid Receptors: properties, distribution and structure of receptors and their subtypes. *Pharmacol Rev* 1994;46:205–229.

Cundell DR, Gerard NP, Gerard C, Idanpaan-Helkklla I, Tuomanen E. *Streptococcus pneumoniae* anchor to activated human cells by the receptor for platelet-activating factor. *Nature* 1995;377:435–438.

Deby C. Metabolism of fatty acids, precursors of eicosanoids. In: Curtis-Prior PB, ed. *Prostaglandins: Biology and Chemistry of Prostaglandins and Related Compounds*. Edinburgh, UK: Churchill Livingstone 1988:11–36.

Eldering JA, Nay MG, Hoberg LM, Longcope C, McCracken JA. Hormonal regulation of endometrial prostaglandin $F_{2\alpha}$ production during luteal phase of the rhesus monkey. *Biol Reprod* 1993; 49:809–815.

Engblom D, et al. Microsomal prostaglandin E synthase-1 is the central switch during immune-induced pyresis. *Nat Neurosci* 2003;6:1137–1138.

Flower RJ. The development of COX2 inhibitors. *Nat Rev Drug Discov* 2003;2:179–191.

Fuchs AR, Helmer H, Chang SM, Fields MJ. Concentration of oxytocin receptors in the placenta and fetal membranes of cows during pregnancy and labor. *J Reprod Fertil* 1992;96:775–783.

Hayaishi O, Matsumura H, Urade Y. Prostaglandin D synthase is the key enzyme in the promotion of physiological sleep. *J Lipid Mediators* 1993;6:429–431.

Hoegy SE, Oh HR, Corcoran ML, Stetler-Stevenson WG. Tissue inhibitor of metalloproteinase-2 (TIMP-2) supresses TKR-growth factor signaling independent of metalloproteinase inhibition. *J Biol Chem* 2001;276:3203–3214.

Klein RF, et al. Regulation of bone mass in mice by the lipoxygenase gene Alox15. *Science* 2004;203:229–232.

Liotta AL, Kohn EC. The microenvironment of the tumor-host interface. *Nature* 2001;411:375–379.

Lui CH, et al. Overexpression of cyclooxygenase-2 is sufficient to induce tumorigenesis in transgenic mice. *J Biol Chem* 2001;276: 18,563–18,569.

McCracken JA, et al. The central oxytocin pulse generator: a pacemaker for luteolysis. *Adv Exper Med Biol* 1995;395:133–154.

McCracken JA, Custer EE, Lamsa JC. Luteolysis: a neuroendocrine-mediated event. *Physiol Rev* 1999;79:263–323.

McCracken JA, et al. Prostaglandin $F_{2\alpha}$ identified as a luteolytic hormone in sheep. *Nat New Biol* 1972;238:129–134.

McCracken JA. Prostaglandin $F_{2\alpha}$: the luteolytic hormone. In: Curtis-Prior P, ed. *The Eicosanoids*. New York, NY: John Wiley & Sons 2004:525–545.

Momma K. Foetal and neonatal ductus arteriosus. In: Curtis-Prior P, ed. *The Eicosanoids*. New York, NY: John Wiley & Sons 2004: 576–590.

Narumiya S, Fitzgerald GA. Genetic and pharmacological analysis of prostanoid receptor function. *J Clin Invest* 2001;108:25–30.

Negeshi M, et al. Signal transduction of the isoforms of mouse prostaglandin E receptor EP3 subtype. *Adv Prosta Thromb Leuk Res* 1995;23:255–257.

O'Flaherty JT, Wykle RL. Biochemical interactions of platelet-activating factor with eicosanoids. In: Curtis-Prior P, ed. *The Eicosanoids*. New York, NY: John Wiley & Sons 2004:585–592.

Piper PF, Letts LG. Biology of leukotrienes. In: Curtis-Prior PB, ed. *Prostaglandins: Biology and Chemistry of Prostaglandins and Related Eicosanoids.* Edinburgh, UK: Churchill Livingstone 1988: 616–624.

Robbiani DF, et al. The leukotriene C4 transporter MRP1 regulates CCL19 (MIP-3B,ELC)-dependent mobilization of dendritic cells to lymph nodes. *Cell* 2000;103:757–786.

Roberts LJ II, Morrow JD. Isoprostanes: novel markers of endogenous lipid peroxidation and potential mediators of oxidant injury. *Ann NY Acad Sci* 1994;744:237–242.

Robinson DS, Campbell D, Barnes PJ. Addition of leukotriene antagonists to therapy in chronic persistent asthma: a double-blind placebo-controlled trial. *Lancet* 2001;235:2007–2011.

Sakamoto K, et al. Cloning and characterization of the novel isoforms for $PGF_{2\alpha}$ receptor in the bovine corpus luteum. *DNA Seq* 2002; 13:307–311.

Samuelsson B, et al. Leukotrienes and lipoxins: structures, biosynthesis, and biological effects. *Science* 1987;2:1171–1176.

Shemesh M, et al. Expression of functional LH receptor and its messenger ribonucleic acid in bovine uterine veins: LH induction of cyclooxygenase and augmentation of prostaglandin production in bovine uterine veins. *Endocrinology* 1997;138:4844–4851.

Skarnes RC, Brown SK, Hull SS, McCracken JA. Role of prostaglandin E in the biphasic fever response to endotoxin. *J Exp Med* 1981;154:1212–1224.

Sorensen PW, Goetz FW. Pheromonal and reproductive function of F prostaglandins and their metabolites in teleost fish. *J Lipid Mediators* 1993;6:385–393.

Stjernschantz J, et al. Microvascular effects of selective prostaglandin analogues in the eye with special reference to latanoprost and glaucoma treatment. *Prog Retin Eye Res* 2000;19:459–596.

Sugimoto Y, Narumiya S, Ichikawa. Distribution and function of prostanoid receptors: studies from knockout mice. *Prog Lipid Res* 2000;39:289-314.

Towle TA, Tsang PCW, Milvae RM, Newbury MK, McCracken JA. Dynamic in vivo changes in tissue inhibitors of metalloproteinase 1 and 2, and in matrix metalloproteinases 2 and 9, during $PGF_{2\alpha}$-induced luteolysis in sheep. *Biol Reprod* 2002;66:1515–1521.

Vanderhoek JY. Regulation of lipoxygenase enzymes in leukocytes. *Immunol Ser* 1992;57:77–86.

von Euler US. Biology of prostanoids. In: Curtis-Prior PB, ed. *Prostaglandins: Biology and Chemistry of Prostaglandins and Related Eicosanoids.* Edinburgh, UK: Churchill Livingstone 1988:1–7.

Watanabe K, et al. Role of prostaglandin E receptor subtype EP1 in colon carcinogenesis. *Cancer Res* 1999;59:5093–5096.

Weggen S, et al. A subset of NSAIDs lower amyloidogenic Aβ42 independently of cyclooxygenase activity. *Nature* 2001;414: 212–216.

Weissmann G. Prostaglandins as modulators rather then mediators of inflammation. *J Lipid Mediators* 1993;6:275–286.

Yokomizo T, et al. A second leukotriene B_4 receptor, BLT2: a new therapeutic target in inflammation and immunological disorders. *J Exp Med* 2000;192:421–431.

Zurier RB. Prostaglandins: then and now and next. *Semin Arthritis Rheum* 2003;33:137–139.

8 The Neuroendocrine–Immune Interface

Michael S. Harbuz, PhD
and Stafford L. Lightman, PhD

CONTENTS

1. INTRODUCTION

In an era of increased specialization where the trend has been for the individual scientist to delve ever deeper into smaller pools, effectively knowing more and more about less and less, one area of research in particular has bucked the trend. The increasing interest in the bidirectional interactions of the immune and the neuroendocrine systems and the importance of these systems in relation to sickness, inflammation, and immune-mediated diseases has required a sea change to the reductionist approach. Susceptibility to a number of autoimmune diseases such as rheumatoid arthritis (RA) and multiple sclerosis (MS) has clear genetic components. However, it is also evident that not all individuals with a genetic predisposition develop these diseases nor are the diseases of equal severity in all individuals. Answering the question, Which factors are responsible for increasing susceptibility to and/or the severity of disease? Has led to the implication of a whole host of neuroendocrine factors. The role of the hypothalamic-pituitary-adrenal (HPA) axis in controlling the release of glucocorticoids from the adrenal cortex together with the antiinflammatory effects of the glucocorticoids, is well established. A proinflammatory role has been proposed for prolactin (PRL), which is itself under the inhibitory control of dopamine released from the hypothalamus. Growth hormone (GH) has also been implicated in regulation of the immune system. The major gender differences associated with many autoimmune diseases have implicated the gonadal steroids. These are under increasing investigation by neuroendocrinologists (interested in the modulation of neuroendocrine systems by the gonadal steroids) and immunologists (interested in the modulation of other immune parameters), in addition to those working at the neuroendocrine-immune interface. Androgens have a generally favorable effect in a number of diseases whereas estrogens appear to have variable effects, depending on the disease.

In this chapter, we address the question of susceptibility to disease and the mechanisms involved particularly at the central and hypothalamic level. We first discuss the system that has been most extensively investigated, the HPA axis.

From: *Endocrinology: Basic and Clinical Principles, Second Edition*
(S. Melmed and P. M. Conn, eds.) © Humana Press Inc., Totowa, NJ

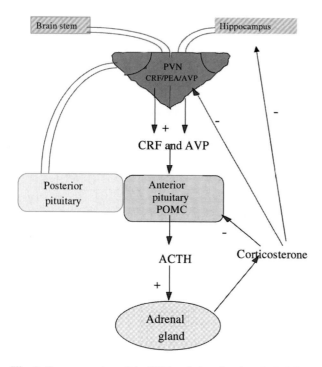

Fig. 1. Representation of the HPA axis (*see* Section 1). Briefly, the major CRFs and AVP are released into the hypophysial portal blood to stimulate the release of ACTH, which stimulates the release of glucocorticoid from the adrenal cortex. The increase in circulating glucocorticoids serves to regulate the system by downregulating the synthesis and release of CRF, AVP, and POMC. Feedback also occurs at the level of the brain stem and the hippocampus.

2. HYPOTHALAMIC-PITUITARY-ADRENAL AXIS

The HPA, or stress, axis is represented in Fig. 1. At the hypothalamic level, corticotropin-releasing factor (CRF) and arginine vasopressin (AVP) are synthesised in the parvocellular cells of the paraventricular nucleus (PVN). In the normal rat, approx 50% of the CRF-positive neurons also contain AVP. The axons of these neurons terminate in the external zone of the median eminence, where CRF and AVP are released into the hypophysial portal blood and carried to the corticotrophs of the anterior pituitary. CRF is generally considered to be the major CRF. It is able to evoke the release of adrenocorticotropin hormone (ACTH) from the anterior pituitary to a greater extent than can AVP alone. However, together these releasing factors act synergistically to evoke the release of ACTH. More important, CRF is currently the only factor that has been demonstrated to induce proopiomelanocortin (POMC) mRNA, the ACTH precursor. The ACTH released from

the anterior pituitary is carried in the general circulation to the adrenal gland, where it stimulates the production and release of glucocorticoid (cortisol in the human; corticosterone in the rat). The glucocorticoid has a negative feedback action at the pituitary and hypothalamic levels (and also at other brain sites), to inhibit the synthesis and release of both ACTH and its hypothalamic releasing factors. To understand the role of the HPA axis in disease, it is first necessary to recapitulate on the mechanisms activated in response to acute and repeated stress.

2.1. HPA Response to Acute Stress

In response to acute stress, CRF and AVP are immediately released into the hypophysial portal blood. These releasing factors are carried to the corticotropes of the anterior pituitary to stimulate the release of ACTH into the blood, which in turn, stimulates the synthesis and release of corticosterone. There is then a subsequent increase in CRF and AVP mRNAs in the PVN and POMC mRNA in the anterior pituitary. The type of stress, the duration of the stress, and the frequency with which it is applied may all influence the HPA axis response. Differential activation of the different components of the HPA axis has been demonstrated. For example, physical stressors such as foot shock, ip hypertonic saline, and naloxone-induced morphine withdrawal increase CRF mRNA and proenkephalin A (PEA) (an opiate precursor) mRNA in the PVN. Predominantly psychologic stressors such as restraint or swim stress activate CRF mRNA but not PEA mRNA. Ether stress, by contrast, results in an increase in PEA mRNA while not affecting CRF mRNA. Oxytocin may be important in the response to psychologic stress. Studies in anesthetized animals have demonstrated that a conscious appreciation of a physical stress is not necessary for a response to occur. These data suggest a subtle control system operating at the hypothalamus integrating signals from other brain areas to coordinate the release of a cocktail of releasing factors into the portal blood. The prevailing steroid milieu is not of primary importance in the mechanism underlying this response because a response to stress can be mounted following adrenalectomy, in which all endogenous steroid negative feedback has been removed, and also in high-dose glucocorticoid-treated animals in which the activity of the HPA axis is maximally suppressed. Therefore, the stress-responsive transsynaptic activation of hypothalamic neurons is able to overcome the level of steroid negative feedback. This is in accord with suggestions that there are mechanisms able to maintain stress responsiveness despite increased glucocorticoid secretion.

2.2. HPA Response to Acute Immune Challenge

It is now evident that factors released from the immune system, such as cytokines, or immune system activators, such as lipopolysaccharide (LPS), are able to stimulate the HPA axis. Injecting these mediators into the periphery, to mimic an infection, can stimulate the HPA axis and initiate a feedback mechanism that damps down the immune response. However, injection directly into the brain can also stimulate a corticosterone response (Fig. 2), and this activation appears more potent than similar injections in the periphery. For example, interleukin-1 (IL-1) injected centrally is 1000-fold more potent than in the periphery. The identification of a range of chemokines, ILs, growth factors, tumor necrosis factors, and interferons within the central nervous system (CNS) together with receptors through which these compounds may act confirms the importance of these so-called immune modulators in CNS function.

IL-1 remains the best studied of these modulators. The actions of IL-1 are exerted through activation of CRF neurons in the PVN. Immunoneutralization of CRF, or ablation of the PVN, can reduce the responsiveness of the HPA axis to IL-1β delivered either centrally or in the periphery. An inability to mount a response to an acute immune stimulus such as IL-1 or LPS can be life-threatening. As argued by Alan Munck, the corticosterone response is not generated against the challenge *per se* but, rather, is an attempt to regulate the response that is generated to the challenge. If the immune system is allowed to rampage unchecked, the effects can be fatal. The interrelationship of corticosteroids and immunologic responses is clearly a complex one, with both permissive and inhibitory effects of corticosteroids.

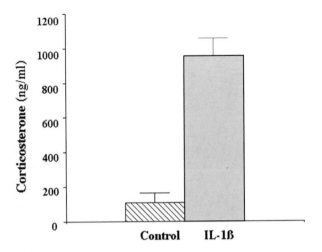

Fig. 2. A single injection of IL-1β directly into the lateral ventricle of the brain of the rat results in a significant increase in plasma corticosterone concentrations 30 min after injection. Values represent means and SEM for *n* = 6 rats per group.

2.3. HPA Axis Response to Repeated Stress

Although the activation of the HPA axis to a single acute stress is relatively well characterized, the response to chronic stress remains less so. In practice, there are few models for chronic stress, and in the literature the term *chronic* usually refers to an experimental paradigm in which an acute stress is repeated for a number of days. In response to repeated stress there may be habituation or adaptation of the HPA axis. Thus, although acute foot-shock, restraint, or ethanol stress will increase circulating ACTH and corticosterone for up to 1 wk with repeated exposure, levels subsequently return to basal levels. At the mRNA level, several days of repeated exposure to a physical stress such as ip injections of hypertonic saline or immobilization results in elevated CRF mRNA levels, whereas repeated exposure to mild predominantly psychologic stressors such

as restraint does not. This presumably reflects the nature and severity of the challenge. In the repeated stress situation, although the animals may not respond to the specific repeated stressor, the system itself has not become refractory to stress; following exposure to a novel stress, a normal or even supranormal response may be observed. This is likely to be mediated by AVP rather than CRF. Exogenous injection of CRF is without effect in repeatedly restrained rats, whereas injection of AVP stimulates ACTH and corticosterone release. It appears, therefore, that in response to chronic or repeated stress, AVP may be essential for sustaining the ability to respond to stress when the axis is refractory to CRF.

2.4. Effects of Stress On Immune Function

There is now considerable literature detailing the bidirectional interactions between the immune and neuroendocrine systems (Fig. 3). Evidence from clinical and preclinical studies has highlighted the impact of stress on immune function. For example, caregivers of patients with a variety of dementias have been shown to have elevated levels of circulating cortisol. This is thought to reflect the constant and chronic stress that caring for a loved one full-time can exert. Not only does this impact on immune measures in vitro, but the ability of these carers to mount suitable antibody titers to, e.g., influenza vaccination is compromised. Stress has been shown to reduce lymphocyte responsiveness to mitogenic stimulation, decrease natural killer (NK) cell activity, increase susceptibility to tumors, and decrease thymus growth and differentiation by inducing apoptosis in immature thymocytes.

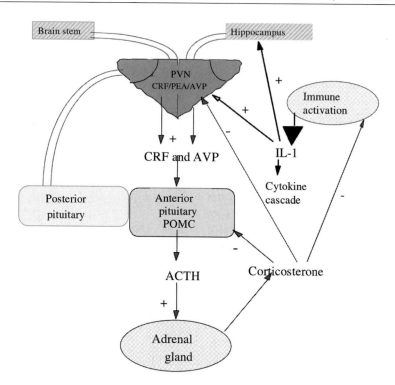

Fig. 3. Representation of the HPA axis demonstrating interrelationship that exists in functioning of neuroendocrine and immune systems. Following immune activation, IL-1 is released and sets in chain a series of cascade systems that results in the increased release of many cytokines and immunomodulators. In addition to exerting effects on the immune system, these immunomodulators are able to stimulate the HPA axis through an action at the PVN and also activate a number of other brain areas. This communication is bi-directional; the endpoint of HPA axis activation is an increase in circulating glucocorticoids, which are able to inhibit the synthesis and release of cytokines. Other hormones released from the pituitary also have immunomodulatory properties.

Table 1
Some Hormones and Neurotransmitters Present in the
Immune Tissues and Immune Modulators Found in Brain [a]

Immune tissues	Brain
CRF	IL-1
AVP	IL-1ra
OT	ICE
LHRH	IL-6
LH	TNF-α
ACTH	IL-3
POMC	IFN-γ
Endorphins	TGF
Enkephalins	and their receptors
TSH	
PRL	
Somatostatin	
GH	
Noradrenaline	
Substance P	

[a] CRF = corticotropin-releasing factor; AVP = arginine vasopressin; OT = oxytocin; LHRH = luteinizing hormone releasing hormone; LH = luteinizing hormone; ACTH = adrenocorticotropin hormone; POMC = pro-opiomelanocortin; TSH = thyrotropin-stimulating hormone; ICE = interleukin-converting enzyme; TNF-α = tumor necrosis factor-α; IFN-γ = interferon-γ; TGF = transforming growth factor.

Not only is the brain able to synthesize a range of immune modulators, but it has also been established that the immune tissues are able to synthesize a wide range of neuropeptides (Table 1). Many of these have already been implicated in modulating the response to stress and immune challenge. The role played by these locally produced peptides remains to be fully elucidated, but they may exert a paracrine or autocrine effect on the functioning of these organs. The temporal changes in these neuroimmunopeptides following stress need to be determined.

There is a wealth of evidence supporting the involvement of a variety of cytokines in autoimmune disease, but a discussion of this evidence is beyond the scope of this chapter. It is clear that there is activation of endogenous cytokines at numerous sites from the brain and pituitary through the immune tissues to local production at the affected sites. The balance of pro- and antiinflammatory effects of these cytokines may be crucial in determining whether the effect is to shift the individual into a proinflammatory Th1 response or an antiinflammatory Th2 response. The realization that there is an active interplay between the neuroendocrine and immune systems that is able to influence disease activity/severity provides novel targets for treatments of individual immune-mediated diseases.

3. NEUROENDOCRINE CHANGES ASSOCIATED WITH ADJUVANT-INDUCED ARTHRITIS

Adjuvant-induced arthritis (AA) is a disease model that shares many characteristics with RA in humans. The model has been used extensively for studies on pain, inflammation and arthritis. This immune-mediated inflammatory disease that is T-cell dependent can be induced in susceptible strains of rat by a single injection into the base of the tail of heat-killed ground *Mycobacterium butyricum* (or synthetic adjuvant) in paraffin oil. Twelve to 14 d after the injection of the adjuvant, the animals begin to develop inflammation of the hind paws. This subsequently spreads to other joints, attaining a maximum severity 21 d after injection.

3.1. Pituitary-Adrenal Response to Disease

The hormonal response to the chronic inflammatory disease model of AA is similar to that seen in chronic stress. The development of hind-paw inflammation results in increased circulating levels of ACTH and corticosterone. POMC mRNA in the anterior pituitary is also increased, reflecting the increased drive to the system. Analysis of the circadian profile of hormone release reveals a flattening in the normal circadian rhythm with higher evening levels apparent throughout the day. This is similar to the situation in humans with RA. The loss of normal circadian rhythm of hormones is associated with a great many diseases, but there are also similar diurnal changes in immune parameters such as variation in total and subset lymphocyte counts, NK cell levels and cytotoxicity, and the expression of cytokines. Whether the hormonal changes result in changes in the immune system or whether the alterations in the immune system result in altered hormonal profiles remains to be determined.

3.2. Alterations in Hypothalamic Control Mechanisms

From our understanding of the regulation of the HPA axis, the activation of the pituitary-adrenal axis seen in AA might be expected to be driven by increases in CRF activity at the level of the PVN. However, no increase in CRF has been reported. Instead, a paradoxical fall in CRF peptide release into the hypophysial portal blood and CRF mRNA in the PVN occurs. This fall is first apparent at the time of onset of inflammation that occurs around d 12–13 and decreases to a nadir at the time of maximum inflammation at d 21

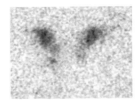
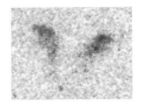

Day 0: Control   **Day 7: Pre-clinical**

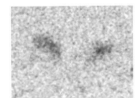
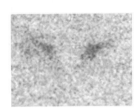

Day 16: Inflamed   **Day 21: Maximum inflammation**

Fig. 4. Representative photomicrographs taken from Hyperfilm MP (Amersham) autoradiography film showing hypothalamic PVN hybridized with ^{35}S-labeled probes complementary to CRF mRNA. With the onset of AA, which occurs at around d 14 following injection of adjuvant, there is a significant decrease in CRF mRNA levels in the PVN. As the disease progresses to a maximum severity at d 21, CRF mRNA levels decrease to a nadir. There is good correlation between the decrease in CRF mRNA levels in the PVN and the increase in severity of inflammation. Levels in d 7 preclinical rats are not significantly different from those of controls.

(Fig. 4). There is also a decrease in CRF binding at the anterior pituitary level, suggesting a decrease in CRF receptor level. The decrease in CRF activity in the PVN in AA is associated with an increase in AVP. Thus, with increasing inflammation, there is an increase in AVP release into the hypophysial portal blood and an increase in AVP mRNA in the parvocellular cells of the PVN. AVP can therefore be considered the major CRF in AA rats. Chikanza and colleagues have recently reviewed the importance of AVP in clinical disease.

3.3. Is the Defective Stress Response Important to Disease Outcome?

The hypothesis that a defect in the regulation of the HPA axis might predispose an individual to autoimmune disease was proposed in the late 1980s and early 1990s. This compelling hypothesis suggested that an inability to mount a suitable corticosterone response to suppress immune activation would allow the immune system to rampage unchecked and attack itself. This arose from observations comparing a stress hyporesponsive Lewis strain of rat with the hyperresponsive Fischer strain. The Lewis rat is susceptible to streptococcal cell wall–induced arthritis whereas the Fischer strain is resistant.

However, evidence has accumulated to question the validity of this hypothesis. First, certain hyperresponsive strains of rat are susceptible to autoimmune disease models. Second, disease susceptibility of a number of different strains of rat does not correlate with their response to stress. Third, a number of laboratories have failed to confirm the differences in stress responsiveness when comparing Lewis and Fischer strains, suggesting that there may be differences within strains derived from different sources. This latter point highlights a flaw in the methodology; comparing different strains of rat will inevitably reflect genetic differences among the strains. These other genetic variations affecting the stress, neuroendocrine, and immune systems are themselves likely to play a major role in determining susceptibility to disease.

Recent studies have attempted to circumvent this problem by investigating a single strain of rat divided into subpopulations on the basis of their response in behavioral tests. Tests such as the Open Field test for anxiety and Learned Helplessness model of depression have effectively identified subpopulations of rats within a larger population. Despite differences in stress responsiveness when comparing these subpopulations, no correlation to susceptibility or severity of inflammation has been determined. Indeed, in the learned helplessness study, the animals with the greater corticosterone response to stress, instead of being relatively protected, actually developed a more severe inflammation than the hyporesponsive group. Together, these data suggest that HPA axis responsivity to stress is not in itself a good predictor of susceptibility to inflammation in the AA model. It is evident that in both animals and humans with immune-mediated disease a functioning HPA axis is crucial, because removing endogenous glucocorticoids or blocking synthesis results in flares of disease activity. Therefore, a functioning HPA axis is important in modulating the severity of disease. It seems likely that there is a balance of pro- and antiinflammatory factors that together determine disease susceptibility and/or severity. Identifying and understanding the interplay of these factors is a challenge for researchers in the twenty-first century.

One feature of the AA rat is an inability to respond to acute stressors such as the predominantly psychologic stressors of noise or restraint or the physical stressor of ip hypertonic saline injection once the inflammation is present, despite a robust response to stress in the PVG strain of rat used. This nonresponsiveness should seriously compromise the animal for, as already noted, an inability to respond to stress or the development of infection that is not terminated could be fatal. A similar inability to mount a cortisol response to the stress of

surgery has also been reported in patients with RA. CRF challenge in RA stimulated ACTH release, suggesting normal pituitary function. However, the cortisol response was found to be impaired, suggesting a defect at the adrenal level. Of course, these findings do not rule out a defect at the hypothalamic level.

One feature of autoimmune disease is that despite the importance of the endogenous glucocorticoids in regulating the immune response, the role of the HPA axis remains to be fully understood. Patients with RA tend not to have significantly different levels of hormones compared with control subjects without AA, despite the increased levels of circulating cytokines that should be stimulating the HPA axis. Recently, in an attempt to identify alterations in HPA axis regulation, the dexamethasone-CRF test was used in patients with autoimmune disease. The dexamethasone-CRF test has been used extensively in patients with psychiatric disorders to investigate alterations in HPA axis regulation. In normal individuals, pretreatment with dexamethasone suppresses the HPA axis and subsequent challenge with CRF fails to stimulate the release of ACTH or cortisol. However, in some psychiatric conditions, such as depression, in which there is impaired glucocorticoid feedback, the dexamethasone is insufficient to suppress the axis and it can escape from the suppression and mount a cortisol response. In patients with MS, the axis is able to escape from dexamethasone suppression in response to CRF challenge in a manner correlated to disease activity. In approximately half of patients with RA who are challenged with CRF, the axis is able to escape the suppression. There was no correlation between disease activity or severity when comparing the responders and nonresponders in these RA patients. Of interest is the observation that approx 50% of MS patients do not suppress cortisol after the administration of dexamethasone, which is similar to what happens in patients with depression and much greater than that found in the general population. These data suggest the existence of subpopulations of patients with differential regulation of the HPA axis. The impact of these differences on disease progression remains to be determined.

4. OTHER DISEASES

4.1. Is There Evidence for Impaired HPA Axis Function in Other Immune-Mediated Diseases?

Evidence against a defect in HPA axis activity predisposing an individual to disease comes from studies in patients with African sleeping sickness. This potentially lethal parasitic disease in humans is caused by the protozoan *Trypanosoma brucei*. In the early stages of infection, the individual may suffer from fever, rash, weight loss, edema, and chronic fatigue. As the disease progresses, it may invade the CNS, resulting in neurologic and psychiatric disturbances. If left untreated, the sickness is usually fatal. Individuals with sleeping sickness have both primary and secondary adrenal insufficiency because they are unable to mount a cortisol response to ACTH or CRF. However, following successful antiparasitic treatment, there is an improvement in their ACTH and cortisol responses to CRF. Following full recovery, they have normal responses indistinguishable from those of control subjects. These data suggest that these people do not have an inherent defect in HPA axis responsivity predisposing them to disease, but, rather, the apparent defect is a response to the development of disease. It may therefore be part of an adaptive, protective mechanism to conserve energy in the presence of disease.

A blunting of the HPA response to exogenous challenge has been noted in the obese strain of chicken with autoimmune thyroiditis, an animal model for Hashimoto disease. These animals show elevated corticosteroid-binding globulin levels and a consequent decrease in free circulating corticosterone. They exhibit a blunted corticosterone response to IL-1 and other stimulants. The alteration in the response has been localized to the hypothalamic-pituitary part of the axis, although the precise locus has yet to be elucidated. The blunted response to challenge is also evident in a number of inbred strains of mice that develop diseases similar to systemic lupus erythematosus (SLE) and Sjögren syndrome. Parallel to the development of the disease in susceptible strains, there is an age-related decline in plasma corticosterone together with a blunted response to challenge with IL-1 and other stimuli.

There are ethical problems to contend with in determining alterations to the HPA axis in humans, particularly at the hypothalamic level. Some patients with MS have elevated levels of plasma cortisol compared with control subjects but, as seen in patients with RA, not all show such an elevation. A commonly used stressor in humans is insulin-induced hypoglycemia, and the cortisol response to this challenge is blunted in MS patients. One can infer changes in hypothalamic regulation by determining the response to the hypothalamic releasing factors CRF and AVP. Studies have revealed a normal response to CRF challenge but a blunted response to AVP, indicating altered release of the endogenous releasing factors. Other studies have noted differential responsiveness of cortisol release dependent on the disease status. Patients with secondary progressive MS had a lower cortisol response to CRF than those with the less severe primary progressive MS that was no different to the normal response seen in control subjects. These findings support those outlined above suggesting

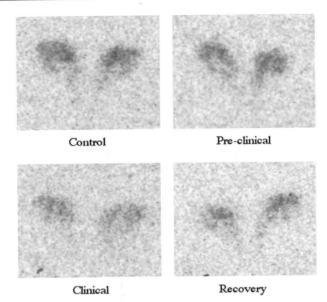

Control

Pre-clinical

Clinical

Recovery

Fig. 5. Representative photomicrographs taken from Hyperfilm MP (Amersham) autoradiography film showing hypothalamic PVN hybridized with ^{35}S-labeled probes complementary to CRF mRNA. With the onset of adoptively transferred EAE, there is a decrease in CRF mRNA that occurs despite activation of the pituitary-adrenal axis. With recovery, levels return to those seen in controls and at the preclinical stage.

that in MS AVP may play a more significant role than CRF in maintaining the activity of the HPA axis. Investigation of postmortem brains from MS patients compared with control subjects has revealed greater activity in the AVP-containing subset of CRF neurons in the PVN, again suggesting an important role for AVP. These data support the notion that associated with autoimmune disease there is an alteration in the responsiveness of the HPA axis. However, when the data are taken together, it appears that the mechanism involved is not simply a predisposition to autoimmune disease secondary to a defect in the HPA axis, but a more complex interaction between the HPA axis and the disease process.

4.2. Do the Changes in Hypothalamic Control Mechanisms Occur in Other Disease Models?

A question worthy of consideration is, are the alterations in the hypothalamic control mechanisms associated with AA a feature of this particular disease model or may a more general mechanism be inferred? In an adoptive transfer model of experimental allergic encephalomyelitis (EAE), which involves injection of activated splenocytes (i.e., no adjuvant is directly used), despite the activation of the pituitary-adrenal axis, there is a similar paradoxical decrease in CRF mRNA in the PVN (Fig. 5).

Supporting the contention that the decrease is separate to the question of susceptibility is the observation that when the animals recover from the disease, the decreased CRF mRNA levels return to normal and the elevated levels of plasma corticosterone and POMC mRNA in the anterior pituitary decline to basal control levels.

Eosinophilia myalgia syndrome (EMS) was originally identified in humans on the West Coast of the United States in the summer and fall of 1989, when the cases of the syndrome reached epidemic proportions. EMS is characterized by eosinophilia, muscle pain, and edema in the early stages, followed by inflammation of the muscles and connective tissues, hardening of the skin, and peripheral neuropathy. In a number of cases the disease proved fatal. The disease was identified as being T-cell mediated. Painstaking detective work identified the culprit, which turned out to be a rogue batch of the amino acid L-tryptophan produced by genetically modified bacteria intended for the health food market, where it was sold to treat insomnia, depression, and other disorders. To confirm the cause-and-effect relationship the suspected compound was fed to Lewis rats, which later developed histologic features consistent with the human disease. Investigation of the HPA axis revealed a tendency to lower plasma corticosterone concentrations in the affected rats. More pertinent for the present discussion, examination of the PVN of the rats with EMS revealed a decrease in CRF mRNA in the PVN related to the disease state.

These changes in hypothalamic regulation are not confined to rat models. In the MRL strain of mouse, animals develop symptoms similar to SLE as they age. As the animals age and the disease progresses, CRF mRNA in the PVN decreases. Leishmaniasis is a parasitic disease endemic in the Third World that infects the liver. This infection is T-cell mediated as well. Mice infected with *Leischmania donovani* also demonstrate a decrease in CRF mRNA in the PVN. Histocompatible mice that are resistant to infection show no change in CRF mRNA following inoculation with the parasite.

Together, these data demonstrate that this alteration in hypothalamic regulation of the HPA axis in response to the development of T-cell-mediated diseases is an adaptive change. This paradoxical decrease in CRF mRNA occurs irrespective of the nature of the challenge or of the species investigated.

4.3. What Are the Effects of Stress on the Development and Severity of Disease?

The role of stress in relation to disease is a complex one. It is generally accepted that in humans major life events such as the death of a spouse or divorce can precipitate autoimmune disease (e.g., RA, insulin-dependent diabetes, Crohn's disease, uveitis, or Graves' disease) in susceptible individuals or exacerbate symptoms in individuals with preexisting disease. Attempts to investigate these observations in experimental models have been less straightforward. Numerous studies have reported that stress can suppress the development or severity of AA, collagen-induced arthritis, and EAE in the rat. However, other studies have demonstrated an increase in severity and accelerated onset of both collagen-induced arthritis and EAE. These discrepancies may be owing to a number of factors. It is likely that the response is going to be altered depending on the type of stress, its duration, and its frequency. The timing of the stressor in relation to the initiation or onset of the disease is likely to be important as well. Also of relevance is likely to be the coping ability of the animals. As noted, the behavioral responses of rats can influence the severity of disease. What has been less well studied are the immune consequences of the acute stressors that have been employed and the relationship between timing of the stressor and the subsequent immune activation. It is likely that the cytokine profile released in response to stress together with the timing and duration of the anti-inflammatory glucocorticoid release may be crucial.

5. GONADAL STEROIDS

There is a clear link between the HPA axis and the hypothalamic-pituitary-gonadal (HPG) axis. Activation of the HPA axis inhibits the HPG axis at multiple levels, and glucocorticoids also inhibit the tissue effects of sex steroids. Sex steroids are also able to modulate the activity of the HPA axis, reflecting the bidirectional interaction of these systems. The involvement of CRF in the sexually dimorphic response to HPA activation has been proposed because of the estrogen response element in the 5´ regulatory region of the CRF gene. Females (mice, rats, and humans) have a more active HPA axis response than males and are also more prone to autoimmune diseases such as autoimmune thyroiditis (19:1), SLE (9:1), and RA (4:1). These findings suggest that gonadal steroids have a major role in autoimmune disease (Table 2). Gonadal competence may also be a factor because young females are many times more susceptible to RA than young males. With increasing age, the ratio is reduced; under age 60 the ratio is about 3:1, but with later onset the female:male ratio approaches parity. These changes may reflect the decrease in testosterone associated with increasing age in males, and it has been suggested that androgens may have a role in protecting males from developing autoimmune diseases in both humans and animal models. For example, castration increases the incidence, time of onset, and severity of streptococcal cell wall–induced arthritis and AA in

Table 2
Circulating Hormones and Their Effects on Immune Function

Hormone	Effect on inflammation	Effects on the immune system
ACTH	Antiinflammatory?	Receptors present on immune tissues ± effects on lymphocyte proliferation Suppresses antibody production Implicated as growth factor
Glucocorticoids	Antiinflammatory	Receptors present on immune tissues Regulates thymocyte maturation and differentiation Decreases thymic mass Inhibits IL-1 synthesis and secretion Inhibits immunoglobulin production Stimulates neutrophil egress
PRL (also GH)	Proinflammatory	Receptors present on immune tissues Stimulates thymocyte maturation and differentiation Increases thymic mass Immunocompetence compromised by hypophysectomy, returned with hormone replacement
Androgens	Antiinflammatory	Receptors present on immune tissues Immunosuppressive on both T- and B- cells Decrease thymic mass Suppress antibody response Increase TGF-β (inhibitor of Th1-mediated functions)
Estrogens	Pro-/antiinflammatory depending on disease	Receptors present on immune tissues Decrease thymic mass Inhibit suppressive T-cells Facilitate T-helper lymphocyte maturation Stimulate B-cell mediated antibody response
DHEA	Antiinflammatory	DHEA-receptor-binding complex present on tissues Inhibits thymic atrophy induced by glucocorticoids Suppresses IL-6 production Enhances IL-2 production Inhibits formation of autoantibodies

males. These effects can be reversed by testosterone treatment in AA. Serum androgen concentrations are reduced in males and females with RA and also in rats with AA. Female NZB/NZW mice usually die following the development of SLE, but this can be prevented by treatment with the androgen dihydrotestosterone. Intact males have a greater chance of survival, but castration results in increased mortality. In general, it appears that in males castration increases the severity of the disease and this can be suppressed by androgen treatment.

The role of estrogens in the female is complex and appears to depend on the type of disease. In SLE, estrogen accelerates the progress of the disease and the influence of estrogen has been suggested as one of the most important contributors to the female preponderance of the disease. By contrast, estrogen suppresses EAE, collagen-induced arthritis and AA. One suggestion for this apparent discrepancy concerns the effects of estrogen on B- and T-cell-mediated immune responses. Estrogen enhance the antibody response (B-cell), while suppressing cell-mediated immunity (T-cell). EAE, collagen-induced arthritis and AA are all considered to be primarily T-cell-mediated disease models. Testosterone acts to suppress both B- and T-cell responses and, hence, suppresses the severity of disease.

The mechanism(s) and site of action by which the actions of the gonadal steroids are exerted is not fully established. The interactions among the HPA, gonadal, and other neuroendocrine systems is complex. Whether the changes reflect the actions of the gonadal steroids themselves or metabolites is not known. Androgen and estrogen receptors are found on lymphocytes and androgen receptors are also expressed by synovial cells, suggesting the possibility of direct effects at the site of inflammation.

Further evidence supporting the important role of the gonadal steroids comes from observations that changes in activity of autoimmune diseases occur at times of change in gonadal axis function, such as puberty, pregnancy, and menopause and following parturition. At these times the hormonal milieu is dramatically altered with not only changes in the gonadal axis but also with changes in other hormones such as PRL and GH.

6. OTHER NEUROENDOCRINE SYSTEMS

Although the HPA and the gonadal axes are the best studied of the neuroendocrine systems in relation to immune interactions, a number of other hormones have also been implicated.

6.1. Dihydroepiandrostenedione

Dihydroepiandrostenedione (DHEAS) is the most abundant adrenal steroid in the circulation of humans and yet its precise function remains a question of debate. A number of actions on the immune system have been ascribed to DHEAS. Specific receptors for the free hormone (Dihydroepiandrostesterone [DHEA]) are found on T-cells, and DHEA can prevent the action of dexamethasone both in inducing apotosis on thymocytes and in unresponsiveness of peripheral T-cells. DHEA directly enhances proinflammatory Th1 T-cell activity and it has been shown that DHEA sulfatase activity regulates the Th1 and Th2 cytokine balance of mouse lymphoid tissue in response to anti-CD3. DHEA levels fall markedly with aging in all species. DHEA supplements have been shown to correct many of the immunologic deficits seen in aged mice. A fall in serum DHEAS has also been reported to herald the progression of human immunodeficiency virus to aquired immunodeficiency syndrome. These observations have resulted in considerable use of DHEA in heroic concentrations as diet supplements.

Stress, such as examination time for students, results in a marked fall in the ratio of DHEAS to cortisol together with a loss of delayed hypersensitivity but a sparing of humoral immunity. This infers that stress drives a shift in the Th1/Th2 balance away from the proinflammatory Th1 profile toward Th2 and implicates the fall in DHEA as a likely candidate factor in modulating this immunologic change.

6.2. Prolactin

PRL is synthesized and released from the anterior pituitary and is under the inhibitory control of dopamine released from the hypothalamus. PRL receptors have a widespread distribution in neuroendocrine organs as well as in immune tissues. PRL is important for IL-2 activation of T-cells and also stimulates B-cells. The release of PRL from the pituitary can be stimulated by IL-1 and IL-6. PRL is therefore ideally suited to play a role in the bidirectional communication between the neuroendocrine and immune systems. A proinflammatory role for PRL has been proposed in AA. Removal of the pituitary prevents the development of AA in the rat. Implanting the pituitary under the kidney capsule, which results in hyperprolactinemia, or treatment with either exogenous PRL or GH (but not any other pituitary hormones), reinstates the susceptibility. Treatment with bromocriptine, which inhibits PRL release, also prevents AA. It is not clear whether this is a direct or an indirect effect of PRL. What is surprising is that in neither RA nor AA are plasma PRL concentrations altered from controls. There is evidence in AA that treatments that increase the severity of disease are associated with a decrease in circulating PRL, thus opposing the proinflammatory view. It may, however, be the balance between circulating levels of the proinflammatory PRL and antiinflammatory glucocorticoids that has greater relevance.

7. SUMMARY

The interactions of the neuroendocrine and immune systems are complex, more so in relation to autoimmune/inflammatory disease. These interactions can occur at many levels. Cytokines exert effects on immune tissues but, in addition, are able to stimulate the HPA axis, inhibit the gonadal axis, acting both in the brain and on the gonads; suppress thyroid function; suppress appetite; and induce fever. Adrenal and gonadal steroids are important in the regulation of the immune system. Glucocorticoids suppress the host immune response and as such are essential for survival. Other hormones such as PRL, GH, and thyroid hormones are also able to influence the immune system and have been implicated in autoimmune disease and disease models. The recent finding of many neuropeptides and transmitters together with their receptors in the immune tissues and cytokines and their receptors in neuroendocrine tissues, including the brain, has added a further level of complexity. It is becoming evident that there is a complex interaction of a variety of systems that together are able to influence the overall balance regulating the switch from a predominantly proinflammatory (Th1) status to an antiinflammatory (Th2) status. Under normal circumstances this switch occurs on a regular circadian basis between predominantly Th1 and Th2 throughout the day and night. We are only beginning to understand how these systems interact and their implications for disease. Dysregulation of these systems and the loss of the normal circadian rhythms are likely to be of crucial importance. Identifying the initiating factors and their regulation will provide targets for novel therapies.

SELECTED READINGS

Buckingham JC, Cowell A-M, Gillies G, Herbison AE, Steel JH. The neuroendocrine system: anatomy, physiology and responses to stress. In: Buckingham JC, Cowell A-M, Gillies G, eds. *Stress, Stress Hormones and the Immune System*. Chichester, UK: John Wiley & Sons, 1997:9–47.

Chikanza IC. Perturbations of arginine vasopressin secretion during inflammatory stress. Pathophysiologic implications. *Ann NY Acad Sci* 2000;917:825–834.

Elenkov IJ. Systemic stress-induced Th2 shift and its clinical implications. *Int Rev Neurobiol* 2002;52:163–186.

Harbuz M. Neuroendocrinology of autoimmunity. *Int Rev Neurobiol* 2002;52:133–161.

Harbuz MS, Jessop DS. Is there a defect in cortisol production in rheumatoid arthritis? *Rheumatology* 1999;38:298–302.

Harbuz MS, Jessop DS. Stress and inflammatory disease: widening roles for serotonin and substance P. *Stress* 2001;4:57–70.

Li XF, Mitchell JC, Wood S, Coen CW, Lightman SL, O'Byrne KT. The effect of oestradiol and progesterone on hypoglycaemic stress-induced suppression of pulsatile luteinising hormone release and on corticotropin releasing hormone mRNA expression in the rat. *J Neuroendocrinol* 2003;15:468–476.

Lightman SL, Windle RJ, Ma X-M, Harbuz MS, Shanks N, Julian MD, Wood SA, Kershaw YM, Ingram CD. Dynamic control of HPA function and its contribution to adaptive plasticity of the stress response. In: Yamashita Y, et al., eds. *Control Mechanisms of Stress and Emotion: Neuroendocrine-Based Studies*. Amsterdam, The Netherlands: Elsevier, 1999:111–125.

Munck A, Guyre PM, Holbrook NJ. Physiological functions of glucocorticoids in stress and their relation to pharmacological actions. *Endocr Rev* 1984;5:25–44.

Tilders FJ, Schmidt ED, Hoogendijk WJ, Swaab DF. Delayed effects of stress and immune activation. *Baillieres Best Pract Res Clin Endocrinol Metab* 1999;13:523–540.

PART III | INSECTS/PLANTS/COMPARATIVE

9 Insect Hormones

Lawrence I. Gilbert, PhD

CONTENTS

1. INTRODUCTION

Recent estimates place the number of insect species at 2–20 million, more by far than the total of all other animals and plants on Earth. Although insects affect the human condition in a variety of ways, primarily as pollinators, competitors for agricultural products, and vectors of disease, their sheer diversity and numbers make this class of arthropods worthy of study. Indeed, insects have become the model of choice for a variety of research endeavors in genetics, biochemistry, developmental biology, endocrinology, and so forth. Because they are encased in a semirigid exoskeleton (cuticle), insects and other arthropods must shed this cuticle periodically (molt) in order to grow and undergo metamorphosis. Although insect molting and metamorphosis have been scrutinized since the time of Aristotle, the exact control mechanisms have remained elusive. However, research on insect hormones has contributed significantly to the general field of endocrinology.

The now accepted dogma that the nervous system not only controls target organs via action potentials and neurotransmitters, but is also, in a sense, an endocrine system (hence, the term *neuroendocrinology*) was first conceptualized on the basis of data derived from studies on insect development. It was more than eight decades ago that Stefen Kopeć (1922), working on larvae (cat-

erpillars) of the gypsy moth, demonstrated that the insect brain released a substance (hormone) that controls insect molting, i.e., the secretion of a new and larger cuticle, to allow growth, and the digestion and shedding of the old cuticle (ecdysis). When the brain was extirpated 10 d or more after the final larval–larval molt, pupation ensued, and brainless but otherwise normal moths emerged. If brain extirpation occurred <10 d after the last larval molt, the larvae failed to metamorphose to the pupal stage, although they survived for weeks. These and other studies led Kopeć to conclude that the brain liberated some substance into the hemolymph (blood) that is essential for the larval-pupal molt and that it is released about 10 d after the last larval molt. This was the cornerstone of the field of neuroendocrinology.

In the 1930s and 1940s, the giants of the field extended research on this brain factor, and the source of the factor was shown to be specific protocerebral neurosecretory cells. We now know that the brain factor acts on glands in the prothorax of the insect to elicit synthesis and secretion of a steroidal prohormone, an ecdysteroid, that is ultimately responsible for eliciting the molting process. The current name for this neurohormone is prothoracicotropic hormone (PTTH) (Fig. 1).

On the basis of subsequent microsurgical studies, it was shown that glands attached to the brain, the corpora allata, were the source of a hormone (juvenile hormone [JH]) that controls the quality of the molt, i.e., whether

From: *Endocrinology: Basic and Clinical Principles, Second Edition*
(S. Melmed and P. M. Conn, eds.) © Humana Press Inc., Totowa, NJ

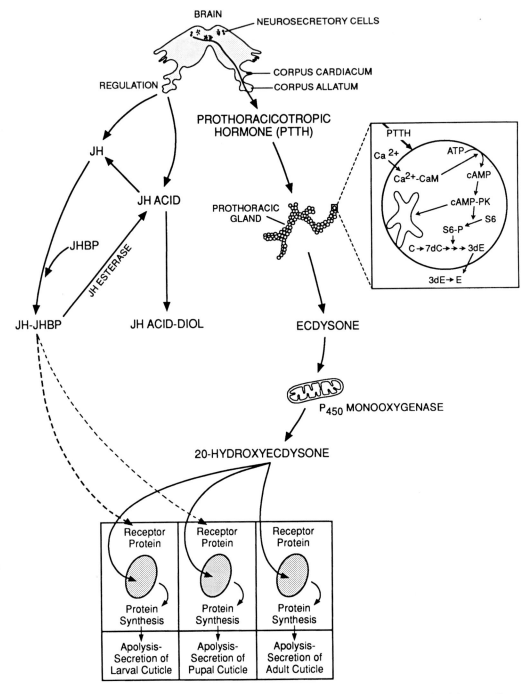

Fig. 1. Endocrine control of metamorphosis. Most of the data contributing to this scheme were derived from studies on silkworms and the tobacco hornworm, *Manduca sexta*, although the scheme applies to all insects in a general sense. Note that in the case of *Manduca*, JH acid rather than JH is released from the corpus allatum toward the end of the last larval stage.

it be larval–larval, larval–pupal, or pupal–adult. Its role is to favor the synthesis of larval (juvenile) structures and inhibit differentiation (metamorphosis) to the pupal and/or adult stages. Although the action of JH is connected to that of the molting hormone and it therefore does not, in a sense, act as an independent agent in con-

trolling growth processes, it does act alone in many adult insects as a gonadotropic hormone. Thus, the three major glands controlling insect growth and development are the brain, prothoracic glands, and corpora allata, their respective secretions being a neuropeptide, a steroid, and sesquiterpenoid compounds (Fig. 2).

A

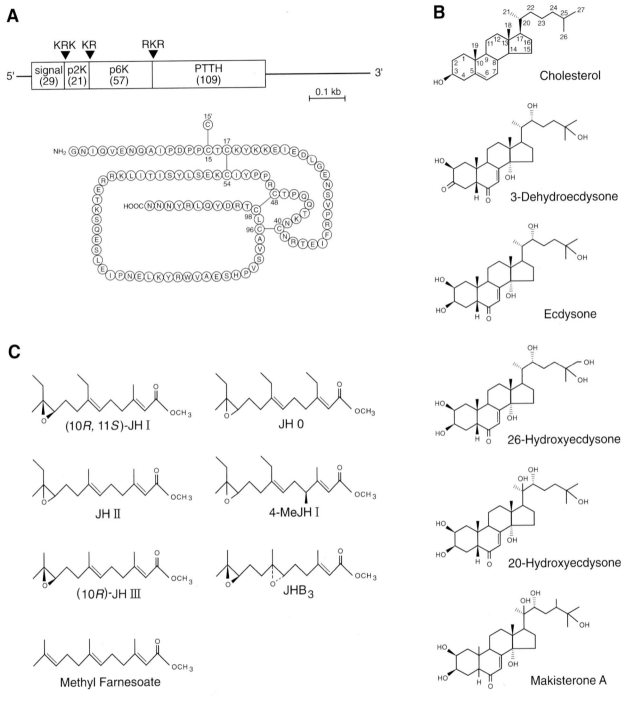

Fig. 2. Hormones and related molecules that play critical roles in control of molting and metamorphosis. (**A**) The structure of *Bombyx* PTTH. The upper diagram indicates the predicted organization of the initial translation product. The lower diagram shows the location of inter- and intracellular disulfide bonds. (**B**) Structure of cholesterol and some major ecdysteroids. (**C**) Structure of various JHs and methyl farnesoate. JH I and JH II are almost entirely restricted to the Lepidoptera, JHB₃ to the cyclorraphan Diptera, whereas JH III is ubiquitous in insects.

Figure 1 is a generalized scheme for the Lepidoptera (moths and butterflies) and the details may not pertain to all insects. Specific neurosecretory cells (the prothoracicotropes) synthesize PTTH as a prohormone that is cleaved to the true PTTH as it is transported along the axons to the corpora allata, where it is stored in axon endings and ultimately released into the hemolymph. Once released, PTTH acts on the prothoracic glands to stimulate ecdysteroid synthesis. In the Lepidoptera, this stimulation results in the enhanced biosynthesis of 3-dehydroecdysone (3dE), which is converted into ecdysone (E) by a hemolymph ketoreductase and from that into 20-hydroxyecdysone (20E) in target cells, 20E being the principal molting hormone of insects. Additionally, as Fig. 1 notes, the corpora allata synthesize and secrete JH, which is bound to a hemolymph-binding protein (JHBP), transported to target tissues, and acts in concert with 20E to determine the quality of the molt. Although this process typifies the endocrine control of molting in most insects, the exact molecular mechanisms are conjectural, although great strides have been made in recent years and are the subject of the remainder of this chapter.

2. PTTH AND PROTHORACIC GLAND ACTIVATION

2.1. Chemistry and Role

Almost all studies on PTTH action have been performed on larvae and pupae of the tobacco hornworm, *Manduca sexta*. This PTTH structure, as well as that of four other lepidopteran PTTHs, has been elucidated by direct sequencing or by deducing the structure after having cloned the gene. The first of these was the PTTH of the commercial silkworm, *Bombyx mori*. After more than 30 yr of study using several million *Bombyx* brains, Ishizaki and Suzuki (1992) purified and characterized the *Bombyx* PTTH (Fig. 2) and showed that it is synthesized as a prohormone of 224 amino acids and then cleaved to form the mature neurohormone, a homodimer (approx 26 kDa) containing inter- and intramonomer disulfide binds, the latter requisite for hormone activity. The *Bombyx* PTTH antibody reacts with putative prothoracicotropes in a variety of insects, including *Manduca* and *Drosophila*, as judged by immunocytochemical and immunogold analyses, but it is physiologically inactive in these species. Thus, there is likely high specificity in the epitopes of the PTTH neuropeptide that are required for interaction with a putative cell membrane receptor in the target glands (i.e., the prothoracic glands).

Correlations have been reported between PTTH levels in the hemolymph and the molting hormone titer for both *Manduca* and *Bombyx* and, in both cases, reflect subsequent increases in the ecdysteroid titer. In *Manduca*, there are two PTTH peaks during the fifth (final) larval stage as well as two ecdysteroid surges. The first is responsible for a small increase in ecdysteroid titer at about d 3.5 of the 9-d fifth instar (stage) when the JH titer is at its nadir and also for a change in commitment (reprogramming), so that when challenged by a larger ecdysteroid surge 4 d later, tar-

get cells respond by synthesizing pupal rather than larval structures. Thus, these two ecdysteriod (and PTTH) peaks are primarily responsible for metamorphosis, and they must be elicited in a very precise manner in the absence of JH. Indeed, the precision of the molting process has contributed significantly to the success enjoyed by insects on this planet during the past half billion years.

The prothoracicotropes apparently receive, directly or indirectly, information from the insect's external (photoperiod, temperature) and internal environment (state of nutrition), and when the appropriate conditions are met, they release PTTH from their termini in the corpus allatum. How and where these influences are sensed and then "transmitted" to the neurons that synthesize PTTH is not known.

2.2. Action via Second-Messenger Systems

The only confirmed targets of PTTH are the paired prothoracic glands, which have been well studied in *Manduca*, each gland composed of about 220 monotypic cells surrounded by a basal lamina. Although no candidate PTTH receptor(s) has yet been reported in the prothoracic glands of any insect, the PTTH-prothoracic gland axis has many similarities to vertebrate steroid hormone–producing pathways, such as the adrenocorticotropic hormone (ACTH)-adrenal gland system. By analogy, it is probable that PTTH binds to a receptor that spans the plasma membrane multiple times, contains an extracellular ligand-binding domain, and has an intracellular domain that binds G protein heterotrimers.

PTTH stimulates increased ecdysteroid production in the prothoracic glands via a cascade of events that has yet to be elucidated completely (Fig. 3). Studies in the 1960s revealed a correlation between circulating ecdysteroid titers and adenylate cyclase activity in the prothoracic gland, suggesting a role for cyclic adenosine monophosphate (cAMP), and also that at some developmental periods a cAMP-independent pathway might be involved. In the *Manduca* prothoracic gland, calcium is clearly pivotal in the response to PTTH. Glands incubated in Ca^{2+}-free medium with a calcium chelator or a calcium channel blocker exhibit a greatly attenuated production of cAMP and ecdysteroids in response to PTTH. More recent studies have implicated the mobilization of internal as well as external Ca^{2+} stores in the PTTH response and have demonstrated a striking rise in the Ca^{2+} levels of prothoracic gland cells within a few seconds of PTTH administration in vitro.

Composite observations suggest that PTTH-dependent cAMP production by prothoracic glands is generated by a Ca^{2+}-calmodulin-sensitive adenylate cyclase.

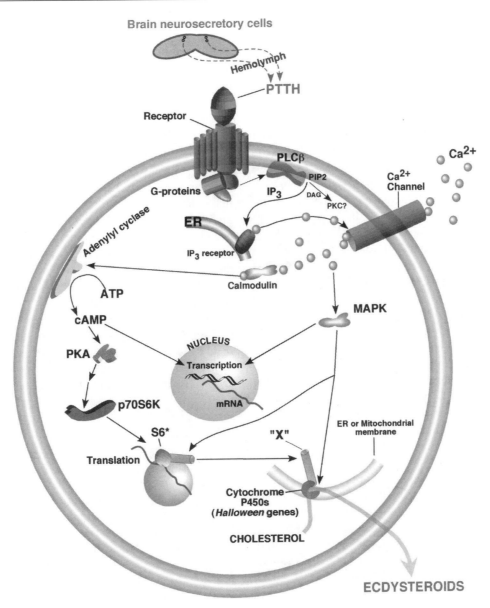

Fig. 3. A signal transductory cascade in the prothoracic glands of *M. sexta* is elicited by PTTH and results in enhanced synthesis and secretion of ecdysteroid, namely, 3-dehydroecdysone. ER = Endoplasmic reticulum; IP_3 = inositol triphosphate; PLCβ = phospholipase Cβ; PIP2 = phosphatidylinositol-4,5-bisphosphate; DAG = diacylglycerol; PKC = protein kinase C; ATP = adenosine triphosphate. (Graphics by R. Rybczynski reproduced with permission.)

The interaction between calmodulin and G protein (presumably $G_{s\alpha}$) is complicated and varies during the final instar. In the first half of this period, calmodulin activates prothoracic gland adenylate cyclase and facilitates G protein activation of adenylate cyclase. Subsequently, prothoracic gland G protein activation of adenylate cyclase is refractory to the presence of calmodulin in such assays. Calcium still apparently plays a role in the PTTH transductory cascade after the first half of the fifth instar, since incubation of pupal glands in Ca^{2+}-free medium inhibits PTTH-stimulated ecdysteroidogenesis, and higher levels of Ca^{2+}-calmodulin can still activate adenylate cyclase in prothoracic gland membrane preparations. Regardless of the complicated, developmentally dynamic relationships among calcium, calmodulin, G proteins, and adenylate cyclase, it is clear that PTTH elicits increased cAMP formation in prothoracic glands leading to activation of a cAMP-dependent protein kinase (protein kinase A [PKA]) and subsequent protein phosphorylation.

PTTH-stimulated PKA activity appears to be necessary for PTTH-stimulated ecdysteroidogenesis, because such ecdysteroid synthesis by prothoracic glands challenged with a PKA-inhibiting cAMP analog is substantially inhibited. Several PTTH-dependent protein phosphorylations have been described for *Manduca* prothoracic glands including a mitogen-activated protein kinase (MAPK), such as extracellular-regulated kinase (ERK), as well as S6 kinase, the most striking and consistent of these phosphoproteins being the ribosomal protein S6, the phosphorylation of which has been correlated with increased translation of specific mRNAs in several mammalian cell types. In *Manduca*, rapamycin inhibits both PTTH-stimulated S6 phosphorylation and ecdysteroidogenesis, suggesting that S6 is an integral player in the PTTH transductory cascade. Consistent with this view are the observations that PTTH-stimulated S6 phosphorylation can be readily detected before the PTTH-stimulated increase in ecdysteroid synthesis occurs and that S6 is phosphorylated multiple times in a dose- and time-dependent manner.

Over the last several years, a number of studies have revealed that PTTH preparations or cAMP analogs stimulate general protein synthesis in the *Manduca* prothoracic gland via a branch of the transductory cascade that is distinct from that leading to the activation of ecdysteroidogenesis. PTTH may, therefore, modulate or control the growth status of the prothoracic gland, perhaps independently of its ability to elicit ecdysteroidogenesis, and could play a role in regulating the levels of ecdysteroidogenic enzymes, analogous to peptide regulation of enzymes responsible for vertebrate steroid hormone synthesis. Additional factors, such as JH, could determine whether PTTH stimulates or inhibits gland growth, ecdysteroid synthesis, or both.

Protein synthesis is required for ACTH stimulation of steroidogenesis in the adrenal cortex as well as for the *Manduca* prothoracic gland response to PTTH. It is therefore likely that in both the adrenal cortex and prothoracic glands, the phosphorylation state of ribosomal S6 is critical to the relationship between protein synthesis and steroidogenesis. Presumably, the PKA-promoted multiple phosphorylation of ribosomal S6 imparts information to the translational machinery to synthesize specific proteins, which, in turn, regulate some rate-limiting step in ecdysteroid biosynthesis.

An interesting outcome of this work is the close analogy observed between control of the insect and mammalian steroidogenic systems. It is obviously a "successful" system in an evolutionary sense, since insects appeared on Earth several hundred million years before mammals, and the ancestors of both groups diverged at least

100 million yr before that. Although it is interesting that such divergent groups of animals use the same types of molecules as hormones (peptides, steroids), it is extraordinary that they regulate the synthesis of their steroid hormones in an almost identical manner.

3. ECDYSTEROIDS
3.1. Structure-Activity Relationships

That ecdysteroids, particularly 20E, elicit the molt is no longer in question and has been established as a central dogma of the field. What may not be so obvious is that in contrast to vertebrate systems, almost the entire insect is the target of ecdysteroids, e.g., regulation of the growth of motor neurons, control of choriogenesis, stimulation of the growth and development of imaginal disks, initiation of the breakdown of larval structures during metamorphosis, and induction of the deposition of cuticle by the epidermis.

Just recently microarray and computational analyses demonstrated that the 20E regulatory network reaches far beyond the molting process in *Drosophila melanogaster*. The data are based on mutations of the 20E (EcR) receptor and indicate that in the metamorphosis of the midgut, genes that encode a variety of factors are activated by this network and that genes involved in cell cycling are also dependent on 20E for their activation.

It is fitting that recent breakthroughs on the mechanism of action of ecdysteroids (*see* Section 3.3.) were accomplished using *Drosophila*, because it was a bioassay developed with another fly that was so well utilized for the initial crystallization of E and then 20E four decades ago. Since that time, a host of ecdysteroids (Fig. 2B), their precursors, and their metabolites have been identified. We know that the *cis*-A-B ring junction is essential for molting hormone activity regardless of whether a hydrogen atom or a hydroxyl group is the 5β substituent, as is the 6-oxo-7-ene system in the B ring. The 3β- and 14α-hydroxyl groups are required for high activity in vivo, whereas the presence or absence of hydroxyls at C-2, C-5, or C-11 does not appear to affect biologic activity. The only essential feature of the side chain appears to be the $22\beta_F$-hydroxyl.

Although E was the first of the ecdysteroids to be crystallized and characterized and thought to be the insect molting hormone 40 yr ago, it is actually converted into the principal molting hormone, 20E, by tissues peripheral to the prothoracic glands (Fig. 1), a reaction mediated by an E 20-monooxygenase. In some insects, particularly the Lepidoptera, as exemplified by *Manduca*, the major if not sole ecdysteroid synthesized and secreted by the prothoracic glands is 3dE (Fig. 2B), which is converted into E by a ketoreductase in the hemolymph, with the resulting E then hydroxylated to 20E in target tissues.

3.2. Biosynthesis

In most organisms, every carbon atom in cholesterol (Fig. 2B) is derived from either the methyl-or carboxylol-carbon of acetate, but insects (and other arthropods) are incapable of this synthesis owing to one or more metabolic blocks between acetate and cholesterol. Thus, sterols are required in the diet.

The first step in the conversion of cholesterol into E via 3dE is the stereospecific removal of the 7β-hydrogen to form 7-dehydrocholesterol (7dC), a sterol relegated to the prothoracic glands of *Manduca* and other Lepidoptera. This cholesterol 7,8-desaturating activity in the prothoracic glands of *Manduca* is cytochrome P-450 dependent, perhaps via 7β-hydrocholesterol. When [^{3}H]7dC is incubated with prothoracic glands in vitro, there is excellent conversion into both 3dE and E, with the kinetics of conversion highly dependent on developmental stage and experimental paradigm. The desaturation to 7dC is probably not PTTH dependent, but the neuropeptide (via S6) may initiate the modulation of enzyme activity responsible for the transformation of 7dC to the next, yet unidentified sterol in the E biosynthetic pathway.

There are a number of postulated intermediates between 7dC and 3dE, such as 5α-sterol intermediates, 3-oxo-Δ^4 intermediates, and Δ^7-5α-6α-epoxide intermediates, but their intermediacy remains conjectural. By contrast, more is known about the terminal hydroxylations necessary for the synthesis of the polyhydroxylated ecdysteroids. The enzymes responsible for mediating the hydroxylations at C-2, C-22, and C-25 appear to be classic cytochrome P-450 enzymes, the former two being mitochondrial and the latter microsomal. The sequence of hydroxylation is C-25, C-22, and C-2.

Very recently, studies on a series of *Drosophila* embryonic lethal mutations have allowed the cloning and characterization of those genes encoding the P-450 enzymes responsible for the terminal hydroxylations leading to the production of E and the monooxygenase that mediates the conversion of E into 20E (Gilbert, 2004). In those studies, advantage was taken of the availability of the fly database (*Drosophila* genome project), and the fact that these so-called Halloween genes (*disembodied, shade, shadow, phantom*) were mapped in the 1980s to specific chromosome loci, and had been shown to regulate embryonic processes that may be attributed to low titers of molting hormone. By identifying these genes in the fly database, sequencing them, transfecting coding regions into a cell line, and using these cell lines for more classic biochemical

analysis, all four genes that encode P-450 enzymes that mediate the last four hydroxylations in 20E biosynthesis have been identified and characterized (see the structure of cholesterol and 20E in Fig. 2B; hydroxylations at C-2, C-20, C-22, and C-25).

Once formed, 3dE is converted into E through the mediation of a hemolymph ketoreductase in the Lepidoptera, and the E is then transformed into 20E at peripheral (target) tissues. In the case of flies such as *Drosophila*, the prothoracic gland cells produce E rather than 3dE, and the intermediary step mediated by the ketoreductase is not needed in these insects. The evolutionary significance of this difference in the product of the prothoracic gland cells is not known. The complete biosynthetic scheme has not been elucidated owing to the difficulty of identifying the extremely short-lived intermediates from minute quantities of tissues and the less than handful of laboratories actively engaged in such investigations; however, perhaps with an extension of the paradigms utilized for the a forementioned Halloween genes, the details of the complete E biosynthetic pathway may be known in the near future. Without the entire sequence of reactions in hand, it is not yet possible to identify those rate-limiting reactions that may be controlled by hormones (PTTH), neuromodulators, or the nervous system.

3.3. Ecdysteroid Receptors

Several cell types in the higher flies and other insects contain polytene (giant) chromosomes, whose structure and ease of examination led to the field of *Drosophila* cytogenetics. At specific developmental stages, discrete regions of these chromosomes undergo puffing, a phenomenon now known to be the morphologic manifestation of gene activity, i.e., mRNA synthesis. Forty-four years ago Clever and Karlson (1960) showed that 20E could elicit a stage-specific puffing pattern in the salivary gland chromosomes of the midge *Chironomus tentans*, the first unequivocal demonstration that steroid hormones act at the level of the gene. This discovery was followed by an exhaustive analysis of salivary gland polytene chromosome puffing during the development of *Drosophila* by Ashburner and colleagues, which involved the testing of E and 20E on the puffing pattern. This led to the "Ashburner Model" of ecdysteroid hormone action. In this model, an intracellular receptor-20E complex elicits elevated transcription of "early puff" genes and, at the same time, represses the transcription of the "late puff" genes. Subsequently, the gene products of the "early puff" genes act on the "late puff" genes to stimulate transcriptional activity while feeding back on the "early puff" genes, resulting in puff regression. This model

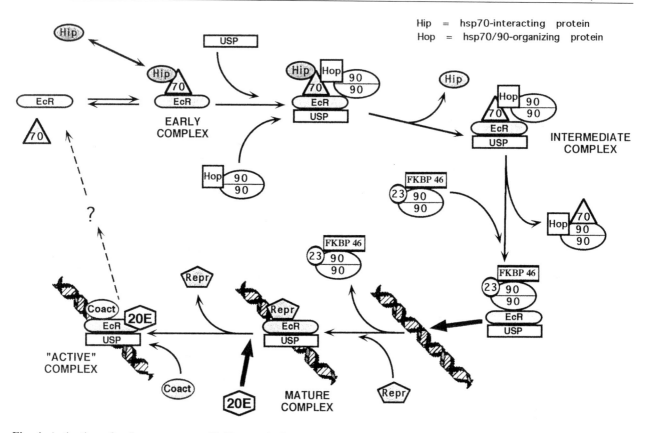

Fig. 4. Activation of ecdysone receptor (EcR), mostly factual but some theoretical (e.g., hsp 90). (Graphics by R. Rybczynski reproduced with permission.)

has withstood the test of time, and several of the "early puff" gene products have been shown to be transcription factors and members of the steroid/thyroid hormone receptor superfamily (nuclear receptor superfamily; *see* Chapters 2 and 4). Indeed, one gene product, E75, was the probe utilized that led to the isolation of the *Drosophila* ecdysone receptor gene (*EcR*) by the Hogness Laboratory a few years ago.

The gene product of *EcR* binds to the proper response elements and to radiolabeled ecdysteroid but requires a heterodimeric partner to fulfill its function (Fig. 4). This critical element is also a member of the nuclear receptor superfamily, ultraspiracle (*Usp*), which is the *Drosophila* homolog of retinoid × receptor (RXR) which forms heterodimers with a variety of mammalian hormones. The *Drosophila* heterodimer is stabilized by endogenous 20E, and there are indications that the application of exogenous hormone will increase the amount or affinity of EcR in target cells, although it is not known if this effect is at the level of transcription or translation.

It is of interest that EcR exists in at least three isoforms that differ from one another in the transactivation domain, and there is some tissue and developmental specificity, although the exact reason for the existence of isoforms remains conjectural. Their presence certainly suggests that there are as yet unidentified *trans*-acting factors with roles in ecdysteroid action. Indirect evidence also suggests that EcR is not monogamous (i.e., can form heterodimeric relationships with gene products other than Usp). Finally, there is a plethora of data indicating that 20E is not the only ecdysteroid with molting hormone activity, and that certain prohormones and "metabolites" of 20E may be hormones in their own right and perhaps interact with specific isoforms of EcR in the EcR-USP complex. As in the field of steroid hormone receptors in general, little is known about the "docking" of the ecdysteroid-receptor complex with the hormone response element and enhanced gene activity in the form of specific mRNA synthesis (puffing).

4. JUVENILE HORMONES
4.1. Chemistry

The development of structures that distinguish adult forms from larval forms is regulated by a complex interaction between JH and the ecdysteroids. The JHs are a unique group of sesquiterpenoid compounds that have been identified definitively only in insects (Fig. 2C) and one plant species, although their structural proximity to retinoids is obvious. At least six JHs have been identified from various insect orders (Fig. 2C). JH III appears to occur in all orders and is the principal product of the corpus allatum in most, with the notable exceptions of the Lepidoptera, in which JH I and JH II may have significant roles, and the Diptera. In *Drosophila*, the bisepoxide of JH III, JHB$_3$, is predominant and the sole JH in some species of flies.

The absolute configurations of the epoxide group of only some of the JHs have been resolved (Fig. 2). There are chiral centers at the 10 position of JH III and at the 10 and 11 positions of the other JHs. In addition, JHB$_3$ from Diptera possesses two chiral centers, at positions 6, 7, and 10. At present, the absolute configurations are known only for JH I, 4-Me-JH I, JHB$_3$, and JH III. This is important because the unnatural enantiomers appear to be less biologically active or are degraded at different rates by esterolytic enzymes than are the natural enantiomers.

JH acids are also produced by the corpora allata of *Manduca* larvae. The glands lose their ability to methylate JH I and II acid during the final larval stage as a result of the disappearance or inactivation of the methyl transferase enzyme, and thus produce large quantities of these JH acids, which are released into the hemolymph (*see* Section 4.3., discussion of methoprene acid).

4.2. Biosynthesis and Degradation

The JHs are synthesized in the corpora allata from acetate (JH III) and/or propionate (higher JH homologs). The biosynthetic pathway for JH III is identical to that for vertebrate sterol biosynthesis until the production of farnesyl pyrophosphate. As noted previously, insects do not produce cholesterol and related steroids *de novo*; rather, JH is the product of this pathway. It is noteworthy that there is significant sequence similarity between the HMGCoA reductase, the enzyme responsible for the conversion of HMGCoA into mevalonate, of the insect corpus allatum and that of vertebrate liver, a principal site of *de novo* sterol biosynthesis, suggesting that this pathway to farnesyl pyrophosphate is of ancient origin.

The formation of the side chains in the "modified" homologs involves differential utilization of substrates, including propionate and acetate, to give rise to both C-5 and C-6 pyrophosphate intermediates. Condensation of two C-6 units plus one C-5 unit results in the formation of JH I, whereas that of one C-6 unit plus two C-5 units produces JH II.

The hemolymph JH titer must reflect both the rate of production and the rate of degradation. This estimate is clouded by the presence of JH-specific-binding proteins in the hemolymph, whose function has been hypothesized to be the protection of JH from degradation by both general and specific hemolymph esterases. JH-specific epoxide hydrolases, capable of hydrating the epoxide function to the diol, also play a role in the catabolism of JH.

4.3. Postulated Action

The JH titer is believed to be the primary endocrine factor influencing the "quality" of developmental events during metamorphosis (e.g., in Lepidoptera, the nature of the molt-larval-larval, larval-pupal, or pupal-adult) (Fig. 1). It is generally assumed that the absence (or near absence) of JH is required for metamorphosis in holometabolous insects (Fig. 1). Therefore, JH defines the outcome of molts, both metamorphic and nonmetamorphic, and can therefore be regarded as the metamorphic hormone of insects.

Although there are still no unequivocal data showing the existence of a JH receptor, there is a multitude of observations that JH can modulate larval and pupal gene activity elicited by the molting hormone (i.e., does not act in the absence of ecdysteroids). There is increasing evidence that JH also acts at the level of the cell membrane via a classic second-messenger system (*see* Chapter 3), as it modulates the uptake of vitellogenin from the hemolymph into the developing oocyte. Therefore, JH may have multivalent roles and modes of action, as does, e.g., progesterone. In preadult stages, JH has an obvious role in preventing precocious development and eliciting larval or pupal syntheses. The prevailing opinion is that JH acts as a "competency determinant;" that is, it affects the target cell's competence to respond to 20E. The mechanism by which JH accomplishes this task is unknown, but it is surely one of the most intriguing problems in endocrinology and developmental biology. Further, very recent work has established that a well-known JH analog, methoprene, as well as its acid metabolite, can activate RXR in vertebrate cells, but that only the metabolite can bind RXR, indicating that methoprene must be metabolized before it is active in this system. This suggests that perhaps in the case of JH, it is a metabolite (JH acid?) that binds to the receptor, whereas past failures in the search for a receptor utilized the native JH.

5. CONCLUSION

In this abbreviated review, only the essence of the field could be discussed, and there was no opportunity to detail the >50 peptide hormones or hormone-like peptides that have been described in recent years, several of which appear to be identical to vertebrate hormones (e.g., insulin) and others that deal with a variety of homeostatic mechanisms (e.g., hypo- and hypergly-cemic, hypolipemic, adipokinetic). For the most part, every vertebrate peptide hormone has an immunocyto-chemically similar (or identical) counterpart in insects, as have estrogens, progesterone, and so on. Therefore, these hormones that play such strategic roles in the life of higher organisms were "discovered" by insects or ancestors of the insects. Thus, the hormones, second-messenger systems, receptor mechanisms, neuroendo-crine axis, biosynthetic mechanisms, and so forth are all of very ancient lineage, and their basic essence has been well preserved. With the current use of a genetic organism (*Drosophila*) to study endocrine paradigms, we can look forward to future findings that should allow insights into the myriad of endocrine mechanisms that have survived severe evolutionary pressures.

ACKNOWLEDGMENTS

I thank Megan Edwards for clerical work, Susan Whitfield for reproducing the figures, and Dr. Robert Rybczynski for the graphics for Figs. 3 and 4.Research from the Gilbert Laboratory was supported by grants from the National Science Foundation and the National Institutes of Health. The Halloween gene work is being supported by NSF grant IBN 0130825.

REFERENCES

Clever U, Karlson P. Induktion von Puff Veränderungen in der Speicheldrüsenchromosomen von *Chironomus tentans* durch ecdson. *Exp Cell Res* 1960;20:623–626.

Gilbert LI, Iatrou K, Gill S, eds. *Comprehensive Molecular Insect Science*, vol. 3. Amsterdam, The Netherlands: Elsevier, 2004.

Gilbert LI, Rybczynski R, Tobe S. Endocrine cascade in insect metamorphosis. In: Gilbert LI, Tata JR, Atkinson BG, eds. *Metamorphosis: Post-Embryonic Reprogramming of Gene Expres-sion in Amphibian and Insect Cells*. San Diego, CA: Academic, 1996:59–107.

Ishizaki H, Suzuki A. Brain secretory peptides of the silkmoth *Bombyx mori*: prothoracicotropic hormone and bombyxin. In: Joose J, Buijs RM, Tilders FJH, eds. *Progress in Brain Research*, vol. 92, Amsterdam, The Netherlands: Elsevier, 1992:1–14.

Kopec´ S. Studies on the necessity of the brain for the inception of insect metamorphosis. *Biol Bull* 1922;42:323–342.

Li T-R, White KP. Tissue-specific gene expression and ecdysone-regulated genomic networks in *Drosophila*. *Dev Cell* 2003; 5:59–71.

SELECTED READINGS

Gilbert LI. Halloween genes encode P450 enzymes that mediate steroid hormone biosynthesis in *Drosophila melanogaster*. *Mol Cell Endocrinol*. 2004;215:1–10.

Gilbert LI, Combest WL, Smith WA, Meller VH, Rountree DB. Neuropeptides, second messengers and insect molting. *BioEssays* 1988;8:153–157.

Gilbert LI, Rybczynski R, Warren JT. Control and biochemical nature of the ecdysteroidogenic pathway. *Ann.Rev. Entomology* 2002;47,883–916.

Harmon MA, Boehm MF, Heyman RA, Mangelsdorf DJ. Activation of mammalian retinoid x receptors by the insect growth regulator methoprene. *Proc Natl Acad Sci USA* 1995;92:615–619.

Henrich V, Rybczynski R, Gilbert LI. Peptide hormones, steroid hormones and puffs: Mechanisms and models in insect develop-ment. In: Litwack G., ed. *Vitamins and Hormones*, vol. 55. San Diego, CA: Academic, 1999:73–125.

Koelle MR, Talbot WS, Segraves WA, Bender MT, Cherbas P, Hogness DS. The *Drosophila* EcR gene encodes an ecdysone receptor, a new member of the steroid receptor superfamily. *Cell* 1991;67:59–77.

Riddiford LM. Cellular and molecular actions of juvenile hormone. I. General considerations and prematamorphic actions. *Adv Insect Physiol* 1994; 24:213–274.

Song Q, Gilbert LI. Multiple phosphorylation of ribosomal protein S6 and specific protein synthesis are required for prothor-acicotropic hormone-stimulated ecdysteroid biosynthesis in the prothoracic glands of *Manduca sexta*. *Insect Biochem Mol Biol* 1995;25:591–602

10 Phytohormones and Signal Transduction Pathways in Plants

William Teale, PhD, Ivan Paponov, PhD, Olaf Tietz, PhD, and Klaus Palme, PhD

CONTENTS

INTRODUCTION

Since the divergence of plants and animals about 1.5 billion yr ago, the signal transduction pathways in both kingdoms have been subjected to very different selection pressures. These fundamental differences have influenced the evolution of both the signaling molecules themselves and the mechanisms by which signals are relayed. Among these differences, a plant's ability to continuously form new organs during its postembryonic development, the increased frequency of high degrees of both ploidy and gene duplication in many higher plants, and the multicellular haploid gametophytes of more primitive plants could be particularly significant. Particular developmental processes, such as totipotency (the ability of a plant to regenerate itself from vegetative tissue), have enabled

plants to increase their reproductive potential and are consequences of the idiosyncrasies of a plant's cellular signaling mechanisms.

2. SIGNAL TRANSDUCTION PATHWAYS OF PLANTS

The emergence of complete genome sequences from strategic eukaryotic models has allowed the comparative analysis of plant and animal signal transduction pathways. In both cases, this analysis has offered insight into the features of specific signaling pathways that were not achievable at the time the previous edition of this book was published. It is now hoped that by looking closely at the emerging differences between analogous signaling pathways in plants and animals, it will be possible to identify their relationship to the divergence of the two lineages. Excellent recent reviews on this

From: *Endocrinology: Basic and Clinical Principles, Second Edition*
(S. Melmed and P. M. Conn, eds.) © Humana Press Inc., Totowa, NJ

topic have been published over the past 5 yr (Cock et al., 2002; Wendehenne et al., 2001). Here we give a brief overview of selected examples in order to illustrate some interesting features of plant signaling pathways and then discuss these pathways in the context of novel developments in plant evolution.

As a result of photoautotrophism, the evolution of plants has been constrained by the absence of mobility and the presence of relatively rigid cell walls. The capture and integration of chloroplasts from bacterial progenitors profoundly influenced the signaling mechanisms of modern plants. Not surprisingly, for sessile photosynthetic organisms able to sense carefully their fluctuating environment, the developmental pathways of plants are irrevocably and necessarily linked to the perception of external cues. Temperature, light, touch, water, and gravity can all activate endogenous developmental programs. Of these, light has an especially important role, not only as the energy source for photosynthesis, but also as a stimulus for many developmental processes throughout the life cycle of plants, from seed germination to flowering. Consequently, plants have the richest array of light-sensing mechanisms of any group of organisms. These photoreceptors are able to measure not only the intensity but also the quality of light available to the plant. Phytochromes, e.g., are the photoreceptors for red and far-red light responses (Nagy and Schäfer, 2002). They are red-light-activated serine/threonine kinases that exist in two photointerconvertible forms. On stimulation with red light, they move from the cytosol to the nucleus, where they interact with proteins such as the helix-loop-helix transcription factor phytochrome-interacting factor (PIF3; Martinez-Garcia et al., 2000). These proteins then bind to light-responsive promoter elements leading to transcription, thereby achieving light-regulated gene activation (Tyagi and Gaur, 2003). Thus, phytochrome signaling involves both nuclear and cytosolic interactions.

Comparative genomic analysis of plant genomes from species such as *Arabidopsis thaliana* (thale cress) and *Oryza sativa* (rice) has revealed many signaling compounds that are highly conserved between animals and plants. The reiteration of core signaling mechanisms in plants and animals suggests that overall differences between the two kingdoms evolved via the modification of basic ancestral pathways. However, this basic similarity is found in combination with many novel elements or motifs. Overall organizational principles are shared among plants and animals, indicating that a core of conserved signaling genes and pathways is used repeatedly in many different developmental contexts. *RAS* genes are a good example to illustrate this argument. *RAS* genes belong to the small guanosine

5′-triphosphatase protein family. They are master regulators of numerous cellular processes including signaling, cargo transport, and nuclear transport. They are regarded as molecular switches that alternate between an active and an inactive state, thereby ensuring the flow of information at the expense of guanosine 5′-triphosphate. This molecular switch appears to have been developed early, and throughout evolution, it has been adapted to a variety of tasks. Small G proteins are classified in five families: the RAS (according to the oncogene Ras from <u>ra</u>t <u>s</u>arcoma virus), the RAB (<u>Ras</u> <u>o</u>f <u>b</u>rain), the ARF (<u>A</u>DP <u>r</u>ibosylation <u>f</u>actor), the RAN (<u>Ra</u>s-related <u>n</u>uclear protein), and the RHO (<u>Ra</u>s <u>ho</u>mologous) family. They interact with partner proteins (effectors) to form dynamic complexes regulating a plethora of crucial cellular processes. In plants, however, no *RAS* genes, but only members of the *RAB*, *ARF*, and the *RAN* families have been found. An additional plant-specific family of small G proteins is named ROP, for <u>R</u>HO <u>o</u>f <u>p</u>lants (Vernoud et al., 2003). Apparently, only members of those families that play intricate roles in metabolite transport and cell polarity control have been conserved in plants. It is conceivable that the sessile nature of plants demands tight control over secretory pathways to enable and precisely adjust the cell elongation processes. In this case, homeostatic control of cellular membrane compartments, transport of macromolecules between intracellular compartments and the extracellular space, and nuclear transport would have added importance for the evolutionary success of plants.

Despite conservation of the basic secretory machinery between plants and other eukaryotes, several recent findings suggest distinct structural and functional differences in plants. It is therefore expected that the systematic functional analysis of key players of plant secretion will uncover novel insights into the processes by which the formation of transport vesicles and intracellular trafficking by internal and external cues are controlled, and by which vesicles are delivered to target membranes.

Ultimately, from analysis of these processes, researchers will learn important lessons on how plant cells control apical and basal cell polarity. Moreover, such approaches will not only uncover important aspects of the organizational blueprint of the plant secretory pathway, but also reveal fundamental functional differences between plants and other eukaryotes and indicate how these differences relate specifically to the relationship between form and function in plants. Analysis of the plant cargo delivery system provides privileged views not just into unique aspects of secretion control, but also into many other plant-specific processes, such as hor-

Growth factor	Structure	Active concentration	Site of synthesis	Transport	Biological response
Auxin (IAA)	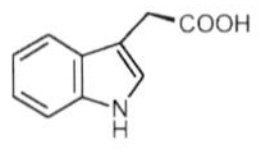	10^{-11} M – 10^{-5} M	meristems, leaf primordia, developing seeds	phloem, cell to cell	cell division, elongation and differentiation, rooting, repression of lateral bud growth, leaf senescence, fruit development, gravitropism, phototropism
Gibberellin (GA$_4$)	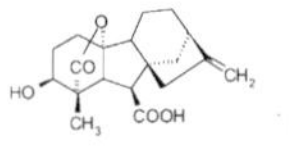	10^{-6} M – 10^{-5} M	young shoot tissue, developing seeds	phloem, xylem	shoot elongation, flower initiation, seed germination,
Cytokinin (trans-zeatin)	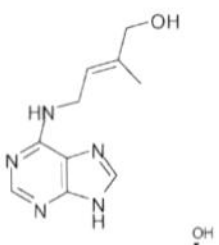	10^{-8} M – 10^{-5} M	root tips, developing seeds	xylem	cell division and differentiation, shooting, growth of lateral buds, delay of leaf senescence, fruit development, chloroplast development, morphogenesis
Brassinosteroid (BR)	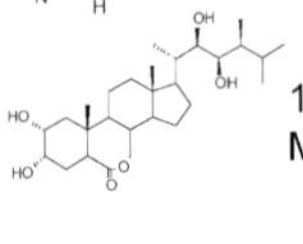	10^{-11} M – 10^{-5} M	most tissues	diffusion	cell division and elongation, leaf bending, inhibition of root growth, differentiation of vascular tissue
Abscisic acid	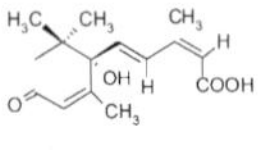	10^{-9} M – 10^{-7} M	mature leaves, roots	phloem, xylem	senescence, water stress, inhibition of shoot growth, defence gene activation upon wounding induction of storage protein synthesis in seeds

Fig. 1. Phytohormones: chemical structure and properties.

monal control of growth, gravitropic and phototropic responses, establishment and maintenance of cell polarity, cell differentiation, mediation of disease resistance, and fruit ripening. In the long term, insight into these fundamental processes will be important for many biotechnological applications.

3. ROLE OF PHYTOHORMONES

Auxin, cytokinin, abscisic acid (ABA), gibberellin (GA), and ethylene are the five classic hormone pathways that appear very early in plant evolution and have been adapted to functional uses in many contexts of plant development (Fig. 1). Brassinosteroids are a relatively recent addition to this list, but must also be considered as potent plant growth regulators. These phytohormones are secondary metabolites that play physiological roles at specific stages of a plant's lifecycle. They are typically considered in terms of three sequential events: their biosynthesis, their perception, and the signals that are subsequently initiated as a consequence. The effects of a phytohormone are commonly demonstrated either by their exogenous application to a growing plant, or by the inhibition or exaggeration of their influence in mutant plants. Such plants may be affected in the rate of biosynthesis of a particular hormone, in the sensing of a hormone's presence, or in the subsequent transduction of a downstream signaling cascade. Phytohormones represent integral components of the mechanisms by which a plant regulates both its own

development and its response to the wide variety of stimuli it receives from its environment. Since Charles and Francis Darwin first attributed the bending of a grass coleoptile toward light to the action of a growth mediator, research into the biosynthesis and mode of action of phytohormones has developed into one of the most widely studied aspects of plant biology (Davies, 1995).

We now give an overview of the current understanding of both how higher (seed-bearing) plants perceive phytohormones and how this perception is translated into a physiological response. Plants, owing to their sessile nature, cannot move autonomously in response to environmental stimuli in the same way as many animals can. As already inferred, this restraint has been overcome, at least in part, by the extension of the role of hormones from that of regulator (either metabolic or developmental) into the means by which a response to environmental stimuli are elicited. For example, Darwin's first experiments on coleoptile bending represent the attempt of a young grass shoot to increase its photosynthetic capacity. It was subsequently demonstrated that the response is mediated by production of indole-acetic acid (IAA) (a member of the auxin class of phytohormones) in the shoot tip, followed by asymmetrical redistribution throughout the growing plant. Cells respond to the concentration of IAA by elongating in a dose-responsive manner, producing a physiologic response.

4. AUXINS

Auxins are vital mediators of developmental and physiological responses in plants and a paradigm for plant growth regulators. They regulate apical-basal polarity in embryonic development; apical dominance in shoots; induction of lateral and adventitious roots; vascular tissue differentiation; and cell growth in both stems and coleoptiles, including the asymmetric growth associated with phototropic and gravitropic responses (Davies, 1995).

Concentration, perception, and the effect that signaling has on gene expression are central issues when considering the phytohormone signaling pathways that affect growth and regulation. In relation to auxin, it has been suggested that efflux-mediated gradients are the underlying driving force for the formation of all plant organs, regardless of their developmental origin and fate. An attractive theory is therefore that the relative concentration of auxin is particularly important in plant development. Both the concentration of auxin in any one cell and the steepness of the auxin concentration gradient over a group of cells are determined by the rate of auxin synthesis in source cells, the rate of its transport through a tissue, and the overall rate of its degradation or conjugation (the majority of auxin present in any one cell exists as biologically inactive conjugate).

Auxin is transported from the shoot downward. However, the prevailing model of the initiation of auxin gradients in the apical meristem has been questioned by the demonstration that all parts of young plants can synthesize IAA, thus potentially diminishing the importance of polar auxin transport (Ljung et al., 2001).

In the 1920s, Cholodny and Went independently suggested the chemiosmotic hypothesis of auxin transport, which was later refined by Rubery and Sheldrake (1974) and Raven (1975). The theory predicts the existence of an auxin efflux carrier that actively and asymmetrically redistributes auxin in root and stem tissue on gravitropic or phototropic stimulation.

Auxin movement both into and out of cells requires specialized carriers (Friml and Palme, 2002). Several Arabidopsis genes encoding putative auxin carriers have been identified during the past decade. The amino acid permease-like gene *AUX1* and the family of bacterial transporter-like *PIN* genes encode putative auxin influx (Bennett et al., 1996) and efflux carriers, respectively. Characterization of the first putative auxin efflux carrier PIN1 (Gälweiler et al., 1998) gave context to auxin's asymmetric localization. PIN1 encodes a 622-amino-acid protein with 12 predicted transmembrane-spanning segments (Fig. 2). It shares similarity with a group of transporters from bacteria of the major facilitator class, evidence supporting a transport function (Gälweiler et al., 1998; Pao et al., 1998). A search of the

Arabidopsis genome for genes with homology to PIN1 revealed another seven genes belonging to the same family. Similar sequences have been found in all other plants now sequenced, but not in animals, indicating that PIN proteins have evolved exclusively in plants. Based on genetic evidence, PIN proteins are strong candidates for either the auxin efflux carrier itself or an important regulatory component of the efflux machinery (Palme and Gälweiler, 1999). More important, the distributions of PIN1 and other PIN proteins in the plasma membrane of auxin-transporting cells of stems and roots were found to be dynamic and asymmetric according to the direction of auxin flux (Friml et al., 2002b; Gälweiler et al., 1998; Geldner et al., 2001; Müller et al., 1998; Steinmann et al., 1999) (Fig. 3). Auxin gradients in plant tissue appear to be sink driven; gradient formation seems to be regulated by auxin transport (rather than degradation) machinery. For example, the formation of a maximum auxin concentration at the Arabidopsis root apex depends on the activity of PIN4 (Friml et al., 2002a).

It is likely that the activity of the efflux complex is regulated by phosphorylation (Delbarre et al., 1998). Auxin efflux was found to be more sensitive to the specific transport inhibitor *N*-1-naphthylphthalamic acid (NPA) in seedlings of an Arabidopsis mutant named *rcn1* ("root curl in NPA") than in the wild type. The *RCN1* gene encodes a subunit of protein phosphatase 2A (Garbers et al., 1996). Furthermore, the mutant can be phenocopied with a phosphatase inhibitor (Deruere et al., 1999). The protein kinase PINOID enhances polar auxin transport (Benjamins et al., 2001) and is another potential component of the hypothetical auxin-efflux complex.

5. AUXIN PERCEPTION

According to the widely accepted theory, phytohormone signaling begins with the perception of free hormone by a specific receptor. In the case of auxin, there is evidence for multiple sites of auxin perception. It therefore appears that, at least initially, the auxin signal can transduce through more than one signaling pathway.

To date, the best-characterized auxin-binding protein is ABP1 (Napier et al., 2002), which was originally identified, purified, and cloned from maize (Hesse et al., 1989; Löbler and Klämbt, 1985). The high binding constant of auxin and ABP1 has inspired much research, however, the protein has no homology to any other known receptor family, and it is ubiquitous in vascular plants, including the pteridophytes and bryophytes (Napier et al., 2002). A KDEL retention motif at the C-terminus of ABP1 ensures an ER loca-

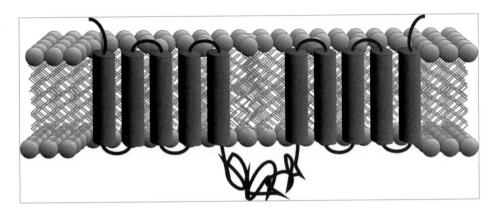

Fig. 2. Predicted AtPIN1 protein structure.

tion (Henderson et al., 1997; Tian et al., 1995); however, some ABP1 does pass along the constitutive secretion pathway to the plasma membrane and cell surface (Diekmann et al., 1995; Henderson et al., 1997). The ER location makes the characterization of ABP1 more complex because most of the physiological data demonstrate activity of ABP1 on the plasma membrane. Here, auxin is able to control several cellular responses, including tobacco mesophyll protoplast hyperpolarization (Leblanc et al., 1999a, 1999b), tobacco mesophyll protoplast division (Fellner et al., 1996), expansion of tobacco and maize cells in culture (Jones et al., 1998), and maize protoplast swelling (Steffens et al., 2001). These effects can be inhibited by the application of anti-ABP1 antibodies, which are unable to enter the cell. It has therefore been concluded that ABP1 is able to elicit a physiological response in the presence of auxin at the surface of the plasma membrane. A functional role of ABP1 inside the ER has not been shown; these data may be reconsidered, however, because auxin efflux carriers are now known to cycle continuously in membrane vesicles between the plasma membrane and the endosome (Geldner et al., 2001). There is considerable speculation about the possible role of auxin transporters in auxin signaling. It is possible that measurement of the flux of auxin through either influx or efflux carriers (or both) monitors auxin level in the cell. It is also possible that specific transporter family members no longer act as transporters but have evolved a receptor function (Friml and Palme, 2002). Sugar sensing is important for plants and yeast to report the carbohydrate status within cells and outside of cells. It has been demonstrated that some proteins that show transporter topology do not transport sugars but sense sugar outside of cells and control transcription of sugar transporters that control the sugar homeostasis in cells (Lalonde et al., 1999). A similar mechanism for auxin perception is conceivable.

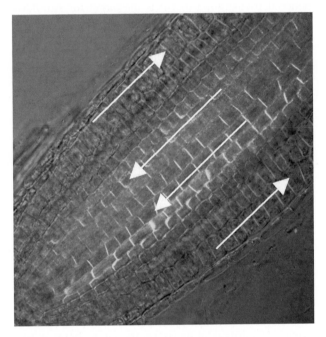

Fig. 3. AtPIN1 (inner arrows) and AtPIN2 (outer arrows) in Arabidopsis root tip. Arrows indicate the direction of Auxin fluxes in marked cell files.

6. EFFECT OF AUXIN SIGNALING ON GENE EXPRESSION

Auxin-dependent transcriptional activation can occur within minutes of a signal being perceived (Abel and Theologis, 1996). In the nucleus, the regulation of gene expression by auxin can be mediated by the action of two families of auxin-induced proteins: the Aux/IAA proteins and the auxin response factors (ARFs) (Hagen and Guilfoyle, 2002). ARFs bind to auxin response promoter elements upstream of genes and activate or repress their transcription. Aux/IAA proteins can dimerize with ARF proteins, thus inhibiting their activity (Tiwari et al.,

2003). However, they have very short half-lives, ranging from a few minutes to a few hours (Abel et al., 1994; Gray et al., 2001). A normal auxin response is dependent on this rapid turnover of Aux/IAA proteins, as it lowers the concentration of the inhibitory ARF-Aux/IAA dimer (Ulmasov et al., 1997; Worley et al., 2000).

Aux/IAA proteins are found in all higher plants and are characterized by four highly conserved domains (Abel and Theologis, 1996; Guilfoyle et al., 1998). In yeast two-hybrid assays, their dimerization with ARF proteins has been shown to involve two of these domains (which are similar to those of the ARF proteins) (Ulmasov et al., 1997). Another domain, domain II, is crucial for Aux/IAA function, with many lines of evidence demonstrating that it is the target for Aux/IAA protein destabilization, ensuring the rapid turnover required for a normal auxin response. The fusion of Aux/IAA proteins to reporter proteins, such as luciferase or β-glucuronase (GUS), results in the destabilization of the reporter protein (Gray et al. 2001; Worley et al., 2000). This indicates that Aux/IAA proteins contain a transferable destabilization sequence. A nonfunctional domain II, as found in the auxin-resistant mutants *axr3-1*, *axr2-1*, and *shy2*, dramatically increases the protein's half-life and prevents the ARF proteins from functioning (Gray et al., 2001; Ouellet et al., 2001; Worley et al., 2000). The stabilization of an Aux/IAA-reporter fusion by inhibitors of the 26S proteasome indicates that auxin signaling requires SCF^{TIR1}-mediated turnover of Aux/IAA proteins.

7. GIBBERELLINS

GAs are a large group of diterpenes comprising well over a hundred members. However, only a handful can elicit a physiological response, the others being representative of a large and complicated web of biosynthetic pathways from *ent*-kaurene, the product of the first dedicated step of GA biosynthesis. These biosynthetic pathways are now well understood. GAs regulate a wide range of physiological processes, including cell division and cell elongation, and are crucial to the control of processes as diverse as germination, stem elongation, flowering, fruit ripening, and senescence.

The last 5 yr have seen a dramatic increase in our understanding of the processes involved in GA signal transduction (Gomi and Matsuoka, 2003), however, the exact mechanisms by which a plant's response to GA is brought about remain unclear. A class of transcription factors, the DELLA proteins, has emerged as a central mediator of many GA responses, although they probably do not bind DNA directly (Dill et al., 2001). It was decided that these proteins (named after a five-amino-acid N-terminal motif) are important

components of the GA signal transduction pathway after the analysis of a number of dwarfed mutants from a range of species (Sun, 2000). An important example (and the mutant from which the first member of the family was cloned) is the gai1-1 mutant of Arabidopsis. Plants with a dominant mutation at the GAI allele display a semidwarf phenotype, insensitive to the exogenous application of GA (Peng and Harberd, 1993). All results indicate that the DELLA proteins are negative regulators of GA signaling.

Altogether there are five DELLA proteins in Arabidopsis (GAI, RGA, RGL1, RGL2, and RGL3), but only one in rice (SLR1) and barley (SLN1). They share a high degree of sequence homology and belong to a wider group of plant transcription factors called the GRAS family. All of these proteins share the same basic structure, with an N-terminal GA-signal-perception domain, a serine/threonine-rich domain, a leucine zipper, and a C-terminal regulatory domain conserved among GRAS proteins. This structure has been used to suggest a model for the mode of action of SLR1 where the protein exists as a dimer, the subunits linked by the leucine zipper (Itoh et al., 2002). The active form (receiving no GA signal) represses the GA response via the C-terminus, which is deactivated when a GA signal is bound by the DELLA domain.

As is the case for auxin, the GA receptor is still unknown. However, there is evidence that the transduction of the GA signal from the plasma membrane to the nucleus involves G proteins (Ueguchi-Tanaka et al., 2000). A range of secondary messengers have also been shown to be involved in this process, but the exact role of many remains unclear (Sun, 2000). As in animals, it has recently emerged that the post-translational modification of proteins by the addition of O-linked *N*-acetylglucosamine could be involved in signaling processes (Thornton et al., 1999). Analysis of two mutants of Arabidopsis, partially rescued by the application of exogenous GA, has revealed two putative O-GlcNAc transferases (by homology with known enzymatic sequences) thought to be involved in the GA signaling pathway (Hartweck et al., 2002). In animals, the transferase ability has been shown to compete with phosphorylation of serine and threonine residues, suggesting a possible mechanism for their mode of action in plants, and a link to DELLA protein function.

8. CYTOKININS

Cytokinins play a major role in many different developmental and physiological processes in plants, such as cell division, regulation of root and shoot growth and branching, chloroplast development, leaf senescence, nutrient mobilization, biomass distribution, stress response, and pathogen resistance. In contrast to our understanding of auxin and GA signal transduction, proteins have been identified that function as cytokinin receptors. Activation tagging experiments in *Arabidopsis* identified *CKI1*, a gene encoding a receptor histidine kinase, whose overexpression was seen to induce typical cytokinin responses (Kakimoto, 1996). Although *CKI1* is able to activate the cytokinin signaling pathway, it does not bind cytokinins directly (Hwang and Sheen, 2001). Nevertheless, the discovery of *CKI1* suggested that the cytokinin transduction pathway in higher plants could be similar to the prokaryotic two-component system. This hypothesis was proved by the identification of CRE1/AHK4, another histidine kinase, as the first cytokinin receptor (Inoue et al., 2001; Suzuki et al., 2001; Ueguchi et al., 2001). The availability of the Arabidopsis genomic sequence led to the identification of two further cytokinin receptors (AHK2 and AHK3).

After cytokinin perception, the resulting signal is transmitted by a multistep phosphorelay system through a complex form of the two-component signaling pathways that has been well characterized in prokaryotes and lower eukaryotes. Functional evidence for cytokinin sensing by the receptor CRE1/AHK4 was obtained in elegant complementation experiments in yeast and *Escherichia coli*, which rendered these heterologous hosts cytokinin sensitive. Two other histidine kinases, AHK2 and AHK3, have been shown to be active in the same complementation test system and to give protoplasts cytokinin sensitivity (Hwang and Sheen, 2001; Yamada et al., 2001), indicating that these two proteins are also cytokinin receptors. Each receptor comprises an N-terminal extracellular domain, a membrane anchor, and a C-terminal transmitter domain, capable of autophosphorylation. The three cytokinin receptor genes differ in their expression pattern. *CRE1/AHK4* is mainly expressed in the roots, whereas *AHK2* and *AHK3* are present in all major organs (Inoue et al., 2001; Ueguchi et al., 2001). This tissue-specific expression of cytokinin receptors could be an additional layer of control to the perception of cytokinin.

Considering the large number of response-regulator genes associated with the two-component signaling sytem (22 in Arabidopsis), it has been suggested that they could both have different functions, using different targets in addition to participating in cross talk with other hormones. There are accumulating data demonstrating that in order to understand the growth responses to cytokinins, it is important to understand such cross talk between cytokinins and nutrients as well as cytokinins and other phytohormones. Moore et al. (2003)

showed that application of cytokinins as well as the use of transgenic *Arabidopsis* lines with constitutive cytokinin signaling could overcome the glucose repression response. The insensitivity of *Arabidopsis glucose insensitive2 (gin2)* to auxin and hypersensitivity to cytokinin could be the clue to understanding the antagonistic interaction between cytokinins and auxin and its dependency on the glucose status of tissues.

9. BRASSINOSTEROIDS

Steroids are important signaling molecules in plants as well as in animals. Since the discovery of brassinolide in 1979, brassinosteroids (BRs) have been shown to be important at a number of stages of a plant's development, including stem elongation, germination and senescence. BRs retain the basic four-ring structure of many steroid hormones; like animal steroid hormones, they are synthesized from cholesterol. Two mutants deficient in the biosynthesis of BRs, *DET2* and *CPD*, develop as if grown under light when grown in the dark (Chory et al., 1991; Li and Chory, 1997). This demonstrates that, in addition to these other crucial processes, BRs play an important role in photomorphogenesis. The identification of a BR receptor has been a recent significant advance in phytohormone biology; this section focuses on the mechanism by which BRs are initially sensed by the cell, before highlighting some interesting similarities between the perception and mode of action of BRs and the regulation of development in animals. In animals, steroids receptors are nuclear located (Marcinkowska and Wiedlocha, 2002); in plants, no nuclear steroid receptors have been found, indicating that plant cells have evolved a different method to receive the BR signal.

The *bri* mutant of Arabidopsis shows a dwarfed phenotype similar to that of mutants deficient in the biosynthesis of BRs. BRI1 was thought to be involved in signaling owing to the mutant plants' unresponsiveness to applied brassinolide. Cloning of the bri1 gene revealed a leucine-rich repeat (LRR) receptor-like kinase, an immediate candidate for the BR receptor (Li and Chory, 1997). BRI1 was subsequently shown to be located at the plasma membrane (Friedrichsen et al., 2000), and to have a relatively high affinity for bioactive BR (Wang et al., 2001). LRR receptor kinases contain three domains: an extracellular domain comprising several leucine-rich repeating sections (in the case of BRI1, 25), a transmembrane section and a cytoplasmic kinase domain. BRI1 also contains a 70-amino-acid island in the LRR domain, necessary for the protein's function (Li and Chory, 1997). The use of chimeric proteins has demonstrated that the BRI1 extracellular domain was both necessary and sufficient for the translation of a specific set of genes. When fused to the intracellular kinase domain of a similar receptor-like kinase, a protein involved triggering a plant's defensive response to pathogens, activation of the extracellular BRI1 domain and, hence, defense-related gene expression could be induced by BR (He et al., 2000). The LRR-receptor kinases are members of a very large class of proteins in Arabidopsis comprising 174 members with diverse function. Only a small number have been ascribed a function, including CLAVATA (involved in meristem development) and ERECTA (involved in organogenesis) (Dievart and Clark, 2003). The functions of LRR-receptor kinases are diverse. In Arabidopsis, three BRI-like proteins share high homology and are similar to protein sequences found in monocotyledonous species. Of these, BRL1 and BRL3 are able to rescue the *bri1* mutation, suggesting a closely related function.

The cloning of a homolog of BRI1 in tomato revealed an intriguing overlap of function of the tBRI1 (BRI of tomato) protein. Systemin is a peptide signal important in pathogen-defense responses in plants, acting by amplifying the induction of the jasmonate signaling pathway. It was discovered that the same receptor (called SR160 in the context of systemin) was responsible for both BR and systemin signaling (Montoya et al., 2002; Szekeres, 2003). This dual receptor function has also been observed in animals, with the hormone progesterone able to inhibit specifically the peptide oxytocin from binding to its receptor, a uterine G protein–coupled receptor (Grazzini et al., 1998). It has been suggested that BR could bind to its receptor while simultaneously bound to a specific protein, owing to sequence homology to animal steroid-binding proteins being found in the Arabidopsis genome (Li and Chory, 1997), and the fact that, in general, LRRs mediate protein-protein interactions rather than smaller ligand binding.

10. ABSCISIC ACID

Plants control water balance with a range of strategies. For most land plants, the anatomy of leaves is centered on a balance between minimizing water loss and maximizing both exposure to the sun and the rate of diffusion of molecular oxygen away from and carbon dioxide into photosynthetic cells. This balance is essential for maintaining the flux of electrons that pass through the light-dependent reactions of photosynthesis. The leaf is an organ that is necessarily exposed to relatively high levels of sunlight and, therefore, of water loss through evaporation from pores (stomata). ABA is the phytohormone which regulates the opening and closing of stomata. It does this by controlling the turgor pressure inside the two surrounding banana-shaped guard cells. Much of the work on ABA signaling has been focused on guard cells and mutants affecting their function. However, ABA influences both physiological (gene expression in response to salt stress and drought) and developmental (e.g., germination and seedling development) processes. ABA seems to affect many different signaling pathways, sometimes with a high degree of redundancy; the extent to which it mediates cross talk between environmental and developmental stimuli is currently the subject of concentrated research.

The amount of free ABA able to elicit a response is thought to be dependent on many factors. These include movement of ABA through the plant, the relative rates of ABA synthesis and catabolism, and the concentration of ABA in the leaf symplast.

It has become clear that the ABA signal is transduced through a number of secondary messengers, among them lipid-derived signals, H_2O_2, G proteins, and nitric oxide (Himmelbach et al., 2003). The varying cellular concentrations of these compounds unite to influence indirectly the cytosolic concentration of Ca^{2+}, the central factor in many ABA signals (McAinsh et al., 1997). It is thought that ABA has two modes of action: the first "nongenomic" effect is able to change the turgor pressure in guard cells by altering the plasma membrane's permeability to ions, and the second acts via changing the transcription levels of ABA-responsive genes. It is thought that both processes are reliant on alterations in the intracellular concentration of Ca^{2+}; however, it is not yet fully understood to what extent the pathways are separated.

Despite a long history of research, the nature of the initial ABA receptor remains elusive. However, it is widely believed that the initial event in the signaling cascade is the binding of ABA to either a membrane-bound or a cytosolic receptor. In many cases, this binding results in the activation of Ca^{2+}-influx channels resulting in the ABA-mediated increase in intracellular Ca^{2+} concentration (Murata et al., 2001). Another important factor in this process is the altering permeability of the tonoplast to Ca^{2+}; this is influenced by intracellular lipid-derived signals and cyclic adenosine 5′-diphosphate–ribose concentration, the latter dependent on the Ca^{2+} concentration itself (Wu et al., 2003). The overall increase in intracellular Ca^{2+} results first in the inhibition of K^+-influx channels and, second, in the activation of K^+-efflux channels and the inhibition of H^+-adenosine triphosphatase. Therefore it can be seen that ABA initiates a complicated mesh of interconnecting signals, resulting in a physiologic response (Finkelstein et al., 2002).

11. ETHYLENE

It has long been known that exposure to ethylene elicits a well-characterized response in seedlings. The so-called triple response, a signature of ethylene signaling, comprises an increase in the girth of hypocotyl and root as well as the formation of an apical hook. This well-defined phenotype has been the basis of ethylene research, which is used to identify mutants in the ethylene signaling pathway. Ethylene has been shown to be important in a wide range of processes including fruit ripening, senescence, and defense response. The ethylene signaling pathway is relatively well characterized, and it has also been shown that ethylene signaling is intrinsically linked to many other phytohormonal signaling pathways.

There are five ethylene receptors in Arabidopsis: ETR1, ETR2, ERS1, ERS2, and EIN4 (Stepanova and Ecker, 2000). They are all histidine kinases, the same class of two-component regulatory system as is found in the cytokinin signaling pathway. The ethylene receptors can be most easily classified in two ways. In the first, they are grouped into those with (ETR1, ETR2, and EIN4) and without (ERS1 and ERS2) a receiver domain, the domain that receives the phosphotransfer from the histidine kinase. It is thought that a signal could be transduced via a dimer of receptors (Hall et al., 2000); it has been suggested that the proteins without a receiver domain operate in a receptor complex. The second and more common classification groups the ethylene receptors according to their structure. Subfamily I (ETR1 and ERS1) has three membrane-spanning regions, whereas subfamily II (ETR2, ERS2, and EIN4) has four membrane-spanning regions and lacks conserved residues in the histidine kinase domain. Interestingly, the phenotype of receptor-deficient mutants can be rescued with an ETR1 protein with an inactivated histidine kinase domain. This work suggests that the ethylene receptor complex can transduce a signal by a mechanism other than histidine kinase–dependent phosphotransfer (Wang et al., 2003). Although it can also homodimerize (Schaller and Bleecker, 1995), ETR1 has been shown to interact directly with CTR, a protein similar to the Raf family of mitogen-activated protein kinase (MAPK) kinases . The receptor complex has been shown to be located at the endoplasmic reticular membrane (Gao et al., 2003), and negative regulation by a MAPK signaling cascade has been demonstrated in Arabidopsis and *Medicago* (Ouaked et al., 2003). This provide another hint as to the complex relationship between what have been traditionally regarded as discrete phytohormone signaling pathways. Understanding the significance of such integration will be a major challenge in the coming years.

12. PERSPECTIVE

Over the last decade, tremendous progress has been made using genetic analysis of the model plant Arabidopsis. This has allowed researchers to dissect developmental programs as well as hormonal and environmental responses, including light regulation and plant-pathogen interactions. This postgenomic era, in which numerous other plant genomes will be fully sequenced (e.g., rice, *Medicago*, poplar), will bring both comparative genomic analysis and biosystems-oriented approaches likely to uncover the regulatory pathways underlying the amazing biosynthetic capacity of plants. This will enable not only basic research but also plant biotechnology to increase the range of plant products available to researchers, providing the potential to create a safer environment.

REFERENCES

Abel S, Oeller PW, Theologis A. Early auxin-induced genes encode short-lived nuclear proteins. *Proc Natl Acad Sci USA* 1994;91: 326–330.

Abel S, Theologis A. Early genes and auxin action. *Plant Physiol* 1996;111:9–17.

Benjamins R, Quint A, Weijers D, Hooykaas P, Offringa R. The PINOID protein kinase regulates organ development in Arabidopsis by enhancing polar auxin transport. *Development* 2001;128:4057–4067.

Bennett MJ, Marchant A, Green HG, May ST, Ward SP, Millner PA, Walker AR, Schulz B, Feldmann KA. Arabidopsis AUX1 gene: a permease-like regulator of root gravitropism. *Science* 1996; 273:948–950.

Chory J, Nagpal P, Peto CA. Phenotypic and genetic analysis of DET2 a new mutant that affects light-regulated seedling development in Arabidopsis. *Plant Cell* 1991;3:445–460.

Cock JM, Vanoosthuyse V, Gaude T. Receptor kinase signalling in plants and animals: distinct molecular systems with mechanistic similarities. *Curr Opin Cell Biol.* 2002;14:230–236.

Davies PJ. The plant hormones: their nature, occurrence, and functions. In: Davies PJ., ed. *Plant Hormones: Physiology, Biochemistry and Molecular Biology*, 2nd Ed. Dordrecht, Netherlands: Kluwer Academic Publishers, 1995:1–12.

Delbarre A, Muller P, Guern J. Short-lived and phosporylated proteins contribute to carrier-mediated efflux, but not to influx, of Auxin in suspension-cultured Tobacco cells. *Plant Physiol* 1998; 116:833–844.

Deruere J, Jackson K, Garbers C, Soll D, DeLong A. The RCN1-encoded A subunit of protein phosphatase 2A increases phosphatase activity in vivo. *Plant J* 1999;20:389–399.

Dievart A., Clark SE. Using mutant alleles to determine the structure and function of leucine-rich repeat receptor-like kinases. *Curr Opin Plant Biol.* 2003;6:507–516.

Dill A, Jung HS, Sun TP. The DELLA motif is essential for gibberellin-induced degradation of RGA. *Proc Natl Acad Sci USA* 2001; 98:14,162–14,167.

Fellner M, Ephritikhine G, Barbierbrygoo H, Guern J. An antobody raised to a maize auxin-binding protein has inhibitory effects on cell division of tobacco mesophyl protoplasts. *Plant Physiol Biochem* 1996;34:133–138.

Finkelstein RR, Gampala SSL, Rock CD. Abscisic acid signaling in seeds and seedlings. *Plant Cell* 2002;14:15–45.

Friml J, Benkova E, Ikram, Blilou I, Wisniewska J, Hamann T, Ljung K, Wood S, Sandberg G, Scheres B, Palme K. AtPIN4 mediates sink-driven gradients and root patterning in Arabidopsis. *Cell* 2002b;108:661–673.

Friml J, Palme K. Polar auxin transport—old questions and new concepts? *Plant Mol Biol* 2002;49:273–284.

Friml J, Wisniewska J, Benkova E, Mendgen K, Palme K. Lateral relocation of auxin efflux regulator PIN3 mediates tropism in Arabidopsis. *Nature* 2002a;415:806–809.

Gälweiler L, Guan C, Müller A, Wisman E, Mendgen K, Yephremov A, Palme K. Regulation of polar auxin transport by AtPIN1 in Arabidopsis vascular tissue. *Science* 1998;282:2226–2230.

Gao ZY, Chen YF, Randlett MD, Zhao XC, Findell JL, Kieber JJ, Schaller GE. Localization of the Raf-like kinase CTR1 to the endoplasmic reticulum of Arabidopsis through participation in ethylene receptor signaling complexes. *J Biol Chem* 2003; 278:34,725–34,732.

Garbers C, Delong A, Deruere J, Bernasconi P, Soll D. A mutation in Arabidopsis 2A phosphatase regulatory subunit affects auxin transport in Arabidopsis. *EMBO J* 1996;15:2115–2124.

Geldner N, Friml J, Stierhof YD, Jürgens G, Palme K. Auxin transport inhibitors block PIN1 cycling and and vesicle trafficking. *Nature* 2001;413:425–428.

Gomi K, Matsuoka M. Gibberellin signalling pathway. *Curr Opin Plant Biol* 2003;6:489–493.

Gomi K, Matsuoka M. Gibberellin signalling pathway. *Curr Opin Plant Biol* 2003;6:489–493.

Gray WM, Kepinski S, Rouse D, Leyser O, Estelle M. Auxin regulates SCFTIR1-dependent degradation of AUX/IAA proteins. *Nature* 2001;414:271–276.

Grazzini E, Guillon G, Mouillac B, Zingg HH. Inhibition of oxytocin receptor function by direct binding of progesterone. *Nature* 1998;392:509–512.

Guilfoyle T, Hagen G, Ulmasov T, Murfett J. How does auxin turn on genes? *Plant Physiol.* 1998;118:341–347.

Hagen G, Guilfoyle T. Auxin-responsive gene expression: genes, promoters and regulatory factors. *Plant Mol Biol* 2002;49: 373–385.

Hall AE, Findell JL, Schaller GE, Sisler EC, Bleecker AB. Ethylene perception by the ERS1 protein in Arabidopsis. *Plant Physiol* 2000;123:1449–1457.

Hartweck LM, Scott CL, Olszewski NE. Two O-linked N-acetylglucosamine transferase genes of *Arabidopsis thaliana* L. Heynh. Have overlapping functions necessary for gamete and seed development. *Genetics* 2002;161:1279–1291.

He Z, Wang ZY, Li J, Zhu Q, Lamb C, Ronald P, Chory J. Perception of brassinosteroids by the extracellular domain of the receptor kinase BRI1. *Science* 2000;288:2360–2363.

Henderson J, Bauly JM, Ashford DA, Oliver SC, Hawes CR, Lazarus CM, Venis MA, Napier RM. Retention of maize auxin-binding protein in the endoplasmic reticulum: Quantifying escape and the role of auxin. *Planta* 1997;202:313–323.

Hesse T, Feldwisch J, Balshuesemann D, Bauw G, Puype M, Vandekerckhove J, Löbler M, Klämbt D, Schell J, Palme K. Molecular cloning and structural analysis of a gene from *Zea mays L.* coding for a putative receptor for the plant hormone auxin. *EMBO J* 1989;8:2453–2462.

Himmelbach A, Yang Y, Grill E. Relay and control of abscisic acid signaling. *Curr Opin Plant Biol* 2003;6:470–479.

Hwang I, Sheen J. Two-component circuitry in Arabidopsis cytokinin signal transduction. *Nature* 2001;413:383–389.

Inoue T, Higuchi M, Hashimoto Y, Seki M, Kobayashi M, Kato T, Tabata S, Shinozaki K, Kakimoto T. Identification of CRE1 as a cytokinin receptor from Arabidopsis. *Nature* 2001;409:1060–1063.

Itoh H, Ueguchi-Tanaka M., Sato Y, Ashikari M, Matsuoka M. The gibberellin signaling pathway is regulated by the appearance and disappearance of SLENDER RICE1 in nuclei. *Plant Cell* 2002; 14:57–70.

Jones AM, Im KH, Savka MA, Wu MJ, DeWitt NG, Shillito R, Binns AN. Auxin-dependent cell expansion mediated by overexpressed auxin-binding protein 1. *Science* 1998;282:1114–1117.

Kakimoto T. CKI1, a cystidine kinase homolog implicated in cytokinin signal transduction. *Science* 1996;274:982–985.

Lalonde S, Boles E, Hellmann H, Barker L, Patrick JW, Frommer WB, Ward J. The dual function of sugar carriers: transport and sugar sensing. *Plant Cell* 1999;11:707–726.

Leblanc N, David K, Grosclaude J, Pradier JM, Barbier-Brygoo H, Labiau S, Perrot-Rechenmann C. A novel immunological approach establishes that the auxin-binding protein, Nt-abp1, is an element involved in auxin signaling at the plasma membrane. *J Biol Chem* 1999b;274:28,314–28,320.

Leblanc N, Perrot-Rechenmann C, Barbier-Brygoo H. The auxin-binding protein Nt-ERabp1 alone activates an auxin-like transduction pathway. *FEBS Lett* 1999a;449:57–60.

Li JM. Brassinosteroids signal through two receptor-like kinases. *Curr Opin Plant Biol* 2003;6:494–499.

Li JM, Chory J. A putative leucine-rich repeat receptor kinase involved in brassinosteroid signal transduction. *Cell* 1997;90: 929–938.

Li JM, Nam KH. Regulation of brassinosteroid signaling by a GSK3/SHAGGY-like kinase. *Science* 2002;295:1299–1301

Li J, Wen JQ, Lease KA, Doke JT, Tax FE, Walker JC. BAK1, an Arabidopsis LRR receptor-like protein kinase, interacts with BRI1 and modulates brassinosteroid signaling. *Cell* 2002;110:213–222.

Ljung K, Bhalerao RP, Sandberg G. Sites and homeostatic control of auxin biosynthesis in Arabidopsis during vegetative growth. *Plant J.* 2001;28:465–474.

Löbler M., Klämbt D. Auxin-binding protein from coleoptile membranes of corn Zea mays cultivar Mutin 1. Purification by immunological methods and characterization. *J Biol Chem* 1985;260: 9848–9853.

Marcinkowska E, Wiedlocha A. Steroid signal transduction activated at the cell membrane: from plants to animals. *Acta Biochem Pol* 2002;49:735–745.

Martinez-Garcia JF, Huq E, Quail PH. Direct targeting of light signals to a promoter element-bound transcription factor. *Science* 2000;288 (5467):859–863.

McAinsh MR, Brownlee C, Hetherington AM. Calcium ions as second messengers in guard cell signal transduction. *Physiol Plant* 1997;100:16–29.

Montoya T, Nomura T, Farrar K, Kaneta T, Yokota T, Bishop GJ. Cloning the tomato curl3 gene highlights the putative dual role of the leucine-rich repeat receptor kinase tBRI1/SR160 in plant steroid hormone and peptide hormone signaling. *Plant Cell* 2002; 14:3163–3176.

Moore B, Zhou L, Rolland F, Hall Q, Cheng WH, Liu YX, Hwang I, Jones T, Sheen J. Role of the Arabidopsis glucose sensor HXK1 in nutrient, light, and hormonal signaling. *Science* 2003;300: 332–336.

Müller A, Guan C, Gälweiler L, Tänzler P, Huijser P, Marchant A, Parry G, Bennett M, Wisman E, Palme K. AtPIN2 defines a locus of Arabidopsis for root gravitropism control. *EMBO J* 1998;17: 6903–6911.

Murata Y, Pei ZM, Mori IC, Schroeder J. Abscisic acid activation of plasma membrane Ca2+ channels in guard cells requires cytosolic NAD (P)H and is differentially disrupted upstream and downstream of reactive oxygen species production in abi1-1 and abi2-1 protein phosphatase 2C mutants. *Plant Cell* 2001;13:2513–2523.

Nagy F, Schäfer E. Phytochromes control photomorphogenesis by differentially regulated, interacting signaling pathways in higher plants. *Ann Rev Plant Biol* 2002;53:329–355.

Napier RM, David KM, Perrot-Rechenmann C. A short history of auxin-binding proteins. *Plant Mol Biol* 2002;49:339–348.

Ouaked F, Rozhon W, Lecourieux D, Hirt H. A MAPK pathway mediates ethylene signaling in plants. *EMBO J* 2003;22:1282–1288.

Ouellet F, Overvoorde PJ, Theologis A. IAA17/AXR3: biochemical insight into an auxin mutant phenotype. *Plant Cell* 2001;13: 829–842.

Pao S, Paulsen I, Saier MH Jr. Major Facilitator Supperfamily. *Microbiol Mol Biol Rev* 1998;62:1–34.

Peng JR, Harberd NP. Derivative alleles of the Arabidopsis Gibberellin-insensitive (Gai) mutation confer a wild-type phenotype. *Plant Cell* 1993;5:351–360.

Schaller GE, Bleecker AB. Ethylene-binding sites generated in yeast expressing the Arabidopsis ETR1 gene. *Science* 1995; 270:1809–1811.

Sheen J. Mutational analysis of protein phosphatase 2C involved in abscisic acid signal transduction in higher plants. *Proc Natl Acad Sci USA* 1998;95:975–980.

Steinmann T, Geldner N, Grebe M, Mangold S, Jackson CL, Paris S, Gälweiler L, Palme K, Jürgens G. Coordinated polar localisation of auxin efflux carrier PIN1 by GNOM ARF GEF. *Science* 1999;286:316–318.

Steffens B, Feckler C, Palme K, Christian M, Böttger M, Lüthen H. The auxin signal for protoplast swelling is perceived by extracellular ABP1. *Plant J.* 2001;27:591–599.

Stepanova AN, Ecker JR. Ethylene signaling: from mutants to molecules. *Curr Opin Plant Biol* 2000;3:353–360.

Sun TP. Gibberellin signal transduction. *Curr Opin Plant Biol* 2000; 3:374–380.

Suzuki T, Miwa K, Ishikawa K, Yamada H, Aiba H, Mizuno T. The Arabidopsis sensor His-kinase, AHK4, can respond to cytokinins. *Plant Cell Physiol* 2001;42 :107–113.

Szekeres M. Brassinosteroid and systemin: two hormones perceived by the same receptor. *Trends Plant Sci* 2003;8:102–104.

Tian HC, Klambt D, Jones AM. Auxin-binding protein 1 does not bind auxin within the ER despite this being the predominant subcellular location for this hormone receptor. *J Biol Chem* 1995; 270:26,962–26,969.

Tiwari SB, Hagen G, Guilfoyle T. The roles of auxin response factor domains in auxin-responsive transcription. *Plant Cell* 2003;15: 533–543.

Thornton TM, Swain SM, Olszewski NE. Gibberellin signal transduction presents ... the SPY who O- GlcNAc'd me. *Trends Plant Sci* 1996;4:424–428.

Tyagi AK, Gaur T. Light regulation of nuclear photosynthetic genes in higher plants. *Crit Rev Plant Sci* 2003;22:417–452.

Ueguchi C, Sato S, Kato T, Tabata S. The AHK4 gene involved in the cytokinin-signaling pathway as a direct receptor molecule in *Arabidopsis thaliana*. *Plant Cell Physiol* 2001;42:751–755.

Ueguchi-Tanaka M, Fujisawa Y, Kobayashi M, Ashikari M, Iwasaki Y, Kitano H, Matsuoka M. Rice dwarf mutant d1, which is defective in the alpha subunit of the heterotrimeric G protein, affects gibberellin signal transduction. *Proc Natl Acad Sci USA* 2000; 97:11,638–11,643.

Ulmasov T, Murfett J, Hagen G, Guilfoyle TJ. AUX/IAA proteins repress expression of reporter genes containing natural and highly active synthetic auxun response elements. *Plant Cell* 1997;9:1963–1971.

Vernoud V, Horton AC, Yang ZB, Nielsen E. Analysis of the small GTPase gene superfamily of Arabidopsis. *Plant Physiol* 2003; 131:1191–1208.

Wang ZY, Seto H, Fujioka S, Yoshida S, Chory J. BRI1 is a critical component of a plasma-membrane receptor for plant steroids. *Nature* 2001;410:380–383.

Wang WY, Hall AE, O'Malley R, Bleecker AB. Canonical histidine kinase activity of the transmitter domain of the ETR1 ethylene receptor from Arabidopsis is not required for signal transmission. *Proc Natl Acad Sci USA* 2003;100:352–357.

Wendehenne D, Pugin A, Klessig DF, Durner J. Nitric oxide: comparative synthesis and signaling in animal and plant cells. *Trends Plant Sci* 2001;6:177–183.

Worley CK, Zenser N, Ramos J, Rouse D, Leyser O, Theologis A, Callis J. Degradation of Aux/IAA proteins is essential for normal auxin signalling. *Plant J* 2000;21:553–562.

Wu Y, Sanchez JP, Lopez-Molina L, Himmelbach A, Grill E, Chua NH. The abi1-1 mutation blocks ABA signaling downstream of cADPR action. *Plant J* 2003;34:307–315.

11 Comparative Endocrinology

Fredrick Stormshak, PhD

CONTENTS

1. INTRODUCTION

Comparative endocrinology encompasses research on the roles of hormones in regulating biological functions in a wide range of diverse vertebrate and invertebrate species. Thus, it becomes an impossibility to adequately describe and discuss within the confines of a single chapter the many endocrine control systems that exist in the animal kingdom. Consequently, an attempt is made in this chapter to present some unique and novel aspects of endocrine function that contribute to behavior, growth and reproduction in a few select species. Although much similarity in endocrine organization and function exists among species, there are differences, which will become apparent in this chapter.

2. ENDOCRINE CONTRIBUTIONS TO BEHAVIOR

2.1. Maternal Behavior

Humans, nonhuman primates, and some species as diverse as elephants exhibit spontaneous maternal behavior. However, as a general rule, this type of spontaneous behavior is relatively rare among most mammalian species. Perhaps because of confinement and human

From: *Endocrinology: Basic and Clinical Principles, Second Edition*
(S. Melmed and P. M. Conn, eds.) © Humana Press Inc., Totowa, NJ

intervention more is known about the endocrinologic basis of maternal behavior in laboratory and domestic mammals than other animals. Domestic sheep (ewes) are but one example of a species whose maternal behavior is hormonally regulated. Ewes become maternally responsive toward a lamb only after parturition. Nonparturient ewes aggressively reject approaches of lambs by head butting the lamb into retreat. Maternal behavior by the parturient ewe, however, consists of licking the lamb, voicing low-pitched bleats, and willingly to suckle the lamb. Usually within 2 h of parturition, an exclusive bond is formed between the dam and her offspring. Strange lambs are rejected by the ewe should they attempt to suckle, and this occurs even after loss of her own lamb.

In the pregnant ewe, the placenta near term is the major site of progesterone and estrogen synthesis. In fact, after d 55 of gestation, ovariectomy of ewes does not result in termination of pregnancy. Progesterone and estrogen are essential in facilitating the changes in the chemistry of the central nervous system (CNS) required for normal maternal behavior in this species. As term approaches, the increase in systemic concentrations of estrogen and reduced concentrations of progesterone induce expression of the oxytocin (OT) gene in the CNS. Concentrations of OT mRNA are increased in cells in the paraventricular and supraoptic nuclei, posterior portion of the medial preoptic area (MPOA), and the bed nucleus of the stria terminalis of the hypothalamus immediately after parturition and during subsequent lactation. In the ewe, exogenous estrogen is more effective than exogenous progesterone in increasing OT mRNA in the bed nucleus of the stria terminalis and MPOA whereas the reverse is true for the supraoptic and paraventricular nuclei. The ability of exogenous progesterone to stimulate significant increases in OT mRNA in several hypothalamic nuclei has not been observed for other species. However, based on immunocytochemical study, estrogen appears to increase storage of OT in the supraoptic and paraventricular nuclei as well as in the olfactory bulb.

The actual process of the young passing through the birth canal, resulting in vaginocervical stimulation, is what is believed to induce the release of OT. In multiparous ewes, OT is the only peptide, when infused via an intracerebral cannula, that promotes all acceptance behaviors of the ewe toward the lamb.

It must not be assumed, however, that maternal behavior is a phenomenon simply regulated by changing systemic ratios of placental steroids and efferent neural stimuli inducing synthesis and release of OT. There is evidence in the ewe that opiates play a role in promoting maternal behavior. Intracerebroventricular (icv) infusion of naltrexone, an opiate antagonist, reduced the ability of vaginocervical stimulation to induce maternal behavior and ewes continued to be aggressive to the lamb. Furthermore, icv infusion of morphine into ewes does not by itself induce significant changes in cerebrospinal or plasma concentrations of OT but markedly potentiates the ability of vaginocervical stimulation to increase concentrations of this nonapeptide in these biologic fluids.

Although there no doubt are other endocrine components that underlie activation of maternal behavior in this species, existing data clearly demonstrate the essentiality of OT in this phenomenon.

The role of OT in promoting maternal behavior in the rat is comparable with its role in sheep. Against rising systemic concentrations of estrogen and decreasing concentrations of progesterone, such as occurs as a prelude to parturition, icv administration of OT to rats rapidly promotes maternal behavior. As in the ewe, the increase in placental secretion of estrogen prior to parturition stimulates synthesis and secretion of OT at parturition. It is not surprising that estrogen can induce increased synthesis of OT in the rat because in this species the 5′-flanking region of the OT gene has been

found to contain estrogen response elements. Administration of OT antiserum to the rat via icv cannula blocked the onset of maternal behavior as did lesioning of the paraventricular nucleus in the hypothalamus. Although secretion of OT from the posterior pituitary occurs during parturition and the onset of suckling, it is not this source of the hormone that evokes maternal behavior. This is supported by experimental evidence demonstrating that intravenous infusion of OT failed to stimulate maternal behavior in rats. It has been demonstrated that oxytocinergic neurons projecting from the MPOA to the ventral tegmental area may be important for initiation of maternal behavior in the rat. Indeed, lesioning of the MPOA in the rat completely prevents the initiation of maternal behavior. Additionally, oxytocinergic neurons have been found to terminate in the amygdala, substantia nigra, olfactory bulb, and ventral hippocampus in rats and sheep. Projection of oxytocinergic neurons to intra- and extrahypothalamic sites is consistent with the detection of OT receptors (OTRs) in the following subsystems of the CNS: the olfactory system, the basal ganglia, the limbic system, the thalamus, the hypothalamus, some cortical regions, the brain stem, and the spinal cord. Thus, it is not surprising that icv rather than iv infusions of OT are more effective in promoting maternal behavior in rats and sheep.

2.2. OTR Expression in the CNS: Role in Regulation of Sexual Behavior and Stress Response

As mentioned in the previous section, OTRs have been detected in many brain regions, including the central nucleus of the amygdala and the ventromedial nucleus of the hypothalamus (VMH). These two regions of the brain are critical elements of neural pathways that regulate distinct behavioral responses. In particular, the VMH has been shown to be an important mediator of female sexual behavior, and the amygdala is that part of the limbic system that coordinates fear and anxiety responses as well as mother-infant interactions.

Expression of female sexual behavior requires the action of estrogen in the brain, including the induction of OTR in the VMH. By contrast, OTR levels in the amygdala are unaffected by estrogen despite the presence of dense collections of estrogen-concentrating neurons. Thus, there are apparent differences among regions of the brain in terms of the signal transduction pathways that activate OTR gene expression. In ovariectomized estrogen-primed rats, infusion of OT into the VMH increased expression of sexual behavior (lordosis) but had no effect on lordosis when infused into the amygdala. The VMH OT-induced increase in lordosis was blocked by previous treatment with a protein kinase C (PKC) inhibitor, suggesting that the effect of this nonapeptide may be dependent on activation of this kinase. Indeed, experiments conducted to measure the binding of OT in the VMH of ovariectomized rats demonstrated that estradiol-induced upregulation of OTR in the VMH was blocked by infusion of a PKC inhibitor. On the other hand, in vehicle-injected rats, infusion of a phorbol ester (an activator of PKC) into the VMH elicited an increase in OT binding comparable with that detected in estradiol-treated rats infused with saline. Infusion of an inhibitor or an activator of PKA into the VMH failed to alter estradiol-induced upregulation of OTR, as determined by binding of OT. These data indicate that estradiol increases OTR binding in the VMH via a PKC-dependent mechanism. The facts that infusion of phorbol ester mimicked the effect of estradiol and that infusion of a PKC inhibitor suppressed OT binding in the VMH suggest that estradiol acts nongenomically to upregulate OTR in the VMH of the rat.

The central nucleus of the amygdala receives direct dopaminergic innervation from the midbrain. In response to stress, there is an increase in the activity of dopamine neurons projecting to the amygdala. Evidence suggests that increased release of dopamine to the amygdala results in maintenance and/or an increase in OTR expression. Experimental evidence indicates that upregulation of OTR in the central nucleus of the amygdala occurs as a result of dopamine binding to D1 receptors to activate PKA. Binding of OT in the amygdala was suppressed in ovariectomized rats in which the amygdala was infused with a PKA inhibitor or dopamine D1 receptor antagonist. OT is also released centrally in response to a variety of stressors and is generally believed to be anxiolytic. Thus, it has been proposed that OT and dopaminergic systems may act in concert to reduce anxiety in response to social and environmental stressors.

In summary, interpretation of the results of research suggests that differences exist in underlying mechanisms for OTR expression among brain regions and that this type of heterologous regulation of OTR is critical for the different behavioral responses evoked by OT. Although estrogen-dependent OTR expression in the VMH is mediated via activation of PKC, the receptors in the amygdala are dependent on PKA, which is activated by dopamine D1 receptors. In the amygdala, OT acts to suppress anxiety, whereas in the VMH, this nonapeptide acts to stimulate sexual behavior.

2.3. A Mouse in the Ointment

As described, OT has been reported to promote maternal as well as sexual behavior and to have anxiolytic and antidepressant actions in most mammalian species. This was presumed to include mice as well. However, recent studies involving the use of mice that are homozygous for deletion of exon 1 of OT gene, i.e., the OT nonapeptide sequence, may lead one to question the role of OT as a modulator of various social and sexual behaviors, at least in this animal. These "OT knockout mice" (OTKO mice) reach sexual maturity, exhibit sexual behavior, deliver their young, and display normal maternal behavior at parturition. Because the milk ejection reflex is absent in these OTKO mice, they are unable to rear their young. The mouse may be unique among mammalian species relative to the role of OT in regulating various behaviors and physiologic phenomena. On the other hand, it is possible that vasopressin (which is still produced by OTKO mice) assumes some of the functions of OT.

3. STRESS AND THE AMPLECTIC CLASP

The endocrinology of sexual behavior has been studied in a wide range of vertebrate species, and from this research has emerged some common concepts. For example, it is central dogma that estrogen and progesterone in females and testosterone in males are essential for promoting sexual behavior. Similarly, in both females and males these steroids stimulate secretion of various neuropeptides with which they act in concert to bring about the full complement of physical responses that allow successful reproduction of the particular species.

As in any field of biologic study, there occasionally emerges a model that greatly expands researchers' base of knowledge. The rough-skinned newt (*Taricha granulosa*) has proven to be an excellent model for understanding the endocrine basis of sexual behavior. In this amphibian species, reproduction usually extends from late winter through spring. Reproductively active males usually congregate in shallow waters of ponds or lakes, awaiting the arrival of gravid females. The male initiates courtship by grasping the female in an amplectic clasp (Fig. 1). Amplexus usually persists for many hours before the male releases the female and deposits a spermatophore on the bottom of the pond or lake. The female then positions herself over the spermatophore and presses the sperm cap of the spermatophore into her cloaca. Females begin to ovulate about 2 wk after being inseminated and clasp underwater objects to which they attach their eggs.

The unique and novel display of reproductive behavior by this amphibian, which can readily be studied in the laboratory, has resulted in new and exciting data about the endocrine regulation of sexual receptivity. In female and male rats, sexual activity is mediated by steroid-induced synthesis of OT and OTRs in the hypo-

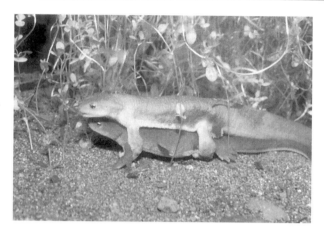

Fig. 1. Rough-skinned male newt (*T. granulosa*) displaying courtship behavior by grasping female in an amplectic clasp. (Photograph courtesy of F. Moore, PhD, Oregon State University, Corvallis, OR.)

thalamus and extrahypothalamic regions of the CNS. In female rats, OT appears to increase the frequency and duration of lordosis as well as stimulate uterine and oviductal contractions. In male rats, this nonapeptide promotes penile erection, and contractions of the seminiferous tubules and vas deferens. By contrast, in the rough-skinned newt the reproductive behaviors are mediated by arginine vasotocin, a peptide that, like OT, is believed to have evolved from a common ancestral peptide. Like other vertebrate species, reproductive activity in male *T. granulosa* requires secretion of testosterone and dihydrotestosterone, which attain peak concentrations in early spring. In females, estrogen is the primary steroid involved in promoting reproductive activity. As demonstrated by results of gonadectomy/steroid-replacement studies, in both male and female newts, gonadal hormones act to maintain the behavioral actions induced by arginine vasotocin. Also in both male and female newts, administration of arginine vasotocin provokes characteristic changes in sexual behavior of either intact or steroid-treated gonadectomized animals. Administration of arginine vasotocin to males promotes initiation of courtship behavior (amplexus), and injection of females with this peptide induces oviposition. In males, several brain regions contain measurable quantities of arginine vasotocin, but during the breeding season only changes in the optic tectum levels of this peptide and courtship behavior are positively correlated. As might be anticipated, changes in optic tectum concentrations of arginine vasotocin are also highly correlated with seasonal changes in plasma steroid concentrations, further suggesting that gonadal steroids modulate synthesis and/or secretion of this peptide. Additionally,

gonadal steroids have been shown to regulate the number of arginine vasotocin receptors in a site-specific manner in the male and female newt brain. It should be mentioned that newts are not the only species in which reproductive behaviors are modulated by vasotocin. For example, administration of vasotocin has been shown to enhance spawning behaviors in fish, sexual receptivity in female frogs, singing in male frogs and birds, and egg-laying behaviors in reptiles and birds.

When males of a given species court and mate, they must be able to recognize conspecific females as potential mates and respond in a species-specific manner to sensory information of various forms telegraphed by the female. Vasotocin in male newts may be responsible for enhancing sensory responsiveness to courtship-related stimuli. Application of cloacal pressure to the male newt causes a contraction of flexor muscles in the hind legs referred to as "reflexive clasping response," which is particularly enhanced in breeding males. This response is mediated via rostral medullary neurons, which on cloacal pressure, exhibit increased firing. Vasotocin applied to the medulla markedly potentiates the magnitude of neuronal responses to cloacal pressure and increases the spontaneous discharge of rostral medullary neurons. Vasotocin also enhances neuronal responses to light pressure on the jaw such as occurs during courtship behavior when the male repeatedly contacts the female's snout with his mandible during amplectic clasping. In conclusion, in male newts the androgen-induced increase in arginine vasotocin enhances sensory responsiveness to courtship-related stimuli.

It should not be inferred from the previous discussion that reproductive behaviors, and especially those of newts, are based solely on the integrated functions of a single neuropeptide and gonadal steroids. On the contrary, reproductive behaviors in all classes of animals are controlled by a vast array of hormones and neurotransmitters that exert either stimulatory or inhibitory actions. The previous discussion focused on those chemical messengers that stimulate sexual behavior in the rough-skinned newt. This stimulated sexual behavior is easily visualized because of the amplectic clasp of the male and the somewhat comparable ovipository clasp of the female. Exposure of male newts to a harsh stimulus markedly reduces courtship behavior as reflected by a reduction in amplexus. Such harsh stimuli are stressful and evoke within minutes a marked increase in plasma concentrations of corticosterone. Similarly, it was found, through laboratory behavioral testing of sexually active males, that administration of corticosterone totally suppressed amplexus. Increased systemic concentrations of corticosterone apparently act to modify brain neuronal activity. In particular, results of neurophysiologic studies indicate that exogenous corticosterone rapidly depresses spontaneous activity and sensory responses of the medullary neurons, which normally fire in response to tactile stimuli of the cloaca or mandible. These observations indicate that the suppressive effects of corticosterone on neuronal processing of sensory stimuli may underlie the ability of this inter renal gland steroid to inhibit reproductive behavior.

Perhaps one of the more important contributions to neuroendocrinology has come from studies of sexual behavior in the rough-skinned newt. Because the effect of exogenous corticosterone in suppressing reproductive behavior was evident within minutes, it was difficult to accept that the action of this steroid was mediated via classic genome transcription pathways. Consequently, studies were undertaken to determine, by use of radioligand binding assays, whether neuronal membranes contained specific binding sites for corticoids. Indeed, in highly purified preparations of neuronal membranes labeled corticosterone specifically bound to sites with high affinity and in a saturable manner. Specific binding of [³H]corticosterone reached equilibrium rapidly and was reversible. Competition studies revealed that the binding sites in neuronal membranes of the newt were highly specific for corticosterone. No other steroid, except cortisol, could compete for the binding sites. The location of the specific high-affinity binding site for corticosterone was subsequently confirmed by autoradiography, which revealed binding of the labeled steroid over synaptic neuropil and not over the cell bodies where intracellular steroid receptors are located. Collectively, the results of these studies indicated that the corticosterone receptor in neuronal membranes was distinguishable from the intracellular corticosteroid receptors. Although membrane receptors for progesterone in *Xenopus* oocytes were known to exist, the research with this species was the first to demonstrate that plasma membrane receptors for steroids could exist in the CNS. Existing data suggest that the rapid response of newts to corticosterone is mediated via G protein–coupled mechanisms. In *T. granulosa*, the results of radioligand binding assays revealed that [³H]corticosterone binding in neuronal membranes is negatively modulated by nonhydrolyzable guanine nucleotide analogs, especially GTPγS. In addition, specific binding of [³H]corticosterone to neuronal membranes is enhanced in a concentration dependent manner by the addition of Mg²⁺ to the assay buffer. These results are consistent with known data for G protein–coupled receptors (GPCRs).

Using nonionic detergents, the membrane glucocorticoid receptor (mGR) has been solubilized from synaptosomes of the newt (*T. granulosa*) brain. The solubi-

lized receptor has been shown to retain high-affinity binding of corticosterone and to have an identical rank-order potency for other steroid ligands as the membrane-bound GR (i.e., corticosterone > cortisol > aldosterone > dexamethasone). However, unlike the membrane-bound receptor, the solubilized receptor is insensitive to negative modulation by guanyl nucleotides and only modestly sensitive to Mg²⁺. Biochemical characterization of the solubilized receptor has revealed it to be an acidic glycoprotein with an apparent mol wt of 63 kDa. This is in contrast to the nuclear GR that is a nonglycosylated protein with a mol wt of approx 96 kDa. The mGR and nuclear GR therefore appear to be distinct receptor proteins. More recently, it has been reported that in addition to corticosterone, administration of various κ-selective opioid agonists could suppress male *T. granulosa* sexual behavior. Thus, results of additional studies to define further the nature of the receptor have revealed that certain opioid ligands could effectively compete with labeled corticosterone for binding. These findings are unique because, for the first time, in any species, it has been shown that specific opioid ligands can displace [³H]-corticosterone binding to neuronal membranes. These data therefore support the hypothesis that the [³H]-corticosterone binding site is located on a κ opioid-like receptor.

4. ENDOCRINE BASIS OF MALE-ORIENTED SEXUAL BEHAVIOR

Male homosexual behavior is quite widespread among mammals. At least 63 mammalian species have been identified in which male homosexual behavior occurs to some extent. Expression of male homosexual behavior has, in general, been attributed to the social environment to which the individual is exposed either prepubertally or as an adult and to the influence of hormones on sexual differentiation of the brain. As an example, male-male mounting of prepubertal domestic animals is believed to be important in the development of normal rear orientation in mount interactions. Even adult males of some species that are restricted from contact with females often exhibit homosexual behavior primarily because they have no choice for interaction with the opposite sex.

Sexual differentiation of the female brain of mammals is generally believed to proceed in the absence of hormonal imprinting. Consequently, as adults, most female mammals exhibit a characteristic cyclical pattern of luteinizing hormone (LH) secretion and feminine sexual behavior. However, sexual differentiation of the male brain of mammals is dependent on an interaction of brain cells with testosterone, which can be aromatized to estrogen, during a critical prenatal and/or postnatal period. Male mammals are characterized by an acyclical pattern of LH secretion and a form of sexual behavior characteristic for the species. Sexual differentiation of the brain has received considerable attention from the standpoint of the role of hormones in regulating the development and function of the neuroendocrine system. Comparatively less effort has been devoted to investigate the basis for sexual behavior. Nevertheless, the few studies that have been conducted provide compelling evidence that hormones do function at the level of the brain to establish patterns of sexual behavior. Male rats castrated 24–36 h after birth and treated with testosterone propionate (TP) on d 2 and 4 after birth when tested for sexual preference at 100 d of age preferred females if injected with TP at this time, but males if injected with estradiol benzoate (EB). Similar responses in terms of sexual preference to those observed for male rats have been recorded for male hamsters and pigs castrated shortly after birth and then as adults treated with TP or EB alone or in combination with progesterone. Collectively, these data seem to indicate that postnatal testosterone secretion may be more important than prenatal secretions of gonadal steroids in masculinizing the brain of the male with respect to sexual orientation as an adult. This is also supported by data on sexual preference of male ferrets castrated at various ages after birth. As adults, male ferrets castrated on d 5 after birth chose males in sexual preference tests more often than males castrated on d 20 or 35 after birth. Although the role of testosterone in masculinizing the brain and promoting female oriented sexual behavior seems fairly well established, it is also quite clear, based on experimental data, that estrogen can induce male homosexual behavior. Perhaps there are other factors produced by the testes of heterosexuals that protect against estrogen-induced homosexual behavior. For example, consider the response of male nonhuman primates to exogenous estrogen. In these males, the hypothalamic-hypophyseal axis responds to exogenous estradiol by releasing surge amounts of LH (ordinarily considered a female response) when the testes are removed but not when the male is left intact. Treatment of castrated males with testosterone or dihydrotestosterone, or testosterone in combination with physiologic levels of estradiol, does not suppress the estradiol-induced LH surge. These observations suggest that the testes of heterosexual males may produce some other substance that interferes with the actions of estradiol in the brain.

Much has been learned about the hormonal induction of homosexual behavior through experimentation, yet in actuality virtually nothing is known about the endocrinology of male subjects that normally express this behavior. Such a deficiency in researchers' knowledge stems from the inability to identify an adequate number of natural homosexual animals of one species that can be utilized in appropriately planned experiments. From this standpoint, domestic male sheep, hereafter referred to as rams, may serve as a useful model for studying the endocrine aspects of the homosexual. Homosexual behavior in domestic rams is quite common and even exists in the wild Bighorn and Dall sheep. In these latter populations, rams continue to mature for 5 or 6 yr after puberty and segregate into groups of their own away from females and juvenile rams. Those rams acting like mature males form all male societies in which dominant rams act the role of courting males and subordinate rams behave as "estrous" males. Studies of these populations have led to the conclusion that mountain sheep societies are basically homosexual.

Researchers at the U.S. Sheep Experiment Station in Dubois, Idaho, have, through rigorous sexual preference testing, identified an adult population of domestic rams consisting predominantly of heterosexuals but with a smaller percentage (<10%) of the population consisting of true homosexuals. Those rams exhibiting homosexual behavior were born as singlets or as a co-twin with either a male or female and all were reared prepubertally as a mixed population of males and females. Exposure of homosexual rams to receiver rams for a prolonged period of time (8 h) failed to provoke any change in plasma LH pulse frequency or basal concentration. By contrast, systemic concentrations of LH in heterosexual rams are markedly increased during prolonged exposure of the rams to estrous females. Sexual partner preference by rams does not appear to be regulated by hormonal status in adulthood. This is exemplified by the fact that variations in basal concentrations of testosterone in adult rams do not correspond with differences in mate preference. Further, castration, although reducing mounting behavior in heterosexual and homosexual rams, does not alter their choice of sexual partners.

The apparent absence of discernible social or hormonal factors that can explain the observed variations in sexual partner preferences of rams suggests the possibility that neural mechanisms are involved. Homosexual rams compared with contemporary heterosexual rams have been found to be deficient in hypothalamic MPOA aromatase activity. This is significant because the preoptic area of the hypothalamus is believed to mediate male reproductive behaviors in most vertebrate species. In rodents, the activity of aromatase (which converts androgens into estrogens) in the MPOA is relatively high compared with other parts of the brain. Within the MPOA/anterior hypothalamus (AH) of several species, including humans, sexually dimorphic cell groups have been identified that are significantly larger in males than in females. A sexually dimorphic nucleus in the preoptic area (SDN-POA) has been identified in rats. This SDN-POA has been found to be correlated with male copulatory patterns and sexual partner preference. In male rats treated perinatally with the aromatase inhibitor 1,4,6-androstatriene-3,17-dione, the volume of SDN was positively correlated with male-typical sexual behavior and female-directed partner preference. In humans, the third interstitial nucleus of the anterior hypothalamus (INAH3), which possesses positional and morphologic similarities to the SDN-POA of the rat, has been found to be significantly larger in heterosexual than in homosexual men and women. However, the extent of the difference has been recently questioned. Based on animal studies, it appears that masculinization of the SDN depends primarily on testosterone and/or estrogenic metabolites acting during early development. Research has been conducted to determine whether sexual partner preferences in rams are associated with morphologic differences in the MPOA/AH. This research has led to identification of a putative SDN in the sheep MPOA/AH. This ovine SDN (oSDN) is situated bilaterally in the caudal portion of the MPOA. The oSDN of heterosexual rams was found to be significantly greater in volume than in homosexual rams and ewes (female sheep). Similarly, by autoradiographic analysis it was demonstrated that aromatase mRNA levels in oSDN were significantly greater in heterosexual rams than in ewes, whereas intermediate levels of the enzyme were present in the oSDN of homosexual rams.

These data do not establish whether the observed differences in the size of the oSDN are the cause or effect of the animal's sexual partner preference. Nevertheless, to the extent that cross-species comparisons are valid, the acquired data regarding the morphologic and biochemical characteristics of the oSDN are in support of research demonstrating the human INAH3 to be more than twice as large in heterosexual men as in homosexual men and women. Moreover, the presence of aromatase in the oSDN suggests that testosterone metabolism to estradiol occurs in this nucleus and may be important for both its development and adult function. Further study of the homosexual ram may provide additional insight regarding the endocrine basis for this form of sexual behavior.

5. GROWTH AND DEVELOPMENT
5.1. Characteristics of Prenatal and Postnatal Growth

Body growth in mammals represents a response of the animals to a combination of genetic, nutritional and endocrine factors. In species such as rats, cattle, sheep and pigs males at birth and maturity are heavier than females. The novice might immediately attribute the weight advantage in males to testicular secretion of androgens. Indeed, if male rats are castrated at birth, they do not attain as great a weight as males castrated at 21 d of age. By contrast, ovariectomized female rats grow to a greater extent than intact females because estrogens have an inhibitory effect on body growth of rats. In both cattle and sheep, castrated males (steers and wethers, respectively) exhibit superior growth rates characterized by enhanced muscle-to-fat ratios over intact females. Unlike the positive effects of ovariectomy on the growth rate of rats, ovariectomy of heifers or ewes has either no effect or a negative effect on growth and body composition. In fact, in these species, exogenous estrogens in appropriate dosages are growth promotants, and the responses that they evoke are more consistent in castrated males than in intact females.

These descriptions of the effects of gonadectomy on body growth of mammals might give one the illusion that gonadal hormones are central in regulating growth. However, it should be recognized that they represent only one of the endocrines involved in this biologic process. Endocrine regulation of growth involves interactions among several hormones and growth factors, acting both systemically and locally. In addition to gonadal hormones, pituitary growth hormone (GH) and insulin-like growth factors (IGFs) are crucial for normal postnatal growth.

5.2. Patterns of GH Secretion

GH secretion in humans and a wide variety of mammals such as baboons, monkeys, cattle, sheep, goats, pigs and rats is pulsatile in nature. GH secretion in ruminants is asynchronous and episodic. In domestic animals, there is no relationship between sleep phases and GH secretion, as has been reported to be the case for higher primates. As a general rule, systemic concentrations of GH are greatest in prenatal and/or neonatal mammals and then decrease with age. The rat seems to be an exception to this rule. In fetal lambs, GH secretion is pulsatile as early as d 110 of gestation, and systemic concentrations of this hormone are greater than in the postnatal animal. Within 24 h of birth, GH concentrations decline 10-fold, with a reduction in both pulse amplitude and basal concentration values, to a secretory pattern not different from that of the adult. Similarly, in fetal pigs, serum GH concentrations increase from 40 d of a 110-d gestation period to concentrations of nearly 100 ng/mL at parturition. Mean serum concentrations of GH in postnatal pigs decrease with age owing mainly to secretory surges of reduced amplitude. In rats, episodic

GH secretion occurs prior to puberty and becomes maximal during early adulthood, after which secretion of the hormone decreases. The pattern of GH secretion is sexually dimorphic in adult male and female rats. Males exhibit a low-frequency, high-amplitude pattern of GH secretion. By contrast, GH secretion in females is characterized by high-frequency, low-amplitude secretory pulses.

It is well established that GH secretion is primarily regulated by two hypothalamic peptides: somatostatin, which suppresses pituitary secretion, and growth hormone releasing hormone (GHRH), which stimulates secretion. GHRH has been shown to stimulate GH secretion in cattle, goats, sheep, and poultry in a dose-dependent manner. There is convincing evidence that gonadal steroids modulate GH secretion. For example, in rats steroids appear to modulate basal GH levels as well as the frequency and amplitude of secretory pulses. Administration of testosterone to adult female rats produced male typical secretory patterns of GH and, after withdrawal of treatment, patterns of secretion of GH returned to those typical of female rats. As already alluded to, gonadal steroids are regulators of growth and development in domestic animals. GH secretion in rams and bulls is characterized by discrete episodic release that continues even after puberty. Castration increases the frequency of episodic release of GH and reduces the amplitude of the pulses. In prepubertal heifers, the pattern of GH secretion is qualitatively similar to that observed in bulls, whereas after puberty GH secretion in heifers is no longer characterized by discrete episodes of release. A pronounced activational effect of gonadal steroids on GH secretion has been observed in castrated male sheep (wethers). Administration of diethylstilbestrol or TP to wethers increased mean basal plasma concentrations of GH, reduced the frequency of episodic release of the hormone, but did not alter the amplitude of pulses compared with untreated control wethers.

In conclusion, some generalities can be drawn regarding patterns of GH secretion in nonprimate mammals. GH secretion in a wide variety of mammals appears to be greater during fetal development than after birth. GH secretion is sexually dimorphic in the rat but apparently not in other species. Patterns of GH secretion are modulated in part by gonadal steroids.

5.3. Regulation of GH Receptors

Two classes of GH receptors defined by affinity (high and low) have been detected in the liver of several species including the rat, rabbit, cattle, sheep, and pig. In ruminants and pigs, the number of high-affinity sites in the liver correlates with growth rate and plasma IGF-1 levels, whereas there is no such correlation for the low-affinity site. Using ligand binding assays, little or no binding of GH to liver membranes could be demonstrated until after birth in the calf or lamb. In pig hepatic membranes, binding of GH at birth is very low and gradually increases over 6 mo. Scatchard analysis has revealed a 10-fold increase in the capacity of the high-affinity GH receptor over this period. Chronic treatment of pigs and sheep with GH upregulates the high-affinity receptor found in hepatocytes but, at least in sheep, there is no effect of treatment on the low-affinity receptor. Little information is available about the effects of GH on its receptor concentrations in other tissues.

5.4. Insulin-Like Growth Factors

IGFs are important mediators of GH action in mammalian species. Ontogenic development of plasma concentrations of IGF-1 has been studied in rats, sheep, cattle, and pigs. Plasma levels of IGF-1 in rats, sheep, and cattle are low at birth and increase postnatally concomitant with the appearance of GH receptors in the liver, reflecting perhaps the onset of GH-dependent IGF-1 secretion. Similar data exist for systemic concentrations of IGF-1 in pigs, but there are also conflicting data suggesting that serum concentrations of IGF-1 are greater at birth and then decline steadily. In rats and pigs, serum concentrations of IGF-2 are greater at birth and decrease with age. In the bovine, IGF-1 and -2 are not only detectable in serum but also in colostrum and milk.

Plasma concentrations of IGF-1 in cattle are dependent on nutritional status through both GH-dependent and -independent mechanisms. In mature cattle, the ability of GH to maintain plasma IGF-1 is impaired when nutrient intake is markedly reduced. Both basal IGF-1 concentrations and the increment in plasma IGF-1 after administration of GH to cattle are most consistently affected by reduced dietary protein intake.

GH acting on the liver stimulates production of IGF-1, which, by vascular transport, affects distant target cells. Additionally, it is now well established that GH can act directly on the "distant" target cells to stimulate production of IGF-1, which acts in an autocrine or paracrine fashion. In recent years, bovine somatotropin has received much attention in the popular press because of its commercialization for use in stimulating milk production in dairy cows. Based on the mechanism by which GH promotes production of IGF-1, it is not surprising that when this pituitary hormone is administered daily to cows, systemic concentrations of IGF-1 increase dramatically. Concentrations of IGF-1 in mammary tissue and milk are also increased, but the increase in milk is minor and concentrations remain within the range of values detected in milk from untreated cows. The effects of exogenous bovine GH on the plasma concentration of IGF-2 in cattle are equivocal.

5.5. IGF Receptors

Not much is known about receptors for IGF in various species of mammals. Receptors for IGF-1 and -2 are present in bovine mammary gland tissue, bone, capillaries, retina, and adrenals. The receptors for IGF-1 are most abundant in mammary tissue during lactogenesis and decline during lactation. Receptors for IGF-2 predominate in mammary tissue in both the nonlactating and lactating glands, but abundance does not change in response to initiation of lactation.

5.6. IGF-Binding Proteins

Presently, six mammalian IGF-binding proteins (IGFBPs) have been cloned. Within a species, the IGFBPs share an overall protein sequence homology of 50%, and between species up to 80% nucleotide sequence homology in corresponding IGFBP is observed. No IGFBP genes have been cloned in nonmammalian vertebrates, yet their likely conservation among vertebrates is attested to by the ability of IGFBP from fish, amphibians, reptiles, birds, and metatherian mammals to specifically bind isotopically labeled mammalian IGF-1. The functional role of IGFBPs has not been determined with certainty, but it is obvious that these proteins have become, at least in mammals, complex players in growth and development processes. The IGFBPs do prolong the half-life of circulating IGF and separate the activities of these hormones from those of insulin. Additionally, there is now mounting evidence that the IGFBPs may play a functional role not only in delivery, but on a local basis, in ensuring that IGFs secreted by a cell are retained in the vicinity and therefore exert their action on the same (autocrine) or adjacent (paracrine) cell populations.

In mature sheep and cattle, the majority of circulating IGF is bound to IGFBP-3, which is comparable to the situation in humans. There is evidence from studies with domestic animals that treatment with GH significantly increases systemic concentrations of IGFBP-3. In sheep, an increase in systemic IGFBP-3 coincides with the marked increase in hepatic GH receptor that occurs during postnatal development. Reduced nutrient intake causes a reduction in plasma concentrations of IGFBP-3, which are markedly increased after refeeding in the rat and pig. On the other hand, in nutritionally restricted animals, an increased hepatic expression of genes for IGFBP-1 and -2 occurs. The physiologic significance of this increased gene expression for these IGFBPs is not completely understood.

6. PUBERTY

The phenomenon of puberty has been extensively studied in mammals. Compared to the human, the interval from birth to puberty is of short duration for most mammals. Puberty in the human occurs at a time when growth (weight) is 80–90% complete, whereas in most other mammals puberty is achieved when the young animal has attained only 30–70% of its adult weight. The Chinese Meishan pig is an example of one mammal that may attain puberty precociously. In this particular breed of pigs' puberty occurs at the age of 3 mo, when its body weight is only about 25% of its adult weight.

Puberty represents that stage in life when the hypothalamic-hypophyseal axis and the gonads have achieved a coordinate state of functional maturation sufficient to allow an individual to reproduce. Changes in hypothalamic, pituitary, and gonadal function that characterize this maturational process from before birth to puberty have been well documented for the rat, sheep, and primate. However, in this presentation, those similarities and differences in endocrine function and certain environmental factors that contribute to the onset of puberty in the rat and sheep are highlighted. When relevant, information on other mammalian species is included.

6.1. Rats

6.1.1. Prenatal Hypothalamic and Hypophyseal Function

In male and female rat fetuses, hypothalamic concentrations of gonadotropin-releasing hormone (GnRH) are low until about d 17 and 18 of gestation, after which concentrations increase to the day of birth. Receptors for GnRH are already detectable in the anterior pituitaries of male rats on d 16 of gestation. Pituitary LH and follicle-stimulating hormone (FSH) have been detected in rat fetuses of both sexes on and after d 17 of gestation. Pituitary LH content in female rats may be greater than in male rats during the late days of gestation.

6.1.2. Ovarian Development

In humans, ewes, and cows, at birth the ovary contains antral follicles. This is not the situation for female rats, mice, and pigs, in which antral follicles develop only after birth. In the rat, a marked increase in primordial follicles is observed between 24 and 48 h after birth. Apparently, the formation of these primordial follicles in the rat is independent of any kind of endogenous gonadotropin stimulation. Neither administration of equine chorionic gonadotropin nor of FSH is able to stimulate follicular development during the first few days postnatally. Furthermore, receptors of LH and FSH have not been detected in the rat ovary during the first 4 or 5 d after birth.

6.1.3. PREPUBERTAL CHANGES IN HYPOTHALAMIC-HYPOPHYSEAL FUNCTION

In female rats, the first ovulation occurs around 38 d of age. Secretion of FSH in the female increases from birth up to 12 d of age and thereafter declines so that by about 5 to 6 d prior to ovulation plasma concentrations of this gonadotropin are markedly reduced. Secretion of LH also increases up to approx 3 wk of age, but the increase is not as dramatic as for FSH. During the remaining 2 to 2.5 wk of the prepubertal period, systemic concentrations of LH are low but quite noticeably pulsatile, with the interpulse interval being about 30 min. These changes in FSH and LH secretion during the prepubertal period are believed to reflect the secretion of GnRH. Infrequent release of GnRH is believed to favor a sustained high level of FSH secretion and only generate transient bursts of LH release. However, as frequency of GnRH pulses increases with resultant increased pulsatile secretion of LH, there occurs a decrease in systemic concentrations of FSH. The increased systemic concentrations of gonadotropins evident during the early prepubertal period may also be owing in part to reduced sensitivity of the anterior pituitary to estradiol negative feedback and to greater responsiveness of the pituitary to GnRH. The anterior pituitary during the early prepubertal period contains a greater percentage of gonadotropins. Additionally, the systemic concentrations of α-fetoprotein that bind endogenous estrogens with relatively high affinity remain elevated until at least d 16 of age. Rat milk contains a GnRH-like substance that is chromatographically indistinguishable from hypothalamic GnRH. During the first 2 wk after birth, this milk GnRH is believed to cross the gastrointestinal epithelium of the pup in sufficient quantities to bind to GnRH receptors in the ovary with a consequent inhibition of gonadotropin-induced estrogen and progesterone production. Such a phenomenon would theoretically suppress ovarian function and hence preclude any type of hormonal feedback on the hypothalamic-hypophyseal system of the young female.

During the latter half of the prepubertal period, the ovary grows in response to the low systemic levels of FSH and LH. Waves of follicles begin to develop and undergo atresia, but it should be emphasized that none attain the ovulatory stage. Concomitantly, there is an increase in the number of gonadotropin receptors, especially the receptors for LH, and a decrease in GnRH receptors, which continues until the first proestrus. Two additional pituitary hormones play a role in regulating prepubertal ovarian function in the

rat. Both prolactin (PRL) and GH have been shown to contribute to ovarian maturation by facilitating the effects of gonadotropins. PRL enhances ovarian steroidogenesis in response to exogenous human chorionic gonadotropin (hCG) and FSH. Although GH may act directly on the ovary, there is considerable evidence that the actions of GH are mediated by IGF-1. IGF-1 is produced by granulosa cells and facilitates FSH induction of aromatase activity, progesterone secretion, and formation of LH receptors. Approximately 8 to 9 d prior to the first proestrus, the diurnal pattern of LH release changes in the female rat. Both basal LH levels and LH pulse amplitude become greater in the afternoon than in the morning. Some peripubertal females also exhibit a more sustained midafternoon episode of LH secretion, which has been termed a minisurge. These minisurges of LH may promote increased synthesis of estrogen by the ovary. However, the afternoon increase in LH pulse amplitude is not estradiol induced, whereas the minisurges of LH do appear to be caused by increases in systemic concentrations of estradiol.

The ovary of the rat during the transition to proestrus produces increasing quantities of estradiol, progesterone, and testosterone and reduced quantities of 3α-androstanediol. Reduction in the synthesis and secretion of the latter steroid may be elicited in part by the rising levels of PRL. It has been proposed that 3α-androstanediol may be involved in delaying the onset of puberty, but this has not been substantiated experimentally. The secretion of estradiol is the key event that ultimately triggers the onset of puberty in the rat. Estradiol acts on both the anterior pituitary and the hypothalamus to promote the proestrous surge of LH that causes ovulation. In the hypothalamus, estradiol evokes a release of GnRH, and in the pituitary, it sensitizes the gonadotropes to the stimulatory effect of GnRH. The increase in ovarian progesterone production prior to proestrus may have a role in facilitating the stimulatory effect of estradiol on GnRH release. Perhaps this effect of progesterone on GnRH release may be owing in part to the ability of this steroid to increase GnRH gene expression.

Hypothalamic concentrations of GnRH in the male rat increase throughout postnatal development and even into adulthood. Pituitary concentrations of GnRH receptors and LH are maximal at about 30 d of age; then receptor levels, decline to adult levels detected at about 60–70 d of age. This reduction in GnRH receptors is inversely related to testicular testosterone feedback action on the hypothalamic-hypophyseal axis.

During neonatal development serum concentrations of gonadotropins in males are increased but are significantly lower than levels detected in females. Subsequently the systemic levels of these gonadotropins decrease. The nature of LH secretion during the peripubertal period in the male rat is equivocal. Some reports suggest that LH secretion increases, whereas other reports indicate a decrease or no change. The onset of puberty in the male is, however, associated with an increase in FSH secretion. Serum FSH levels rise postnatally and attain maximum levels usually between 30 and 40 d of age. Thereafter, serum concentrations of FSH decline as serum levels of testosterone increase.

During the interval between 1 and 4 wk of age, testosterone is not the primary androgen produced by the rat testes. During this time, the activity of 5α-reductase in the testes is markedly increased. Consequently, the primary androgens produced by the immature rat testes are androstenedione, 5 α-androstanediol, and 5 α-dihydrotestosterone. After d 40 of age, 5 α-reductase activity decreases, and because of enhanced activity of 17 α-hydroxylase, C_{17-20} lyase, and 17 α-hydroxysteroid dehydrogenase, testosterone becomes the major androgen synthesized and secreted. As in males of other species, actual testosterone secretion is highly correlated, but phase delayed, with pulses of LH release.

6.2. Sheep

6.2.1. Puberty in Females

In most North American breeds of sheep, the females born in late winter and early spring usually attain puberty at about 7 mo of age. The ovaries of ewe lambs, although possessing antral follicles at birth, do not respond to exogenous gonadotropins until after 2–4 wk of age. After 5 to 6 wk, exogenous gonadotropins can induce ovulation and formation of corpora lutea. In the prepubertal ewe lamb, pulsatile secretion of LH has been detected as early as the second week after birth. The amplitude of the LH pulses is similar to that detected in the adult ewe, but the frequency is lower, on the order of 90–120 min apart. From the time of birth to puberty, systemic concentrations of FSH are greater than basal or pulsatile concentrations of LH. Changes in systemic concentrations of FSH are, however, positively correlated with pulsatile releases of LH in the intact and ovariectomized ewe lamb. A functional ovarian negative feedback system is apparently not operational in the ewe lamb during the first few weeks after birth. This is supported by data demonstrating that ovariectomy of ewe lambs is followed by a lag period of 2 to 3 wk or more before pulsatile secretion of LH occurs with a frequency and an amplitude resembling that found in ovariectomized mature ewes. This is similar to the situation in the neonatal female rat in which ovariectomy during the first few postnatal days of life fails to activate gonadotropin release. The fact that ovariectomy of ewe lambs results in high-frequency LH pulses during prepuberty may also be interpreted as indirect evidence that the pituitary is able to respond accordingly to GnRH. Indeed, it has been demonstrated that each LH pulse in ovariectomized prepubertal lambs is preceded by a GnRH pulse. In the ewe lamb, onset of puberty appears to be dictated by the sensitivity of the hypothalamic-hypophyseal axis to the negative feedback of ovarian estradiol. This sensitivity decreases with the age of the ewe lamb, thus allowing increased gonadotropin secretion, which, in turn, stimulates the ovary to produce sufficient estrogen to provoke the preovulatory surge of LH. This role of estradiol in regulating gonadotropin secretion in the ewe lamb has been demonstrated experimentally. Chronic treatment of ovariectomized ewe lambs with estradiol beginning at an early age suppressed high-frequency pulsatile secretion of LH up until the time that intact controls began exhibiting pubertal estrus. At this time, pulsatile secretion of LH began occurring in the ovariectomized ewe lambs.

In ewe lambs approaching puberty, the frequency of pulsatile LH secretion increases and the amplitude of the pulses decreases. This is similar to the pattern of LH secretion during the follicular phase of the cycle of mature ewes. Ultimately, this pattern of LH secretion promotes increased synthesis of estradiol by ovarian follicles, which then feeds back positively to trigger the first ovulatory surge of LH. However, this ovulatory surge of LH is rarely accompanied by expression of behavioral estrus. In most cases, the corpus luteum or luteinized follicle developing from the first ovulatory surge is short-lived, resulting in a so-called short luteal phase of about 6 to 7 d of duration, and characterized by a transient increase in systemic concentrations of progesterone. This short luteal phase may be followed by an ovulatory surge of LH accompanied by expression of behavioral estrus, which results in a cycle of normal duration (15–17 d) in ewes, or the ovulatory surge may result in another short luteal phase before ovulation with estrus occurs. In mature ewes that are seasonal breeders, short luteal phases also precede the expression of estrus with ovulation during the transition from anestrus to cyclic activity. A short luteal phase, or at least a transient increase in systemic concentration of progesterone, has been found to precede first ovulation with estrus in prepubertal heifers. In female pigs, pubertal estrus and ovulation is not preceded by a transient increase in progesterone secretion. It appears that prepubertal short luteal phases may be a characteristic common to ruminants.

6.2.2. Photoperiod Can Affect Puberty in Female Sheep

In seasonal breeding sheep, changes in sensitivity of the hypothalamic-hypophyseal axis to estradiol that characterize the onset of puberty are modulated by photoperiod signals to which the animal is exposed. In sheep, changes in the photoperiod (hours of light and hours of darkness) are perceived by the retina, and the information is telegraphed via a neuronal pathway ultimately to affect synthesis of melatonin by the pineal gland. During darkness, the pineal gland of sheep secretes rather copious quantities of melatonin in a pulsatile fashion. The pattern of melatonin secretion constitutes a form of neuroendocrine record of changes in the photoperiod that modulates the frequency of GnRH secretion and, hence, pulsatile LH secretion required for the onset of puberty. For puberty to be attained in the correct season for mating (autumn in the northern hemisphere), the lamb must be born in late winter or spring. In other words, these lambs must be exposed to long days (long hours of daylight) followed by short days. Lambs born out of season (i.e., born in autumn or winter) are exposed to short days followed by long days. Although these lambs attain a state of maturity and somatic development commensurate with attainment of puberty during the following spring, puberty is delayed until autumn. The reason for the delay in puberty arises from continued hypersensitivity of the hypothalamic-hypophyseal axis to estradiol negative feedback. Consequently, tonic LH secretion is low in autumn-born lambs during the spring and summer, thus preventing preovulatory follicular development. In conclusion, the photoperiod regulates the onset of puberty in some breeds of sheep through changes in hypothalamic-hypophyseal sensitivity to estradiol inhibition of LH secretion.

6.2.3. Onset of Puberty in Males

Spring-born male lambs begin reproductive development at about 10 wk of age, as evidenced by the onset of the spermatogenic cycle. In ram lambs, the first pulsatile release of LH occurs on average at about 3 wk of age but can occur as early as 1 wk of age. The frequency of pulsatile LH release increases with age, reaching a maximum near 8 wk and decreasing thereafter. Serum concentrations of LH increase concomitantly with the frequency of pulses, attaining maximum levels at 8 wk and then decreasing. Pulsatile release of LH in ram lambs stimulates a rise in systemic concentrations of testosterone that are maximal by 1 h after the pulse of LH. The testes of the neonatal lamb are responsive to stimulation by gonadotropins. The administration of hCG to a 2-d-old ram lamb provoked an increase in testosterone secretion. It has been proposed that during prenatal development, androgens from the testes both masculinize (male traits) and defeminize (female traits) mechanisms controlling LH secretion in the male sheep. Presumably, the androgens would act to alter the neural components that process and relay information about the photoperiod to the neural network governing GnRH secretion. Consequently, tonic secretion of LH would be masculinized and defeminization of the LH surge mechanism would occur, thus preventing activation of the GnRH surge in response to estradiol. In essence, this would prevent the preovulatory gonadotropin surge from becoming operative in the male. The pattern of melatonin secretion in the ram and ewe in response to a changing photoperiod is similar. However, unlike the ewe, the ram's GnRH pulse generator appears to be rather insensitive to changes in the photoperiod. Precisely why males do not respond to the photoperiod whereas females do is unknown.

7. ENDOCRINOLOGY OF THE ESTROUS CYCLE

7.1. Patterns of Hormone Secretion

The sequences of neuroendocrine and gonadal hormones secreted during the course of the estrous or menstrual cycles of mammals are coordinated to promote successful reproduction of the species. Characteristics of the estrous cycle of a number of mammalian species are presented in Table 1. As can be appreciated from these data, the time of spontaneous ovulation occurs coincident with the expression of behavioral estrus thus ensuring that mating will occur when a viable ovum is available to be fertilized. In the primate, ovulation occurs midway in the menstrual cycle (duration of 28 d) and is not overtly associated with expression of mating behavior, as occurs in other mammals. In contrast to the protracted follicular phase of the menstrual cycle, the follicular phase during the estrous cycle is of relatively

Table 1
Characteristics of Estrous Cycles of Some Mammals

Species	Duration of cycle (d)	Duration of estrus (h)	Time of ovulation relative to onset or end of estrus
Cow	19–23	13–18	10–12 h after end
Elephant	120	96	Not defined
Goat	21	30–40	30–36 h after beginning
Guinea pig	16–19	12	8–10 h after beginning
Hamster	4	24	8–12 h after beginning
Mare	19–25	96–192	24–48 h before end
Mouse	4	10	2–3 h after beginning
Pig	18–22	48–72	36–46 h after beginning
Rat	4–5	13–15	8–10 h after beginning
Sheep	15–17	24–48	24–30 h after beginning

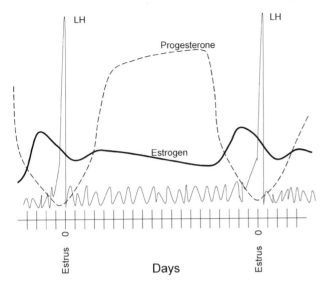

Fig. 2. Temporal patterns of pituitary and ovarian hormones secreted during estrous cycle of domestic animals. Although variable among species, serum concentrations of progesterone and LH are in nanograms/milliliter and those of estrogen are in picograms/milliliter.

short duration (1–3 d) and occurs during proestrus. The granulosa and theca cells of the ovulated follicle luteinize to form one or more corpora lutea, depending on whether the animal is monovular or polyovular. The formation and growth of the corpus luteum that occurs during metestrus and diestrus, respectively, and the progesterone produced by this gland dictate, in part, the duration of the cycle. For most domestic and laboratory animals, the duration of the estrous cycle is long compared with that of rats, mice, and hamsters, whose cycles are 4 to 5 d in duration. Hence, during the estrous cycles of rats and mice, in which no mating occurs, corpora lutea develop rapidly after ovulation but produce little progesterone, and within 2 to 3 d the corpora lutea undergo functional regression. A typical pattern of hormone secretion that occurs during the estrous cycle of domestic animals is presented in Fig. 2.

7.2. Folliculogenesis

Ovulatory-size follicles do not develop during the luteal phase of the primate menstrual cycle, but a cohort of growing follicles emerges during the early follicular phase. Toward the end of the follicular phase, only one follicle usually continues to become the ovulatory follicle and the others undergo atresia. Although follicular development occurs during the luteal phase of the estrous cycle of pigs, no follicles attain ovulatory size. Similarly, during the luteal phase of the cycle of sheep,

follicular development in polyovular ewes apparently occurs as a continuum, with no clear evidence for follicular dominance until corpora lutea regress. By contrast, in cows, waves of follicular development occur during the luteal phase of the cycle. Usually animals have only two waves that begin developing on d 2 and 11. In some, three waves of follicles develop beginning on d 2, 9, and 16 of the cycle. Each wave consists of three to six follicles. The duration of the luteal phase of the cycle appears to determine, at least in part, the number of follicular waves during the cycle. After several days, one follicle grows to near ovulatory size to become a dominant follicle whereas the subordinate follicles regress. Eventually the dominant follicle in each wave, except the last one, also regress. In the last wave, the dominant follicle becomes the ovulatory follicle. Mares usually have one wave of follicular development that occurs during the midluteal phase of the cycle, but about one-third of mares have two waves, one beginning shortly after ovulation and the other during the mid- to late luteal phase.

Recruitment of follicles is owing to secretion of FSH. For example, in rats a secondary surge of FSH occurs on the day of estrus, just before the next cohort of ovulatory follicles is recruited. In the cow, there is not only a secondary surge of FSH on the day of ovulation (d 1) that precedes the first follicular wave of the cycle, but also slight increases in systemic FSH that precede the second and third follicular waves.

In most mammalian species, follicular estradiol synthesis requires the coordinated function of both follicular endocrine cell types and both LH and FSH: theca cells producing androgens in response to LH and granulosa cells aromatizing the androgens to estradiol in response to FSH and later in follicular development in response to both FSH and LH. Theca cells from dominant follicles secrete significantly more androgen, and granulosa cells possess a greater capacity to convert androgens to estradiol than follicular cells from subordinate follicles. Subordinate follicles destined for atresia usually are characterized by the presence of follicular fluid containing high concentrations of androgens. The increased production of estradiol by the dominant preovulatory follicle(s) feeds back to the hypothalamic-pituitary axis to stimulate the pulsatile secretion of LH, which ultimately constitutes the ovulatory surge of this gonadotropin.

7.3. Characteristics of Corpus Luteum

The mature corpus luteum varies in size, depending on the species of mammal. In the rat, the corpus luteum weighs a few milligrams, whereas in the cow one corpus luteum may weigh in excess of 5 g. Corpora lutea of the rat, cow, ewe, sow, monkey, and rabbit have been found to consist of two steroidogenic cell types, referred to most commonly as small and large cells. This designation is based primarily on cell diameter along with distinguishing morphologic characteristics. Large luteal cells possess both rough and smooth endoplasmic reticula, whereas small luteal cells possess only the smooth endoplasmic reticulum characteristic of steroidogenic cells. The major secretory product of the corpus luteum is progesterone, but, in addition, this endocrine gland produces other steroids, the nature and quantity of which vary among the mammalian species. This variation in steroid secretory products indicates that differences do exist in the complexity of luteal steroidogenic pathways. Extremes in steroidogenesis are exemplified, on the one hand, by the bovine corpus luteum, which secretes progesterone, 20β-hydroxy-4-pregnen-3-one, and pregnenolone, and on the other hand, by the human corpus luteum, which secretes progesterone, 20α-hydroxy-4-pregnen-3-one, pregnenolone, 17β-hydroxyprogesterone, 4-androstenedione, estrone, and estradiol. In bovine and ovine corpora lutea, although large cells are fewer in number than small cells, they account for the majority of progesterone synthesized and secreted.

7.3.1. LUTEOTROPINS

Large and small luteal cells are endowed with LH receptors. Therefore, it is not surprising that LH is luteotropic during the estrous cycle of such species as the cow, ewe, mare, and primate. Tonic secretion of LH that occurs during the cycle of these animals is apparently able to sustain the maintenance and function of the corpus luteum until the response to the gonadotropin is overridden by the endogenous luteolysin. The designation of this gonadotropin as a luteotropin is based on research demonstrating that exogenous LH prolongs the luteal life-span and that LH is able to stimulate luteal progesterone synthesis in vivo and in vitro. Interestingly, the stimulation of progesterone production in response to LH is based on its effect on small luteal cells. Large luteal cells, at least in the cow and ewe, are unresponsive to stimulation by LH, although, as mentioned, these cells do possess LH receptors as well as adenylyl cyclase capable of being activated by forskolin and cholera toxin. Steroidogenesis in the large luteal cell appears to be "free running" until induced to undergo apoptosis.

Whether LH is luteotropic in the sow is debatable because hypophysectomy shortly after the onset of estrus allows ovulation and development of corpora lutea that are slightly smaller in size by d 13 to 14 of the cycle but otherwise fully functional. However, an injection of hCG administered to the sow near the midluteal phase of

Table 2
Duration of Pseudopregnancy and Pregnancy in Select Mammals

Species	Type of ovulation	Duration of pseudopregnancy (d)	Duration of pregnancy (d)
Cat	Induced	30–40	65
Dog	Spontaneous	~ 60 [a]	58–63
Fox	Spontaneous	40–50 [a]	52
Hamster	Spontaneous	7–13	16–19
Mink	Induced	Variable	Variable [b]
Mouse	Spontaneous	10–12	19
Rabbit	Induced	16–17	30–32
Rat	Spontaneous	12–14	22

[a] Pseudopregnancy follows even without copulation.
[b] Variable owing to delayed implantation; the duration depending on time of mating during the breeding season.

the cycle prolongs the functional life-span of the corpora lutea.

Some species of mammals that ovulate spontaneously and have relatively short estrous cycles will on cervical stimulation at estrus resulting from an infertile mating or experimental manipulation become pseudopregnant. Similarly, some mammals become pseudopregnant if ovulation is induced as a result of an infertile mating or if injected with LH or hCG. Characteristics of pseudopregnancy in a select group of spontaneous and induced ovulators are presented in Table 2. Corpora lutea of pseudopregnancy have unique requirements for luteotropic support. The rabbit is one species in which the maintenance and function of corpora lutea during pseudopregnancy as well as during pregnancy are dependent on estrogen. In the northern hemisphere, mink, an induced ovulator, mate only in late February to March. The corpora lutea that form remain nonfunctional until after the vernal equinox, when the lengthening hours of daylight to which the animal is exposed promote increased secretion of PRL. This pituitary hormone serves as a luteotropin in mink and activates the corpora lutea to begin producing large quantities of progesterone in the pseudopregnant or pregnant animal. In the pseudopregnant or pregnant rat the stimulus of mating results in PRL being secreted as two daily surges for the first 8 d and as a single nocturnal surge on d 9. PRL is luteotropic in the rat and also functions to suppress the activity of 20α-hydroxysteroid dehydrogenase, whose activation is associated with luteal regression in this species. Pituitary LH is also luteotropic in the pseudopregnant and pregnant rat and is required from d 8 to 12 for the synthesis of ovarian estrogen, the third luteotropic hormone. If the rat is pregnant, additional luteotropic support in the form of decidual and placental lactogens is provided throughout gestation. After d 12, hormones of the pituitary gland are no longer required. The placenta of the rat also synthesizes androgens, which are aromatized to estrogens by the corpora lutea.

7.3.2. Luteal Peptide Hormones

OT and the related peptide, vasopressin, are synthesized in the large luteal cells and granulosa cells in the ovaries of humans, nonhuman primates, cattle, sheep, goats, and pigs. In cattle and sheep, the ovulatory surge of LH initiates OT gene transcription and OT synthesis and secretion by granulosa cells. After ovulation and luteinization of granulosa cells, mRNA for this nonapeptide continues to increase dramatically, attaining maximal luteal concentrations by about d 3 of the cycle. Thereafter, luteal concentrations of OT mRNA decrease, whereas luteal concentrations of the hormone actually increase, reaching maximal levels by the midluteal phase of the estrous cycle and then gradually decreasing. Why OT levels in the corpora lutea of domestic animals increase early in the cycle is not known. It has been suggested that OT may serve as an autocrine or paracrine modulator of luteal cell function in the developing corpus luteum.

7.4. Luteolysis

It is well established that regression of the corpus luteum in most mammals is initiated by exposure of the gland to endogenous prostaglandin $F_{2\alpha}$ ($PGF_{2\alpha}$) synthesized and secreted by the uterus or the corpus luteum itself. In the cow and ewe, with two distinct uterine horns, the uterine vein draining each horn lies in close apposition to the ovarian artery. Regression of the corpus luteum in these species during the estrous cycle is the consequence of a functional interrelationship between the ovary and adjacent uterine horn. At the end of the estrous cycle, uterine concentrations of OTRs are increased in the cow and ewe. OT, most probably of pituitary origin, binds to uterine OTRs to stimulate endometrial synthesis and secretion of $PGF_{2\alpha}$, which is transferred via a countercurrent mechanism from the uterine vein to the ovarian artery (Fig. 3). This pulsatile release of $PGF_{2\alpha}$ acts on the corpus luteum to stimulate secretion of OT, which acts back on the uterus to provoke another pulse of $PGF_{2\alpha}$ release. This double positive feedback system between the adjacent ovary and uterine horn ensures the generation of several pulsatile releases of $PGF_{2\alpha}$ that ultimately cause luteal regression. In species in which the anatomic arrangement of the vascular system precludes a local effect of the uterus on ovarian function, such as in the mare, the $PGF_{2\alpha}$ generated by the uterus must travel via the gen-

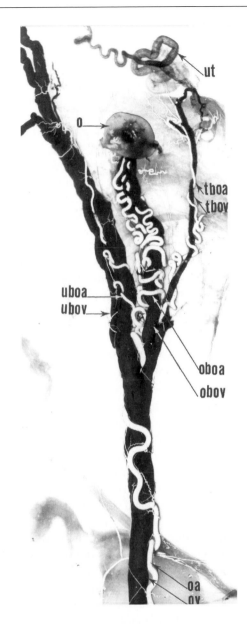

Fig. 3. Arteries (light) and veins (dark) of right uterine horn and ovary from sheep. $PGF_{2\alpha}$ secreted by the uterus is transferred from the uterine branch of the ovarian vein (ubov) by a countercurrent mechanism to the ovarian artery (oa). The tortuous nature of the ovarian artery and its close apposition to the uteroovarian vein increase the surface area by which transfer of $PGF_{2\alpha}$ can occur. o = ovary; oboa = ovarian branch of ovarian artery; obov = ovarian branch of ovarian vein; ov = ovarian vein; tboa = tubal branch of ovarian artery; tbov = tubal branch of ovarian vein; uboa = uterine branch of ovarian artery; ut = uterine tube. (Reproduced with permission from the American Journal of Veterinary Research and Dr. O. J. Ginther, University of Wisconsin.)

eral systemic route to reach the ovary. In primates, it is believed that the corpus luteum brings about its own demise through the synthesis of $PGF_{2\alpha}$.

7.4.1. ENDOTHELINS: MEDIATORS OF PGF$_{2\alpha}$ ACTION IN LUTEOLYSIS

Endothelin-1 (ET-1) is a vasoactive peptide that was first isolated from porcine vascular endothelial cells. This peptide is a member of a structurally homologous family that includes ET-2, ET-3, and sarafotoxins. ET-1 is synthesized from a 212-amino acid precursor referred to as prepro ET-1 (ppET-1) that is proteolytically cleaved into big ET-1 (38 amino acids) and then further processed into the active form of ET-1 (21 amino acids) by ET-converting enzyme-1 (ECE-1). This enzyme is a membrane-bound protein that belongs to the zinc-binding metalloendopeptidases. Several isoforms of this enzyme differ in their N-terminal sequence.

ETs bind two major receptor subtypes designated ETA (for aorta) and ETB (for bronchus) that belong to the serpentine GPCR superfamily. The ETA receptor binds ET-1 with the highest affinity, and ETB binds all three ETs with equal affinity.

7.4.2. ET-1 RECEPTORS AND CONVERTING ENZYME IN LUTEAL TISSUE

Interest in ET-1 as a potential agent involved in regulating the function of the corpus luteum stemmed from the initial reports that ET-1 inhibited cyclic adenosine monophosphate (cAMP)– and LH- or FSH-stimulated progesterone production by rat and porcine granulosa cells. Subsequent research demonstrated that ET-1 inhibited basal as well as LH-stimulated progesterone production by bovine luteal cells in vitro. The use of a selective ETA receptor antagonist (BQ123) established that the inhibitory actions of ET-1 were exerted via ETA receptor–binding sites in bovine, ovine, rat and human corpora lutea. The ETA receptor was found to be expressed in both the large and small steroidogenic cells of the bovine corpus luteum. In theca-derived luteal cells, LH and forskolin downregulated the ETA receptor mRNA, and in granulosa-derived luteal cells, downregulation of ET-1 mRNA was caused by exposure to IGF-1. The results of these in vitro experiments are of physiologic significance. The results of subsequent research demonstrated that concentrations of ETA mRNA were lowest in the LH-stimulated developing corpus luteum and maximal by the end of the estrous cycle.

Two different isoforms of ECE-1 exist in the bovine corpus luteum. Both isoforms possess comparable enzymatic activity but differ in N-terminal sequence. More interesting was the finding that one form, ECE-1b, is found in the plasma membrane, and the other form, ECE-1a, is an intracellular enzyme. Both steroidogenic and endothelial cells of the corpus luteum can synthesize ECE. However, whereas endothelial cells in the mature corpus luteum express both ECE-1a and -1b mRNAs, the luteal cells express only ECE-1b. This finding was confirmed by the observation that steroidogenic luteal cells cleaved the big ET-1 and therefore must express the membrane-bound form of the enzyme.

Apparently, the expression of ECE-1 might vary during the estrous cycle because levels of mRNA and protein are greater in the mature than in the developing corpus luteum. This is supported by the finding that concentrations of big ET-1 in the developing corpus luteum are greater than in the mature gland, and the luteal ratio of ET-1 to big ET-1, reflecting ECE-1 activity, increased from the early to the midluteal phase of the cycle.

7.4.3. ROLE OF ET-1 IN CORPUS LUTEUM REGRESSION

In the highly vascular corpus luteum, the endothelium is the primary source of ET-1. The concentration of ppET-1 mRNA is maximal in the bovine corpus luteum on d 18 of the estrous cycle and much less on d 5 and 10 of the cycle. As might be expected, luteal concentrations of ET-1 were found to be highest on d 17–21 of the bovine estrous cycle, about 30 times greater than on d 5 of the cycle. Because regression of the bovine corpus luteum normally is under way on or about d 17 of the cycle, it was surmised that the luteolytic hormone PGF$_{2\alpha}$ induced the expression of ppET-1. Indeed, research has confirmed that exposure of luteal tissue to PGF$_{2\alpha}$ results in increased expression of ET-1 mRNA and its translation product. In the bovine, exogenous PGF$_{2\alpha}$ is effective in inducing luteal regression only after d 5 of the cycle. The ineffectiveness of PGF$_{2\alpha}$ in causing luteal regression prior to d 5 is consistent with the observation that the developing corpus luteum contains minimal levels of ET-1 and ETA receptor compared with levels present in the mature gland. The ineffectiveness of PGF$_{2\alpha}$ in causing luteolysis of the developing corpus luteum cannot be attributed to a lack of functional F2 receptors. This is evident from the observation that administration of PGF$_{2\alpha}$ to the bovine prior to d 5 induces secretion of luteal OT.

As a consequence of the research on luteal characteristics of the ET system, a model has been proposed to account for the mechanisms of action of PGF$_{2\alpha}$ and ET-1 in causing luteal regression (Fig. 4). It is proposed that PGF$_{2\alpha}$, in addition to binding to its luteal cell receptor, also binds to its receptor in endothelial cells to stimulate the production of big ET-1 and ET-1. Steroidogenic luteal cells expressing the membrane form of ECE-1b and no ppET-1 cleave the increasing quantities of big ET-1, thus further increasing the extracellular levels of ET-1 to which the cell is exposed. This ET-1 is then able to bind to the ETA receptor and act in concert with PGF$_{2\alpha}$

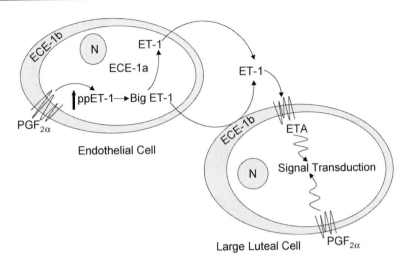

Fig. 4. Proposed functional relationship between endothelial and large steroidogenic cells during $PGF_{2\alpha}$-induced regression of bovine corpus luteum. Binding of $PGF_{2\alpha}$ to receptors in the endothelial cell stimulates an increase in ppET-1, which is enzymatically cleaved to form big ET-1. The big ET-1 is acted on by intracellular ECE-1a to form ET-1, which is then secreted. Big ET-1 can also be secreted from endothelial cells to be converted to ET-1 by ECE-1b located in the plasma membrane of luteal cells. The available ET-1 binds to its receptor (ETA) in the plasma membrane of the large luteal cell. The combined actions of ET-1 and $PGF_{2\alpha}$ on the luteal cell result in luteolysis.

to provoke the regression of the corpus luteum. This latter premise is supported in part by the observation that intraluteal injection of the ETA receptor antagonist (BQ123) prior to administration of $PGF_{2\alpha}$ delayed the luteolytic effect of $PGF_{2\alpha}$ compared to pretreatment with saline.

7.4.4. Nitric Oxide: Another Factor in Luteal Regression

Nitric oxide (NO) is a vasodilator produced by endothelial cells. Intraluteal administration of Nω-nitro-L-arginine methyl ester, an inhibitor of NO synthase, was shown to prolong luteal life-span in the bovine. Endothelial cells of the corpus luteum may contain ETB receptors that bind ET-1, -2, or -3 to stimulate the release of NO in response to $PGF_{2\alpha}$. It is obvious that NO is somehow involved in promoting luteolysis, but whether NO is a mediator of $PGF_{2\alpha}$ or acts in concert with $PGF_{2\alpha}$ is unknown.

8. LEPTIN IN DOMESTIC ANIMALS
8.1. Discovery and Significance

Several single-gene obesity mutations in rodents have been identified during the past half-century, but none has provoked more interest in the scientific community than the mouse ob gene discovered in 1950. The recessive ob/ob mouse is excessively obese owing to hyperphagia and suffers from hyperinsulinemia, hypercorticism and hypothermia. Subsequently, another

closely related mutant mouse (db/db) was discovered that exhibited a similar phenotype. This latter obese mouse was hyperphagic, had decreased energy expenditure, and was hyperglycemic. The results of elegant parabiotic experiments in which ob/ob mice were paired with db/db mice led to hypotheses that the ob gene encoded a satiety hormone and the db gene, the corresponding receptor. Subsequent research proved the hypotheses to be correct. In 1994, the encoded product of the ob gene was reported to be a 16-kDa protein that was named leptin (from the Greek *leptos*, meaning thin). In all species studied, leptin is synthesized primarily by adipose tissue. Shortly thereafter, in 1995, the leptin receptor was cloned and genetically mapped to the db locus on mouse chromosome 4. Further research established that in rodents there are at least six variants of the leptin receptor owing to alternative splicing of the mRNA. In the db/db mouse, the long form of the leptin receptor was found to be abnormal. Hence, although this mouse produced leptin, the abnormal receptor prevented its ability to respond to the satiety hormone. The leptin receptor belongs to the class I family of cytokine receptors, which include receptors for interleukin-6, leukemia inhibitory factor (LIF), granulocyte colony-stimulating factor, and glycoprotein 130. The six leptin receptor isoforms share a common extracellular amino terminus to which the leptin binds but differ in their carboxy terminus. Five receptor isoforms possess transmembrane domains, but only the long form contains an intracellular motif sufficient to activate signal transduction via the JAK-STAT or mitogen-activated protein kinase pathway. It is known that leptin binds to receptor homodimers with high affinity. One form of the leptin receptor lacks a transmembrane domain and may serve to transport leptin in the systemic circulation.

In the fed rodent and human, at steady-state energy balance, leptin secretion and body fat mass are positively correlated. This fact coupled with the reports that administration of recombinant leptin to ob/ob mice reduced feed intake and body weight became of intense interest to clinicians and scientists with visions of using leptin therapy to combat obesity in humans. These reports also became of interest to animal scientists who have labored for years to discover biologic or pharmaceutical compounds capable of altering body composition through repartitioning of nutrients to enhance lean protein accretion over fat deposition. The report that exogenous leptin reversed infertility in ob/ob mice by stimulating the secretion of gonadotropins was also of interest from the standpoint of its potential use in improving reproductive efficiency in domestic animal species.

8.2. Characteristics of Leptin Secretion

Leptin is secreted in a pulsatile manner in humans, and in both humans and rodents the leptin concentrations in blood are diurnally regulated with the maximal level attained at night. In rodents, but not in humans, peak levels of leptin coincide with the initiation of feeding behavior. In sheep and pigs, as in humans, secretion of leptin appears to be in a pulsatile manner. The reason for the pulsatile nature of secretion of leptin from adipocytes is unknown but suggests the existence of some factor that regulates leptin secretion and/or clearance. Because adipocytes contain β-adrenergic and insulin receptors, it is conceivable that the pulsatile nature of leptin secretion reflects, at least in part, the exposure of the adipocyte to neural releases of catecholeamine or changing systemic concentrations of insulin. Diurnal changes in systemic concentrations of leptin are not present in sheep or in periparturient dairy cows, as is evident in rodents and humans.

8.3. Regulation of Food Intake in Domestic Animals

The hypothalamus has long been recognized as playing a central role in regulating food intake. In rats, ablation of the VMH caused hyperphagia and morbid obesity whereas lateral hypothalamic lesions led to inanition and starvation. Consequently, the ventromedial hypothalamus is considered to be the site of a satiety center, and the lateral hypothalamus contains the feeding cen-

ter. Evidence exists suggesting that the regulation of food intake in mammals is owing to the action of leptin on these hypothalamic centers. In sheep, leptin binds primarily to the ventromedial and arcuate nuclei. Fasting of sheep for 3 wk caused an increase in the expression of the mRNA for the long form of the leptin receptor in these hypothalamic nuclei compared with those of well-fed sheep. Intracerebroventricular injections of leptin cause marked reductions in food intake and fat reserves in ob/ob mice, wild type mice, rats, monkeys and pigs. Similarly, icv administration of human leptin for 3 d markedly reduced voluntary dry-matter food intake by ovariectomized sheep. Neuropeptide Y (NPY) is believed to be a major mediator of the effects of leptin on feed intake and gonadotropin secretion. NPY is a potent stimulator of food intake in rodents, and hypothalamic concentrations of this neurotransmitter reflect the nutritional status of the animal; for example, concentrations are increased in fasting animals. Furthermore, the long form of the leptin receptor has been shown to be colocalized with NPY receptors in the arcuate nucleus of the rat and sheep. Intracerebroventricular administration of leptin reduces NPY expression and synthesis in the hypothalamus of obese and fasted rodents and sheep (ewes). By contrast, NPY secretion in the arcuate nucleus increases during fasting and decreases during feeding in the rat. It should be recognized that other neuropeptides, such as galanin, corticotropin-releasing hormone, agouti-related protein, α-melanocyte-stimulating hormone (MSH), proopiomelanocortin, and orexins A and B, also may play a role in regulating food intake. This is supported by the observation that NPY gene knockout fails to normalize weight in ob/ob mice and is without effect on food intake and body weight in the non-obese mouse.

8.4. Leptin and Reproduction in Domestic Animals

8.4.1. Puberty

The administration of recombinant leptin to ob/ob mice reversed infertility in these animals by stimulating increased secretion of gonadotropins, with a resultant increase in secondary sex organ weight and function. Subsequently, it was reported that exogenous leptin was able to promote early onset of puberty in mice. These were highly significant observations in the minds of scientists who labor to improve reproductive efficiency in domestic animals by inducing early onset of puberty in females. It is not surprising, therefore, that attempts have been made by some to determine the role of leptin relative to the onset of puberty in cattle, sheep, and pigs. In ovariectomized prepubertal gilts, estrogen-induced leptin mRNA expression occurred at the time of expected puberty, as in intact contemporaries, and was associated with greater LH secretion. In prepubertal beef heifers, fasting by restricting intake of food for 48 h decreased leptin gene expression and systemic leptin in association with reductions in the secretion of LH as well as IGF-1 and insulin. Furthermore, in the fasted group of animals, the mean frequency of LH pulses was lower than in the well-fed control group of heifers. Although limited in scope, these studies suggest that leptin is likely involved in regulating gonadotropin secretion and, hence, the onset of puberty in domestic animals.

8.4.2. LEPTIN REGULATION OF LH SECRETION

The lactating postpartum ruminant is generally in a state of negative energy balance, even when provided with adequate nutrition, and is anestrus, at least through the early postpartum period. In lactating sheep, plasma leptin and adipose tissue leptin mRNA concentrations are reduced. Expression of the gene for the long form of the leptin receptor (OB-Rb) was shown to be increased in the hypothalamic arcuate nucleus and ventromedial hypothalamic nucleus. However, NPY was increased in both the arcuate nucleus and dorsomedial hypothalamus, which serves to account, at least in part, for the hyperphagia of these lactating sheep. Restoration of estrous activity in lactating ruminants has been shown to be dictated primarily by the onset of normal LH secretion. Consequently, much interest has focused on the role of leptin in promoting gonadotropin secretion in the mature animal. In mature ovariectomized cows implanted with estradiol to maintain basal secretion of LH, fasting for 60 h significantly reduced serum levels of insulin and leptin. The icv infusion of recombinant leptin into these fasted cows increased serum concentrations of insulin, leptin, and LH compared with concentrations prior to treatment. The mean magnitude of LH pulses (determined by the area under each pulse) was greater in fasted than in control cows. This was apparently owing to extended duration of individual pulses because neither amplitude nor frequency of pulses differed between control and treated animals. However, in fasted castrated ram lambs, the administration of leptin prevented the reduction in LH pulse frequency that occurred in vehicle-treated controls.

It has been generally assumed that the feedback effect of leptin in regulating gonadotropin secretion was manifested at the level of the hypothalamus. In fact, it has been reported that leptin stimulates GnRH release from rat hypothalamic explants. It is believed that the effects of leptin on hypothalamic GnRH release are mediated by NPY. This premise is supported by data demonstrating that icv administration of NPY suppresses LH secre-

tion in pigs and sheep. However, leptin receptors have been shown to be present in gonadotropes of the anterior pituitary of sheep, pigs, mice, and rats, and leptin has been shown to stimulate directly gonadotropin secretion from cultured anterior pituitaries of the rat, steer, and pig. The ability of leptin to act at the level of the gonadotrope in cattle seems to depend on whether the animal is in a negative or positive energy balance. Basal release of LH from anterior pituitary explants of fasted but not normally fed cows was increased in response to leptin. By contrast, leptin-treated explants from normally fed, but not fasted, cows released more LH in response to GnRH than respective control tissues. These latter data suggest that leptin modulates the secretion of LH in mature cows, to a large extent, by its direct actions on the adenohypophysis.

9. ENDOCRINE CONTROL OF PELAGE GROWTH AND REPRODUCTION IN MUSTELIDS

In the order Carnivora, the family Mustelidae encompasses numerous members that abound in the wild as well as some that have been domesticated or, because of their economic value, are reared in captivity. Examples of the latter types are the ferret and mink. Therefore, it is not surprising that more is known about the biology of these two species than all other mustelids.

In this section, emphasis is devoted to describing some of the unique aspects of the endocrine control of pelage growth and reproduction in mink. However, when available and relevant, information about these processes in other species is provided.

Mink, regardless of whether wild or reared in captivity, are photosensitive animals. Pelage growth and reproduction of mink occur, to a large extent, as responses to seasonal changes in hormone secretion by the CNS.

9.1. Pelage Growth Cycle

In the late 1930s, it was first reported that mink exhibited a seasonal fur growth cycle regulated by the photoperiod. Considerable evidence now exists that exposure of mink to decreasing hours of daylight after the summer solstice (June 21–22) stimulates molting of the summer fur and growth of winter fur, whereas the increasing hours of daylight after the vernal equinox (March 21–22) induce molting and growth of the summer fur. Studies on such unrelated species as the weasel, raccoon, snowshoe hare, Djungarian hamster and white-footed mouse have confirmed that changes in the photoperiod are involved in regulating seasonal hair growth cycles.

The possibility that hormones might be responsible for seasonal changes in pelage growth seemed remote until Wisconsin researchers demonstrated that melatonin implanted into another mustelid, the short-tailed weasel, forced molting of their brown summer fur and the growth of white winter fur. Subsequently, similar studies were conducted in which mink were treated with this indoleamine. The results of these studies confirmed that melatonin, when administered as an implant to mink during the summer, induced molting of the summer fur and early growth of winter pelage. This seasonal effectiveness of melatonin became obvious once it was demonstrated that in all vertebrate species examined thus far, the concentrations of melatonin in the pineal gland and plasma are increased during the dark portion of the daily light/dark cycle. It is now well established that the nocturnal rise in melatonin production occurs because norepinephrine released from innervating sympathetic neurons binds to pinealocyte β-adrenergic receptors, resulting in cAMP-mediated induction of N-acetyltransferase, the rate-limiting enzyme in the biochemical pathway leading to melatonin synthesis. Thus, as summer turns to fall, the average daily endogenous levels of melatonin to which mink are exposed increase and are sufficient to promote changes in pelage growth as just described.

It was generally assumed that melatonin acted directly on the hair follicle to evoke molting and regrowth. However, the discovery that seasonal changes in daily systemic levels of PRL occurred that were inversely related to those of melatonin suggested the possibility that this protein hormone might actually mediate the apparent effect of melatonin on the pelage cycle. Indeed, in mink, the spring and autumn molts were found to be correlated with increasing and decreasing daily plasma concentrations of PRL, respectively. Proof that photoperiod-related changes in prolactin secretion in mink are regulated, at least in part, by melatonin was provided by results of research demonstrating that the administration of melatonin to mink prior to the spring molt reduced systemic PRL levels and delayed the molt. Further evidence that PRL played an important role in controlling the pelage growth cycle was provided by data of studies in which mink were treated with bromocriptine. This ergot alkaloid suppresses PRL secretion and when given to mink during the summer induces molting of the summer pelage and rapid out-of-season growth of winter fur, just as in response to exogenous melatonin. Collectively, the available data suggest that PRL secretion as regulated by the seasonal changes in melatonin production stimulates fur growth of mink during the spring molt and may inhibit the autumn molt until mean daily levels become markedly suppressed owing to increased production of melatonin.

Although it is apparent that melatonin and PRL are primary regulators of the seasonal changes in hair growth, it should be noted that hormones such as MSH, adrenocorticotropic hormone, and even gonadal steroids have also been shown to be involved in this process, but perhaps more so in species other than mustelids.

9.2. Delayed Implantation

Delayed implantation is a form of diapause during which development of the embryo is retarded at the blastocyst stage. There are two types of delayed implantation: facultive (lactational) delay, as occurs in mice and rats, and obligate delay, as occurs in bats, roe deer, and various carnivores. The endocrinology of delayed implantation has been extensively studied in mink and the Western spotted skunk. Mink generally begin mating during late February or early March in the northern hemisphere. Ova fertilized at these early matings undergo development to the blastocyst stage and enter a diapause state. Interestingly, although diapaused embryos resulting from an early mating may be in residence in the uterus, the female may mate again. Fertilized ova from this second mating may also only develop to the blastocyst stage, with further development being arrested. Mating of the female to different males at the first and subsequent matings, which might occur as much as 1 wk later, can result in superfetation in this species.

The duration of delayed implantation in mink is variable, depending on the time of mating. After ovulation, corpora lutea are formed, but these structures appear to be almost translucent and devoid of complete vascularization during diapause. In both mink and spotted skunks, the corpora lutea apparently produce low quantities of progestins, but neither administration of progesterone nor of estrogens will induce implantation in intact or ovariectomized mink and skunks. Yet, the small amount of progestin produced by corpora lutea or perhaps some unknown ovarian protein hormone is essential to maintain embryo viability. Bilateral ovariectomy of mink during the delayed implantation period prevents implantation and results in death of the blastocysts.

As with the endocrine regulation of pelage growth, research has established that seasonal changes in the photoperiod act as the "zeitgeber" that times implantation in mustelids. Implantation of embryos occurs shortly after the vernal equinox in the northern hemisphere and coincides with the daily increased quantities of PRL being secreted. The uterus and ovaries of the mink contain relatively high concentrations of PRL receptors. In fact, the ovarian concentration of PRL receptors during diapause is about 30 times greater than the concentration of unoccupied receptors measured after the vernal equinox. The high concentration of PRL receptors in the ovary prior to the increase in PRL secretion reflects the fact that in mink PRL has been shown to be luteotropic and essential for functional activation of the corpora lutea to synthesize and secrete progesterone. As might be expected, treatment of mink with bromocryptine (a dopaminergic agonist) or melatonin suppresses PRL and progesterone secretion and prolongs the period of delayed implantation. It is to be noted that exogenous melatonin also decreases uterine concentrations of PRL receptors. Whether this is owing to inhibition of PRL secretion or some other indirect or direct effect of melatonin is not known.

Collectively, these data might be interpreted to suggest that implantation is initiated by activation of corpora lutea to produce progesterone. However, as indicated, progesterone by itself cannot initiate implantation of diapaused mink embryos. Similarly, there is no evidence that increased estrogen secretion is required for renewed blastocyst development or induction of implantation in carnivores as it is in rodents. Although evidence suggests that PRL and progesterone are involved in initiating implantation and maintaining pregnancy, the key biochemical(s) essential for terminating embryonic diapause in mustelids remains an enigma. Expression of LIF (a cytokine) in the endo-metrium of the mink uterus during embryo expression suggests the possibility that this compound may at least be another component of the implantation phenomenon.

SELECTED READING

Adkins-Regan E. Hormonal mechanisms of mate choice. *Am Zool* 1998;38:166–178.

Davis JS, Rueda BR. The corpus luteum: an ovarian structure with maternal instincts and suicidal tendencies. *Front Biosci* 2002;7: 1949–1978.

Foster DL. Puberty in the sheep. In: Knobil E, Neill JD, eds. *The Physiology of Reproduction*, 2nd Ed., vol 2. New York, NY: Raven, 1994:411–451.

Geist V. Mountain Sheep. *A Study in Behavior and Evolution*. Chicago, IL: University of Chicago Press, 1971.

Ginther OJ, Berg MA, Bergfelt DR, Donadeu FX, Kot K. Follicle selection in monovular species. *Biol Reprod* 2001;65:638–647.

Keverne EB, Kendrick KM. Oxytocin facilitation of maternal behavior in sheep. *Ann NY Acad Sci* 1992;652:83–101.

Ojeda SR, Urbanski HE. Puberty in the rat. In: Knobil E, Neill JD, eds., *The Physiology of Reproduction*, 2nd Ed., vol. 2. New York, NY: Raven, 1994:363–409.

Resko JA, Perkins A, Roselli CE, Stellflug JN, Stormshak F. Sexual behavior of rams: male orientation and its endocrine correlates. *J Reprod Fertil* 1999;Suppl 54:259–269.

Straus DS. Nutritional regulation of hormones and growth factors that control mammalian growth. *FASEB J* 1994;8:6–12.

Williams GL, Amstalden M, Garcia MR, Stanko RL, Nizielski SE, Morrison CD, Keisler DH. Leptin and its role in the central regulation of reproduction in cattle. *Dom Anim Endocrinol* 2002;23: 339–349.

Part IV

HYPOTHALAMIC–PITUITARY

12 Hypothalamic Hormones

GnRH, TRH, GHRH, SRIF, CRH, and Dopamine

*Constantine A. Stratakis, MD, DSc
and George P. Chrousos, MD*

CONTENTS

1. INTRODUCTION

Alcmaeon, a sixth-century BC physiologist philosopher, introduced the brain as the center of human thinking, organizer of the senses, and coordinator for survival. However, the need for a visible connection between the brain and the rest of the body to explain a rapid and effective way of communication that would maintain homeostasis led Aristotle to the erroneous conclusion that the heart was the central coordinating organ and blood the means of information transmission. In contemporary medicine, the two ancient concepts are integrated in the exciting field of neuroendocrinology. The traditional distinctions between neural (brain) and hormonal (blood) control have become blurred. Endocrine secretions are influenced directly or indirectly by the central nervous system (CNS), and many hormones influence brain function. The hypothalamic-pituitary unit is the mainstay of this nonstop, interactive, and highly efficient connection between the two systems. Its function is mediated by hypothalamic-releasing or hypothalamic-inhibiting hormones, including gonadotropin-releasing hormone (GnRH), thyrotropin-releasing hormone (TRH), growth hormone–releasing hormone (GHRH), somatostatin (SRIF), corticotropin-releasing hormone (CRH), and the neurotransmitter dopamine.

2. GnRH

2.1. GnRH Protein and Its Structure

The existence of GnRH as a hypothalamic factor was demonstrated in 1960. Systemic injection of acid hypothalamic extracts released LH from rat anterior pituitaries. The structure of GnRH was elucidated in 1971. The decapeptide pyroGlu-His-Trp-Ser-Tyr-Gly-Leu-Arg-Pro-Gly-amide was named luteinizing hormone-releasing hormone (LHRH). The term has been supplanted by GnRH, since this peptide not only releases LH from the gonadotropes, but also follicle-stimulating hormone (FSH). An FSH-specific hypothalamic-releasing hormone, however, may also exist and be similar to the LHRH/GnRH protein, explaining the difficulty researchers have met with its purification.

From: *Endocrinology: Basic and Clinical Principles, Second Edition*
(S. Melmed and P. M. Conn, eds.) © Humana Press Inc., Totowa, NJ

GnRH plays a pivotal role in reproduction. Phylogenetically, this protein has been a releasing factor for pituitary gonadotropins, since the appearance of vertebrates. The structures of its gene and encoded protein have been highly preserved. Only one form of GnRH has been identified in most placental mammals, but six additional highly homologous GnRH forms have been found in other more primitive vertebrates. Only three amino acids vary in these six molecules, which together with the mammalian protein (mGnRH) form a family of molecules with diversity of function, including stimulation of gonadotropin release; regulation of sexual behavior and placental secretion; immuno-stimulation; and, possibly, mediation of olfactory stimuli. In the human brain, placenta, and other tissues, where the gene is expressed, GnRH protein is the same. In other species, however, several GnRH forms are expressed in the various tissues and have different functions. In amphibians, mGnRH releases gonadotropins from the pituitary, but another, nonmammalian GnRH is responsible for slow neurotransmission in sympathetic ganglia.

Marked diversification of function exists within the relatively small GnRH peptide. The residues at the amino (N)- and corboxy (C)-termini appear to be primarily responsible for binding to the GnRH receptor, whereas release of LH and FSH depends on the presence of residues 1–4. These critical residues are conserved in evolution. In addition, residues 5, 7, and 8 form a structural unit, which is important for the biologic activity of GnRH receptors. Thus, the functional unit formed by the side chains of His^2, Tyr^5, and Arg^8 is necessary for full biologic activity of mGnRH. Substitution of the Arg residue reduces potency in releasing both LH and FSH, whereas replacement of the Leu^7 increases the potency for LH release, but does not alter that for FSH. Similar structure-function specificity is present in the remaining GnRH family members. The secondary structure of all GnRH peptides is highly conserved, too. A β-turn, formed by residues 5–8, creates a hairpin loop, which aligns the N- and C-termini of the GnRH molecule and provides the active domain of the hormone.

2.2. GnRH Gene and Its Expression

GnRH is synthesized as part of a larger peptide, the prepro-GnRH precursor. The latter contains a signal sequence, immediately followed by the GnRH decapeptide; a processing sequence (Gly-Lys-Arg) necessary for amidation; and a 56-amino-acid-long fragment, called GnRH-associated peptide, or GAP. Thus, the structure of prepro-GnRH is similar to that of many secreted proteins, in which the active sequence is coded along with a signal and processing sequences, and an "associated" peptide that is cleaved prior to secretion. GAP appears to coexist with GnRH in hypothalamic neurons, but its function remains elusive. Its sequence is considerably less preserved among species, and it does not appear to bind to specific receptors. GAP was initially thought to inhibit the secretion of prolactin (PRL), but this was not confirmed in vivo.

The human GnRH gene is located on the short arm of chromosome 8 (Table 1) and in all mammals consists of four exons. The first exon encodes the 5´-untranslated region (UTR). The second exon encodes prepro-GnRH up to the first 11 amino acids of GAP. The third and fourth exons encode the remaining sequence of the GAP and the 3´-UTR. Interestingly, the opposite strand of DNA is also transcribed in the hypothalamus and the heart. The function of this transcript, named SH, is unknown and may be involved in GnRH gene regulation. Despite the presence of many sequence changes among the GnRH genes of different species, the intro/exon boundaries have been preserved through evolution. The presence of highly homologous other GnRH forms in nonmammalian vertebrates suggests a common evolutionary process, that of the duplication of one common ancestor gene.

Expression of the GnRH gene is subject to significant species- and tissue-specific regulation. One example is the alternative splicing of the first GnRH gene exon in the mammalian brain and placenta. The promoter region of the rat GnRH gene has been sequenced and studied extensively. Sequences that can bind transcription factors, such as Pit-1, Oct-1, and Tst-1, as well as estrogen and other steroid hormone response elements exist in the 5´-flanking region of the rat GnRH gene, suggesting a quite complex and extensive hormonal regulation of its expression.

2.3. GnRH Receptor

The first step in GnRH action is recognition of the hormone by a specific cell membrane receptor (GnRH-R). The latter was recently cloned from several species, including human. It is a member of the seven-transmembrane segment class, characteristic of G protein–linked receptors. Several differences exist, however, between the GnRH-R and the other members of this superfamily of membrane proteins. The highly conserved Asp-Glu, which is essential for function and is found in the second seven-transmembrane segment of many receptors, is replaced in the GnRH-R with Asp. In addition, the GnRH-R lacks a polar cytoplasmic C-terminal region and has a novel phosphorylation site adjacent to the third seven-transmembrane segment.

The concentration of GnRH-Rs in the pituitary gland is tightly regulated and changes with the physiologic

Table 1
Genes, Pathophysiology, and Clinical Use of Hypothalamic Hormones

Hormone	Chromosome	Receptor	Associated disorders	Clinical Use
GnRH	8p	GnRH-R	Kallmann syndrome, precocious puberty, *hpg* mouse.	GnRH test, GnRH superagonists and antagonists
TRH	3	TRH-R	"Hypothalamic" hypothyroidism	TRH test
GHRH	20p	GHRH-R	*lit–, dw–,* and *dwj–* mice, "hypothalamic" GH deficiency	GHRH test, GHRH analogs and antagonists
SRIF	3q	SSTR-1–5		SRIF analogs
CRH	8q	CRH-R 1α, 1β CRH-R2	"Hypothalamic" adrenal insufficiency, chronic fatigue, fibromyalgia, atypical and melancholic depression, stress, autoimmune states	CRH test, CRH analogs and antagonists
Dopamine		D-1R–D-5R (pituitary: D2-R)	Nonadenomatous hyperprolactinemia	D-2R agonists

state of the organism. During the estrous cycle of rats, hamsters, ewes, and cows, the maximum number of receptors is observed just prior to the preovulatory surge of LH; thereafter, the number decreases and may require several days to achieve proestrous levels. Ovariectomy increases the number decreases significantly after exposure to androgens and during pregnancy and lactation. Several in vitro models employing pituitary cell cultures have indicated a biphasic response of GnRH-R to physiologic concentrations of GnRH. An initial desensitization of gonadotropes to GnRH is associated with downregulation of the receptor. This phase followed by an upregulation of the receptor number, which, however, is not associated with increased sensitivity to GnRH, since gonadotropes respond with near-maximal LH release, when only 20% of available GnRH-Rs are occupied.

The regulation of GnRH-R gene expression and protein function by GnRH provides the basis for the effects of constant GnRH infusion of GnRh superagonists on LH and FSH secretion. Whereas low or physiologic concentrations of GnRH stimulate the synthesis of GnRH-R, constantly high concentrations of this hormone downregulate the receptor in a process that involves physical internalization of agonist-occupied receptors. This is accompanied by loss of a functional calcium channel and other mechanisms. Indeed, GnRH regulates pituitary LH and FSH synthesis and release by a Ca^{2+}-dependent mechanism involving GnRH-R-mediated phosphoinositide hydrolysis and protein kinase C (PKC) activation. A G protein or multiple G proteins coupled to GnRH-R also play(s) and intermediatiory role. This protein appears to be dif-

ferent from G_s or G_i, and similar to that hypothesized to be involved in TRH mediation of action. Following GnRH stimulation, an increase in phospholipid metabolism and intracellular Ca^{2+} and accumulation of inositol phosphates occur in pituitary gonadotropes. Calmodulin and its dependent protein system are important intracellular mediators of the Ca^{2+} signal in the gonadotropes.

In addition to its action on the gonadotropes, GnRH exerts a variety of effects in the CNS. Lordosis and mounting behaviors are facilitated by intraventricular and subarachnoid administration of GnRH, or local infusion of this peptide in the rat hypothalamic ventromedial nucleus (VMN) and central gray. GnRh can change the firing patterns of many neurons and is present in presynaptic nerve terminals. These actions are mediated through GnRH-R. The latter has been found to be widely distributed in the rat brain, in areas such as the hypothalamic VMN and arcuate nucleus (but not the preoptic region), the olfactory bulb and the nucleus olfactorius, the septum, and the amygdala and hippocampus. With few exceptions, CNS GnRH-R binds to GnRH analogs with the same affinity as the pituitary GnRH-R does. However, the former may not share the same second-messenger system(s) with the latter, since it is unclear whether Ca^{2+} is needed for hippocampal GnRh action. Aside from the CNS, GnRH-R is present in the gonads (rat and human ovary, rat testis) and rat immune system. GnRH has also been demonstrated to stimulate the production of ovarian steroidogenesis from isolated rat ovaries. The physiologic significance of these actions, however, remains unclear.

2.4. GnRH-Secreting Neurons: Embryology and Expression

Almost all the GnRH in mammalian brains is present in the hypothalamus and regions of the limbic system, hippocampus, cingulate cortex, and olfactory bulb. GnRH-expressing neurons migrate during development from their original place on the medial side of the olfactory placode into the forebrain. The GnRH neurons, which are generated by cells of the medial olfactory pit, do not have a GnRH secretory function before they attain their target sites in the basal forebrain. They do, however, express the GnRH gene, a feature that allowed their detection by *in situ* hybridization. In mice, these cells are first noted in the olfactory epithelium by d 11 of embryonic life. By d 12 and 13, they are seen migrating across the nasal septum toward the forebrain, arriving at the preoptic area (POA) of the developing hypothalamus by d 16–20. GnRh neuron migration is dependent on a neural cell adhesion molecule, a cell-surface protein that mediates sell-to-cell adhesion, is expressed by cells surrounding the GnRH neurons, and appears to be a "guide" for their migration.

By immunocytochemistry, GnRH cell bodies are found scattered in their final destination, the POA, among the fibers of the diagonal band of Broca and in the septum, with fibers projecting not only to the median eminence, but also through the hypothalamus and midbrain. In primates, more anteriorly placed cell bodies in the POA and septum are connected with dorsally projecting fibers that enter extrahypothalamic pathways presumably involved in reproductive behavior, whereas more posteriorly placed cell bodies in the medial hypothalamus itself give rise to axons that terminate in the median eminence. The two types of GnRH neurons are also morphologically different; the former have a smooth cytoplasmic contour, whereas the latter have "spiny" protrusions. Similar anatomic and functional plasticity has been documented at the level of the GnRH neuronal terminal.

GnRH may be present in other areas of the nervous system. In frogs, a GnRH-like peptide in sympathetic ganglia is thought to be an important neurotransmitter. GnRH can enhance or suppress the electrical activity of certain neurons in vitro. GnRH is also present in the placenta, where its mRNA was first isolated. Interestingly, GnRH, like TRH, is secreted into milk.

2.5. GnRH Secretion and Action

Secretion of hypothalamic GnRH is required for reproductive function in all species of mammals studied. Its secretion is subject to regulation by many hormones and neurotransmitters that act on the endogenous GnRH secretory rhythm, the "GnRH pulse generator."

The latter provides a GnRH pulse into the hypophyseal-portal vessels at approx 90 intervals, which can be slowed down or accelerated by gonadal hormones. Testosterone and progesterone in physiologic concentrations and hyperprolactinemia slow the discharge rate of the generator, whereas estrogens have no effect on the frequency of the GnRH pulses. Females of all species respond to estrogens with an acute increase in LH and, to a lesser degree, FSH, a phenomenon that explains the "ovulatory LH surge" via positive estrogen feedback on the pituitary.

The mechanism of the estrogen-induced LH release has yet to be elucidated. The presence of testicular tissue prevents the estrogen-stimulatory effect on GnRH and LH secretion, but testosterone, although it slows down the GnRH pacemaker, does not completely abolish the estrogen effect. Since estrogen releases LH in castrated male monkeys, a nontestosterone testicular hormone other than inhibin may be responsible for this blocking effect in males.

GnRH secretion responds to emotional stress, changes in light-dark cycle, and sexual stimuli through the inputs that GnRH neurons receive from the rest of the CNS. Norepinephrine stimulates LH release through the activation of α-adrenergic receptors, and administration of α-antagonists blocks ovulation. A population of β-adrenergic neurons, which are inhibitory of GnRH secretion, has also been identified. Dopamine has inhibitory effects, but the role of epinephrine, G-aminobutyric acid (GABA), and serotonin is less clear. Acetylcholine may increase GnRH secretion, because it can induce estrus in the rat that is blocked by atropine. Glutamate stimulates GnRH secretion via the *N*-methyl-D-aspartate (NMDA) receptor. Naloxone can stimulate LH secretion in humans, but this effect is modulated by the hormonal milieu. Thus, administration of naloxone increases LH levels in the late follicular and luteal phases, but not in the early follicular phase or in postmenopausal women. It has been postulated that endogenous opioids may mediate the effects of gonadal steroids on GnRH secretion, since β-endorphin levels are markedly increased by administration of estrogen and progesterone.

Disruption of reproductive function in mammals is a well-known consequence of stress. This effect is thought to be mediated through activation of both the central and peripheral stress system. CRH directly inhibits hypothalamic GnRH secretion via synaptic contacts between CRH axon terminals and dendrites of GnRH neurons in the medial POA. The role of CRH regulation of GnRH secretion may be species specific with important differences noted between rodents and primates. Endogenous opioids mediate some of these effects of CRH, but their importance varies with species, as well as with the period of the cycle and the gender of the animals. CNS cytokines also regulate GnRH secretion and function. Central injection of interleukin-1 (IL-1) inhibits GnRH neuronal activity and reduces GnRH synthesis and release. These effects are in part mediated through endogenous opioids and CNS prostaglandins (PGs). IL-1 and possibly other central cytokines may act as endogenous mediators of the inflammatory stress-induced inhibition of reproductive function.

2.6. Gonadotropin Deficiency: Kallmann Syndrome

In 1943, Kallmann and associates described a clinical syndrome of hypogonadism and anosmia affecting both men and women. The pathologic documentation of the characteristic neuroanatomic defects of the syndrome led to the term *olfactory-genital dysplasia* for what is now known as *Kallmann syndrome*. With the discovery of GnRH in 1971, the defect was determined to be hypothalamic in all patients with the syndrome, who subsequently were shown to resume normal gonadotropin secretion after repeated and/or pulsatile administration of GnRH.

The genetic basis of Kallmann syndrome, which has in most cases an X-linked inheritance, was recently elucidated at the molecular level. The earlier evidence that GnRH-secreting neurons migrate to the hypothalamus from the olfactory placode during development, combined with the observation that many patients with the X-linked form of ichthyosis caused by steroid sulfatase deficiency also had deafness and hypogonadotropic hypogonadism, led to identification of the *KAL* gene. The latter maps at chromosomes Xp22.3, is contiguous to the steroid sulfatase gene, and codes for a protein that is homologous to the fibronectins, with an important role in neural chemotaxis and cell adhesion.

Since the identification of the *KAL* gene, several defects have been described in patients with Kallman syndrome. Contiguous gene deletions have been found in patients with other genetic defects, such as ichthyosis, blindness, and/or deafness, whereas smaller deletions of the *KAL* gene are found in patients with anosmia and GnRH deficiency. These patients also demonstrate cerebellar dysfunction, oculomotor abnormalities, and mirror movements. Mutations of the gene that cause only anosmia in some affected patients have been described, and recently, *KAL* gene defects were reported in few patients with isolated gonadotropin deficiency.

Selective, idiopathic GnRH deficiency (IGD) is thought to be caused by various genetic defects that may include the GnRH gene itself. Patients with IGD and hereditary spherocytosis were recently described and are believed to have contiguous gene deletions involving the 8p11-p21.1 locus. In a murine model of hypogonadotropic hypogonadism (the mouse), the defect was found to be caused by a deletion of the GnRH gene and was recently repaired by gene replacement therapy.

2.7. Clinical Uses of GnRH

GnRH and its long-acting agonist analogs are, respectively, used in the treatment of GnRH deficiency, including menstrual and fertility disorders in women and hypothalamic hypogonadism in both sexes, and the treatment of central precocious puberty (CPP) in both boys and girls. Soon after the pulsatile nature of gonadotropin secretion was characterized, the requirement for intermittent stimulation by GnRH to elicit physiologic pituitary responses was determined. This led to the development of long-acting GnRH analogs, which provide the means of medical castration not only in CPP, but in a variety of disorders, ranging from endometriosis to uterine leiomyomas and prostate cancer. GnRH antagonists are currently being developed for the treatment of hormone-dependent cancers, such as prostate cancer, and for potential use of a male contraceptive in combination with testosterone.

GnRH is also used in clinical testing for the identification of CPP in children and the diagnosis of GnRH deficiency in all age groups. The gonadotropin response to 100 μg GnRH (intravenously [iv]) changes from an FSH-predominant response during the prepubertal years to an LH-predominant response during puberty. Significant gender differences exist in the peak hormonal values attained following GnRH stimulation, and the test is used in combination with other criteria for establishment of the diagnosis of precocious puberty. The same test is used in adults with suspected central hypogonadism. The lack of LH and FSH response to 100 μg GnRH iv is compatible with GnRH deficiency or pituitary hypogonadism, and repeated stimulation with GnRH may be needed to distinguish patients with Kallmann syndrome or selective IGD. The GnRH stimulation test is particularly useful in testing the efficacy of medical castration by GnRH agonists.

3. TRH

3.1. Prepro-TRH and Its Structure

TRH was the first hypothalamic-releasing factor to be isolated in 1969. Its discovery was followed by the description of GnRH, somatostatin, CRH, and GHRH, all in the early 1070s. TRH is a tripeptideamide (pGlu-His-Pro-NH$_2$), synthesized as part of a large prohormone termed *prepro-TRH*. The latter contains repeating sequences (Gln-His-Pro-Gly), the number of which

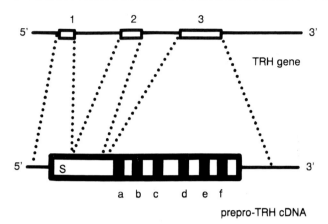

Fig. 1. Schematic representation of human TRH gene and its encoded cDNA. Three exons (1, 2, and 3) code for a transcript that contains a single peptide (S) and six potential copies (a–f) of the TRH tripeptide. This structure is highly preserved in evolution and is considered a model mechanism by which multiple copies of small peptides are produced from a single transcript.

varies from species to species. There are five of these repeats in the rat and six in the human preprohormone, and each can give rise to a TRH molecule after extensive posttranslational processing, which includes enzymatic cleavage of the prepro-TRH transcript, cyclization of the amino-terminal glutamic acid, and exchange of an amide for the carboxy-terminal glycine (Fig. 1). This structure, highly conserved in the mammalian genome, is considered a model of large production of small molecules from a single gene. copy.

The human prepro-TRH gene is on chromosome 3, has three exons, and encodes a cDNA that extends 3.7 kb. Exon 1 encodes the 5′ UTR of the mRNA, exon 2 encodes the signal sequence and part of the amino-terminal peptide, and exon 3 codes for the six potential copies of RH and the C-terminal peptide (Fig. 1). The rat prepro-TRH gene has a similar structure and size, but exon 3 codes for only five potential copies of TRH. The human prepro-TRH protein is smaller than that of the rat (242 amino acids long compared with 255 in the rat) and has a 60% homology to the latter.

Analysis of the rat 5′-flanking sequences has revealed the presence of many regulatory sequences that underline the complex regulation and determine the tissue-specific expression of the gene. A glucocorticoid-responsive element and an SP-1 transcription factor-binding sequence are located 100–200 bp upstream, whereas closer to the start site are sequences that are imperfect copies of the cyclic adenosine monophosphate (cAMP) regulatory element (CRE), and those that bind the triiodothyronine (T_3) receptor (c-*erb* A) and the activating protein-1 (AP-1) transcription factor. As is

the case in other pluripotential prohormone proteins, the connecting sequences between the repeat TRH units in the prepro-TRH transcript have the potential to modulate the biologic activity of TRH and are involved in long-term storage of the uncleaved molecule.

3.2. TRH Receptor

The pituitary TRH receptor (TRH-R) is a member of the seven-transmembrane segment–G protein–coupled receptor (GPCR) family. The gene that codes for the human TRH-R is located on chromosome 8p23. It consists of two exons, and its coded peptide has 398 amino acids. Although highly homologous to the rat and mouse TRH-Rs, the human transcript has a distinct C-terminal. Arg-283 and Arg-306, in transmembrane helices 6 and 7, respectively, appear to be important for binding and activation. A binding pocket formed by the third transmembrane segment domain is also important for binding with TRH. Recently, two TRH-R cDNAs encoding for a long and a short isoform have been identified in the rat. Their regulation of expression and second-messenger systems appears to be cell specific. The exact pattern of their distribution in the brain and elsewhere has not been determined.

Evidence supports a central role for the phosphoinositol/Ca^{2+} system mediating TRH actions. Following binding to TRH, TRH-R stimulates hydrolysis of the membrane lipid phosphatidylinositol 4,5-biphosphate to yield inositol 1,4,5-triphosphate and diacylglycerol. Both function as second messengers of the TRH-R and stimulate pKC. The response is Ca^{2+} dependent and involves a G protein as an intermediary. TRH stimulates a rapid, biphasic elevation of intracellular Ca^{2+}. The early phase is believed to come from intracellular Ca^{2+} stores and the sustained second phase from the influx of extracellular Ca^{2+} through voltage-dependent Ca^{2+} channels. A rapid translocation of pKC to the membrane has also been reported in response to TRH. As a result of TRH-R activation, a series of proteins is phosphorylated.

TRH does not appear to have a primary action on adenylate cyclase activity, despite the unequivocal evidence that cAMP stimulates thyroid-stimulating hormone (TSH) secretion from pituitary thyrotropes. However, cAMP-induced TSH secretion may not e TRH dependent. TRH action is exerted on the membrane and does not depend on internalization of TRH-R, although the latter does take place. The TRH-R C-terminus is important for receptor-mediated endocytosis, a process that is clathrin mediated and acidic pH dependent.

The receptor is specific for TRH and does not bind to any other known peptides. Several TRH analogs have been designed that bind to TRH-R with high affinity and mimic TRH action. The receptor is widely distributed in the CNS and many nonneuronal tissues, but its second-messenger systems in tissues other than the pituitary have not been elucidated. Rat TRH-R mRNA, indistinguishable from that of the pituitary thyrotropes, is found in the hypothalamus, cerebrum, cerebellum, brain stem, spinal cord, and retina. Extraneuronal sites include the immune system and the gonads.

3.3. TRH-Secreting Cells

In addition to anticipated regions of immunostaining for pro-TRH in the hypothalamus, immunoreactivity for this prohormone is detected in many other regions of the rat brain. These include the reticular nucleus of the thalamus, pyramidal cells of the hippocampus, cerebral cortex, external plexiform layers of the olfactory bulb, sexually bimorphic nucleus of the POA, anterior commissural nucleus, caudate-putamen nucleus, supraoptic nucleus, substania nigra, pontine nuclei, external cuneate nucleus, and dorsal motor nucleus of the vagus. TRH is also present in the pineal gland and the spinal cord. The extensive extrahypothalamic distribution of TRH, its localization in nerve endings, and the presence of TRH receptors in brain tissue suggest the TRH serves as a neurotransmitter or neuromodulator in many areas of the brain. There is also evidence that posttranslational processing of the prepro-TRH transcript is not identical throughout the CNS. In many areas of the rat brain, C- but not N-terminal extensions of the TRH are found, indicating that the dibasic residues of the latter are subject to enhanced cleavage compared to the former. Differential processing of the prepro-TRH transcript amplifies the biologic significance of its gene product and is similar to that of other potent propeptides with wide distribution and array of action in the mammalian brain, such as the preproenkephalins (-A and -B) and propiomelanocortin (POMC).

In extraneuronal tissues, prepro-TRH mRNA that is identical to that of the hypothalamus is found in mammalian pancreas, normal thyroid tissue, and medullary thyroid carcinoma cell lines. In the rabbit prostate, a TRH-related peptide was found that is believed to be derived from a precursor distinct from the hypothalamic TRH prohormone. In nonmammals and as the phylogenetic scale is descended, TRH concentration in nonhypothalamic areas of the brain and extraneural tissues increases. TRH is present and functions solely as a neurotransmitter in primitive vertebrates that do not synthesize TSH. The peptide is also found in the skin of some species of frogs, which provides testimony to the common embryologic origin of the brain and skin from the neuroectoderm.

3.4. Regulation of TRH Synthesis and Secretion

TSH secretion by the anterior pituitary thyrotropes is characterized by a circadian rhythm with a maximum around midnight and a minimum in the later afternoon hours. Superimposed to the basic rhythm are smaller, ultradian TSH peaks occurring every 2–4 h. TRH appears to be responsible for the ultradian TSH release that is also regulated by somatostatin. Imput from the suprochiasmatic nucleus and potentially other circadian pacemakers is required for this part of hypothalamic TRH secretion. Several other brain regions have been implicated in the regulation of TRH secretion, including the limbic system, the pineal gland, and CNS areas involved in the stress response.

Hypothyroidism, induced either pharmacologically or by thyroidectomy, increases the concentration of prepro-TRH mRNA at least twofold in the medial and periventricular parvocellular neurons of experimental animals. This response occurs shortly after levorotatory thyroxine (T_4) falls to undetectable levels, and parallels the gradual rise in serum TSH. This response is not TSH mediated, because hyphysectomy has not effect, whereas the administration of T_4 completely prevents it and supraphysiologic doses of T_4 cause an even further decline. Interestingly, the increase in prepro-TRH mRNA levels in hypothyroid animals occurs over several weeks, whereas its decline following administration of T_4 is faster, occurring within 24 h. Because of the absence of Type II deiodinase in the paraventricular nucleus (PVN), the feedback regulation of prepro-TRH gene expression is mediated by circulating levels of free T_3 rather than by intracellular conversion of T_4 into T_3. This serves to increase the sensitivity of TRH neurons to declining levels of thyroid hormone. The hypothalamic TRH neuron thus determines the set point of the thyroid hormone feedback control.

The dramatic feedback effects of thyroid hormone on TRH synthesis appear to be limited to the TRH-synthesizing neurons of the hypothalamic PVN. In contrast to the medial and periventricular parvocellular PVN neurons, no increase in prepro-TRH mRNA was observed in the anterior parvocellular subdivision cells of hypothyroid animals, a hypothalamic region that is functionally diverse. Similarly, no change was detectable in any other TRH neuronal population in the hypothalamus or the thalamus. Thus, the nonhypophysiotropic TRH neurons of the CNS may not be subject to thyroid hormone control. Their function is regulated via a variety of neurotransmitters, including catecholamines, other neuropeptides, and perhaps excitatory amino acids.

Catecholamines have an important regulatory role in the secretion of hypothalamic TRH. The stimulation of ascending α_1-adrenergic neurons from the brain stem causes activation of hypothalamic TRH neurons, and norepinephrine induces TRH secretion in vitro. Dopamine inhibits TSH release and the administration of α-methyl-*p*-tyrosine, a tyrosine hydroxylase inhibitor, diminishes the cold-induced TSH release. The action of serotonin is unclear, because both stimulatory and inhibitory responses have been found.

Endogenous opioids inhibit TRH release and so does somatostatin, which inhibits TSH secretion as well. Glucocorticoids decrease hypothalamic prepro-TRH mRNA synthesis both directly and indirectly via somatostatin. However, in vitro studies have shown upregulation of the prepro-TRH transcript by dexamethasone in several cell lines. This discrepancy may be explained by the in vivo complexity of prepro-TRH gene regulation vs the deafferentiated in vitro system. Thus, even though the direct effect of glucocorticoids on hypothalamic TRH synthesis is stimulatory, the in vivo effect is normally overridden by inhibitory neuronal influences, such as those emanating from the hippocampus via the fornix.

3.5. Endocrine and Nonendocrine Action of TRH

The iv administration of TRH in humans if followed by a robust increase in serum TSH and PRL levels. TRH is the primary determinant of TSH secretion by the pituitary thyrotropes, but its physiologic role in PRL secretion is unclear. PRL, but not TSH, is elevated in nursing women. The administration of anti-TRH antibody does not block the physiologic PRL rise during pregnancy or suckling. On the other hand, the PRL response to TRH is dose dependent and suppressible by thyroid hormone pretreatment. Hyperprolactinemia and galactorrhea have been observed in primary hypothyroidism.

Normally, TRH does not stimulate secretion of other pituitary hormones. However, GH release is stimulated by administration of TRH in many subjects with acromegaly, occasionally in midpuberty, and in patients with renal failure, anorexia nervosa, and depression. TRH can also stimulate adrenocorticotrophic hormone (ACTH) release by corticotropinomas in Cushing disease and Nelson syndrome, and FSH and α-subunit by pituitary gonadotropinomas and clinically nonfunctioning adenomas.

As a neurotransmitter, TRH has a general stimulant activity, with its most significant roles being thermoregulation and potentiation of noradrenergic and dopaminergic actions. Directly, TRH regulates temperature homeostasis, by stimulating the hypothalamic pre-optic region, which is responsible for raising body temperature in response to signals received from the skin and elsewhere in the brain. Indirectly, TRH elevates body temperature by activating thyroid gland function and regulation sympathetic nerve activity in the brain stem and spinal cord. TRH participates in regulation of the animal stress response by increasing blood pressure and spontaneous motor activity. Other TRH actions include potentiation of NMDA receptor activation, by changing the electrical properties of NMDA neurons, and alteration of human sleep patterns.

TRH appears to function as a neurotrophic factor in addition to being a neurotransmitter. Its administration in animals decreases the severity of spinal shock and increases muscle tone and the intensity of spinal reflexes. Recently, TRH was found to play an important role in fetal extrathymic immune cell differentiation and, thus, appears to be involved in the neuroendocrine regulation of the immune system.

In the CNS, a TRH-degrading ectoenzyme (TRH-DE) degrades TRH to acid TRH and cyclic dipeptide (cycled His-Pro). The former has some of the TRH actions, but the latter may function as a separate neurotransmitter with its own distinct actions, such as increase in stereotypical and inhibition of eating behaviors. TRH-DE is regulated in a manner that is the mirror image of that of TRH-R; thus, its mRNA levels are increased by thyroid hormone and decreased by antithyroid agents.

3.6. Clinical Uses of TRH

Oral, im, or iv administration of TRH stimulates the immediate secretion of TSH and PRL from the anterior pituitary. The maximal response is obtained after a 400 µg iv injection of TRH, but the most frequently administered dose is 200–550 µg. The peak serum TSH concentration is achieved 20–30 min after the iv bolus of TRH, but in individuals with central (hypothalamic) hypothyroidism, this response is delayed and prolonged. In primary hypothyroidism, the TSH response to TRH stimulation is accentuated, and in patients with isolated TSH deficiency, TRH fails to elicit an increase in serum TSH, whereas the PRL response is normal. In thyrotoxicosis, because even minute amounts of supraphysiologic thyroid hormone suppress the hypothalamic-pituitary-thyroid axis, TSH response to TRH are blunted. However, owing to the wide variation in TRH-induced increases in serum TSH levels in normal individuals, interpretation of the test is difficult, and the latter is seldom necessary in clinical practice.

The most frequent use of TRH testing, prior to the advent of third-generation TSH assays, was in patients with mild or borderline thyrotoxicosis and equivocal levels of thyroid hormone. Another application of the TRH test was in the diagnosis of central hypothyroidism, caused by lesions of the hypothalamic-pituitary area. However, the loss of circadian TSH variation is a far more sensitive test than TRH stimulation for the diagnosis of secondary (central) hypothyroidism and has replaced the latter in clinical practice. Currently, the TRH stimulation test is mot useful in the differential diagnosis of TSH-secreting adenomas and thyroid resistance with determination of the plasma α-subunit vs intact TSH concentration ratio. A ratio > 1 suggests the presence of a TSH-secreting adenoma. The test is also useful in the identification of gonadotropinomas and clinically nonfunctioning pituitary adenomas, which respond to TRH with an FSH and/or a glycoprotein α-subunit predominant gonadotropin response, whereas healthy individuals do not have a gonadotropin or an α-subunit response to TRH. The observation that patients with acromegaly respond to TRH with an increase in their GH levels has been in clinical use of a diagnostic provocative test and as a way to monitor the therapeutic response of patients with acromegaly to transsphenoidal surgery, pituitary radiation, or somatostatin analog treatment.

4. GHRH

4.1. Prepro-GHRH Gene and Its Product

In contrast to GNRH and TRH, a deca- and tripeptide, respectively, GHRH is larger and exists in more than one isoform in the human hypothalamus. The first evidence for a hypothalamic substance with GH-releasing action because available in 1960, when it was shown that rat hypothalamic extracts could release GH from pituitary cells in vitro. It was not until 1980 that part of the peptide was purified from a nonhypothalamic tumor in a patient with acromegaly. Subsequently, three isoforms of the peptide were identified and sequenced from pancreatic islet cell adenomas with ectopic GHRH production. Two of the three isoforms were also present in human hypothalamus (GHRH-[1–44]NH$_2$ and GHRH[1–40]OH) and differ only by four amino acids at the C-terminus. GHRH-(1–44)NH$_2$ is the most abundant form and homologous to the GHRH of other species, but the shorter, 40-amino-acid isoform has equipotent bioactivity and is physiologically important. The third form, HGRH(1–37)OH, has only been found in neuroendocrine tumors from patients with acromegaly and is less potent in releasing GH. The shortest prepro-GHRH sequence with GH-releasing activity consists of the first 29 amino acids of the intact GHRH, whereas the GHRH(1–27) form has no biologic activity.

The human *GHRH* gene is on chromosome 20p12 (Table 1). It is 10 kb long and consists of five exons. The mRNA transcript is 750 bp long and generates on GHRH molecule but exhibits heterogeneity owing to an alternative splice site present in the fifth exon. Like the other hypothalamic peptides, GHRH is coded in a larger prohormone molecule. Prepro-GHRH contains a 30-residue signal peptide and the GHRH(1–44) sequence, followed by an amidation signal and a 30- or 31-residue C-terminus peptide (GCTP). The prepro-GHRH peptide undergoes extensive posttranslational processing during which the signal peptide is removed and the rest of the molecule is cleaved by endopeptidases to GHRH(1–45)-glycine and GCTP. GHRH(1–45) is then converted into GHRH(1–44)NH$_2$ by peptidylglycine α-amidating monooxygenase. In the human hypothalamus, pituitary, extrahypothalamic brain, and several other normal and tumor tissues, endopeptidases convert GHRH(1–44)NH$_2$ into GHRH(1–40)OH, a form that is absent in other species studied to date.

The human prepro-GHRH transcript has been identified in hypothalamus, nonhypothalamic areas of the brain, testicular germ cells, and a variety of neuroendocrine tissues and tumors. The hypothalamic expression of the gene is primarily under the control of GH. Deficieincy of the latter, caused by hypophysectomy or defects in the GH gene, is associated with increased GHRH mRNA steady-state levels. Conversely, GH treatment decrease the synthesis of GHRH. These effects are exerted directly on the GHRH-secreting neurons, since GH receptor mRNA has been colocalized with prepro-GHRH mRNA in many areas of the brain, including the hypothalamus and thalamus, septal region, hippocampus, dentate gyrus, and amygdala. Preliminary results also indicate an inhibitory effect of insulin-like growth factor-1 (IGF-1) on prepro-GHRH mRNA.

Baseline GHRH mRNA levels are greater in hypothalami of male rats compared with hypothalami of female rats. This sexually bimorphic expression of the prepro-GHRH gene in the rat is significantly regulated by gonadal steroids. Administration of dihydrotestosterone to ovariectomized rates masculinizes their GH-secretion pattern and increases hypothalamic prepro-GHRH mRNA content. Conversely, administration of estrogens to male rats decreases GHRH synthesis, although this is not a consistent finding. In addition, GH-feedback inhibition of GHRH synthesis appears to be sex specific. Furthermore, after caloric deprivation of genetically obese and/or diabetic animal models, GHRH synthesis is decreased in a GH-independent fashion.

Tissue-specific regulation is exhibited by the prepro-GHRH gene in the mouse placenta. The transcript in this tissue contains a first exon that is approx 8–12 kb upstream from the mouse hypothalamic first exon,

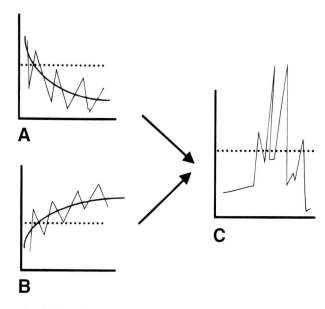

Fig. 2. Regulation of GH secretion. The theory proposed by Tannenbaum and Ling suggests that every secretory pulse of GH (**C**) is the product of a GHRH pulse (**B**) and an SRIF trough (**A**).

indicating a different transcription start site. The human placenta does not contain the prepro-GHRH transcript. A GHRH-like mRNA and peptide have been detected in rat and human testes.

4.3. GHRH Secretion

GHRH-containing nerve fibers arise from neurons of the ventromedial and arcuate nuclei of the hypothalamus. These neurons receive a variety of inputs from diverse areas of the CNS. Signals from sleep centers are excitatory and linked to the sleep cycle, whereas signals from the amygdala and ascending noradrenergic neurons from the brain stem are linked to activation of the stress system and responsible for stress-induced GH release. The VMN integrates the secretion of glucoregulatory hormones and also influences GHRH release in response to hypoglycemia.

The secretion of GH is regulated by the excitatory GHRH and the inhibitory somatostatin (SRIF) (Fig. 2). Functional and anatomic reciprocal interactions exist between GHRH and SRIF neurons, in the ventromedial/ arcuate and periventricular nuclei, respectively. Endogenous SRIF blocks GHRH release from the median eminence, whereas intracerebral administration of SRIF stimulates GHRH secretion from the specific neurons. The importance of SRIF in the regulation of GHRH secretion is demonstrated by the presence of high-affinity SRIF receptors in the GHRH neurons of the ventro-

lateral portion of the arcuate nucleus. Regulation of SRIF and the endogenous zeitgeber in the suprachiasmatic nucleus and elsewhere are responsible for the ultradian GHRH secretion. The latter, along with the tonic pulses of SRIF, defines the GH-circadian release, which is synchronized with the sleep cycle.

Neuronal inputs to the GHRH-secreting neurons are transmitted via a variety of neurotransmitters. Sleep-induced GH release is mediated mainly by serotoninergic and cholinergic fibers. The spontaneous ultradian pulses of GH, caused by GHRH or transient inhibition of SRIF, can be blocked by α-antagonists or drugs that inhibit catecholamine biosynthesis. β_2-Agonists stimulate GH secretion, presumably by inhibiting SRIF release. Anticholinergic substances block all GH-stimulatory responses, with the exception of that of hypoglycemia. L-dopa and dopamine stimulate GH release in humans, though in vitro dopamine inhibits GH secretion by normal pituitary or somatotropinomas. It has been postulated that the in vivo stimulatory effect of L-dopa and dopamine is owing to their local conversion into norepinephrine.

In addition to SRIF, many other CNS peptides interact with GHRH and affect GH secretion. Endogenous opiates, particularly β-endorphin, stimulate the GHRH neuron and induce GH release. Vasoactive intestinal peptide (VIP) and peptide histidine isoleucine (PHI) stimulate rat GH and PRL secretion. Since VIP and PHI do not bind to GHRH-R, it is not clear whether these effects of GH secretion are mediated at the hypothalamic or the pituitary level, or both. In humans, VIP-induced GH secretion has been observed only in acromegaly. PACAP has been shown to stimulate GH release in rats in vitro; however, this action may not be specific, since it also enhances the secretion of PRL, ACTH, and LH. Central administration of TRH induces GH release by Ca^{2+}-dependent, cAMP-independent mechanism that is modified by the presence of GHRH and is species specific. In humans, TRH-induced GH secretion is observed only in acromegaly. Galanin, motilin, and neuropeptide (NPY) enhance GHRH-induced GH release from rat pituitary cells. NPY and a structurally similar hormone, the pancreatic polypeptide, have opposite effects on GH secretion, depending on the dose and the route of administration. A subset of GHRH neurons contains NYP, which appears to enhance GH secretion in vitro. After intracerebroventricular (ICV) administration, however, NPY inhibits GH release, demonstrating additional function at the level of the GHRH or SRIF neuron. This may be via inhibition of ascending noradrenergic neurons from the brain stem, which normally stimulates GH secretion via GHRH.

4.4. Pathophysiology of GHRH Action

GHRH secretion and GHRH-R binding to its ligand in rodents are decreased with aging. The GH response to GHRH stimulation is similarly decreased in elderly humans. Studies in children with short stature have failed to demonstrate deficiency in either GHRH synthesis or action, although GHRH-induced GH secretion may be augmented in young adults with idiopathic tall stature. The human prepro-GHRH gene was recently excluded as a cause for short stature in familial GH deficiency by linkage and single-strand conformation analysis. Nevertheless, mutations in this gene and those of the GHRH-R and its second messengers are still candidates for familial disorders of human growth. In support of the latter is a well-studied rodent model of GHRH deficiency. GHRH-R of the *lit* mouse contains a missense mutation in the extracellular domain that disrupts receptor function. Another animal model, the *dw* rat, demonstrates a defect in the ability of GHRH-activated $G_s\alpha$ to stimulate adenylate cyclase, which results in low or undetectable GH levels. In contrast to the *dw* (Snell) and *dwJ* (Jackson) dwarf mice with similarly low GH levels, in which mutations are present in the Pit-1 pituitary transcription factor, the *dw* rat defect has not been elucidated. Recent studies have shown normal Pit-1 and GHRH mRNA levels, and a normal $G_s\alpha$ sequence, indicating that another or other proteins are responsible for this phenotype.

Hypersecretion of GHRH causes sustained GH secretion, somatotrope hyperplasia, and adenoma formation. A transgenic mouse expressing the human GHRH gene exhibits GH hypersecretion associated with somatotrope and lactotrope hyperplasia that eventually leads to adenoma formation. Indeed, approximately half of human GH-secreting tumors contain point mutations of the $G_s\alpha$ gene that interfere with the intrinsic guanosine triphosphate activity of G_s and lead to constitutive activation. A similar pathophysiologic mechanism explains the presence of somatotropinomas in patients with McCune-Albright syndrome.

4.5. Clinical Uses of GHRH and Its Analogs

The GHRH stimulation test is rarely used in clinical practice because of the wide variability of GH responses in healthy individuals. In the diagnosis of GH deficiency, pharmacologic agents, such as clonidine, arginine, and l-dopa, provide more sensitive and specific GH stimulation tests.

GH-releasing peptides (GHRPs) are oligopeptides with GH-releasing effects that bind to receptors different from the GHRH-R in the hypothalamus and elsewhere in the CNS. The original GHRP was a synthetic, met-enkephalin-derived hexapeptide (His-D-Trp-Ala-Trp-D-Phe-Lys-NH$_2$), which was a much more potent GH secretagogue than GHRH both in vivo and in vitro. When administered in large doses, GHRPs enhance ACTH and PRL release from the pituitary, whereas in smaller doses and/or after prolonged oral administration, only GH is secreted. Recently, a peptide analog (hexarelin) has been shown to be a relatively specific and potent GH secetagogue after oral administration in GH-deficient adults and children. Nonpeptide, equipotent analogs were subsequently synthesized that could be administered orally. Their use is still investigational.

5. SRIF

5.1. Somatostatin Gene and Protein

The first evidence for the existence of SRIF was provided in 1968, when hypothalamic extracts were shown to inhibit GH secretion from pituitary cells in vitro. A tetradecapeptide was isolated a few years later in parallel to the discovery of a factor in pancreatic islet extracts that inhibited insulin secretion. The term *somatostatin* was applied to the originally described cyclic peptide (S-14), but today it is used for other members of this family of proteins, which in mammals include the 28-amino-acid form (S-28) and a fragment corresponding to the first 12 amino acids of S-28 (S-28[1–12]). S-14 contains two cysteine residues connected by a disulfide bond that is essential for biologic activity, as are residues 6–9, which are contained within its ring structure.

The mammalian SRIF gene is located on chromosome 3q28 (Table 1), spans a region of 1.2 kb, and contains two exons. The SRIF mRNA is 600 nucleotides long and codes for a 116-amino-acid precursor, preprosomatostatin. Unlike GHRH, the sequence of the SRIF gene is highly conserved in evolution. Single-cell protozoan organisms have a somatostatin-like peptide, whereas the mammalian and one of the two anglerfish somatostatins are identical. A total of seven genes coding for the somatostatin family of peptides have been described in the animal kingdom. Posttranslational processing of preprosomatostatin by a number of peptidases/convertases is also conserved and results in various molecular forms with some degree of functional specificity. S-14 is the predominant form in the brain, whereas S-28 predominates in the gastrointestinal (GI) tract, especially the colon. Specificity of somatostatin form appears to be determined by the presence of different convertases in the various tissues and cell lines examined.

The 5′-UTR of the SRIF gene contains several cAMP and other nuclear transcription factor–responsive elements. Administration of GH increases SRIF mRNA levels in the hypothalamus, whereas GH deficiency does not always cause a decrease in the level of

SRIF gene expression. Glucocorticoids enhance hypothalamic somatostatin expression, but the effect may be indirect through the activation of β-adrenergic neurons. T_3 also regulates brain somatostatin mRNA levels in vitro. Extensive SRIF gene tissue-specific regulation has been described, a necessary phenomenon for a gene that is so widely expressed and has so many functions.

5.2. Somatostatin Receptors

In 1992, five different somatostatin receptor genes (SSTR- 1–5) were identified, which belong to the seven-transmembrane segment domain receptor family. The tissue expression of these receptors matches with the distribution of the classic binding sites of somatostatin in the brain, pituitary, islet cells, and adrenals. The pituitary SRIF receptor appears to be SSTR-2, but other actions of the different forms of somatostatin have not yet been attributed to a single receptor subtype. The clinically useful somatostatin agonists (octreotide, lanreotide, and vapreotide) bind specifically to SSTR-2 and less to SSTR-3 and are inactive for SSTR-1 and SSTR-4.

All five SRIF receptors are expressed in rat brain and pituitary, whereas the exact distribution of the receptor subtypes is not known for the periphery. In the fetal pituitary, SSTR-4 is not expressed. SSTR-4 is coexpressed with SSTR-3 in cells of the rat brain, in the hippocampus, in the subiculum, and in layer IV of the cortex. SSTR-3 alone is expressed in the olfactory bulb, dentate gyrus, several metencephalic nuclei, and cerebellum, whereas SSTR-4 is primarily in the amygdala, pyramidal hippocampus, and anterior olfactory nuclei. Human pituitary adenomas express multiple SSTR transcripts from all five genes, although SSTR-2 predominates. SSTR-5 mRNA, which has not been reported in other human tumors, is expressed in neoplastic pituitary tissues, including GH-secreting adenomas.

The main pituitary SRIF receptor, SSTR-2, demonstrates heterogeneity by alternative splicing. Two isoforms (SSTR-2A and SSTR-SB) have been identified, and their expression is subject to tissue-specific regulation. In human tumors, the predominant form is SSTR-2A. In the mouse brain, SSTR-2A was mainly present in cortex, but both mRNAs were found in hippocampus, hypothalamus, striatum, mesencephalon, cerebellum, pituitary, and testis. The promoter region of the human SSTR-2 gene shares many characteristics with the promoters of other GPCR-encoding genes, including a number of GC-rich regions, binding sites for several transcription factors, and the absence of coupled TATAA and CAAT sequences.

SRIF inhibits adenylate cyclase activity on binding to the SSTRs. The latter are coupled to the adenylate cyclase–inhibitory G protein, G_i, which is activated in a manner similar to that for G_s. Additionally, SRIF induces a dose-dependent reduction in the basal intracellular Ca^{2+} levels. Ca^{2+} channel agonists abolish this effect, indicating that SRIF acts by reducing Ca^{2+} influx through voltage-sensitive channels. Voltage on either side of the cell membrane is altered via K^+ channels that are stimulated by SRIF, resulting in hyperpolarization of the cell and a decrease in the open Ca^{2+} channels. The role of the inositol phosphate–diacylglycerol–pKC and arachidonic acid–eicosanoid pathways in mediating SRIF action is uncertain.

Recently, evidence was presented that the widespread inhibitory actions of somatostatin may be mediated by its ability to inhibit the expression of the c-fos and c-jun genes. Interference with in effects of AP-1 results in inhibition of cellular proliferation, but this could be important for the control of tumor growth. It is not clear how the SSTRs mediate this action of somatostatin, but one way may be the stimulation of several protein phosphatases that inhibit AP- 1 binding and transcriptional activity.

5.3. SRIF Secretion

Somatostatin-secreting cells, in contrast to GHRH-secreting cells, are widely dispersed throughout the CNS, peripheral nervous system, tissues of neuroectodermal origin, placenta, GI tract, and immune system. Those neurons secreting SRIF and involved in GH regulation are present in the periventricular nuclei of the anterior hypothalamus. The axonal fibers sweep laterally and inferiorly to terminate in the outer layer of the median eminence. SRIF neurons are also present in the ventromedial and arcuate nuclei, where they contact GHRH containing perikarya providing the anatomic basis for the concerted action of the two hormones on the pituitary somatotropes.

The secretory pattern of GH is dependent on the interaction between GHRH and SRIF at the level of the somatotrope (Fig. 2). Both hormones are required for pulsatile secretion of GH, since GHRH and/or SRIF antibodies can abolish spontaneous GH pulses in vivo. The manner by which the two proteins maintain GH secretion has been the subject of intense investigation for more than two decades. The prevailing theory is that proposed by Tannenbaum and Ling, who suggested that GH pulses are the consequence of GHRH pulses together with troughs of SRIF release (Fig. 2). Additional factors, however, appear to contribute to this basic model of GH secretion, such as the regulation of the SSTRs, the IGFs (particularly IGF- 1), other hypothalamic hormones (CRH and perhaps TRH), the glucocorticoids, and gonadal steroids.

GH stimulates SRIF secretion, and SRIF mRNA levels are increased by GH and/or IGF- 1. Hypothalamic SRIF mRNA levels are decreased by gonadectomy in both male and female rats, whereas estradiol (E_2) and testosterone reverse these changes in female and male rats, respectively. In humans, GH-pulse frequency does not appear to be different in the two genders, but GH trough levels are higher and peaks lower in women than men. Pulsatile GH secretion in the rat is diminished in states of altered nutrition (diabetes, obesity, deprivation). In vivo administration of SRIF antiserum restores GH secretion in food-deprived rats. During stress, CRH-mediated SRIF secretion provides the basis for inhibition of GH secretion observed in this state. TRH appears to stimulate SRIF release, whereas galanin increases hypothalamic SRIF secretion. Acetylcholine inhibits SRIF release and induces GHRH secretion. Similarly, the other neurotransmitter-mediated regulation of hypothalamic SRIF secretion mirrors that of the GHRH, although studying SRIF neurons has been proven to be a task of considerable difficulty, because of their multiple connections and widespread presence.

In the pituitary, SRIF inhibits GH and TSH secretion and occasionally that of ACTH and PRL. In the GI tract, pancreas, and genitourinary tract, somatostatin inhibits gastrin, secretin, gastric inhibitory peptide, VIP, motilin, insulin, glucagon, and renin. These actions are the result of a combined endocrine, autocrine, and paracrine function of somatostatin, which is supported by its widespread gene expression and receptor distribution.

5.4. SRIF Analogs

In view of its ability to affect so many physiologic regulations, SRIF was expected to be of therapeutic value in clinical conditions associated with hyperactivity of endocrine and other systems. The finding that many tumors from neuroendocrine and other tissues expressed the SSTR subtypes raised these expectations, which, however, were hampered by the short half-life need for iv administration and nonspecific activity of the native peptide. These problems were overcome with the introduction of a number of SRIF analogs, which are more potent, have longer action and different activities than somatostatin, and do not require iv administration. The best-studied among these analogs is octreotide (D-Phe-Cys-Phe-D-Trp-Lys-Thr-Cys-Thr[ol]), which is currently used extensively in neuroendocrine tumor chemotherapy, the treatment of acromegaly, and for radioisotopic detection of these and other neoplasms.

6. CRH

6.1. CRH Gene and Prepro-CRH

The idea that the hypothalamus controlled pituitary corticotropin (ACTH) secretion was first suggested in the late 1940s, whereas experimental support for the existence of a hypothalamic CRH that regulates the hypothalamic-pituitary-adrenal (HPA) axis was obtained in 1955. In 1981, the sequence of a 41-amino-acid peptide from ovine hypothalami, designated CRH, was reported. This peptide showed greater ACTH-releasing potency in vitro and in vivo than any other previously identified endogenous or synthetic peptide.

CRH is synthesized as part of a prohormone. It is processed enzymatically and undergoes enzymatic modification to the amidated form (CRH[1–41]NH_2). Mammalian CRH has homologies with nonmammalian vertebrate peptides xCRH and sauvagine in amphibia (from frog brain/spleen and skin, respectively), and urotensin-I in teleost fish. It also has homologies with the two diuretic peptides Mas-DPI and Mas-DPII from the tobacco homworm *Manduca sexta*. The vertebrate homologs have been tested and found to possess potent mammalian and fish pituitary ACTH–releasing activity. In addition, they decrease peripheral vascular resistance and cause hypotension when injected into mammals.

The N-terminal of CRH is not essential for binding to the receptor, whereas absence of the C-terminal amide abolishes specific CRH binding to its target cells. Oxidation of a methionine residue abolishes the biologic activity of CRH, and this may be a mechanism for neutralization of the peptide in vivo. CRH bioavailability is also regulated by binding to CRH-binding protein (CRHBP), with which it partially colocalizes in the rat CNS and other tissues. CRHBP is present in the circulation, where it determines the bioavailability of CRH. In the CNS, CRHBP plays a role analogous to that of enzymes and transporters that decrease the synaptic concentration of neurotransmitters either by breaking it down (acetylcholinesterase) or by taking it up at the presynaptic site (dopamine, serotonin).

The CRH gene is expressed widely in mammalian tissues, including the hypothalamus, brain and peripheral nervous system, lung, liver, GI tract, immune cells and organs, gonads, and placenta. The biologic roles of extraneural CRH have not yet been fully elucidated, although it is likely that it might participate in the auto/paracrine regulation of opioid production and analgesia, and that it may modulate immune/inflammatory responses and gonadal function.

The human *CRH* gene has been mapped to chromosome 8 (8q13) (Table 1). It consists of two exons. The

3′-untranslated region of the hCRH gene contains several polyadenylation sites, which may be utilized differentially in a potentially tissue-specific manner. CRH mRNA polyA-tail length is regulated by phorbol esters in the human hepatoma CRH-expressing cell line NPLC, and this may have potential relevance for differential stability of CRH mRNA in various tissues in vivo. Alignment of the human, rat, and ovine CRH (oCRH) gene sequences has allowed comparison of the relative degree of evolutionary conservation of their various segments. These comparisons revealed that the 330-bp-long proximal segment of the 5′-flanking region of the hCRH gene had the highest degree of homology (94%), suggesting that it may play a very important role in CRH gene regulation throughout phylogeny. A conserved polypurine sequence feature of unknown biologic significance is present at –829 of hCRH (–801 of the oCRH gene) as well as in the –400-bp 5′-flanking region of POMC, rat GH, and other hormone genes. A segment at position 2213–2580 of the 5′-flanking region of the hCRH gene has >80% homology to members of the type-O family of repetitive elements, and another at –2835 to –2972 has homology to the 3′-terminal half of the Alu I family of repetitive elements.

CRH regulation by the PKA pathway is well documented. Administration of cAMP increases CRH secretion from perfused rat hypothalami, and forskolin, an activator of adenylate cyclase, increases CRH secretion and CRH mRNA levels in primary cultures of rat hypothalamic cells. Regulation of the hCRH gene by cAMP has also been demonstrated in the mouse tumorous anterior pituitary cell line AtT-20, stably or transiently transfected with the hCRH gene. The hCRH 5′-flanking sequence contains a perfect consensus CRE element that is conserved in the rat and sheep.

TPA, an activator of pKC and ligand of the TPA-response element that mediates epidermal growth factor (EGF) function and binds AP-l, stimulates CRH mRNA levels and peptide secretion in vitro. TPA also increases CRH mRNA levels by almost 16-fold and CRH mRNA poly-A tall length by about 100 nucleotides in the human hepatoma cell line NPLC. The proximal 0.9 kb 5′-flanking the hCRH gene confers TPA inducibility to a CAT reporter in transient expression assays. In the absence of a clearly discernible perfect TRE in this region, it has been suggested that the CRE of the CRH promoter may, under certain conditions, elicit TRE-like responses, thus conferring TPA responsivity to the CRE site. Further upstream into the 5′-flanking region of the hCRH gene, eight perfect consensus AP-1-binding sites have been detected. Their ability to mediate TPA-directed enhancement of

hCRH gene expression has not yet been tested by conventional reporter gene assays. EGF, however, has been shown to stimulate ACTH secretion in the primate and to stimulate directly CRH secretion by rat hypothalami in vitro.

Glucocorticoids play a key regulatory role in the biosynthesis and release of CRH. They downregulate rat and ovine hypothalamic CRH content. However, adrenalectomy and administration of dexamethasone in the rat elicit differential CRH mRNA responses in the PVN and the cerebral cortex, respectively, stimulating and suppressing it in the former, but not influencing it in the latter. Glucocorticoids can also stimulate hCRH gene expression in other tissues, such as the human placenta and the central nucleus of the amygdala. A construct containing the proximal 900 bp of the 5′-flanking region of the hCRH gene was found to confer negative and positive glucocorticoid effects, depending on the coexpression of a glucocorticoid receptor (GR)–containing plasmid. The molecular mechanism by which glucocorticoids regulate IICRH gene expression is somewhat obscure. Suppression might be mediated by the inhibitory interaction of the activated GR with the *c-jun* component of the AP-1 complex. On the other hand, glucocorticoid enhancement of hCRH gene expression might be mediated by the potentially active half-perfect glucocorticoid-responsive elements (GREs) present in the 5′-flanking region of the gene, since half-GREs have been shown to confer delayed secondary glucocorticoid responses in other genes.

Gonadal steroids may modulate hGRH gene expression. Human female hypothalami have higher CRH content than the male ones. E_2 stimulates rat PVN CRH mRNA levels. A bidirectional interaction between the HPA and gonadal axes has been suggested on the basis of hCRH gene responsiveness to gonadal hormones. A direct E_2 enhancement of the CAT reporter was found by using two overlapping hCRH 5′-flanking region-driven constructs. Furthermore, the two perfect half-palindromic estrogen-response elements (EREs) present in the common area of both CRH constructs bound specifically to a synthetic peptide spanning the DNA-binding domain of the human estrogen receptor, suggesting that hCRH gene is under direct E_2 regulation.

Tissue-specific regulation of hCRH gene expression has been suggested for the human decidua and placenta. In rodents, such regulation was absent, which probably accounts for the differences in placental CRH expression between these species and primates. Differential distribution of short and long hCRH mRNA transcripts has been detected in several tissues and under varying physiological conditions. Tissue-specific and/or stress-dependent differential utilization of the two hCRH promoters may explain these observations. Differential mRNA stability would then be a particularly important feature in CRH homeostasis, primarily in conditions of chronic stress, since in the latter case, sustained production of CRH would be required, and the long stable mRNAs produced by activation of the distal promoter would be beneficial to the organism.

6.2. CRH Receptors

In the pituitary, CRH acts by binding to membrane receptors (CRH-Rs) on corticotropes, which couple to guanine nucleotide–binding proteins and stimulate the release of ACTH in the presence of Ca^{2+} by a cAMP-dependent mechanism. CRH stimulation of cAMP production increases in parallel with the secretion of ACTH in rat pituitary corticotropes and human corticotrope cells. In addition to enhancing the secretion of ACTH, CRH stimulates the *de novo* biosynthesis of POMC. CRH regulation of POMC gene expression in mouse AtT-20 cells involves the induction of *c-fos* expression by cAMP- and Ca^{2+}-dependent mechanisms.

Sequence analysis of hCRH-R cDNAs isolated from cDNA libraries prepared from human corticotropinoma or total human brain mRNA revealed homology to the GPCR superfamily. The hCRH-R cDNA sequences of the tumor and normal brain were aligned and found to be identical. The hCRH-R gene has been assigned to 17q12-qter. Human/rodent CRH-R protein sequences differ primarily in their extracellular domains. In particular, positively charged arginine amino acids are present in the third and fourth positions of the extracellular amino-terminal domain sequences of the rodent, but not the hCRH-R peptide. This might be responsible for the differential activity of the α-helical 9–41 CRH antagonist between rodents and primates.

Central sites of CRH-R expression include the hypothalamus, the cerebral cortex, the limbic system, the cerebellum, and the spinal cord, consistent with the broad range of neural effects of CRH administered intracerebroventricularly, including arousal, increase in sympathetic system activity, elevations in systemic blood pressure, tachycardia, suppression of the hypothalamic component of gonadotropin regulation (GnRH), suppression of growth, and inhibition of feeding and sexual behaviors characteristic of emotional and physical stress.

A splice variant of the hypothalamic hCRH-R, referred to as hCRH-R1A$_2$, was identified in a human Cushing disease tumor cDNA library, in which 29 amino acids were inserted into the first intracellular loop. This protein has a pattern of distribution similar to that of the hypothalamic hCRH-R (hCRH-R1A). A different

CRH-R, designated CRH-R2, was recently cloned from a mouse heart cDNA library. It is expressed in the heart, epididymis, brain, and GI tract and has its own splice variant expressed in the hypothalamus. The pattern of expression of the CRH-R2 protein differs from that of CRH-R1A, but its functional significance is currently unknown. Apparently, both rodents and humans express the CRH-R2 type.

6.3. CRH Neurons:
Regulation and the Central Stress System

CRH is the primary hormonal regulator of the body's stress response. Exciting information collected from anatomic, pharmacologic, and behavioral studies in the past decades has suggested a broader role for CRH in coordinating the stress response than had been suspected previously (Fig. 3). The presence of CRH-R in many extrahypothalamic sites of the brain, including parts of the limbic system and the central arousal-sympathetic systems in the brain stem and spinal cord, provides the basis for this role. Central administration of CRH was shown to set into motion a coordinated series of physiologic and behavioral responses, which included activation of the pituitary–adrenal axis and the sympathetic nervous system, enhanced arousal, suppression of feeding and sexual behaviors, hypothalamic hypogonadism, and changes in motor activity, all characteristics of stress behaviors. Factors other than CRH also exert major regulatory influences on the corticotropes.

It appears that there is a reciprocal positive interaction between CRH and arginine vasopression (AVP) at the level of the hypothalamic-pituitary unit. Thus, AVP stimulates CRH secretion, whereas CRH causes AVP secretion in vitro. In nonstressful situations, both CRH and AVP are secreted in the portal system in a pulsatile fashion, with approx 80% concordance of the pulses. During stress, the amplitude of the pulsation increases, whereas if the magnocellular AVP-secreting neurons are involved, continuous elevations of plasma AVP concentrations are seen.

Both CRH and AVP are released following stimulation with catecholamines. Indeed, the two components of the stress system in the brain, the CRH/AVP and the locus cerulus/noradrenergic (LC/NE) neurons, are tightly connected and are regulated in parallel by mostly the same factors. Reciprocal neural connections exist between the CRH and noradrenergic neurons, and there are autoregulatory ultrashort neg\ative-feedback loops on the CRH neurons exerted by CRH and on the catecholaminergic neurons exerted by NE via collateral fibers and presynaptic receptors. Both CRH and noradrenergic neurons are stimulated by serotonin and acetylcholine and inhibited by glucocorticoids, by the GABA/

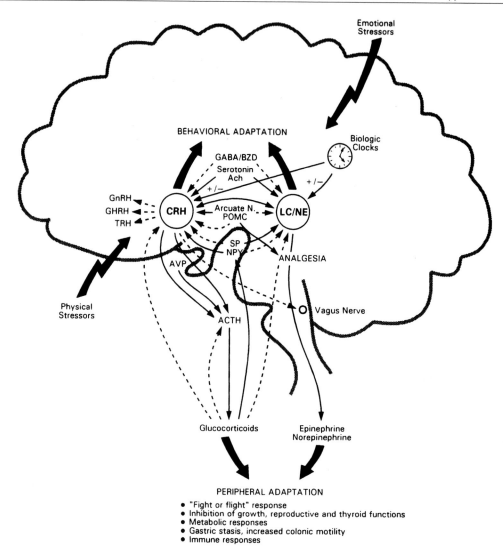

Fig. 3. Simplified representation of central and peripheral components of stress system, their functional interrelations, and their relations to other CNS systems involved in stress response. Solid lines represent direct or indirect activation, and dashed lines represent direct or indirect inhibition. Ach acetylcholine; ACTH = corticotropin; Arcuate N = arcuate nucleus; AVP = vasopressin; GABAIBZD = γ-aminobutyric acid/benzodiazepine receptor system; GHRH = growth hormone–releasing hormone; GnRH = gonadotropin-releasing hormone; LC = locus cerulus; NE = norepinephrine; NPY neuropeptide Y; PAF = platelet-activating factor; POMC = proopiomelanocortin; RH = corticotropin-releasing hormone; SP substance P; TRH = thyrotropin-releasing hormone.

benzodiazepine receptor system and by POMC-derived peptides (ACTH, α-melanocyte-stimulating hormone, β-endorphin) or other opioid peptides, such as dynorphin. Intracerebroventricular administration of NE acutely increases CR11, AVP, and ACTH concentrations, whereas NE does not affect pituitary ACTH secretion. Thus, catecholamines act mainly on suprahypophyseal brain sites and increase CR11 and AVP release.

Activation of the stress system stimulates hypothalamic POMC-peptide secretion, which reciprocally inhibits the activity of the stress system, and, in addition, through projections to the hindbrain and spinal cord, produces analgesia. CR11 and AVP neurons cosecrete dynorphin, a potent endogenous opioid derived from the cleavage of prodynorphin, which acts oppositely at the target cells. NPY- and substance P (SP)–secreting neurons also participate in the regulation of the central stress system by resetting the activity of the CRH and AVP neurons. Activation of the central NPY system overrides the glucocorticoid negative feedback exercised at hypothalamic and other suprahypophyseal areas, since icy administration of NPY causes sustained hypersecretion of CRH and AVP, despite high plasma cortisol levels. NPY, on the other hand, suppresses the LCINE sympathetic system through central actions on these neurons. The importance of NPY lies in the fact that it is the most potent appetite stimulant known in the organism and may be involved in the regulation of the HPA axis in malnutrition, anorexia nervosa, and obesity. SP is an 11-amino-acid peptide that belongs to the tachykinin family, together with neurokinins A and B. SP is present in the median eminence and elsewhere in the central and peripheral nervous systems. In the hypothalamus, it exerts negative effects on the CRH neurons, whereas it regulates positively the LC/NE neurons of the brainstem. SP plays a major role in the neurotransmission of pain and may be involved in the regulation of the HPA axis in chronic inflammatory or infectious states. NPY, somatostatin, and galanin are colocalized in noradrenergic vasoconstrictive neurons, whereas VIP and SP are colocalized in cholinergic neurons.

CRH neurons may be affected during stress by other factors, such as angiotensin II, the inflammatory cytokines, and lipid mediators of inflammation. The latter two are particularly important, because they may account for the activation of the HPA axis observed during the stress of inflammation. In the human, interleukin-6 (IL-6) is an extremely potent stimulus of the HPA axis. The elevations of ACTH and cortisol attained by IL-6 are well above those observed with maximal stimulatory doses of CRH, suggesting that parvocellular AVP and other ACTH secretagogues are also stimulated by this cytokine. In a dose response, maximal levels of ACTH are seen at doses at which no peripheral AVP levels are increased. At higher doses, however, IL-6 stimulates peripheral elevations of AVP, indicating that this cytokine is also able to activate magnocellular AVP-secreting neurons. The route of access of the inflammatory cytokines to the central CRH and AVP-secreting neurons is not clear, given that the cellular bodies of both are protected by the blood-brain barrier. It has been suggested that they may act on nerve terminals of these neurons at the median eminence through the fenestrated endothelia of this circumventricular organ. Other possibilities include stimulation of intermediate neurons located in the organum vasculosum of the lamina terminalis, another circumventricular organ. In addition, crossing the blood-brain barrier with the help of a specific transport system has not been excluded. Furthermore, and quite likely, each of these cytokines might initiate a cascade of paracrine and autocrine events with sequential secretion of local mediators of inflammation by nonfenestrated endothelial cells, glial cells, andlor cytokinergic neurons, finally causing activation of CR11 and AVP-secreting neurons.

In addition to setting the level of arousal and influencing the vital signs, the stress system interacts with two other major CNS elements; the mesocorticolimbic dopaminergic system and the amygdala/hippocampus. Both of these are activated during stress and, in turn, influence the activity of the stress system. Both the mesocortical and mesolimbic components of the dopaminergic system are innervated by the LC/NE sympathetic system and are activated during stress. The mesocortical system contains neurons whose bodies are in the ventral tegmentum, and whose projections terminate in the prefrontal cortex and are thought to be involved in anticipatory phenomena and cognitive functions. The mesolimbic system, which also consists of neurons of the ventral tegmentum that innervate the nucleus accumbens, is believed to play a principal role in motivational/reinforcement/reward phenomena.

The amygdala/hippocampus complex is activated during stress primarily by ascending catecholaminergic neurons originating in the brain stem or by inner emotional stressors, such as conditioned fear, possibly from cortical association areas. Activation of the amygdala is important for retrieval and emotional analysis of relevant information for any given stressor. In response to emotional stressors, the amygdala can directly stimulate both central components of the stress system and the mesocorticolimbic dopaminergic system. Interestingly, there are CRH peptidergic neurons in the central nucleus of the amygdala that respond positively to glucocorticoids and whose activation leads to anxiety. The hippocampus exerts important, primarily inhibitory influences on the activity of the amygdala, as well as on the PVN/CRH and LC/NE sympathetic systems.

6.4. CRH Secretion and Pathophysiology

ACTH, a 39-amino-acid peptide-proteolytic product of POMC, is the key effector of CRH action, as a regulator of glucocorticoid secretion by the adrenal cortex. The regulatory influence of CRH on pituitary ACTH secretion varies diurnally and changes during stress. The highest plasma ACTH concentrations are found at 6 AM to 8 PM, and the lowest concentrations are seen around midnight, with episodic bursts of secretion appearing throughout the day. The mechanisms responsible for the circadian release of CRH, AVP, and ACTH are not completely understood but appear to be controlled by one or more pacemakers, including the suprachiasmatic nucleus. The diurnal variation of ACTH secretion is disrupted if a stressor is imposed and/or changes occur in zeitgebers, e.g., lighting and activity. These changes affect CRH secretion, which, in turn, regulates ACTH responses.

Glucocorticoids are the final effectors of the HPA axis and participate in the control of whole-body homeostasis and the organism's response to stress. They play a key regulatory role in CRH secretion and the basal activity of the HPA axis, and in the termination of the stress response by exerting negative feedback at the CNS components of the stress system. The other component of the peripheral stress system is the systemic sympathetic and adrenomedullary divisions of the ANS. It widely innervates vascular smooth muscle cells, as well as the adipose tissue and the kidney, gut, and many other organs. In addition to acetylcholine, norepinephrine, and epinephrine, both the sympathetic and the parasympathetic divisions of the ANS secrete a variety of neuropeptides, including CRH itself.

Several states seem to represent dysregulation of the generalized stress response, normally regulated by the CRH neurons and the stress system. In melancholic depression, the cardinal symptoms are the hyperarousal (anxiety) and suppression of feeding and sexual behaviors (anorexia, loss of libido), and excessive and prolonged redirection of energy (tachycardia, hypertension), all of which are extremes of the classic manifestations of the stress reaction. Both the HPA axis and the sympathetic system are chronically activated in melancholic depression. In a postmortem study, individuals who have had depression were found to have had a three- to fourfold increase in the number of hypothalamic PVN CRH neurons, when compared with normal age-matched control subjects. This could be an inherent feature of melancholic depression or a result of the chronic, although intermittent, hyperactivity of the HPA axis that is known to occur in these patients.

Chronic activation of the HPA axis has been shown also in a host of other conditions, such as anorexia nervosa; panic anxiety; obsessive-compulsive disorder; chronic active alcoholism, alcohol and narcotic withdrawal, excessive exercising; malnuthtion; and, more recently, in sexually abused girls. Animal data are rather confirmatory of the association between chronic activation of the HPA axis and affective disorders. Traumatic separation of infant rhesus monkeys and laboratory rats from their mothers causes behavioral agitation and elevated plasma ACTH and cortisol responses to stress that are sustained later in life. Such activation of the CRH system was originally thought to be an epiphenomenon, as a result of stress. Administration of CRH to experimental animals, however, with its profound effect on totally reproducing the stress response suggested that CRH is a major participant in the initiation and/or propagation of a vicious cycle.

Interaction of CRH with the other hormone regulatory systems provides the basis for the various endocrine manifestations of CRH hypersecretion/ chronic hyperactivity of the stress system. CRH suppresses the secretion of GnRH by the arcuate neurons of the hypothalamus either directly or via the stimulation of arcuate POMC peptide-secreting neurons, whereas glucocorticoids exert inhibitory effects at all levels of the reproductive axis, including the gonads and the target tissues of sex steroids (Fig. 4A). Suppression of gonadal function caused by chronic HPA activation has been demonstrated in highly trained runners of both sexes and ballet dancers. These subjects have increased evening plasma cortisol and ACTH levels, increased urinary free cortisol excretion, and blunted ACTH responses to exogenous CRH; males have low LH and testosterone levels, and females have amenorrhea. Obligate athletes go through withdrawal symptoms and signs if, for any reason, they have to discontinue their exercise routine. This syndrome is possibly the result of withdrawal from the daily exercise-induced elevation of opioid peptides and from similarly induced stimulation of the mesocorticolimbic system. The interaction between CRH and the gonadal axis appears to be bidirectional. The presence of EREs in the promoter area of the human CRH gene and direct stimulatory estrogen effects on CRH gene expression implicate CRH, and, therefore, the HPA axis, as a potentially important target of ovarian steroids and a potential mediator of gender-related differences in the stress response.

In parallel to its effects on the gonadal axis, the stress system suppresses thyroid axis function via a number of known pathways, including SRIF-induced suppression of TRH and TSH secretion and glucocorticoid-mediated suppression of TSR secretion and the 5′-deiodinase enzyme (Fig. 4B). Thus, during stress, there is suppressed secretion of TRH and TSH and decreased conversion of T_4 into T_3 in peripheral tissues. This situation is similar to what is observed in the "euthyroid sick" syndrome, a phenomenon that serves to conserve energy during stress. The mediators of these changes in thyroid function include the CRH neurons, glucocorticoids, somatostatin, and cytokines. Accordingly, patients with melancholic depression; patients with anorexia; highly trained athletes; and patients with chronic, inflammatory diseases have significantly lower thyroid hormone concentrations than healthy control subjects.

Prolonged activation of the HPA axis leads to suppression of GH and inhibition of IGF-1 effects on target tissues (Fig. 4B). CRH-induced increases in somatostatinergic tone have been implicated as a potential mechanism of stress-induced suppression of GH secretion. In several stress system–related mood disorders, GH and/or IGF-1 levels are significantly decreased in

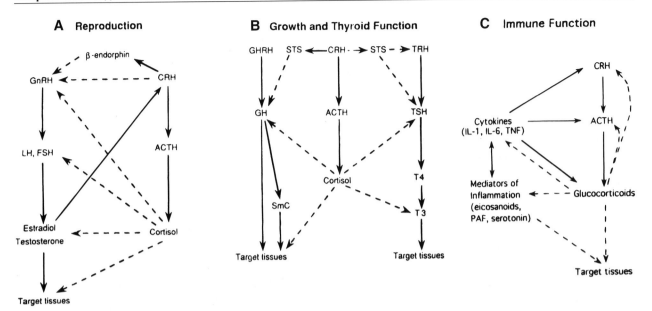

Fig. 4. Interactions of HPA axis and systems that subserve reproduction, growth, and metabolism. (**A**) Interactions between the HPA and reproductive axes; (**B**) interactions between HPA and and growth and thyroid axes; (**C**) interactions between HPA axis and immune system. Solid lines represent direct or indirect activation, and dashed lines, direct or indirect inhibition: Abbreviations are the same as those in Fig. 3; in addition, SmC = somatomedin C (insulin-like growth factor 1); STS = somatostatin (SRIF); TNF-α = tumor necrosis factor-α. (Modified with permission from Chrousos and Gold, 1992.)

animals and humans. Nervous pointer dogs, an animal model of anxiety with mixed panic and phobic features, were found to have low IGF- 1 levels and lower body growth than nonaffected animals. Patients with panic disorder, compared with healthy control subjects, had blunted GH responses to clonidine administered intravenously, and children with anxiety disorders can be short in stature.

The association between chronic, experimentally induced psychosocial stress and a hypercortisolism/ metabolic syndrome-X–like state, with increased incidence of atherosclerosis, was recently reported in cynomolgus monkeys. In these animals, chronic psychosocial stress-induced activation of the HPA axis led to hypercortisolism, dexamethasone nonsuppression, visceral obesity, insulin resistance, hypertension, suppression of GH secretion, and osteoporosis.

GI function is also affected by chronic CRH hypersecretion. During stress, gastric emptying is delayed, whereas colonic motor activity increases in animals and humans. Innervations by the vagus nerve and the LCINE sympathetic system provide the network for the rapid responses of the GI system to stress. CRH microinjected into the PVN was shown to reproduce the stress responses of the GI system in an animal model, including inhibition of gastric emptying and stimulation of colonic transit and fecal excretion. This effect was abolished by the intrathecal administration

of a CRH antagonist. CRH may be implicated in mediating the gastric stasis observed during the stress of surgery and/or anesthesia. IL- 1β, a potent cytokine that is found increased during surgery and in the immediate postoperative period, also inhibits gastric motility. Intrathecal administration of a CRH antagonist prevented surgery-induced rises in IL-1β in rats, thus suggesting that CRH may be an important mediator of IL-1β-induced gastric stasis. CRH hypersecretion could be the hidden link between the symptoms of chronic GI pain and history of abuse, since young victims of abuse demonstrate CRH hypersecretion.

A large infrastructure of anatomic, chemical, and molecular connections allows communication within and between the neuroendocrine and immune systems (Fig. 4C). In addition to the HPA axis, which via glucocorticoids exerts major immunosuppressive and antiinflammatory effects, the efferent sympathetic/adrenomedullay system participates in the restraint immune/inflammatory reaction by transmitting neural signals to the immune system. This is mediated through a dense innervation of both primary and secondary lymphoid organs, and by reaching all sites of inflammation via postganglionic sympathetic neurons. The sympathetic system, when activated, causes systemic secretion of IL-6, which by inhibiting the other two inflammatory cytokines, tumor necrosis factor-α (TNF-α) and IL-1, and by activating the HPA axis, participates in the stress-induced suppression of the immune inflammatory reactions. Stress-associated CRH hypersecretion, and the resultant glucocorticoid- , catecholamine-, and IL-6-mediated immunosuppression correlate well with such clinical observations as the suppression of the immune and inflammatory reaction during chronic psychologic and physical stress, the reactivation of autoimmune diseases during the postpartum period or following cure of Cushing syndrome, and the decreased ability of the stressed organism to fight viral infections and neoplasms.

In contrast to states with a hyperactive stress system, there is a host of different conditions, such as atypical or seasonal depression in the dark months of the year, the postpartum period, the period following the cessation of smoking, rheumatoid arthritis, and the chronic fatigue and fibromyalgia syndromes, that represent hypoarousal states. In these conditions, CRH secretion is decreased and symptoms, such as increase in appetite and weight gain, somnolence, and fatigue are seen.

6.5. Clinical Uses of CRH

The CRH stimulation test (1 μg/kg intravenously) is used clinically in the differential diagnosis of Cushing syndrome alone or in combination with inferior petrosal sinus sampling (IPSS). More than 80% of patients with CD respond to iv oCRH with an increase in ACTH and cortisol in the first 30–45 mm of the test. Most patients with ACTH-independent Cushing syndrome do not respond to this test, whereas ectopic ACTH-producing tumors occasionally respond. IPSS is the best available test for the diagnosis of CD, because >95% of the patients with CD respond to intravenously administered oCRH with a twofold increase in their petrosal sinus over peripheral ACTH levels in the first 3–10 min of the test, and 100% of the patients with Cushing syndrome from other causes do not respond. The administration of dexamethasone prior to the oCRH test has been suggested for the differential diagnosis of Cushing syndrome vs pgeudo-Cushing states. In primary adrenal insufficiency, patients respond to oCRH with markedly elevated ACTH levels, whereas two patterns have been described in patients with secondary arterial insufficiency: a pituitary pattern with absence of an ACTH response, and a hypothalamic pattern with a delayed and prolonged ACTH response to oCRH.

In the clinical investigation of depression and other disorders of the HPA axis, including anorexia nervosa, panic anxiety, abuse, malnutrition, addiction, and withdrawal syndromes and autoimmune diseases, the oCRH-stimulation test, as a sensitive indicator of corticotrope function, has been proven to be an invaluable tool. A variety of CRH analogs have been synthesized but not used in clinical trials. They bind specifically to the CRH-Rs, and in vitro studies have suggested that they might find therapeutic use in the treatment of disorders of the HPA axis.

Recently, two groups of substances were discovered that might be therapeutically useful. Nonpeptide CRH antagonists might prove useful in the treatment of melancholic depression, anorexia nervosa, panic anxiety, withdrawal from addiction agents, and other conditions associated with hyperactivation of the HPA axis. Conversely, CRFI-BP antagonists might provid~ a means of increasing levels of CRH in states characterized by low CRH, such as atypical depression, chronic fatigue/fibromyalgia syndromes, and autoimmune disorders.

7. DOPAMINE

7.1. Dopamine Synthesis and Dopaminergic Neurons

Dopamine is a catecholamine neurotransmitter and a hormone with a wide distribution and array of functions in the animal kingdom. It differs from the other catecholamines in that it is present in many nonneuronal tissues, but in relatively limited areas of the brain. It is a hypothalamic hormone directly involved in the regulation of PRL secretion from pituitary lactotropes, where, unlike other neurotransmitters, it forms its own short-feedback loop and is released in great quantities.

Dopamine is endogenously synthesized by hydroxylation of L-tyrosine (by tyrosine hydroxylase [TH]) and subsequent decarboxylation of the product (L-dopa) by the aromatic- L-amino acid decarboxylase.

The TH step is the rate-limiting step in the synthesis of dopamine. An increase in hydroxylation of tyrosine can be demonstrated rapidly after the stimulation of catecholaminergic neurons. Tetrahydrobiopterin is an important cofactor in the TH reaction, and its availability plays a regulatory role in the in vivo stimulation of TH activity. TH exhibits product inhibition by catecholamines and is stimulated by acetylcholine and by phosphorylation from a cAMP-dependent kinase. The TH gene is located on chromosome lip and codes for a cDNA that is approx 1900 bp long. Multiple mRNA species have been identified, indicating that tissue-specific regulation of TH gene expression is extensive. Unlike TH, which is only located in catecholamine-producing neurons and neuroendocrine cells, the L-dopa decarboxylase is expressed in many neuronal and nonneuronal tissues. It is not substrate specific and decarboxylates a variety of amino acids.

There are four major dopamine pathways in the mammalian forebrain. Nerve cell bodies of origin are clustered in nuclei in the rostral midbrain of three of these pathways, with the borders between the nuclei not always well defined. These nuclei have been shown to contain dopamine neurons. Anatomically, the most distinctive nuclei are the paired substantia nigra neurons, whose axons ascend rostrally in the nigrostriatal pathway to provide dopaminergic innervation of the corpus striatum (caudate and putamen). The substantia nigra neurons selectively degenerate in Parkinson disease. A closely paired nucleus, the ventral tegmental area, lies medially and dorsally to the substantia nigra, and its dopamine neurons provide two ascending pathways: (1) the mesolimbic, which provides dopamine innervation to forebrain limbic structures, especially the nucleus accumbens in the ventral striatum; and (2) the mesocortical, which provides dopamine innervation to the frontal and cingulate cortex. The fourth dopamine nucleus, the arcuate, is in the hypothalamus, projects to the median eminence through the tuberoinfundibular pathway and the intermediate lobe (in species that have this structure) through the tuberohypophyseal pathway, and releases dopamine directly into the hypophyseal portal circulation.

Although all of these groups of neurons synthesize dopamine by identical mechanisms, they are not identical functionally. Alterations in pituitary function related to changes in dopamine secretion by tuberoinfundibular neurons do not necessarily reflect alterations in other central dopaminergic systems. Tuberoinfundibular neurons are components of the short-loop feedback control of PRL secretion by the pituitary lactotrophs, and they possess PRL receptors but not dopamine receptors. Thus, dopaminergic drugs and their antagonists act directly on the mesolimbic and nigrostriatal systems and on the pituitary, but not on the tuberoinfundibular system.

7.2. Dopamine Regulation of PRL Secretion

The synthesis and release of PRL from lactotropes have been extensively studied over the past two decades. Unlike other anterior pituitary cells, lactotropes release their hormone at a high rate in the absence of hypothalamic regulation. Lesioning the median eminence, transecting the pituitary stalk, and grafting the pituitary beneath the kidney capsule all result in hyperprolactinemia. The incubation of pituitary fragments or dispersed cells in vitro is also associated with a sustained release of PRL.

Dopamine is the long-sought hypothalamic PRL-release inhibiting factor and the main modulator of the pleiotropic regulation of PRL secretion. Concentrations of dopamine in portal blood are maintained at physiologically active levels, and lactotropes contain dopamine receptors. PRL levels increase after treatment with dopamine antagonists and when dopamine is removed from the perfusion medium of cultured pituitary cells. Neither dopamine nor hypothalamic function is necessary for the pulsatile release of PRL from the pituitary, but tonic inhibition by the former synchronizes PRL secretion.

Both TRH and VIP stimulate PRL release, although only the former appears to be affected by dopamine. Part of the suckling-induced release of PRL appears to be mediated by TRH, and this effect can be prevented by the administration of a dopamine agonist. A trough in vivo or removal of dopamine secretion in vitro appears to enhance PRL release by TRH. By contrast, the transient removal of dopamine has no effects on VIP-induced PRL release, and blockade of dopamine receptors does not potentiate VIP or oxytocin-stimulated PRL release. Significant reduction of the rat portal concentrations of dopamine is observed immediately before large releases of PRL, such as during the last day of pregnancy and in response to suckling and estradiol, the latter on the afternoon of proestruS.

7.3. Dopamine Receptors

Pituitary lactotrope regulation by dopamine is primarily through dopamine type-2 receptors (D2-R). Five DRs exist (D-1R–5R) and all their genes were cloned before 1991. They belong to the seven-transmembrane segment domain GPCR family and have common structural organization and some homology with serotoninergic and adrenergic receptors. D-IR and D-5R activate, whereas D-2R, D-3R, and D-4R inhibit adenylate cyclase. The third cytoplasmic loop is short in the former and long in the latter. It is generally believed that receptors with a short third cytoplasmic loop couple to stimulatory G proteins (G_s) and, thus, activate adenylate cyclase, whereas those with a long third cytoplasmic loop react with G_i and G_o, which inhibit adenylate cyclase, and G_q, which couples with PLC. Although the structures of the extra- and intracellular loops of the DRs vary with each receptor, the transmembrane domains are highly homologous. The genes for these receptors are located on different chromosomes in humans ($5q3^4$, 11q22, 3q13, 4pl6, and 4p16 for the D-1R, D-2R, D-3R, D-4R, and D-5R, respectively) and are intronless for the activating D-1R and D-5R but contain 6, 5, and 4 introns for the inhibitory D-2R, D-3R, and D-4R, respectively. Posttranslational processing is extensive for the latter three receptors, resulting in a greater number of receptor isoforms.

The action of dopamine on pituitary PRL release is mediated through D-2R, the first DR to be cloned, and a receptor that is abundant in the pituitary, striatum, nucleus accumbens, olfactory tubercle, and substantia nigra. There are two isoforms of the D-2R that differ in length by 29 amino acids owing to an insertion in the third cytoplasmic loop. Both forms are expressed in all the tissues in which D-2Rs are present, including the pituitary, and are equipotent in inhibiting adenylate cyclase and activating K^+ channels, the latter an action unique to D-2Rs among the dopamine receptors.

Administration of dopamine decreases cAMP concentration in pituitary cells in vitro. It also inhibits the Ca^{2+} second-messenger system and decreases intracellular Ca^{2+} concentration. PRL release is inhibited in Ca^{2+}-deficient medium and by Ca^{2+} channel blockers. The effects of dopamine on Ca^{2+} are mediated by a G protein–dependent mechanism or by direct coupling to Ca^{2+} channels. The effects of dopamine on PLC are less clear, and although PKC is involved in regulating PRL secretion, the evidence that dopamine regulates PKC activity is scant. Basal activity of PLC in the lactotropes is low, but dopamine dissociation from its receptor is associated with its activation. The latter is not dependent on adenylate cyclase activity, which is also significantly activated on dissociation of dopamine from the pituitary D-2R.

7.4. Hyperprolactinemia and the Use of D-2R Agonists

The anatomic (by surgery, or mass effects of a large pituitary or hypothalamic tumor) or functional (by the use of dopamine antagonists) uncoupling of the pituitary lactotropes from hypothalamic dopaminergic control results in hyperprolactinemia. The latter is a manifestation of a number of disorders of the hypothalamic-pituitary unit and leads to hypogonadism, decreased libido, and/or galactorrhea. It can also develop from the administration of neuroleptic drugs, such as reserpine (a catecholamine depletor), and phenothiazines, such as chlorpromazine and haloperidol. The PRL response to the latter is an excellent predictor of their antipsychotic effects.

Dopamine agonists have been developed and in clinical use for the management of hyperprolactinemia. Bromocriptine and, recently, pergolide and cabergoline are D-2R agonists that effectively restore PRL inhibition and are used in the medical management of pituitary prolactinomas. Only 10% of the latter are resistant to the action of bromocriptine; the rest respond with significant reduction of their size and resolution of hyperprolactinemia. Although dopamine agonists are useful for the reduction of PRL levels induced by disruption of hypothalamic function by other pituitary tumors, they are not effective in decreasing the size of non-PRL-secreting tumors.

The response to dopamine receptor stimulation and blockade is not specific for the central, pituitary, or peripheral actions of dopamine. Indeed, bromocriptine can induce schizophrenic psychosis in a small proportion of individuals with no prior history of mental disorders. In general, however, dopamine agonists have few side effects, and bromocriptine can be safely used during pregnancy, if needed.

REFERENCE

Chrousos GP, Gold PW. The concepts of stress and stress system disorders: an overview of physical and behavioral homeostasis. *JAMA* 1992;267:1244–1252.

SELECTED READING

Ben-Jonathan N, Hnasko R. Dopamine as a prolactin (PRL) inhibitor. *Endocr Rev* 2001;22:724–763.

Chrousos GP. The hypothalamic-pituitary-adrenal axis and immune-mediated inflammation. *N Engl J Med* 1995;332: 1351–1362.

Chrousos GP. The role of stress and the hypothalamic-pituitary-adrenal axis in the pathogenesis of the metabolic syndrome: neuro-endocrine and target tissue-related causes [review]. *Int J Obesity* 2000;24:S50–S55.

Conn PM, Janovick JA, Stanislaus D, Kuphal D, Jennes L. Molecular and cellular bases of GnRH action in the pituitary and central nervous system. *Vitam Horm* 1995;50:151–214.

De La Escalera GM, Weiner RI. Dissociation of dopamine from its receptor as a signal in the pleiotropic hypothalamic regulation of prolactin secretion. *Endocr Rev* 1992;13:241–255.

Frohman LA, Downs TR, Chomzynski P. Regulation of growth hormone secretion. *Front Neuroendocrinol* 1992;13:344–405.

Gold PW, Chrousos GP. Organization of the stress system and its dysregulation in melancholic and atypical depression: high vs. low CRH/NE states. *Mol Psychiatry* 2002;254–275.

Grammatopoulos D, Chrousos GP. Structural and signaling diversity of corticotropin-releasing hormone (CRH) and related peptides and their receptors: potential clinical applications of CRH receptor antagonists. *Trends Endocrinol Metab* 2002;13: 436–444.

Jackson IMD, Lechan RM, Lee SL. TRH-prohormone: biosynthesis, anatomic distribution and processing. *Front Neuroendocrinol* 1990;11:267–283.

Kalantaridou SN, Chrousos GP. Monogenic disorders of puberty. *J Clin Endocrinol Metab* 2002;87:2481–2494.

King JC, Rubin BS. Dynamic changes in LHRH neurovascular terminals with various endocrine conditions in adults. *Horm Behav* 1994;28:349–356.

Korbonits M, Grossman AB. Growth hormone–releasing peptide and its analogues: novel stimuli to growth hormone release. *Trends Endocrinol Metab* 1995;6:43–49.

Makrigiannakis A, Zoumakis E, Kalantaridou S, Mitsiadis N, Margioris N, Chrousos G, Gravanis A. Corticotropin-releasing hormone (CRH) and immunotolerance of the fetus. *Biochem Pharmacol* 2003;65:917–921.

Rivest S. Rivier C. The role of corticotropin-releasing factor and interleukin-1 in the regulation of neurons controlling reproductive functions. *Endocr Rev* 1995;16:177–199.

Schwanzel-Fukuda M, Jorgenson KL, Bergen HT, Weesner GD, Pfaff DW. Biology of normal LHRH neurons during and after their migration from olfactory placode. *Endocr Rev* 1992;13: 623–634.

Sherwood NM, Lovejoy DA, Coe IR. Origin of mammalian gonadotropin-releasing hormones. *Endocr Rev* 1993;14:241–254.

Spada A, Faglia G. G-proteins and hormonal signalling in human pituitary tumors: genetic mutations and functional alterations. *Front Neuroendocrinol* 1993;14:214–232.

Vamvakopoulos NC, Chrousos GP. Hormonal regulation of human corticotropin-releasing hormone gene expression: implications for the stress response and immune/inflammatory reaction. *Endocr Rev* 1994;15:409–420.

Vgontzas AN, Chrousos GP. Sleep, the hypothalamic-pituitary-adrenal axis, and cytokines: multiple interactions and disturbances in sleep disorders. *Endocrinol Metab Clin in North Am* 2002;31:15–36.

Viollet C, Prevost G, Maubert E, et al. Molecular pharmacology of somatostatin receptors. *Fundam Clin Pharmacol* 1995;9:107–113.

Wehrenberg WB, Giustina A. Basic counterpoint: mechanisms and pathways of gonadal steroid stimulation of growth hormone secretion. *Endocr Rev* 1992;13:299–308.

13 Anterior Pituitary Hormones

Ilan Shimon, MD and Shlomo Melmed, MD

CONTENTS

1. INTRODUCTION

The human anterior pituitary gland contains at least five distinct hormone-producing cell populations, expressing six different hormones (Table 1): proopiomelanocortin (POMC), growth hormone (GH), prolactin (PRL), thyroid-stimulating hormone (TSH), follicle-stimulating hormone (FSH), and luteinizing hormone (LH).

2. PROOPIOMELANOCORTIN

2.1. Embryology and Cytogenesis of Corticotropes

The corticotrope is the first cell type to develop in the human fetal pituitary, as early as 6 wk of gestation, and 2 wk later adrenocorticotropic hormone (ACTH) is detectable by radioimmunoassay (RIA) of both the fetal pituitary and fetal blood. The corticotropes constitute between 15 and 20% of the adenohypophyseal cell population, are initially identified by their basophilic staining, and express strong granular cytoplasmic immunopositivity for ACTH and for other fragments of the POMC molecule. By electron microscopy (EM) the cells are oval with spherical eccentric nuclei, and a large membrane-bound lysosomal structure, the "enigmatic body."

From: *Endocrinology: Basic and Clinical Principles, Second Edition*
(S. Melmed and P. M. Conn, eds.) © Humana Press Inc., Totowa, NJ

2.2. POMC Gene

The human POMC gene (Fig. 1) is an 8-kb single-copy gene located on chromosome 2p25. It consists of a 400 to 700-bp promoter, three exons, and two introns. The majority of the 266-amino-acid POMC precursor protein is encoded by exon 3, which contains all the known peptide products of the gene, including the 39-amino-acid adrenocorticotropin (ACTH), α-melanocyte-stimulating hormone (α-MSH), β-MSH, β-lipotropin (β-LPH), β-endorphin, and corticotropin-like intermediate lobe peptide (CLIP). Human POMC is digested at either Lys-Arg or Arg-Arg residues by two endopeptidases: prohormone convertase 1 (PC1), abundant in anterior pituitary corticotropes, and PC2, expressed in the brain as well as in pancreatic islet cells, but absent from the anterior pituitary. This tissue-specific enzyme distribution correlates well with the different enzymatic cleavage of the prohormone to its products. Thus, in the pituitary, corticotrope POMC is cleaved into ACTH, β-LPH, and other peptides including N-terminal glycopeptide and joining peptide, and in the brain, ACTH is further cleaved to α-MSH and CLIP (Fig. 1). Exon 1 is not translated and there is only 45% nucleotide sequence homology in exon 1 and the promoter region of the human, bovine, and other mammals. By contrast, exons 2 and 3 bear 80–95% homology among humans, other mammals, and mice. The

Table 1
Expression of Human Anterior Pituitary Hormone Gene and Protein Action

	POMC	GH	PRL	TSH	FSH	LH
Cell	Corticotrope	Somatotrope	Lactotrope	Thyrotrope	Gonadotrope	Gonadotrope
Fetal appearance	6 wk	8 wk	12 wk	12 wk	12 wk	12 wk
Chromosomal gene locus	2p	17q	6	α: 6q; β: 1p	β: 11p	β: 19q
Protein	Polypeptide	Polypeptide	Polypeptide	Glycoprotein αβ-subunits	Glycoprotein αβ-subunits	Glycoprotein αβ-subunits
Protein length (kDa)	ACTH: 4.5	22	23	28	34	28.5
Amino acid no.	266 (ACTH-39)	191	199	211	210	204
Normal range	ACTH, 4–22 pmol/L	<0.5 µg/L[b]	M < 15; F < 20 µg/L	0.1–5 mU/L	M: 5–20 IU/L; F: (basal) 5–20 IU/L	M: 5–20 IU/L; F: (basal) 5–20 IU/L
Secretion Regulators						
Stimulators	CRH, AVP	GHRH, ghrelin	Estrogen, TRH	TRH	GnRH, estrogen	GnRH, estrogen
Inhibitors	Glucocorticoids	Somatostatin, IGF-1	Dopamine, T₃	T₃, T₄, dopamine, somatostatin, glucocorticoids	Estrogen, inhibin	Estrogen, inhibin
Receptor	GSTD[a]	Single transmembrane	Single transmembrane	GSTD[a]	GSTD[a]	GSTD[a]
Location	Adrenal	Liver, other tissues	Breast, other tissues	Thyroid	Ovary	Testis
Tropic effects	Steroid production	IGF-1 production, growth induction	Milk production	T³, T⁴ synthesis and secretion	Testosterone synthesis, follicle growth	Testosterone synthesis, follicle growth

[a]GSTD = G$_s$ protein coupled with seven transmembrane domains.
[b]Integrated over 24 h.

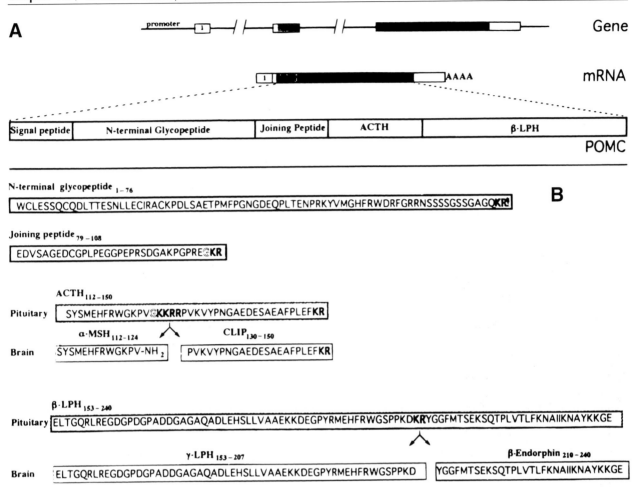

Fig. 1. Schematic structure of POMC gene, mRNA, and protein products. (**A**) The gene (top) contains the promoter, three exons (thick bars; translated regions are stippled), separated by two introns (diagonal lines). The mRNA transcript (middle) consists of the three exons and the polyadenylation site. The POMC precursor protein (bottom) consists of the signal peptide, N-terminal glycopeptide, joining peptide, ACTH, and β-LPH. (**B**) Tissue-specific enzymatic cleavage of POMC to its products. POMC is cleaved into N-terminal glycopeptide and joining peptide in the pituitary coticotropes and the brain. In brain, ACTH is further cleaved to α-MSH and CLIP, and β-LPH is digested into γLPH and β-endorphin. KR = dibasic amino acids at proteolytic cleavage sites. (From Holm and Majzoub [adrenocorticotropin] in Melmed, 1995.)

main regulators of POMC transcription are corticotropin-releasing hormone (CRH) and glucocorticoids, which exert opposite effects on POMC transcription rate. CRH increases POMC mRNA and protein content via cyclic adenosine monophosphate (cAMP), and the glucocorticoid-negative feedback effect is probably mediated through binding of the glucocorticoid receptor complex to *cis*-acting POMC promoter sequences. POMC transcription is also stimulated by β-adrenergic catecholamines and insulin-induced hypoglycemia, but suppressed by arginine vasopressin (AVP).

2.3. Regulation of ACTH Secretion

The endogenous circadian rhythm of ACTH pulsatile secretion leads to a parallel diurnal pattern of gluco-corticoid release. Both ACTH and cortisol are high in the early morning and decline throughout the day, maintaining lower levels during the night. This rhythmicity of ACTH pulse amplitude may be controlled by the concomitant diurnal variation of CRH secretion. CRH and AVP are the main secretagogues of ACTH, and glucocorticoids inhibit its secretion (Fig. 2). CRH, by binding to CRH receptors on the corticotrope, stimulates ACTH synthesis as well as release. In addition, physical stress, exercise, acute illness and hypoglycemia increase ACTH levels. Inflammatory cytokines—tumor necrosis factor-α (TNF-α), interleukin-1 (IL-1), IL-6, and leukemia inhibitory factor (LIF)—stimulate pituitary corticotropin secretion, and oxytocin, opiates, and somatostatin inhibit ACTH release.

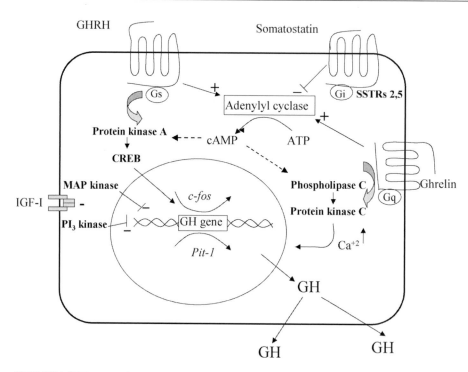

Fig. 2. Regulation of POMC/ACTH expression in pituitary corticotropes. CRH binds to its G_s protein–coupled seven-transmembrane domain receptor and activates adenylyl cyclase and cAMP generation to promote POMC through protein kinase A (PKA) activation. Vasopressin binds to the V_{1b} receptor in the anterior pituitary and via PKC and Ca^{+2} mobilization potentiates the CRH-stimulated increase in cAMP. Inflammatory cytokines, including TNF-α, IL-1, IL-6, and LIF stimulate POMC expression and ACTH secretion. Cortisol binds to its nuclear receptor and suppresses POMC transcription. CREB = CRE binding protein; MAP kinase = mitogen-activated protein kinase; PI_3 kinase = phosphatidylinositol 3-kinase; ATP = adenosine triphosphate; SSTR = somatostatin receptor.

2.4. ACTH Receptor Gene

ACTH receptors have been detected in human adrenal glands, in adrenal tumors, on human mononuclear leukocytes, and on rat lymphocytes. The ACTH receptor gene encodes a 297-amino-acid protein that belongs to the G_s protein–coupled superfamily of receptors containing seven transmembrane domains. The effect of ACTH is mediated by adenylate cyclase activation, cAMP production, and PKA induction in the adrenal.

2.5. ACTH Action

ACTH stimulates steroidogenesis in the adrenocortical cells. Lipoprotein uptake from the plasma is enhanced, and steroid hormone enzyme gene transcription is increased. The prolonged effects of ACTH may promote growth of adrenal size and act with β-LPH on melanocytes to increase skin pigmentation.

2.6. ACTH Hypersecretion

2.6.1. Pituitary Adenoma

ACTH-producing tumors are usually monoclonal, well-differentiated microadenomas. About 10–15% of all pituitary adenomas are clinically active ACTH-pro-

ducing tumors, and 5% are silent corticotrope adenomas. In addition to POMC glycoprotein, secretory granules in tumor cells stain for ACTH, β-endorphin, β-LPH, and N-terminal peptide. Some corticotrope adenomas contain altered forms of gastrin, cholecystokinin, and also vasoactive intestinal peptide (VIP), neurophysin, α-subunit, and chromogranin A. Cell cultures of corticotrope adenomas secrete ACTH in response to CRH and AVP, and ACTH is suppressible by glucocorticoids, but to a lesser extent than with normal corticotropes.

2.6.2. Ectopic ACTH Secretion

Small-cell carcinomas of the lung, and bronchial and thymic carcinoids, can produce ACTH, leading to Cushing syndrome. These tumors express other neuroendocrine markers including chromogranins, synaptophysin, and neurotensin. POMC mRNA from nonpituitary tumors may be longer than normal or pituitary tumor POMC mRNA. In addition, CLIP and β-MSH are detected in ectopic tumors, indicating an alternative POMC processing. POMC mRNA and ACTH are not suppressed in small-cell lung cell lines by glucocorticoids.

2.7. ACTH Hyposecretion

BT:Pituitary failure due to irradiation, hypophysectomy, large macroadenomas, pituitary apoplexy, trauma, postpartum necrosis, hypophysitis, glucocorticoid withdrawal, or CRH deficiency results in ACTH hyposecretion and hypocortisolism. This is usually a late manifestation of pituitary failure and indicates severly compromised pituitary function.

2.8. ACTH Receptor Defects

Familial glucocorticoid deficiency is a rare autosomal recessive disorder of adrenal unresponsiveness to ACTH, characterized by glucocorticoid deficiency in the presence of elevated circulating ACTH and normal mineralocorticoid production. Affected children usually have hypoglycemic episodes, hyperpigmentation, failure to thrive, and chronic asthenia. They have no cortisol or aldosterone responses to exogenous ACTH. Recently, homozygous and compound heterozygous point mutations have been reported in the ACTH receptor gene.

2.9. Clinical Testing

The low-dose (1 mg) overnight dexamethasone suppression test and the measurement of 24-h urinary-free cortisol are the standard screening tests for Cushing syndrome. A 48-h low-dose dexamethasone suppression test (2 mg/d) is usually performed to diagnose Cushing syndrome, and a high-dose (8 mg/d) suppression test will differentiate a pituitary from a nonpituitary tumor source of ACTH. Once the diagnosis of Cushing syndrome is made, measuring ACTH concentration in plasma is important for etiologic evaluation. The normal levels of ACTH are 4–22 pmol/L. In Cushing disease, ACTH is moderately increased, to 10–50 pmol/L, and ectopic ACTH syndrome usually results in highly elevated levels. Patients with adrenal adenoma have low or undetectable ACTH. The CRH stimulation test may serve to differentiate patients with Cushing disease who have exaggerated ACTH and cortisol response to CRH from patients with ectopic ACTH-producing tumors that, in general, do not respond furthur to CRH. To screen the functional adrenal reserve for cortisol production, the rapid cortrosyn (ACTH 1-24, 1–250 µg) stimulation test is used. Patients with ACTH hyposecretion have a blunted cortisol response to administration of cortrosyn.

2.10. Clinical Syndromes

2.10.1. Cushing Syndrome

In 1932, Harvey Cushing described a syndrome resulting from long-term exposure to glucocorticoids. Most patients (70%) have pituitary corticotrope adenomas (Cushing disease). Other etiologies include ectopic ACTH (12%); cortisol-producing adrenal adenoma, carcinoma, and hyperplasia (18%); and the rare ectopic CRH syndrome. Prolonged administration of glucocorticoids produces a similar syndrome. Patients have a typical habitus including "moon facies," "buffalo hump," truncal obesity, and cutaneous striae, as well as muscle weakness, osteoporosis, impaired glucose tolerance, hirsutism, acne, hypertension, depression, and ovarian dysfunction. Usually the clinical presentation is insidious, but the ectopic syndrome associated with small-cell lung carcinoma may be acute, with rapid onset of hypertension, edema, hypokalemia, glucose intolerance, and hyperpigmentation. When a probable diagnosis of Cushing disease is made, the most direct way to demonstrate pituitary ACTH hypersecretion is by catheterization of the inferior petrosal venous sinuses, which drain the pituitary. ACTH measurements in petrosal and peripheral venous plasma before and after CRH stimulation can document a central-to-peripheral gradient of ACTH in blood draining an adenoma. High-resolution magnetic resonance imaging of the sella turcica, enhanced by gadolinium, is useful in determining the location of corticotrope adenomas with a sensitivity of 2 mm. The treatment of choice is transsphenoidal adenomectomy, and the cure rate is 70–80%.

2.10.2 Hypocortisolism

Hypocortisolism can be either primary (Addison disease), secondary to pituitary ACTH deficiency, or tertiary resulting from CRH deficiency. Primary adrenal insufficiency can result from autoimmune adrenocortical destruction, acquired immunodeficiency syndrome, tuberculosis, bilateral hemorrhage, and metastatic disease. Clinically, patients present with fatigue, weakness, nausea and vomiting, weight loss, hypotension, hypoglycemia, and hyperpigmentation (only in primary hypocortisolism). Treatment of patients with Addison disease includes glucocorticoids and mineralocorticoids, whereas patients with secondary adrenal insufficiency do not require mineralocorticoid replacement.

GROWTH HORMONE
3.1. Embryology and Cytogenesis of Somatotropes

Somatotropes that contain GH immunoreactivity are identified at 8 wk of gestation, and circulating GH is measurable in fetal serum at the end of the first trimester. Somatotropes comprise 40–50% of pituitary cells and are located in the lateral wings of the gland. These acidophilic cells reveal intense cytoplasmic immunopositivity for GH.

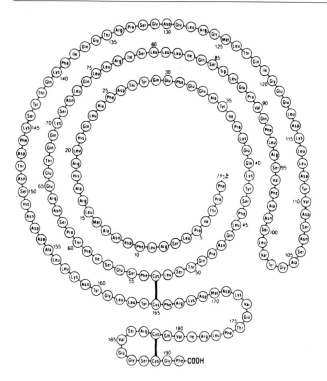

Fig. 3. Primary structure of human GH. GH is a 191-amino-acid single-chain 22-kDa polypeptide with two intramolecular disulfide bonds. (From Fryklund et al., 1986.)

3.2. GH Gene

The human GH genomic locus contains a cluster of five highly conserved genes and spans approx 66 kb on the long arm of chromosome 17 (q22-24). All these genes have the same basic structure consisting of five exons separated by four introns. The hGH gene codes for a 22-kDa protein (Fig. 3) containing 191 amino acids and is exclusively expressed in somatotropes, whereas the others are expressed in placental tissue. The GH promoter, 300 bp of 5'-flanking DNA, contains *cis*-elements that mediate both pituitary- and hormone-specific signaling. *Pit-1*, a 33-kDa tissue-specific transcription factor, binds to specific sites on the promoter. This factor is expressed in lactotropes, somatotropes, and thyrotropes and is critical for GH, PRL, and TSH-β gene transcription. GH-releasing hormone (GHRH) stimulates GH transcription, and insulin-like growth factor-1 (IGF-1) inhibits GH mRNA expression (Fig. 4).

3.3. GH Secretion

GH is secreted as a 22-kDa single-chain polypeptide hormone, or a less abundant 20-kDa monomer, formed by alternative mRNA splicing. The secretion is pulsatile, with low or undetectable basal levels between

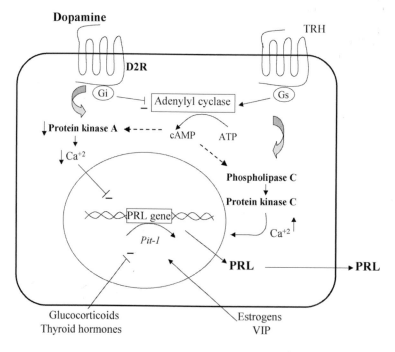

Fig. 4. Regulation of GH expression in the somatotrope. GHRH and somatostain bind to specific G protein–coupled seven-transmembrane domain receptors (GHRH receptor; SSTRs 2 and 5, respectively). GHRH activates adenylyl cyclase to generate cAMP, whereas somatostatin receptor binding suppresses cAMP production. GHRH stimulation activates PKA and CREB phosphorylation. The transcription factors *c-fos* and *Pit-1* then induce GH transcription. Somatostatin, coupled to the G_i protein, suppresses GH secretion. Ghrelin binds to the GH secretagogue receptor, induces adenylyl cyclase to generate cAMP, and activates phospholipase C (PLC) signaling, leading to protein kinase C induction and Ca^{+2} release. IGF-1, through binding to its receptor, exerts negative feedback on GH expression via the phosphatidylinositol 3-kinase and mitogen-activated protein kinase signaling pathways.

peaks. In children, maximum GH secretory peaks are detected within 1 h of the onset of deep sleep. Somatostatin (SRIF) and GHRH interact to generate pulsatile GH release, and SRIF appears to be the primary regulator of GH pulses in response to physiologic stimuli. GHRH stimulates GH synthesis and secretion, whereas SRIF, as well as IGF-1, inhibits GH secretion (Fig. 4). Ghrelin, a recently discovered orexigenic factor, is a potent GH secretagogue produced by the neuroendocrine cells of the stomach. Ghrelin stimulates GH secretion through binding to its specific receptor, the GH secretagogue receptor, in the hypothalamus and pituitary. Thyrotropin-releasing hormone (TRH) does not stimulate GH secretion in normal subjects but induces GH release in patients with acromegaly.

3.4. GH Receptor and Binding Proteins

In addition to the liver, which contains the highest concentration of GH receptors, many other tissues express these receptors. The human GH receptor is a 620-amino-acid protein (130 kDa) with an extracellular hormone-binding domain of 246 amino acids, a single transmembrane region, and a cytoplasmic domain of 350 residues. The human GH receptor gene has been assigned to chromosome 5p13. The GH-binding proteins, soluble short forms (60 kDa) of the hepatic GH receptor and identical to the extracellular domain, bind half of circulating GH. They prolong GH plasma half-life by decreasing the GH metabolic clearance rate and also inhibit GH binding to surface receptors by ligand competition.

3.5. GH Action

GH acts both directly, via its own receptor, and indirectly, via IGF-1, on peripheral target tissues. Longitudinal bone growth–promoting actions on the chondrocytes in the epiphyseal growth plate are probably stimulated indirectly by GH, through local as well as hepatic-derived circulating IGF-1. GH itself has chronic antiinsulin effects that may result in glucose intolerance. When administered to GH-deficient adults, the hormone increases muscle volume and lean body mass, significantly decreases body fat, as well as improves physical performance and psychologic well-being in these patients.

3.6. Clinical Testing

GH immunoradiometric assays (IRMA), employing a double monoclonal antibody sandwich system, are now widely used because of their sensitivity and accuracy, compared with RIAs. Random GH measurements are not helpful in the diagnosis of GH hypersecretory or deficiency states because of the pulsatile nature of pitu-

itary GH secretion, and integrated measurements over time are required. Serum IGF-1 levels are invariably high in acromegaly and correlate better with the clinical manifestations of hypersomatotrophism than single GH measurements. Therefore, high IGF-1 levels are highly specific for diagnosing acromegaly. IGF-1 is less helpful in the evaluation of GH deficiency (GHD), because its levels are low in infancy and the normal range overlaps with values measured in GH-deficient children.

3.6.1. PROVOCATIVE TESTS

Provocative tests are dynamic tests that assess GH reserve in the evaluation of GHD, by pharmacologic stimulation of the somatotropes. The diagnosis of GHD in children is determined by an inadequate GH response to at least two separate provocative tests.

3.6.2. GROWTH HORMONE–RELEASING HORMONE

The GHRH test (1 µg/kg, intravenously) may help in the diagnosis of GH insufficiency, when GH does not increase within 60 min subsequent to injection. If the somatotropes are first primed with intermittent GHRH pulses, the acute GHRH test may sometimes distinguish between hypothalamic and pituitary GH deficiency.

3.6.3. INSULIN-INDUCED HYPOGLYCEMIA

Insulin-induced hypoglycemia is the most reliable provocative stimulus for the diagnosis of GHD. Clonidine, arginine, L-dopa, and propranolol are other stimulants used in the evaluation of GH reserve. The diagnosis of GHD in adults is currently being reevaluated because the sensitive new IRMAs indicate "normal" integrated GH levels of <0.5 µg/L.

3.6.4. SUPPRESSION TESTS

In patients with acromegaly, the elevated GH levels fail to suppress (<1 µg/L) after an oral glucose load.

3.7. GH Hypersecretion: Acromegaly

More than 95% of patients with acromegaly harbor a pituitary adenoma; two-thirds have pure GH-cell tumors; and the others have plurihormonal tumors, usually expressing PRL in addition to GH. These patients have elevated GH and IGF-1 levels and normal GHRH concentrations. Ectopic acromegaly may be central owing to excess GHRH production by functional hypothalamic tumors, or by peripheral rare extrapituitary GH-secreting tumors (pancreas) and the more common tumors secreting GHRH (carcinoid, pancreas, small-cell lung cancer). Patients with ectopic acromegaly disclose normal (central) or elevated (peripheral) GHRH levels. The clinical manifestations of acromegaly include generalized visceromegaly with enlargement of the tongue, bones, salivary glands, thyroid, heart, and soft organs; characteristic facial features of wide spacing of the teeth, large fleshy nose and frontal bossing; and skeletal overgrowth leading to mandibular overgrowth with prognathism, and increased hand, foot, and hat size. Patients present with voice deepening, headaches, arthropathy and carpal tunnel syndrome, muscle weakness and fatigue, oily skin and hyperhydrosis, hypertension and left ventricular hypertrophy, sleep apnea, menstrual abnormalities, depression, and glucose intolerance. Patients with acromegaly have a significant increase in overall mortality owing to cardiovascular disorders, malignancy, and respiratory disease. Selective transsphenoidal resection is the indicated treatment for GH-secreting pituitary adenoma. Octreotide and lanreotide (cyclic somatostatin analogs) significantly attenuates GH and IGF-1 levels in most patients, and chronic administration is accompanied by marked clinical improvement. Pegvisomant (GH antagonist) was shown recently to normalize IGF-1 levels in most patients with acromegaly, when administered daily. However, this drug further increases GH (albeit biologically inactivated) in treated patients, and the long-term effects on adenoma size are still unknown.

3.8. GH Hyposecretion

GHD in children may be isolated or combined with deficiencies of other pituitary hormones. Its incidence approaches 1:5000 to 1:10,000, and only between 25 and 30% of affected children exhibit identifiable underlying disorders. Several types of hereditary GHD with different modes of inheritance have been described. Molecular defects include GH gene deletion or lack of synthesis or secretion of GHRH, and excess somatostatin secretion has also been postulated. A group of children with growth failure may secrete an immunoreactive but a bioinactive GH molecule. Point mutations or major deletion of the *Pit-1* gene results in strains of dwarf mice that fail to develop pituitary somatotrope, lactotrope, and thyrotrope cells. This may be a potential mechanism for human GHD. Children with GHD are short and fail to grow at a normal rate, and this is usually noted by 12–18 mo of age. Patients tend to be overweight for their height but are normally proportioned. These children have low stimulated GH levels and low IGF-binding protein-3 (IGFBP-3). IGF-1 levels are normally very low before 3 yr of age and do not correlate with stimulated GH levels. GH replacement with recombinant human GH (rhGH) should be started as early as possible, because total height gain is inversely proportional to pretreatment chronologic and bone age. Adult GHD may be isolated or owing to panhypopituitarism from several causes. These include pituitary

apoplexy, large pituitary tumors, surgical trauma, hemochromatosis, hypophysitis, and other sellar lesions. GH-deficient adults have altered body composition with increased fat and decreased muscle volume and strength, lower psychosocial achievement, and altered glucose and lipid metabolism. These patients have low stimulated GH, low or normal IGF-1 and low IGFBP-3. The clinical effects of rhGH treatment in adults include changes in body composition and lipid profile and improvement in quality of life.

3.9. GH Receptor Defects (Laron Dwarfism)

GHD may be owing to failure of the liver and peripheral tissues to generate IGF-1 in response to GH. The genetic defect appears to be in the GH receptor itself, but the clinical characteristics of Laron dwarfism are identical to those in GH-deficient children. Basal and stimulated GH levels are high, but IGF-1 values are low and do not respond to GH therapy. Successful response of Laron dwarfs to recombinant IGF-1 therapy has been reported.

4. PROLACTIN

4.1. Embryology and Cytogenesis of Lactotropes

Lactotropes are the last cells to differentiate in the human fetal pituitary. PRL is found only at 12 wk of gestation and until 24 wk is localized in mammosomatotropes. These cells produce both GH and PRL and appear to be the source of differentiated lactotropes, which are found only after that time. The lactotropes are acidophilic cells, contain PRL-immunostained secretory granules, and constitute 15% of adenohypophysial cells. However, in multiparous women they represent up to a third of the cells, and during pregnancy and lactation they may constitute 70% of the pituitary cells.

4.2. Prolactin Gene

The human PRL gene is approx 10 kb long, consists of five exons separated by four large introns, and encodes the 199-amino-acid PRL peptide (23 kDa) (Fig. 5). The gene, located on chromosome 6, has two regions responsible for lactotrope-specific transcription activation— a proximal promoter (–422 to +33) and a distal enhancer element (–1831 to –1530 bp), both containing specific binding sites for *Pit-1*. PRL is homologous to GH and placental lactogen, and they are thought to have arisen from a common original ancestral gene. Sequence homology among human PRL, bovine, and other mammals is in the range of 70–80%. Dopamine, the major PRL inhibitory factor, acts through the D2 dopamine receptor (D2R), to decrease intracellular cAMP, PRL gene transcription, synthesis, and release,

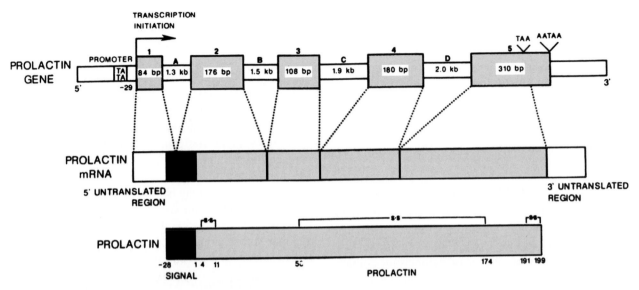

Fig. 5. Schematic structure of PRL gene, mRNA, and protein. The PRL gene (top) consists of the promoter, and five exons (1–5), separated by four introns (A–D). The PRL protein is a 199-amino-acid 23-kDa polypeptide with three intraprotein disulfide bonds. (From Molitch [Prolactin] in Melmed, 1995.)

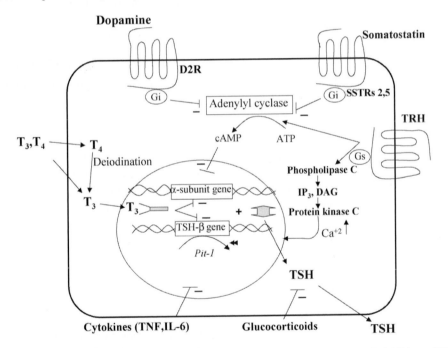

Fig. 6. Regulation of PRL expression in the lactotrope. Dopamine is the predominant physiologic inhibitor of PRL. Dopamine binds to the D2R, coupled to G_i protein, and suppresses cAMP, PKA, and intracellular calcium, thus inhibiting *Pit-1* and PRL expression. Estrogens (stimulation) and glucocorticoids and thyroid hormones (suppression) mediate their effects on PRL via binding of their nuclear receptors to response elements on the PRL promoter. TRH binds a G protein–coupled seven-transmembrane domain receptor, activates the G_s stimulatory protein, increases cAMP, and induces the phosphoinositide-PKC pathway that also increases intracellular calcium concentrations. This may result in increased transcriptional activity of *Pit-1*. IP_3 = inositol triphosphate; DAG = diacylgylcerol.

mediated by the phosphoinositide/calcium pathway (Fig. 6). VIP induces PRL synthesis and secretion, whereas glucocorticoids and thyroid hormones exert an inhibitory effect on PRL transcription and secretion. Estrogens, by binding of the estrogen receptor to the PRL enhancer element, and TRH through the phosphoinositide-PKC pathway, induce PRL transcription and secretion (Fig. 6).

4.3. PRL Secretion

PRL is under tonic inhibitory hypothalamic control and is secreted in pulses with an increase in amplitude during sleep. Basal levels increase throughout the course of pregnancy, up to 10-fold by term. In the postpartum period, basal PRL levels remain elevated in lactating women, and suckling triggers a rapid release of PRL. TRH is a pharmacologic stimulator of PRL release, and dopamine is the predominant physiologic inhibitor factor (Fig. 6).

4.4. PRL Receptor

The human PRL receptor is a 598-amino-acid protein encoded by a gene on chromosome 5 (p13-p14). The receptor contains a long extracellular region, a single transmembrane region, and a short cytoplasmic domain. There is a high sequence homology among the human, rat, and rabbit PRL receptors, and between the human PRL and GH receptors, which are colocalized to the same area on chromosome 5. PRL receptors are widely distributed, and their hormonal regulation is tissue specific. In the mammary gland, high progesterone levels during pregnancy limit PRL receptor numbers, and early in lactation the numbers increase markedly. Testosterone increases and estrogens decrease PRL receptor levels in the prostate. In most organs studied, PRL is able to up- and downregulate the level of its own receptor.

4.5. PRL Action

PRL contributes to breast development during pregnancy, with estrogen, progesterone, and placental lactogen. After delivery PRL stimulates milk production. Hyperprolactinemia suppresses gonadotropin-releasing hormone (GnRH) pulses at the hypothalamus, pulsatile secretion of pituitary gonadotropins, and ovarian release of progesterone and estrogen. In men testosterone levels are low. PRL may induce mild glucose intolerance and has a role as an immune modulator.

4.6. Immunoradiometric Assay

Most assays for human PRL are based on the double-antibody method. Normal concentrations are slightly higher (<20 µg/L) in women than in men (<15 µg/L).

4.7. Hyperprolactinemia

The differential diagnosis of hyperprolactinemia includes PRL-secreting pituitary adenomas, pituitary stalk compression blocking dopamine access (owing to large nonfunctioning adenomas), acromegaly, chronic breast stimulation, pregnancy, hypothyroidism, chronic renal failure, hypothalamic disorders, and medications (estrogens, phenothiazines, methyldopa, metoclopramide, and verapamil). PRL serum levels >200 µg/L are usually associated with prolactinoma. Hyperprolactinemia presents as amenorrhea and galactorrhea in women, and impotence and infertility in men.

4.8. PRL-Secreting Pituitary Adenomas

Prolactinomas are the most common hormone-secreting pituitary adenomas. Many tumors secrete both GH and PRL. These monoclonal tumors are classified as microprolactinomas (<10 mm, 90% occurring in women), or macroprolactinomas (>10 mm, 60% occurring in men). In macroadenomas, the clinical presentation of hyperprolactinemia may be associated with mass effect signs of headaches and visual field disturbances. Most patients (70%) are successfully treated with dopamine agonists (bromocriptine and cabergoline). Transsphenoidal surgery is reserved for drug-resistant tumors.

4.9. Immune System Interaction.

Lymphocytes express PRL receptors. Hypoprolactinemic states are associated with impaired lymphocyte proliferation, decreased macrophage activation, and other manifestations of immunosuppression, which can be restored with PRL treatment in rats.

5. THYROID-STIMULATING HORMONE
5.1. Embryology and Cytogenesis of Thyrotropes

Differentiated thyrotropes are found in the fetal pituitary at 12 wk of gestation, when TSH β-subunits are immunolocalized and also found in the circulation. However, TSH levels remain low until wk 18, when the fetal levels increase significantly. Thyrotropes comprise only 5% of the anterior pituitary cell population.

5.2. TSH Gene

Human TSH is a 211-amino-acid glycoprotein with a molecular mass of 28 kDa, which is structurally related to LH, FSH, and human chorionic gonadotropin (hCG). They are composed of a heterodimer of two noncovalently linked subunits, α and β. The α-subunits of all four glycoproteins are identical and are encoded by a 13.5-kb gene (Fig. 7), located on chromosome 6q21-23, containing four exons and three introns. The α-subunit is expressed in thyrotropes, gonadotropes, and placental cells, but cell-specific expression is dependent on different regions of the promoter. The β-subunits of the glycoproteins define tissue specificity despite a 75% similarity in their primary structure and cysteine residues. The TSH β-subunit gene is 4.9 kb in size, is located on chromosome 1p22, and consists of three exons and two introns. The pituitary transcription factor *Pit-1* binds to the β-subunit promoter but is not required for α-subunit gene expression. Both α- and β-

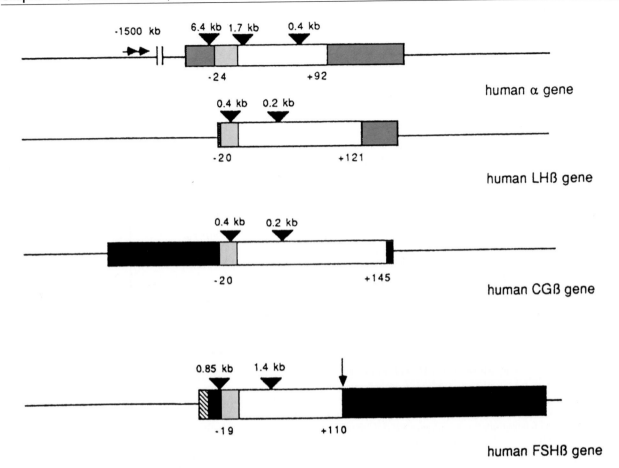

Fig. 7. Schematic structures of human α, hLH-β, hCG-β, and hFSH-β genes: dark areas = untranslated regions; stippled areas = signal peptides; unshaded areas = mature proteins; hatched area = 5' untranslated sequence; solid triangles = introns; pair of arrows in top diagram = cAMP regulatory element; arrow in bottom diagram = polyadenylation site used by some FSH-β transcripts. (From Gharib et al., 1990.)

subunit transcription are induced by TRH and inhibited by triiodothyronine (T$_3$) and dopamine (Fig. 8).

5.3. TSH Secretion

TSH pulsatile secretion occurs every 2–3 h, and is superimposed upon basal hormone release from the pituitary. TSH has a circadian pattern of secretion, with nocturnal levels measured up to twice daytime levels. TSH secretion is enhanced by TRH, while T$_3$, thyroxine (T$_4$), dopamine, SRIF and glucocorticoids suppress TSH secretion (Figure 8).

5.4. TSH Receptor

The TSH receptor is located on the plasma membrane of thyroid follicular cells. It consists of a polypeptide chain of 764 amino acids containing a 398-amino-acid extracellular domain, seven transmembrane segments, and a short intracellular domain of 82 amino acids. Receptor-ligand binding activates Gs protein and adeny-

late cyclase cascade. The TSH receptor gene is located on chromosome 14 (q31) and consists of 10 exons. The extracellular domain and parts of the transmembrane domain contribute to TSH binding, and binding specifity is conferred by the TSH β-subunit, although LH and hCG can activate the human TSH receptor to a certain degree. Germ-line mutations in the transmembrane domain of the TSH receptor gene, resulting in constitutive cAMP activation, were reported in congenital hyperthyroidism, and somatic mutations in this domain were also found in patients with hyperfunctioning thyroid adenomas. Moreover, resistance to thyrotropin, caused by mutations in the extracellular domain of the TSH receptor gene, has been described.

5.5. TSH Action

TSH induces morphologic changes of the follicular cells; causes thyroid gland enlargement owing to hyperplasia and hypertrophy; and stimulates iodide uptake

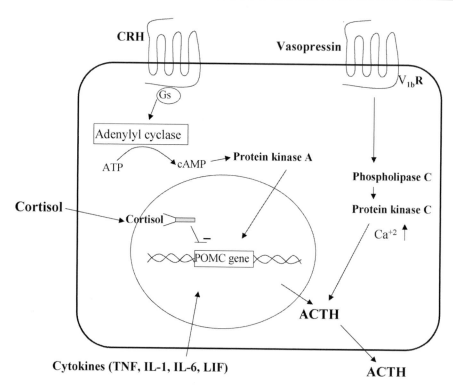

Fig. 8. Regulation of TSH expression in the thyrotrope. Both α- and β-subunit transcription and TSH secretion are induced by TRH and inhibited by thyroid hormones and dopamine. TRH, via binding to a G_s protein–coupled seven-transmembrane domain receptor, activates PLC, which hydrolyzes phosphoinositol 4,5-bisphosphate to DAG and IP_3, activating PKC, and stimulating α-subunit and β-TSH transcription. Increased cAMP also enhances α- and β-subunit transcription. Dopamine and somatostatin decrease TSH by receptors coupling to the G_i protein, reducing adenylyl cyclase activity. Dopamine inhibits TSH transcription, production, and secretion, whereas somatostatin suppresses secretion. Both T_4 and T_3 are potent feedback inhibitors of TSH. The intracellular monodeiodination pituitary of T_4 to T_3 contributes to T_3 content in the thyrotrope, where T_3 binds to specific nuclear receptors, inhibiting transcription of TSH subunit genes. Glucocorticoids and cytokines (TNF, IL-6) also decrease TSH secretion.

and organification, thyroglobulin gene transcription, and thyroid hormone secretion.

5.6. Clinical Testing

RIA for TSH, the "first-generation assay," uses labeled antigen and is useful in distinguishing elevated TSH levels in primary hypothyroidism from normal euthyroid values but is unable to differentiate euthyroid and hyperthyroid subjects. The new sensitive immuno-metric assays employ labeled antibody and a "capture antibody" in sandwich formation and clearly discriminate euthyroid from hyperthyroid patients. TRH (200–500 μg, intravenously or intramuscularly) stimulates TSH release in euthyroid subjects. Hyperthyroid patients have no response, and primary hypothyroid patients demonstrate augmented TSH response to TRH stimulation. However, elevated basal TSH levels in TSH-secreting pituitary tumors fail to respond to TRH, and patients with hypothyroidism secondary to pituitary or hypothalamic disease have attenuated TSH response.

5.7. TSH Hypersecretion

Most cases of elevated serum TSH levels are a result of primary thyroid failure. Thyroid hormone resistance is a rare syndrome that includes clinical euthyroidism, elevated levels of thyroid hormones, and inappropriately normal to slightly increased TSH levels. TSH-producing pituitary adenomas comprise <1% of all pituitary tumors and secrete the TSH α- and β-subunits chractericstic of the normal thyrotropes. However, the α-subunit is synthesized in excess of the β-subunit, a useful characteristic in the diagnosis of these tumors. TSH secretion by these tumors fails to respond to TRH stimulation or to normal thyroid hormone–negative feedback. However, somatostatin suppresses TSH release from the tumors. Most patients present with hyperthyroidism and diffuse goiter. TSH is elevated or inappropriately normal in the presence of elevated thyroid hormones. Cosecretion of other pituitary hormones—GH, PRL, and FSH—is common, resulting in acromegaly, and amenorrhea, galactorrhea, and impotence. Because these tumors are usually large macroadenomas, local intracranial mass effects are common. Transsphenoidal pituitary surgery is the preferred initial approach, but most patients are not cured and require adjuvant medical or radiation therapy. The use of somatostatin analogs, octreotide and lanreotide, is a successful treatment option for these tumors. Thyroid ablation or surgery is not recommended because of the potential risk of pituitary tumor expansion, owing to release of the thyrotrope cells from negative feedback inhibition.

6. FSH AND LH

6.1. Embryology and Cytogenesis of Gonadotropes

Gonadotropes are found in the fetal pituitary at 12 wk of gestation, when β-subunits are immunolocalized and first detected in blood. Gonadotropes represent up to 10% of the pituitary cell population. These basophilic cells reveal cytoplasmic positivity for FSH and LH, usually both in the same cell. However, some cells contain only one of the two hormones.

6.2. FSH and LH Genes

The gonadotropins, FSH and LH, are members of the glycoprotein hormone family and share many structural similarities with TSH and hCG. The α-subunits of all four members of this hormone family are identical, and the β-subunits share considerable amino acid homology with one another, indicating evolution from a common precursor. The FSH- and LH-β-subunits are both expressed in the gonadotropes and possess three exons and two introns (Fig. 7). FSH-β-subunit, located on the short arm of human chromosome 11p13, is highly conserved among different species. LH β-gene, approx 1.5 kb in length, is one of the hCG β-like gene cluster, arranged on human chromosome 19q, and encodes a 121-amino-acid mature protein. Human FSH is a 34-kDa protein with 210 amino acids, and LH is a 28.5-kDa protein consisting of 204 amino acid residues. GnRH pulses increase transcription rates of all three gonadotropin subunits: α, LH-β, and FSH-β. Testosterone increases FSH-β mRNA levels in pituitary cell cultures but has no effect on LH-β mRNA. Estrogen negatively regulates transcription of all three subunits. However, estrogen exerts a positive feedback effect at the pituitary level under several physiologic conditions and increases LH-β mRNA.

6.3. Regulation of Secretion

GnRH is the major regulator of gonadotropin secretion from pituitary cells. The frequency and amplitude of GnRH pulses are critical for stimulating LH and FSH output. Estrogens can exert both stimulatory and inhibitory effects on gonadotropin secretion, depending on the dose, duration, and other physiologic factors. Testosterone inhibits in vivo serum FSH levels, but its direct effects on FSH release at the pituitary level are stimulatory. Another regulator of FSH secretion is inhibin, a gonadal peptide produced by Sertoli cells that inhibits FSH release and, under some conditions, may also regulate LH output.

6.4. Gonadotropin Receptor

FSH, LH, and TSH receptors have similar structure and belong to the subfamily of G_s protein–coupled receptors having seven hydrophobic transmembrane segments. The specific, high-affinity interaction between hormone and receptor is owing to the large extracellular N-terminal domain of the receptor (LH: 340 amino acids). The LH receptor is a single 75-kDa polypeptide of 700 amino acids. FSH receptor is also a single polypeptide, consisting of four subunits of similar mass (60 kDa).

6.5. Gonadotropin Action

In the male, LH binds to receptors on the Leydig cells and stimulates testosterone synthesis. High intratesticular testosterone levels are important for spermatogenesis. FSH is probably essential for the maturation process of the spermatids. In the female, LH and FSH are major regulators of ovarian steroid production. FSH plays a critical role in follicle growth and cytodifferentiation of granulosa cells.

6.6. Clinical Testing

RIAs of FSH and LH suffer from limited sensitivity and specificity owing to crossreactivity of free α-subunits and other pituitary glycoprotein hormones. The two site-directed IRMA and nonisotopic asays are more sensitive measurements with no α-crossreactivity and are extremely useful in studying physiologic events characterized by low gonadotropin levels. The GnRH (25–100 µg, intravenously) stimulation test has limited usefulness in the diagnosis of hypothalamic-pituitary disorders. Patients with primary testicular failure exhibit an exaggerated increase in serum FSH and LH response within 30 min after injection. However, patients with hypothalamic and pituitary disorders cannot be distinguished. Repetitive administration of GnRH pulses may normalize gonadotropin responses in patients with hypothalamic disease, indicating pituitary integrity.

6.7. Gonadotrope-Cell Tumors

Gonadotrope adenomas are the most common pituitary adenomas. In the past, they were called "nonsecreting adenomas," because the gonadotropins and their subunits produced by them are either not released or inefficiently secreted, and they usually do not produce a distinct clinical syndrome. These tumors produce supranormal (up to 10 times normal) serum levels of α- and FSH-β-subunits, but rarely of LH-β. Usually, the subunits are not secreted in the same proportions. Some gonadotrope adenomas produce α-subunits but not intact FSH or LH. Administration of TRH to patients with gonadotrope adenomas usually results in secretion of gonadotropins or their subunits, compared with no stimulation in healthy subjects. Most of the "nonsecreting adenomas" immunostain for intact FSH and LH, or α-, FSH-β-, and LH-β-subunits. Mass effects, including optic chiasm pressure and other neurologic symptoms, may be the first symptoms of large gonadotrope tumors. Excessive secretion of FSH or LH may actually down-regulate the axis.

SELECTED READING

Bertolino P, Tong, WM, et al. Heterozygous MEN1 mutant mice develop a range of endocrine tumors mimicking multiple endocrine neoplasia type 1. *Mol Endocrinol* 2003;17:1880–1892.

Cohen LE, Radovick S. Molecular basis of combined pituitary hormone deficiencies. *Endocr Rev* 2002;23:431–442.

Combarnous Y. Molecular basis of the specificity of binding of glycoprotein hormones to their receptors. *Endocr Rev* 1992;13: 670–691.

Cushman LJ, Watkins-Chow DE, Brinkmeier ML, Raetzman LT, Radak AL, Lloyd RV, Camper SA. Persistent Prop1 expression delays gonadotrope differentiation and enhances pituitary tumor susceptibility. *Hum Mol Genet* 2001;10:1141–1153.

Freeman ME, Kanyicska B, Lerant A, Nagy G. Prolactin: structure, function and regulation of secretion. *Phys Rev* 2000;80:1523–1631.

Goffin V, Binart N, et al. Prolactin: the new biology of an old hormone. *Annu Rev Physiol* 2002;64:47–67.

Guistina A, Veldhuis JD. Pathophysiology of the neuroregulation of growth hormone secretion in experimental animals and the human. *Endocr Rev* 1998;19:717–797.

Heaney AP, Horwitz GA, Wang Z, Singson R, Melmed S. Early involvement of estrogen-induced pituitary tumor transforming gene and fibroblast growth factor expression in prolactinoma pathogenesis. *Nat Med* 1999;5:1317–1321.

Herrington J, Carter-Su C. Signaling pathways activated by the growth hormone receptor. *Trends Endocrinol Metab* 2001;12:252–257.

Horvath E, Kovacs K, Scheithauer BW. Pituitary hyperplasia. *Pituitary* 1999;1:169–179.

Kojima M, Hosoda H, Date Y, Nakazato M, Matsuo H, Kangawa K. Ghrelin is a growth hormone–releasing acylated peptide from stomach. *Nature* 1999;402:656–660.

Lamolet B, Pulichino AM, Lamonerie T, Gauthier Y, Brue T, Enjalbert A, Drouin J. A pituitary cell–restricted T box factor, Tpit, activates POMC transcription in cooperation with Pitx homeoproteins. *Cell* 2001;104:849–859.

Levy A, and Lightman S. Molecular defects in the pathogenesis of pituitary tumours. *Front Neuroendocrinol* 2003;24:94–127.

Liu J, Lin C, Gleiberman A, Ohgi KA, Herman T, Huang HP, Tsai MJ, Rosenfeld MG. Tbx19, a tissue-selective regulator of POMC gene expression. *Proc Natl Acad Sci USA* 2001;98:8674–8679.

Olson LE, Rosenfeld MG. Perspective: genetic and genomic approaches in elucidating mechanisms of pituitary development. *Endocrinology* 2002;143:2007–2011.

Prezant TR, Melmed S. Molecular pathogenesis of pituitary disorders. *Curr Opin Endocrinol Diabetes* 2002;9:61–78.

Shimon I, Melmed S. Management of pituitary tumors. *Ann Intern Med* 1998;129:472–483.

Vassart G, Dumont JE. The thyrotropin receptor and the regulation of thyrocyte function and growth. *Endocr Rev* 1992;13:596–611.

14 Posterior Pituitary Hormones

Daniel G. Bichet, MD

CONTENTS

1. STRUCTURE OF NEUROHYPOPHYSIS: ANATOMY OF VASOPRESSIN-PRODUCING CELLS

The hypothalamus (Fig. 1) embodies a group of nuclei that form the floor and ventrolateral walls of the triangular-shaped third ventricle. A thin membrane called the lamina terminalis forms the anterior wall of this compartment and contains osmoreceptor cells in a structure known as the organum vasculosum. The subfornical organ (SFO) also contains osmoreceptors. The organum vasculosum of the lamina terminalis (OVLT), the SFO, and the pituitary gland lack a blood-brain barrier. The supraoptic nucleus lies just dorsal to the optic chiasm and approx 2 mm from the third ventricle. The paraventricular nucleus lies closer to the thalamus in the suprachiasmatic portion of the hypothalamus, but it borders on the third ventricular space. These well-defined nuclei contain the majority of the large neuroendocrine cell bodies, known as the magnocellular or neurosecretory cells, that manufacture arginine vasopressin (AVP) and oxytocin (OT). The neurohypophysis consists of (1) a set of hypothalamic nuclei, the supraoptic

From: *Endocrinology: Basic and Clinical Principles, Second Edition*
(S. Melmed and P. M. Conn, eds.) © Humana Press Inc., Totowa, NJ

and paraventricular nuclei, which house the pericarya of the magnocellular neurons; (2) the axonal processes of the magnocellular neurons that form the supraoptical hypophyseal tract; and, (3) the neurosecretory material of these neurons, which is carried on to the posterior pituitary gland (Fig. 1).

2. ARGININE VASOPRESSIN
2.1. Synthesis

Nonapeptides of the vasopressin family are the key regulators of water homeostasis in amphibia, reptiles, birds, and mammals. Because these peptides reduce urinary output, they are also referred to as antidiuretic hormones. OT and AVP (Fig. 2) are synthesized in separate populations of magnocellular neurons (cell body diameter of 20–40 μm) of the supraoptic and paraventricular nuclei. OT and vasopressin magnocellular neurons are found intermingled in the magnocellular nuclei. OT is most recognized for its key role in parturition and milk letdown in mammals. The axonal projections of AVP- and OT-producing neurons from supraoptic and

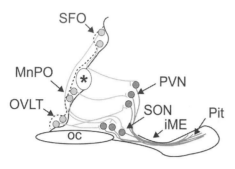

Fig. 1. Schematic representation of osmoregulatory pathway of hypothalamus (sagittal section of midline of ventral brain around third ventricle in mice). Neurons (lightly shaded circles) in the lamina terminalis—consisting of the OVLT, median preoptic nucleus (MnPO), and SFO—that are responsive to plasma hypertonicity send efferent axonal projections (gray lines) to magnocellular neurons of the paraventricular (PVN) and supraoptic (SON) nuclei. The processes (black lines) of these magnocellular neurons form the hypothalamo-neurohypophysial pathway that courses in the median eminence to reach the posterior pituitary, where neurosecretion of vasopressin and OT occurs. (Modified with permission from Wilson et al., 2002.)

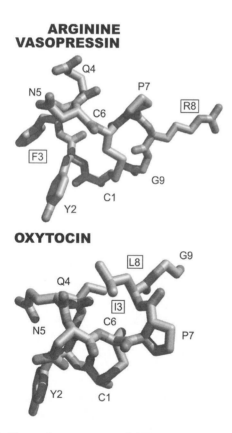

Fig. 2. Contrasting structures of AVP and OT. The peptides differ only by two amino acids (F3 → I3 and R8 → L8 in AVP and OT, respectively). The conformation of AVP was obtained from Mouillac et al. (1995), and the conformation of OT was obtained from the Protein Data Bank (PDB Id 1XY1).

paraventricular nuclei reflect the dual function of AVP and OT as hormones and as neuropeptides, in that they project their axons to several brain areas and to the neurohypophysis. Another pathway from parvocellular neurons (cell body diameter of 10–15 μm) to the hypophysial portal system transports high concentrations of AVP to the anterior pituitary gland. AVP produced by this pathway and the corticotropin-releasing hormone (CRH) are two major hypothalamic secretagogues regulating the secretion of adrenocorticotropic hormone (ACTH) by the anterior pituitary.

More than half of parvocellular neurons coexpress both *CRH* and *prepro-AVP-NPII*. In addition, while passing through the median eminence and the hypophysial stalk, magnocellular axons can also release AVP into the long portal system. Furthermore, a number of neuroanatomic studies have shown the existence of short portal vessels that allow communication between the posterior and anterior pituitary. Thus, in addition to parvocellular vasopressin, magnocellular vasopressin is able to influence ACTH secretion.

AVP and its corresponding carrier protein, neurophysin II, are synthesized as a composite precursor by the magnocellular and parvocellular neurons described previously. In contrast to conventional neurotransmitters (e.g., acetylcholine, excitatory and inhibitory amino acids, monoamines), which are synthesized in nerve terminals and can be packaged locally in recycled small vesicular membranes, the biosynthesis and secretion of neuropeptides such as OT and vasopressin in the hypothalamo-neurohypophysial system requires continual *de novo* transcription and translation of peptide precursor proteins (Fig. 3). The precursor is packaged into neurosecretory granules and transported axonally in the stalk of the posterior pituitary. En route to the neurohypophysis, the precursor is processed into the active hormone. Prepro-vasopressin has 164 amino acids and is encoded by the 2.5-kb *prepro-AVP-NPII* gene located in chromosome region 20p13. The *prepro-AVP-NPII* gene and the *prepro-OT-NPI* gene are located within the same chromosomal locus, at a very short distance from each other (3–11 kb) in head-to-head orientation. Data from transgenic mouse studies indicate that the intergenic region between the OT and VP genes contains the critical enhancer sites for magnocellular neuron cell-specific expression. Exon 1 of the *prepro-AVP-NPII* gene encodes the signal peptide, AVP, and the NH$_2$-terminal region of NPII. Exon 2 encodes the central region of NPII, and exon 3 encodes the COOH-terminal region of NPII and the glycopeptide. Pro-vasopressin is generated by the removal of the signal peptide from prepro-vasopressin and the addition of a carbohydrate chain to the glycopeptide. Additional

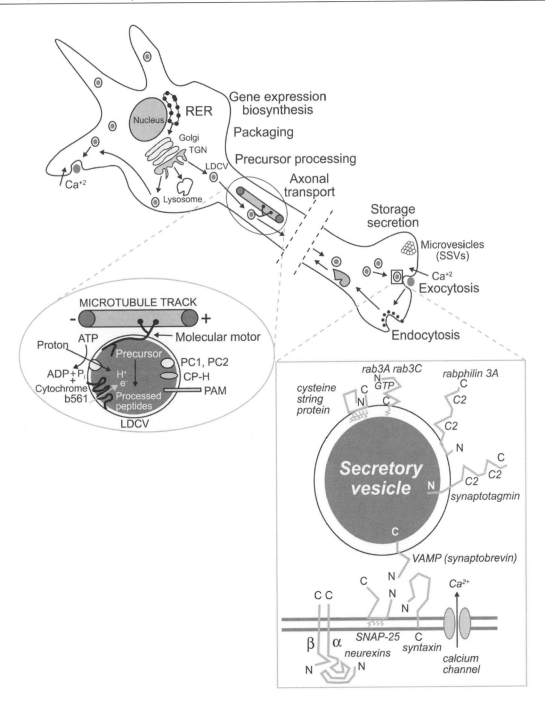

Fig. 3. Peptidergic neuron. Cellular and molecular properties of a peptidergic neuron (neurosecretory cell) are shown. The structure of the neurosecretory cell is depicted schematically with notations of the various cell biologic processes that occur in each topographic domain. Gene expression, protein biosynthesis, and packaging of the protein into large dense-core vesicles (LDCVs) occurs in the cell body, where the nucleus, rough ER (RER), and Golgi apparatus are located. Enzymatic processing of the precursor proteins into the biologically active peptides occurs primarily in the LDCVS (*see* inset), often during the process of anterograde axonal transport of the LDCVS to the nerve terminals on microtubule tracks in the axon. Upon reaching the nerve terminal, the LDCVS are usually stored in preparation for secretion. Conduction of a nerve impulse (action potential) down the axon and its arrival in the nerve terminal cause an influx of calcium ion through calcium channels. The increased calcium ion concentration causes a cascade of molecular events that leads to neurosecretion (exocytosis). Recovery of the excess LDCV membrane after exocytosis is performed by endocytosis, but this membrane is not recycled locally and, instead, is retrogradely transported to the cell body for reuse or degradation in lysosomes. ATP = adenosine triphosphate; ADP = adenosine 5′-diphosphate; GTP = guanosine 5′- triphosphate; TGN = trans-Golgi network; SSV = small secretory vesicles; PC1 or PC2 = prohormone convertase 1 or 2, respectively; CP-H = carboxypeptidase H; PAM = peptiylglycine -amidating monooxygenase. (Reproduced with permission from Burbach et al. [2001].)

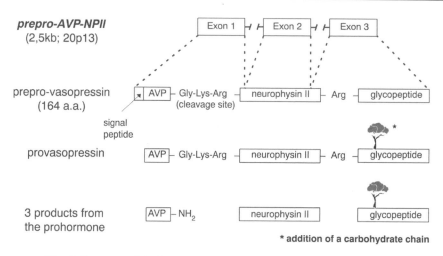

Fig. 4. Structure of the human vasopressin (AVP) gene and prohormone.

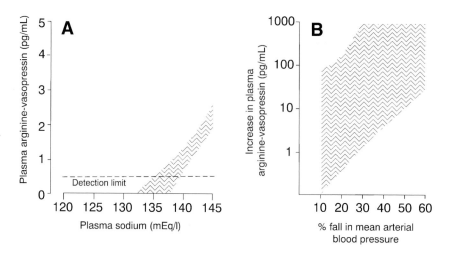

Fig. 5. Osmotic and nonosmotic stimulation of AVP. (**A**) The relationship between plasma AVP (P_{AVP}) and plasma sodium (P_{Na}) in 19 normal subjects is described by the area with vertical lines, which includes the 99% confidence limits of the regression line P_{Na}/P_{AVP}. The osmotic threshold for AVP release is about 280–285 mmol/kg or 136 meq of sodium/L. AVP secretion should be abolished when plasma sodium is lower than 135 meq/L (Bichet et al., 1986). (**B**) Increase in plasma AVP during hypotension (vertical lines). Note that a large diminution in blood pressure in healthy humans induces large increments in AVP. (Reproduced with permission from Vokes and Robertson, 1985.)

posttranslation processing occurs within neurosecretory vesicles during transport of the precursor protein to axon terminals in the posterior pituitary, yielding AVP, NPII, and glycopeptide (Fig. 4). The AVP-NPII complex forms tetramers that can self-associate to form higher oligomers. Neurophysins should be seen as chaperone-like molecules serving intracellular transport in magnocellular cells.

In the posterior pituitary, AVP is stored in vesicles. Exocytotic release is stimulated by minute increases in serum osmolality (hypernatremia, osmotic regulation) and by more pronounced decreases in extracellular fluid (hypovolemia, nonosmotic regulation). OT and neuro-

physin I are released from the posterior pituitary by the suckling response in lactating females.

2.2. Osmotic and Nonosmotic Stimulation

The regulation of antidiuretic hormone (ADH) release from the posterior pituitary is dependent primarily on two mechanisms involving the osmotic and nonosmotic pathways (Fig. 5). Vasopressin release can be regulated by changes in either osmolality or cerebrospinal fluid Na^+ concentration.

Although magnocellular neurons are themselves osmosensitives, they require input from the lamina terminalis to respond fully to osmotic challenges. Neu-

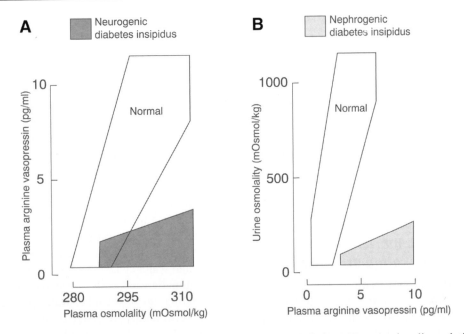

Fig. 6. (A) Relationship between plasma AVP and plasma osmolality during infusion of hypertonic saline solution. Patients with primary polydipsia and NDI have values within the normal range (open area) in contrast to patients with neurogenic diabetes insipidus, who show subnormal plasma ADH responses (stippled area). **(B)** Relationship between urine osmolality and plasma ADH during dehydration and water loading. Patients with neurogenic diabetes insipidus and primary polydipsia have values within the normal range (open area) in contrast to patients with NDI, who have hypotonic urine despite high plasma ADH (stippled area). (Reproduced with permission from Zerbe and Robertson, 1984.)

rons in the lamina terminalis are also osmosensitive and because the SFO and the OVLT lie outside the blood-brain barrier, they can integrate this information with endocrine signals borne by circulating hormones, such as angiotensin II (Ang-II), relaxin, and atrial natriuretic peptide (ANP). While circulating Ang-II and relaxin excite both OT and vasopressin magnocellular neurons, ANP inhibits vasopressin neurons. In addition to an angiotensinergic path from the SFO, the OVLT and the median preoptic nucleus provide direct glutaminergic and GABAergic projections to the hypothalamo-neuro-hypophysial system. Nitric oxide may also modulate neurohormone release.

The cellular basis for osmoreceptor potentials has been characterized using patch-clamp recordings and morphometric analysis in magnocellular cells isolated from the supraoptic nucleus of the adult rat. In these cells, stretch-inactivating cationic channels transduce osmotically evoked changes in cell volume into functionally relevant changes in membrane potential. In addition, magnocellular neurons also operate as intrinsic Na^+ detectors. The transient receptor potential channel (TRPV4) is an osmotically activated channel expressed in the circumventricular organs, the OVLT, and the SFO.

Vasopressin release can also be caused by the nonosmotic stimulation of AVP. Large decrements in blood volume or blood pressure (>10%) stimulate ADH release (Fig. 5). A fall in arterial blood pressure produces a secretion of vasopressin owing to an inhibition of baroreceptors in the aortic arch and activation of chemoreceptors in the carotid body. Afferent from these receptors terminates in the dorsal medulla oblongata of the brain stem, including the nucleus of the tractus solitarus.

The osmotic stimulation of AVP release by dehydration, hypertonic saline infusion, or both is regularly used to determine the vasopressin secretory capacity of the posterior pituitary. This secretory capacity can be assessed *directly* by comparing the plasma AVP concentrations measured sequentially during the dehydration procedure with the normal values and then correlating the plasma AVP values with the urine osmolality measurements obtained simultaneously (Fig. 6).

AVP release can also be assessed *indirectly* by measuring plasma and urine osmolalities at regular intervals during the dehydration test. The maximal urine osmolality obtained during dehydration is compared with the maximal urine osmolality obtained after the administration of vasopressin (Pitressin, 5 U subcutaneously in adults, 1 U subcutaneously in children) or 1-desamino[8-d-arginine]vasopressin (desmopressin [dDAVP], 1–4 μg intravenously over 5–10 min).

The nonosmotic stimulation of AVP release can be used to assess the vasopressin secretory capacity of the posterior pituitary in a rare group of patients with the essential hypernatremia and hypodipsia syndrome. Although some of these patients may have partial central diabetes insipidus, they respond normally to nonosmolar AVP release signals such as hypotension, emesis, and hypoglycemia. In all other cases of suspected central diabetes insipidus, these nonosmotic stimulation tests will not provide additional clinical information.

2.3. Clinically Important Hormonal Influences on Secretion of Vasopressin

Angiotensin is a well-known dipsogen and has been shown to cause drinking in all the species tested. Ang-II receptors have been described in the SFO and OVLT. However, knockout models for angiotensinogen or for angiotensin-1A (AT1A) receptor did not alter thirst or water balance. Disruption of the AT2 receptor only induced mild abnormalities of thirst postdehydration. Earlier reports suggested that the iv administration of atrial peptides inhibits the release of vasopressin, but this was not confirmed by later studies. Vasopressin secretion is under the influence of a glucocorticoid-negative feedback system, and the vasopressin responses to a variety of stimuli (hemorrhage, hypoxia, hypertonic saline) in healthy humans and animals appear to be attenuated or eliminated by pretreatment with glucocorticoids. Finally, nausea and emesis are potent stimuli of AVP release in humans and seem to involve dopaminergic neurotransmission.

2.4. Cellular Actions of Vasopressin

The neurohypophyseal hormone AVP has multiple actions, including the inhibition of diuresis, contraction of smooth muscle, aggregation of platelets, stimulation of liver glycogenolysis, modulation of ACTH release from the pituitary, and central regulation of somatic functions (thermoregulation, blood pressure). These multiple actions of AVP could be explained by the interaction of AVP with at least three types of G protein–coupled receptors (GPCRs); the V_{1a} (vascular hepatic) and V_{1b} (anterior pituitary) receptors act through phosphatidylinositol hydrolysis to mobilize calcium, and the V_2 (kidney) receptor is coupled to adenylate cyclase.

The first step in the action of AVP on water excretion is its binding to AVP type 2 receptors (V_2 receptors) on the basolateral membrane of the collecting duct cells (Fig. 7). The human V_2 receptor gene, *AVPR2*, is located in chromosome region Xq28 and has three exons and two small introns. The sequence of the cDNA predicts a polypeptide of 371 amino acids with a structure typical of guanine nucleotide (G) protein–coupled receptors with seven transmembrane, four extracellular, and four cyto-plasmic domains (Fig. 8). Activation of the V_2 receptor on renal collecting tubules stimulates adenylate cyclase via the stimulatory G protein (G_s) and promotes the cyclic adenosine monophosphate (cAMP)–mediated incorporation of water channels (aquaporins) into the luminal surface of these cells. This process is the molecular basis of the vasopressin-induced increase in the osmotic water permeability of the apical membrane of the collecting tubule. Aquaporin-1 (AQP1, also known as CHIP, a channel-forming integral membrane protein of 28 kDa) was the first protein shown to function as a molecular water channel and is constitutively expressed in mammalian red cells, renal proximal tubules, thin descending limbs, and other water-permeable epithelia. At the subcellular level, AQP1 is localized in both apical and basolateral plasma membranes, which may represent entrance and exit routes for transepithelial water transport. The 2003 Nobel Prize in Chemistry was awarded to Peter Agre and Roderick MacKinnon, who solved two complementary problems presented by the cell membrane: (1) How does a cell let one type of ion through the lipid membrane to the exclusion of other ions? and (2) How does it permeate water without ions?

AQP2 is the vasopressin-regulated water channel in renal collecting ducts. It is exclusively present in principal cells of inner medullary collecting duct cells and is diffusely distributed in the cytoplasm in the euhydrated condition, whereas apical staining of AQP2 is intensified in the dehydrated condition or after administration of dDAVP, a synthetic structural analog of AVP. Short-term AQP2 regulation by AVP involves the movement of AQP2 from intracellular vesicles to the plasma membrane, a confirmation of the shuttle hypothesis of AVP action that was proposed two decades ago. In the long-term regulation, which requires a sustained elevation of circulating AVP levels for 24 h or more, AVP increases the abundance of water channels. This is thought to be a consequence of increased transcription of the *AQP2* gene. The activation of PKA leads to phosphorylation of AQP2 on serine residue 256 in the cytoplasmic carboxyl terminus. This phosphorylation step is essential for the regulated movement of AQP2-containing vesicles to the plasma membrane on elevation of intracellular cAMP concentration.

The gene that codes for the water channel of the apical membrane of the kidney collecting tubule has been designated *AQP2* and was cloned by homology to the rat aquaporin of collecting duct. The human *AQP2* gene is located in chromosome region 12q13 and has four exons

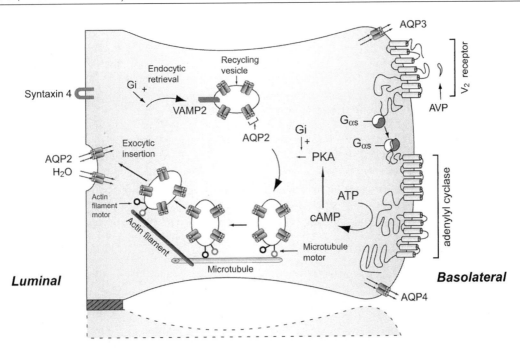

Fig. 7. Schematic representation of effect of AVP to increase water permeability in the principal cells of the collecting duct. AVP is bound to the V$_2$ receptor (a GPCR) on the basolateral membrane. The basic process of GPCR signaling consists of three steps: a hepta-helical receptor detects a ligand (in this case, AVP) in the extracellular milieu, a G protein dissociates into a-subunits bound to guanosine 5′-triphosphate (GTP) and βγ-subunits after interaction with the ligand-bound receptor, and an effector (in this case, adenylyl cyclase) interacts with dissociated G protein subunits to generate small-molecule second messengers. AVP activates adenylyl cyclase, increasing the intracellular concentration of cAMP. The topology of adenylyl cyclase is characterized by 2 tandem repeats of six hydrophobic transmembrane domains separated by a large cytoplasmic loop and terminates in a large intracellular tail. Generation of cAMP follows receptor-linked activation of the heteromeric G protein (G$_s$) and interaction of the free G$_{as}$-chain with the adenylyl cyclase catalyst. Protein kinase (PKA) is the target of the generated cAMP. Cytoplasmic vesicles carrying the water channel proteins (represented as homotetrameric complexes) are fused to the luminal membrane in response to AVP, thereby increasing the water permeability of this membrane. Microtubules and actin filaments are necessary for vesicle movement toward the membrane. The mechanisms underlying docking and fusion of AQP2-bearing vesicles are not known. The detection of the small GTP-binding protein Rab3a, synaptobrevin 2, and syntaxin 4 in principal cells suggests that these proteins are involved in AQP2 trafficking (Valenti et al., 1998). When AVP is not available, water channels are retrieved by an endocytic process, and water permeability returns to its original low rate. AQP3 and AQP4 water channels are expressed on the basolateral membrane.

and three introns. It is predicted to code for a polypeptide of 271 amino acids that is organized into two repeats oriented at 180° to each other and has six membrane-spanning domains, both terminal ends located intracellularly, and conserved Asn-Pro-Ala boxes (Fig. 9). AQP2 is detectable in urine, and changes in urinary excretion of this protein can be used as an index of the action of vasopressin on the kidney.

AVP also increases the water reabsorptive capacity of the kidney by regulating the urea transporter UT1 that is present in the inner medullary collecting duct, predominantly in its terminal part. AVP also increases the permeability of principal collecting duct cells to sodium.

In summary, in the absence of AVP stimulation, collecting duct epithelia exhibit very low permeabilities to sodium urea and water. These specialized permeability properties permit the excretion of large volumes of hypotonic urine formed during intervals of water diuresis.

By contrast, AVP stimulation of the principal cells of the collecting ducts leads to selective increases in the permeability of the apical membrane to water (P$_f$), urea (P$_{urea}$), and Na (P$_{Na}$).

These actions of vasopressin in the distal nephron are possibly modulated by prostaglandins E$_2$ (PGE$_2$s) and by the luminal calcium concentration. High levels of E-prostanoid (EP$_3$) receptors are expressed in the kidney. However, mice lacking EP$_3$ receptors for PGE$_2$ were found to have quasi-normal regulation of urine volume and osmolality in response to various physiologic stimuli. An apical calcium/polycation receptor protein expressed in the terminal portion of the inner medullary collecting duct of the rat has been shown to reduce AVP-elicited osmotic water permeability when luminal calcium concentration rises. This possible link between calcium and water metabolism may play a role in the pathogenesis of renal stone formation.

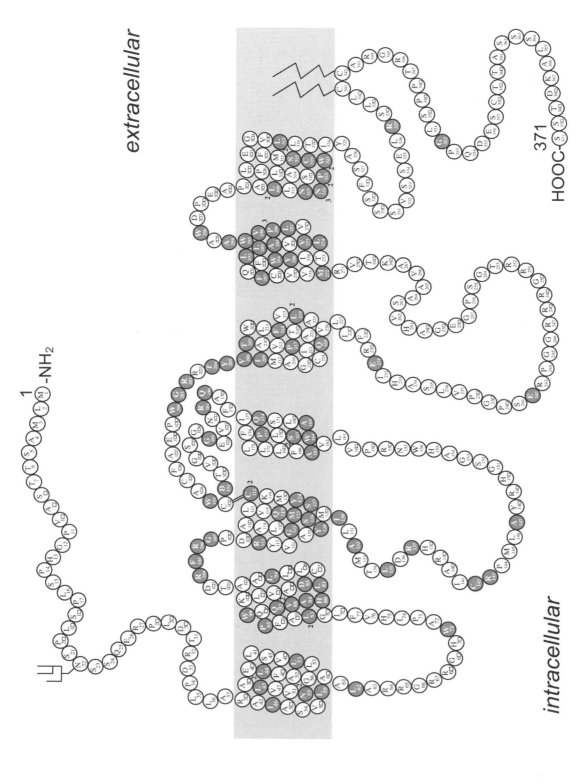

Fig. 8. Schematic representation of V$_2$ receptor and identification of 183 putative disease-causing *AVPR2* mutations. Predicted amino acids are given as the one-letter code. A solid symbol indicates the location (or the closest codon) of a mutation; a number indicates more than one mutation in the same codon. The names of the mutations were assigned according to recommended nomenclature (Antonarakis S. and the Nomenclature Working Group, 1998). The extracellular, transmembrane, and cytoplasmic domains are defined according to Mouillac et al. (1995).

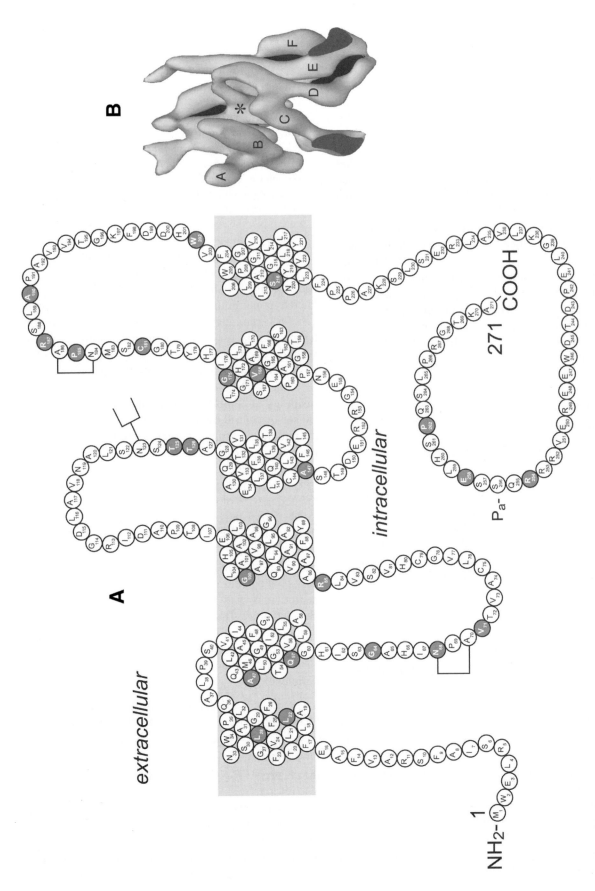

Fig. 9. (A) Schematic representation of AQP2 protein and identification of 24 missense or nonsense putative disease-causing *AQP2* mutations. Seven frameshift and one splice-site mutations are not represented. A monomer is represented with six transmembrane helices. The location of the PKA phosphorylation site (P_a) is indicated. The extracellular (E), transmembrane (TM), and cytoplasmic (C) domains are defined according to Deen et al. (1994). As in Fig. 8, solid symbols indicate the location of the mutations.

3. THE BRATTLEBORO RAT WITH AUTOSOMAL RECESSIVE NEUROGENIC DIABETES INSIPIDUS

The classic animal model for studying diabetes insipidus has been the Brattleboro rat with autosomal recessive neurogenic diabetes insipidus. *di/di* rats are homozygous for a 1-bp deletion (G) in the second exon that results in a frameshift mutation in the coding sequence of the carrier neurophysin II (NPII). Polyuric symptoms are also observed in heterozygous *di/n* rats. Homozygous Brattleboro rats may still demonstrate some V_2 antidiuretic effect since the administration of a selective nonpeptide V_2 antagonist (SR121463A, 10 mg/kg intraperitoneally) induced a further increase in urine flow rate (200 to 354 ± 42 mL/24 h) and a decline in urinary osmolality (170 to 92 ± 8 mmol/kg). OT, which is present at enhanced plasma concentrations in Brattleboro rats, may be responsible for the antidiuretic activity observed. OT is not stimulated by increased plasma osmolality in humans. The Brattleboro rat model is therefore not strictly comparable with the rarely observed human cases of autosomal recessive neurogenic diabetes insipidus.

4. QUANTITATING RENAL WATER EXCRETION

Diabetes insipidus is characterized by the excretion of abnormally large volumes of hypoosmotic urine (<250 mmol/kg). This definition excludes osmotic diuresis, which occurs when excess solute is being excreted, as with glucose in the polyuria of diabetes mellitus. Other agents that produce osmotic diuresis are mannitol, urea, glycerol, contrast media, and loop diuretics. Osmotic diuresis should be considered when solute excretion exceeds 60 mmol/h.

5. CLINICAL CHARACTERISTICS OF DIABETES INSIPIDUS DISORDERS

5.1. Central Diabetes Insipidus

5.1.1. COMMON FORMS

Failure to synthesize or secrete vasopressin normally limits maximal urinary concentration and, depending on the severity of the disease, causes varying degrees of polyuria and polydipsia. Experimental destruction of the vasopressin-synthesizing areas of the hypothalamus (supraoptic and paraventricular nuclei) causes a permanent form of the disease. Similar results are obtained by sectioning the hypophyseal hypothalamic tract above the median eminence. Sections below the median eminence, however, produce only transient diabetes insipidus. Lesions to the hypothalamic-pituitary tract are frequently associated with a three-stage response both in experimental animals and in humans:

1. An initial diuretic phase lasting from a few hours to 5 to 6 d.
2. A period of antidiuresis unresponsive to fluid administration. This antidiuresis is probably owing to vasopressin release from injured axons and may last from a few hours to several days. Since urinary dilution is impaired during this phase, continued administration of water can cause severe hyponatremia.
3. A final period of diabetes insipidus. The extent of the injury determines the completeness of the diabetes insipidus, and, as already discussed, the site of the lesion determines whether the disease will or will not be permanent.

Twenty-five percent of patients studied after transsphenoidal surgery developed spontaneous isolated hyponatremia, 20% developed diabetes insipidus, and 46% remained normonatremic. Normonatremia, hyponatremia, and diabetes insipidus were associated with increasing degrees of surgical manipulation of the posterior lobe and pituitary stalk during surgery.

Table 1 provides the etiologies of central diabetes insipidus in adults and in children are listed in. Rare causes of central diabetes insipidus include leukemia, thrombotic thrombocytopenic purpura, pituitary apoplexy, sarcoidosis, Wegener granulomatosis, progressive spastic cerebellar ataxia and neurosarcoidosis.

Deficits in anterior pituitary hormones were documented in 61% of patients a median of 0.6 yr (range: 01 to 18.0) after the onset of diabetes insipidus. The most frequent abnormality was growth hormone deficiency (59%), followed by hypothyroidism (28%), hypogonadism (24%) and adrenal insufficiency (22%). Seventy-five percent of the patients with Langerhans-cell histiocytosis had an anterior pituitary hormone deficiency that was first detected a median of 3.5 yr after the onset of diabetes insipidus. None of the patients with central diabetes insipidus secondary to *prepro-AVP-NPII* mutations developed anterior pituitary hormone deficiencies

5.1.2. RARE FORMS: AUTOSOMAL DOMINANT CENTRAL DIABETES INSIPIDUS AND THE DIDMOAD SYNDROME

Neurogenic diabetes insipidus (OMIM 125700) is a now well-characterized entity, secondary to mutations in the *prepro-AVP-NPII* (OMIM 192340). This disorder is also referred to as central, cranial, pituitary, or neurohypophyseal diabetes insipidus. Patients with autosomal dominant neurogenic diabetes insipidus retain some limited capacity to secrete AVP during severe dehydration, and the polyuropolydipsic symptoms usually appear after the first year of life, when an infant's demand for water is more likely to be understood by adults. Thirty-four *prepro-AVP-NPII* mutations segregating with

Table 1
Etiology of Hypothalamic Diabetes
Insipidus in Children and Adults [d]

	Children (%)	Children and young adults (%)	Adults (%)
Primary brain tumor [a]	49.5	22	30
• Before surgery	33.5	—	13
• After surgery	16	—	17
Idiopathic (isolated or familial)	29	58	25
Histiocytosis	16	12	—
Metastatic cancer [b]	—	—	8
Trauma [c]	2.2	2.0	17
Postinfectious disease	2.2	6.0	—

[a] Primary malignancy: craniopharyngioma, dysgerminoma, meningioma, adenoma, glioma, astrocytoma.

[b] Secondary: metastatic from lung or breast, lymphoma, leukemia, dysplastic pancytopenia.

[c] Trauma could be severe or mild.

[d] Data from Czernichow et al. (1985), Greger et al. (1986), Moses et al. (1985), and Maghnie et al. (2000).

autosomal dominant or autosomal recessive neurogenic diabetes insipidus have been described. The mechanism(s) by which a mutant allele causes neurogenic diabetes insipidus could involve the induction of magnocellular cell death as a result of the accumulation of AVP precursors within the endoplasmic reticulum (ER). This hypothesis could account for the delayed onset and autosomal mode of inheritance of the disease. In addition to the cytotoxicity caused by mutant AVP precursors, the interaction between the wild-type and the mutant precursors suggests that a dominant-negative mechanism may also contribute to the pathogenesis of autosomal dominant diabetes insipidus. The absence of symptoms in infancy in autosomal dominant central diabetes insipidus is in sharp contrast with nephrogenic diabetes insipidus (NDI) secondary to mutations in *AVPR2* or in *AQP2* (vide infra) in which the polyuropolydipsic symptoms are present during the first week of life. Of interest, errors in protein folding represent the underlying basis for a large number of inherited diseases and are also pathogenic mechanisms for *AVPR2* and *AQP2* mutants responsible for hereditary NDI (*vide infra*). Why are *prepro-AVP-NPII* misfolded mutants are cytotoxic to AVP-producing neurons is an unresolved issue. The NDI *AVPR2* missense mutations are likely to impair folding and to lead to the rapid degradation of the affected polypeptide and not to the accumulation of toxic aggregates since the other important functions of the principal cells of the collecting ducts (where *AVPR2* is expressed) are entirely normal. Three families with autosomal recessive neurogenic diabetes insipidus have been identified in which the patients were homozygous or compound heterozygotes for *prepro-AVP-NPII* mutations. As a consequence, early hereditary diabetes insipidus can be neurogenic or nephrogenic.

The acronym DIDMOAD describes the following clinical features of a syndrome: *d*iabetes *i*nsipidus, *d*iabetes *m*ellitus, *o*ptic *a*trophy, sensorineural *d*eafness. An unusual incidence of psychiatric symptoms has also been described in subjects with this syndrome. These included paranoid delusions, auditory or visual hallucinations, psychotic behavior, violent behavior, organic brain syndrome typically in the late or preterminal stages of their illness, progressive dementia, and severe learning disabilities or mental retardation or both. The syndrome is an autosomal recessive trait, the diabetes insipidus is usually partial and of gradual onset, and the polyuria can be wrongly attributed to poor glycemic control. Furthermore, a severe hyperosmolar state can occur if untreated diabetes mellitus is associated with an unrecognized pituitary deficiency. The dilatation of the urinary tract observed in the DIDMOAD syndrome may be secondary to chronic high urine flow rates and, perhaps, to some degenerative aspects of the innervation of the urinary tract. Wolfram syndrome (OMIM 222300) is secondary to mutations in the *WFS1* gene (chromosome region 4p16), which codes for a transmembrane protein expressed in various tissues including brain and pancreas.

5.1.3. THE SYNDROME OF HYPERNATREMIA AND HYPODIPSIA

Some patients with the hypernatremia and hypodipsia syndrome may have partial central diabetes insipidus. These patients also have persistent hypernatremia, which is not owing to any apparent extracellular volume loss; absence or attenuation of thirst; and a normal renal response to AVP. In almost all the patients studied to date, hypodipsia has been associated with cerebral lesions in the vicinity of the hypothalamus. It has been proposed that in these patients there is a "resetting" of the osmoreceptor, because their urine tends to become concentrated or diluted at inappropriately high levels of plasma osmolality. However, by using the regression analysis of plasma AVP concentration vs plasma osmolality, it has been possible to show that in some of these patients the tendency to concentrate and dilute urine at inappropriately high levels of plasma osmolality is owing solely to a marked reduction in sensitivity or a gain in the osmoregulatory mechanism. This finding is compatible with the diagnosis of partial central diabetes insipidus. In other patients, however, plasma AVP concentrations fluctuate randomly, bearing no apparent relationship to changes in plasma osmolality. Such patients frequently display large swings in serum sodium concentrations and frequently exhibit hypodipsia. It appears that most patients with essential hypernatremia fit one of these two patterns. Both of these groups of patients consistently respond normally to nonosmolar AVP release signals, such as hypotension, emesis, or hypoglycemia or all three. These observations suggest that the osmoreceptor may be anatomically as well as functionally separate from the nonosmotic efferent pathways and neurosecretory neurons for vasopressin.

5.2. Nephrogenic Diabetes Insipidus

5.2.1. X-Linked NDI and Mutations in AVPR2 Gene

X-linked NDI (OMIM 304800) is generally a rare disease in which the urine of affected male patients does not concentrate after the administration of AVP. Because it is a rare, recessive X-linked disease, females are unlikely to be affected, but heterozygous females exhibit variable degrees of polyuria and polydipsia because of skewed X chromosome inactivation. X-linked NDI is secondary to *AVPR2* mutations that result in the loss of function or a dysregulation of the V_2 receptor.

5.2.1.1. Rareness and Diversity of AVPR2 Mutations. We estimated the incidence of X-linked NDI in the general population from patients born in the province of Quebec during the 10-yr period, from 1988–1997, to be approx 8.8 per million (SD = 4.4 per million) male live births.

To date, 183 putative disease-causing AVPR2 mutations have been identified in 284 NDI families (Fig. 8) (additional information is available at the NDI Mutation Database at Website: http://www.medincine.mcgill.ca/nephros/). Of these, we identified 82 different muta-

tions in 117 NDI families referred to our laboratory. Half of the mutations are missense mutations. Frameshift mutations owing to nucleotide deletions or insertions (25%), nonsense mutations (10%), large deletions (10%), in-frame deletions or insertions (4%), splice-site mutations, and one complex mutation account for the remainder of the mutations. Mutations have been identified in every domain, but on a per-nucleotide basis, about twice as many mutations occur in transmembrane domains compared with the extracellular or intracellular domains. We previously identified private mutations, recurrent mutations, and mechanisms of mutagenesis. The 10 recurrent mutations (D85N, V88M, R113W, Y128S, R137H, S167L, R181C, R202C, A294P, and S315R) were found in 35 ancestrally independent families. The occurrence of the same mutation on different haplotypes was considered evidence for recurrent mutation. In addition, the most frequent mutations—D85N, V88M, R113W, R137H, S167L, R181C, and R202C— occurred at potential mutational hot spots (a C-to-T or G-to-A nucleotide substitution occurred at a CpG dinucleotide).

5.2.1.2. Benefits of Genetic Testing. The natural history of untreated X-linked NDI includes hypernatremia, hyperthermia, mental retardation, and repeated episodes of dehydration in early infancy. Mental retardation, a consequence of repeated episodes of dehydration, was prevalent in the Crawford and Bode study, in which only 9 of 82 patients (11%) had normal intelligence; however, data from the Nijmegen group suggest that this complication was overestimated in their group of NDI patients. Early recognition and treatment of X-linked NDI with an abundant intake of water allows a normal life-span with normal physical and mental development. Familial occurrence of males and mental retardation in untreated patients are two characteristics suggestive of X-linked NDI. Skewed X-inactivation is the most likely explanation for clinical symptoms of NDI in female carriers.

Identification of the molecular defect underlying X-linked NDI is of immediate clinical significance because early diagnosis and treatment of affected infants can avert the physical and mental retardation resulting from repeated episodes of dehydration. Affected males are immediately treated with abundant water intake, a low-sodium diet, and hydrochlorothiazide. They do not experience severe episodes of dehydration and their physical and mental development remains normal, however, their urinary output is only decreased by 30% and a normal growth curve is still difficult to reach during the first 2 to 3 yr of their life despite the aforementioned treatments and intensive attention. Water should be offered every 2 h day and night, and temperature, appetite, and growth should be monitored.

Admission to hospital may be necessary for continuous gastric feeding. The voluminous amounts of water kept in patients' stomachs will exacerbate physiologic gastrointestinal reflux as an infant and a toddler, and many affected boys frequently vomit and have a strong positive "Tuttle test" (esophageal pH testing). These young patients often improve with the absorption of an H-2 blocker and with metoclopramide (which could induce extrapyramidal symptoms) or with domperidone, which seems to be better tolerated and efficacious.

5.2.1.3. Most Mutant V2 Receptors Are Not Transported to the Cell Membrane and Are Retained in the Intracellular Compartments.

Classification of the defects of mutant V_2 receptors is based on that of the low-density lipoprotein receptor, for which mutations have been grouped according to the function and subcellular localization of the mutant protein whose cDNA has been transiently transfected in a heterologous expression system. Following this classification, type 1 mutant receptors reach the cell surface but display impaired ligand binding and are, consequently, unable to induce normal cAMP production. Type 2 mutant receptors have defective intracellular transport. Type 3 mutant receptors are ineffectively transcribed. This subgroup seems to be rare because Northern blot analysis of transfected cells reveals that most V_2 receptor mutations produce the same quantity and molecular size of receptor mRNA.

Of the 12 mutants that we tested, only three were detected on the cell surface. Similar results were obtained by other groups.

Other genetic disorders are also characterized by protein misfolding. AQP-2 mutations responsible for autosomal recessive NDI are also characterized by misrouting of the misfolded mutant proteins and trapping in the ER. The ΔF508 mutation in cystic fibrosis is also characterized by misfolding and retention in the ER of the mutated cystic fibrosis transmembrane conductance regulator that is associated with calnexin and Hsp70. The C282Y mutant HFE protein, which is responsible for 83% of hemochromatosis in the Caucasian population, is retained in the ER and middle Golgi compartment, fails to undergo late Golgi processing, and is subject to accelerated degradation. Mutants encoding other renal membrane proteins that are responsible for Gitelman syndrome and cystinuria are also retained in the ER.

5.2.1.4. Nonpeptide Vasopressin Antagonists Act as Pharmacological Chaperones to Functionally Rescue Misfolded Mutant V2 Receptors Responsible for X-Linked NDI .

We recently proposed a model in which small nonpeptide V_2 receptor antagonists permeate into the cell and bind to incompletely folded mutant receptors. This would then stabilize a conformation of the receptor that allows its release from the ER quality control apparatus. The stabilized receptor would then be targeted to the cell surface, where on dissociation from the antagonist it could bind vasopressin and promote signal transduction. Given that these antagonists are specific to the V_2 receptor and that they perform a chaperone-like function, we termed these compounds pharmacologic chaperones.

5.2.2. Autosomal Recessive and Dominant NDI Owing to Mutations in AQP2 Gene

To date, 26 putative disease-causing AQP2 mutations have been identified in 25 NDI families (Fig. 9). By type of mutation, there are 65% missense, 23% frameshift due to small nucleotide deletions or insertions, 8% nonsense, and 4% splice-site mutations (additional information is available at the NDI Mutation Database at Website: http://www.medicine.mcgill.ca/nephros/).

Reminiscent of expression studies done with AVPR2 proteins, misrouting of AQP2 mutant proteins has been shown to be the major cause underlying autosomal recessive NDI.

In contrast to the AQP2 mutations in autosomal recessive NDI, which are located throughout the gene, the dominant mutations are predicted to affect the carboxyl terminus of AQP2. The dominant action of AQP2 mutations can be explained by the formation of heterotetramers of mutant and wild type AQP2 that are impaired in their routing after oligomerization.

5.2.3. Acquired Nephrogenic Diabetes Insipidus

The acquired form of NDI is much more common than the congenital form of the disease, but it is rarely severe. The ability to elaborate a hypertonic urine is usually preserved despite the impairment of the maximal concentrating ability of the nephrons. Polyuria and polydipsia are therefore moderate (3–4 L/d). Table 2 provides the more common causes of acquired NDI.

Administration of lithium has become the most common cause of NDI. Nineteen percent of these patients had polyuria, as defined by a 24-h urine output exceeding 3 L. Renal biopsy revealed a chronic tubulointerstitial nephropathy in all patients with biopsy-proven lithium toxicity. The mechanism whereby lithium causes polyuria has been extensively studied. Lithium has been shown to inhibit adenylate cyclase in a number of cell types, including renal epithelia. Lithium also caused a marked downregulation of AQP2 and AQP3, only partially reversed by cessation of therapy, dehydration, or dDAVP treatment, consistent with clinical observations of slow recovery from lithium-induced urinary concentrating defects. Downregula-

Table 2
Acquired Causes of NDI

Chronic renal disease	*Drugs*
• Polycystic disease	• Alcohol
• Medullary cystic disease	• Phenytoin
Pyelonephritis	• Lithium
• Ureteral obstruction	• Demeclocycline
• Far-advanced renal failure	• Acetohexamide
failure	• Tolazamide
Electrolyte disorders	• Glyburide
• Hypokalemia	• Propoxyphene
• Hypercalcemia	• Amphotericin
Blood disease	• Foscarnet
• Sickle cell disease	• Methoxyflurane
Dietary abnormalities	• Norepinephrine
• Excessive water intake	• Vinblastine
• Decreased sodium	• Colchicine
chloride intake	• Gentamicin
• Decreased protein intake	• Methicillin
Miscellaneous	• Isophosphamide
• Multiple myeloma	• Angiographic dyes
• Amyloidosis	• Osmotic diuretics
• Sjögren's disease	• Furosemide and
• Sarcoidosis	ethacrynic acid

tion of AQP2 has also been shown to be associated with the development of severe polyuria due to other causes of acquired NDI: hypokalemia, release of bilateral ureteral obstruction, and hypercalciuria. Thus, AQP2 expression is severely downregulated in both congenital and acquired NDI.

5.3. Primary Polydipsia

Primary polydipsia is a state of hypotonic polyuria secondary to excessive fluid intake. Primary polydipsia was extensively studied by Barlow and de Wardener in 1959; however, the understanding of the pathophysiology of this disease has made little progress over the past 30 yr. Barlow and de Wardener described seven women and two men who were compulsive water drinkers; their ages ranged from 48 to 59 yr except for one patient, 24. Eight of these patients had histories of previous psychologic disorders, which ranged from delusions, depression, and agitation to frank hysterical behavior. The other patient appeared psychologically normal. The consumption of water fluctuated irregularly from hour to hour or from day to day; in some patients, there were remissions and relapses lasting several months or longer. In eight of the patients, the mean plasma osmolality was significantly lower than normal. Vasopressin tannate in oil made most of these patients feel ill; in one, it caused overhydration. In four patients, the fluid intake returned to normal after electroconvulsive therapy or a period of continuous narcosis; the improvement in three was tran-

sient, but in the fourth it lasted 2 yr. Polyuric female subjects might be heterozygous for *de novo* or previously unrecognized *AVPR2* mutations or autosomal dominant *AQP2* mutations and may be classified as compulsive water drinkers. Therefore, the diagnosis of compulsive water drinking must be made with care and may represent ignorance of yet undescribed pathophysiologic mechanisms. Robertson has described, under the term *dipsogenic diabetes insipidus*, a selective defect in the osmoregulation of thirst. Three studied patients had under basal conditions of ad libitum water intake, thirst, polydipsia, polyuria, and high-normal plasma osmolality. They had a normal secretion of AVP, but osmotic threshold for thirst was abnormally low. These cases of dipsogenic diabetes insipidus might represent up to 10% of all patients with diabetes insipidus.

5.4. Diabetes Insipidus and Pregnancy

5.4.1. PREGNANCY IN A PATIENT KNOWN TO HAVE DIABETES INSIPIDUS

An isolated deficiency of vasopressin without a concomitant loss of hormones in the anterior pituitary does not result in altered fertility, and with the exception of polyuria and polydipsia, gestation, delivery, and lactation are uncomplicated. Treated patients may require increasing dosages of desmopressin. The increased thirst may be owing to a resetting of the thirst osmostat.

Increased polyuria also occurs during pregnancy in patients with partial NDI. These patients may be obligatory carriers of the NDI gene.

5.4.2. SYNDROMES OF DIABETES INSIPIDUS THAT BEGIN DURING GESTATION AND REMIT AFTER DELIVERY

Barron et al. in 1984 described three pregnant women in whom transient diabetes insipidus developed late in gestation and subsequently remitted postpartum. In one of these patients, dilute urine was present in spite of high plasma concentrations of AVP. Hyposthenuria in all three patients was resistant to administered aqueous vasopressin. Since excessive vasopressinase activity was not excluded as a cause of this disorder, Barron et al. labeled the disease-vasopressin diabetes insipidus resistant rather than NDI. It is suggested that pregnancy may be associated with several different forms of diabetes insipidus, including central, nephrogenic, and vasopressinase mediated.

6. DIFFERENTIAL DIAGNOSIS OF POLYURIC STATES

Plasma sodium and osmolality are maintained within normal limits (136–143 mmol/L for plasma sodium, 275–290 mmol/kg for plasma osmolality) by a thirst-ADH-renal axis. Thirst and ADH, both stimulated by increased osmolality, have been termed a double-negative feedback system. Thus, even when the ADH limb of this double-negative regulatory feedback system is lost, the thirst mechanism still preserves the plasma sodium and osmolality within the normal range but at the expense of pronounced polydipsia and polyuria. Thus, the plasma sodium concentration or osmolality of an untreated patient with diabetes insipidus may be slightly higher than the mean normal value, but since the values usually remain within the normal range, these small increases have no diagnostic significance.

Theoretically, it should be relatively easy to differentiate among central diabetes insipidus, NDI, and primary polydipsia. A comparison of the osmolality of urine obtained during dehydration from patients with central diabetes insipidus or NDI with that of urine obtained after the administration of AVP should reveal a rapid increase in osmolality only in the central diabetes insipidus patients. Urine osmolality should increase normally in response to moderate dehydration in primary polydipsia patients.

However, these distinctions may not be as clear as one might expect because of several factors. First, chronic polyuria of any etiology interferes with the maintenance of the medullary concentration gradient, and this "washout" effect diminishes the maximum concentrating ability of the kidney. The extent of the blunting varies in direct proportion to the severity of the polyuria and is independent of its cause. Hence, for any given level of basal urine output, the maximum urine osmolality achieved in the presence of saturating concentrations of AVP is depressed to the same extent in patients with primary polydipsia, central diabetes insipidus, and NDI (Fig. 10). Second, most patients with central diabetes insipidus maintain a small, but detectable capacity to secrete AVP during severe dehydration, and urine osmolality may then rise above plasma osmolality. Third, many patients with acquired NDI have an incomplete deficit in AVP action, and concentrated urine could again be obtained during dehydration testing. Finally, all polyuric states (whether central, nephrogenic, or psychogenic) can induce large dilatations of the urinary tract and bladder. As a consequence, the urinary bladder of these patients may contain an increased residual capacity, and changes in urine osmolalities induced by diagnostic maneuvers might be difficult to demonstrate.

6.1. Indirect Test

The measurement of urine osmolality after dehydration or administration of vasopressin is usually referred to as "indirect testing" because vasopressin secretion is indirectly assessed through changes in urine osmolalities. The patient is maintained on a complete fluid restriction regimen until urine osmolality reaches a plateau, as indicated by an hourly increase of <30 mmol/kg for at least three successive hours. After the plasma osmolality is measured, 5 U of aqueous vasopressin is administered subcutaneously. Urine osmolality is measured 30 and 60 min later. The last urine osmolality value obtained before the vasopressin injection and the highest value obtained after the injection are compared. The patients are then separated into five categories according to previously published criteria (Table 3).

6.2. Direct Test

For the direct test, the two approaches of Zerbe and Robertson (1984) are used. First, during the dehydration test, plasma is collected and assayed for vasopressin. The results are plotted on a nomogram depicting the normal relationship between plasma sodium or osmolality and plasma AVP in healthy subjects (Fig. 6). If the relationship between plasma vasopressin and osmolality falls below the normal range, the disorder is diagnosed as central diabetes insipidus.

Second, partial NDI and primary polydipsia can be differentiated by analyzing the relationship between plasma AVP and urine osmolality at the end of the dehydration period (Figs. 6 and 10). However, a definitive differentiation between these two disorders might be impossible because a normal or even supranormal AVP response to increased plasma osmolality occurs in patients with polydipsia. None of the patients with psychogenic or other forms of severe polydipsia studied by Robertson have ever shown any evidence of pituitary suppression.

Table 4 describes a *combined* direct and indirect testing of the AVP function.

6.3. Therapeutic Trial

In selected patients with an uncertain diagnosis, a closely monitored therapeutic trial of desmopressin (10 µg intranasally twice a day) may be used to distinguish partial NDI from partial neurogenic diabetes insipidus and primary polydipsia. If desmopressin at this dosage causes a significant antidiuretic effect, NDI is effectively excluded. If polydipsia as well as polyuria is abolished and plasma sodium does not fall below the normal range, the patient probably has central diabetes insipidus. Conversely, if desmopressin causes a reduction in urine output without a reduction in water intake and hyponatremia appears, the patient probably has primary polydipsia. Because fatal water intoxication is a remote possibility, the desmopressin trial should be carried out with closed monitoring.

Table 3
Urinary Responses to Fluid Deprivation and Exogenous Vasopressin
in Recognition of Partial Defects in Antidiuretic Hormone Secretion [a]

	No. of cases	Maximum U_{osm} with dehydration (mmol/kg)	U_{osm} after vasopressin (mmol/kg)	% Change (U_{osm})	Increase in U_{osm} after vasopressin (%)
Healthy subjects	9	1068 ± 69	979 ± 79	-9 ± 3	<9
Complete central diabetes insipidus	18	168 ± 13	445 ± 52	183 ± 41	>50
Partial central diabetes insipidus	11	438 ± 34	549 ± 28	28 ± 5	>9 <50
NDI	2	123.5	174.5	42	<50
Compulsive water drinking	7	738 ± 53	780 ± 73	5.0 ± 2.2	<9

[a] Data from Miller et al. (1970).

Table 4
Direct and Indirect Tests of AVP Function in Patients With Polyuria [a]

Measurements of AVP cannot be used in isolation but must be interpreted in light of four other factors:

- Clinical history
- Concurrent measurements of plasma osmolality
- Urine osmolality
- Maximal urinary response to exogenous vasopressin in reference to the basal urine flow

[a] Data from Stern and Valtin (1981).

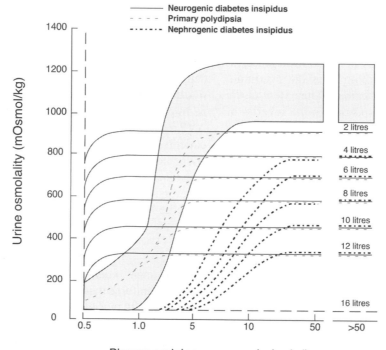

Fig. 10. Relationship between urine osmolality and plasma vasopressin in patients with polyuria of diverse etiology and severity. Note that for each of the three categories of polyuria (neurogenic diabetes insipidus, NDI, and primary polydipsia), the relationship is described by a family of sigmoid curves that differ in height. These differences in height reflect differences in maximum concentrating capacity owing to "washout" of the medullary concentration gradient. They are proportional to the severity of the underlying polyuria (indicated in liters per day at the right end of each plateau) and are largely independent of the etiology. Thus, the three categories of diabetes insipidus differ principally in the submaximal or ascending portion of the dose-response curve. In patients with partial neurogenic diabetes insipidus, this part of the curve lies to the left of normal, reflecting increased sensitivity to the antidiuretic effects of very low concentrations of plasma AVP. By contrast, in patients with partial NDI, this part of the curve lies to the right of normal, reflecting decreased sensitivity to the antidiuretic effects of normal concentrations of plasma AVP. In primary polydipsia, this relationship is relatively normal. (Reproduced with permission from Robertson, 1985.)

Table 5
Differential Diagnosis of Diabetes Insipidus [a]

1. Measure plasma osmolality and/or sodium concentration under conditions of ad libitum fluid intake. If they are >295 mmol/kg and 143 mmol/L, respectively, the diagnosis of primary polydipsia is excluded, and the workup should proceed directly to step 5 and/or 6 to distinguish between neurogenic and NDI. Otherwise,
2. Perform a dehydration test. If urinary concentration does not occur before plasma osmolality and/or sodium reaches 295 mmol/kg and 143 mmol/L, respectively, the diagnosis of primary polydipsia is again excluded, and the workup should proceed to step 5 and/or 6. Otherwise,
3. Determine the ratio of urine to plasma osmolality at the end of the dehydration test. If it is <1.5, the diagnosis of primary polydipsia is again excluded, and the workup should proceed to step 5 and/or 6. Otherwise,
4. Perform a hypertonic saline infusion with measurements of plasma vasopressin and osmolality at intervals during the procedure. If the relationship between these two variables is subnormal, the diagnosis of diabetes insipidus is established. Otherwise,
5. Perform a vasopressin infusion test. If urine osmolality rises by more than 150 mosM/kg above the value obtained at the end of the dehydration test, NDI is excluded. Alternately,
6. Measure urine osmolality and plasma vasopressin at the end of the dehydration test. If the relationship is normal, the diagnosis of NDI is excluded.

[a] Data from Robertson (1981).

6.4. Recommendations

Table 5 provides recommendations for obtaining a differential diagnosis of diabetes insipidus.

6.5. Carrier Detection and Postnatal Diagnosis

As developed earlier in this chapter, the identification, characterization, and mutational analysis of three different genes—*prepro-AVP-NPII*, *AVPR2*, and the vasopressin-sensitive water channel gene (*AQP2*)—provide the basis for the understanding of different hereditary forms of diabetes insipidus: autosomal dominant and recessive neurogenic diabetes insipidus, X-linked NDI, and autosomal recessive or autosomal dominant NDI, respectively. The identification of mutations in these three genes that cause diabetes insipidus enables the early diagnosis and management of at-risk members of families with identified mutations. Some patients with Bartter syndrome may present with severe hypernatremia, hyperchloremia, and a low urine osmolality unresponsive to dDAVP. In these cases, the antenatal period is characterized by polyhydramnios. In my experience, perinatal polyuropolydipsic patients with a mother's pregnancy characterized by polyhydramnios are not bearing *AVPR2* or *AQP2* mutations. We encourage physicians who follow families with X-linked NDI to recommend mutation analysis before the birth of a male infant because early diagnosis and treatment of male infants can avert the physical and mental retardation associated with episodes of dehydration. Early diagnosis of autosomal recessive NDI is also essential for early treatment of affected infants to avoid repeated episodes of dehydration. Detection of mutation in families with inherited neurogenic diabetes insipidus provides a powerful clinical tool for early diagnosis and management of subsequent cases, especially in early childhood when diagnosis is difficult and the clinical risks are the greatest.

7. MAGNETIC RESONANCE IMAGING IN PATIENTS WITH DIABETES INSIPIDUS

Magnetic resonance imaging (MRI) permits visualization of the anterior and posterior pituitary glands and the pituitary stalk. The pituitary stalk is permeated by numerous capillary loops of the hypophyseal-portal blood system. This vascular structure also provides the principal blood supply to the anterior pituitary lobe, for there is no direct arterial supply to this organ. By contrast, the posterior pituitary lobe has a direct vascular supply. Therefore, the posterior lobe can be more rapidly visualized in a dynamic mode after administration of a gadolinium (gadopentetate dimeglumine) as contrast material during MRI. The posterior pituitary lobe is easily distinguished by a round, high-intensity signal (the posterior pituitary "bright spot") in the posterior part of the sella turcica on T1-weighted images. This round, high-intensity signal is usually absent in patients with central diabetes insipidus. MRI is reported to be "the best technique" with which to evaluate the pituitary stalk and infundibulum in patients with idiopathic polyuria. Thus, the absence of posterior pituitary hyperintensity, although nonspecific, is a cardinal feature of central diabetes insipidus. In the five patients who did have posterior pituitary hyperintensity at diagnosis, this feature invariably disappeared during follow-up. Thickening of either the entire pituitary stalk or just the proximal portion was the second most common abnormality on MRI scans.

8. TREATMENT OF POLYURIC DISORDERS

In most patients with diabetes insipidus, the thirst mechanism remains intact. Thus, these patients do not develop hypernatremia and suffer only from the inconvenience associated with marked polyuria and polydipsia. If hypodipsia develops or access to water is limited, severe hypernatremia can supervene. The treatment of choice for patients with severe hypothalamic diabetes insipidus is desmopressin, a synthetic, long-acting vasopressin analog, with minimal vasopressor activity but a large antidiuretic potency. The usual intranasal daily dose is between 5 and 20 µg. To avoid the potential complication of dilutional hyponatremia, which is exceptional in these patients due to an intact thirst mechanism, desmopressin can be withdrawn at regular intervals to allow the patients to become polyuric. Aqueous vasopressin (Pitressin) or desmopressin (4.0 µg/1-mL ampoule) can be used intravenously in acute situations such as after hypophysectomy or for the treatment of diabetes insipidus in the brain-dead organ donor. Pitressin tannate in oil and nonhormonal antidiuretic drugs are somewhat obsolete and now rarely used. For example, chlorpropamide (250–500 mg daily) appears to potentiate the antidiuretic action of circulating AVP, but troublesome side effects of hypoglycemia and hyponatremia do occur.

A low-osmolar and low-sodium diet, hydrochlorothiazide (1 to 2 mg/[kg·d]) alone or with amiloride (20 mg/ [1.73m^2·d]), and indomethacin (0.75–1.5 mg/kg) substantially reduce water excretion and are helpful in the treatment of children. Initial nausea may occur in some patients who start on amiloride but is generally transient and rarely a reason to discontinue therapy. Many adult patients receive no treatment at all.

Patients with acquired NDI secondary to long-term lithium usually benefit from a low sodium intake and, under strict surveillance, of the chronic administration of hydrochlorothiazide or amiloride. A low sodium intake and a distal diuretic will induce a contraction of the extracellular fluid volume, an increase in proximal fluid—and lithium—reabsorption, and a decrease in the volume of water presented to the distal tubule. Plasma lithium should be measured frequently at the initiation of such a treatment. In the postoperative care of polyuric-lithium patients, indomethacin (25 mg three times daily) will decrease glomerular filtration rate and decrease water excretion. The dosage of lithium should be decreased and plasma lithium levels should also be frequently measured if indomethacin is used and only short treatment(s) (4–7 d) is (are) indicated.

Hypernatremic dehydration seen in breast-fed infants could be easily prevented by the simple habit of offering newborns water once a day. In most cases, the newborn refuses the offer, and the mother is advised not to be concerned because it means that the child is getting sufficient water in breast milk. This clinical presentation is easily differentiated from the intense thirst and continuous voiding of newborns with congenital NDI.

9. SYNDROME OF INAPPROPRIATE SECRETION OF THE ANTIDIURETIC HORMONE

Hyponatremia (defined as a plasma sodium <130 meq/L) is the most common disorder of body fluid and electrolyte balance encountered in the clinical practice of medicine, with incidences ranging from 1 to 2% in both acutely and chronically hospitalized patients. Because a defect in renal water excretion, as reflected by hypoosmolality, may occur in the presence of an excess or deficit of total body sodium or nearly normal total body sodium, it is useful to classify the hyponatremic states accordingly (Fig. 11). Moreover, because total-body sodium is the primary determinant of extracellular fluid (ECF) volume, evaluation of the ECF volume allows for a convenient means of classifying patients with hyponatremia.

Since 1957, when Schwartz and coworkers first described syndrome of inappropriate secretion of the antidiuretic hormone (SIADH) in two patients with bronchogenic carcinoma who were hyponatremic, clinically euvolemic with normal renal and adrenal function, and had less than maximally dilute urine with appreciable urinary sodium concentrations (>20 meq/ L), SIADH has been recognized in a variety of pathologic processes. Table 6 provides various diseases that may be accompanied by SIADH. These diseases generally fall into three categories: malignancies, pulmonary disorders, and central nervous system (CNS) disorders.

In spite of the hyponatremia, patients with SIADH have a concentrated urine in which the urinary sodium concentration closely parallels the sodium intake; that is it is usually >20 meq/L. However, in the presence of sodium restriction or volume depletion, these patients can conserve sodium normally and decrease their urinary sodium concentration to <10 meq/L. Serum uric acid has been found to be reduced in patients with SIADH, whereas patients with other causes of hyponatremia have normal concentrations of serum uric acid. Uric acid and phosphate clearances were found to be increased in patients with SIADH as the consequence of volume expansion and decreased tubular reabsorp-

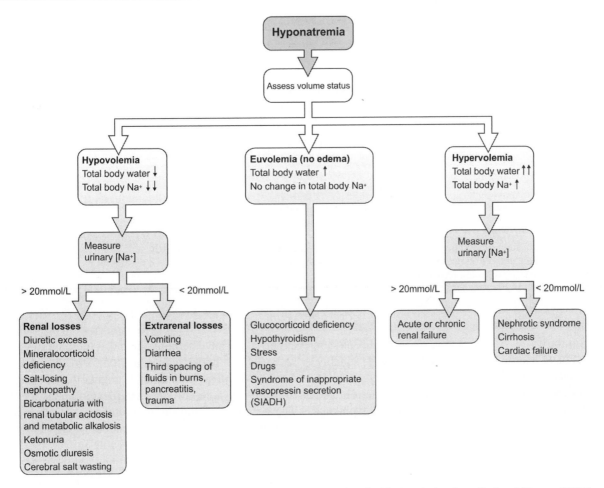

Fig. 11. Approach for diagnosing the patient with hyponatremia. (Reproduced with permission from Berl and Kumar, 2000.)

Table 6
Disorders Associated With SIADH

Carcinomas	*CNS disorders*
• Bronchogenic carcinoma	• Encephalitis (viral or bacterial)
• Carcinoma of duodenum	• Meningitis
• Carcinoma of pancreas	(viral, bacterial, tuberculous, and fungal)
• Thymoma	• Head trauma
• Carcinoma of stomach	• Brain abscess
• Lymphoma	• Brain tumors
• Ewing sarcoma	• Guillain-Barré syndrome
• Carcinoma of bladder	• Acute intermittent porphyria
• Prostatic carcinomaa	• Subarachnoid hemorrhage
• Oropharyngeal tumor	or subdural hematoma
• Carcinoma of ureter	• Cerebellar and cerebral atrophy
Pulmonary disorders	• Cavernous sinus thrombosis
• Viral pneumonia	• Neonatal hypoxia
• Bacterial pneumonia	• Hydrocephalus
• Pulmonary abscess	• Shy-Drager syndrome
• Tuberculosis	• Rocky Mountain spotted fever
• Aspergillosis	• Delirium tremens
• Positive pressure breathing	• Cerebrovascular accident
• Asthma	(cerebral thrombosis or hemorrhage)
• Pneumothorax	• Acute psychosis
• Mesothelioma	• Peripheral neuropathy
• Cystic fibrosis	• Multiple sclerosis

Table 7
Prudent Approach to Treatment of Hyponatremia

Guiding principles in the treatment of hyponatremia

- Neurologic disease can follow both the failure to treat promptly and the injudicious rapid treatment of hyponatremia.
- The presence or absence of significant neurologic signs and symptoms must guide the treatment.
- The acuteness or chronicity of the electrolyte disturbance influences the rate at which the correction should be undertaken.

Acute symptomatic hyponatremia

- The risk of the complications of cerebral edema is greater than the risk of the complications of the treatment.
- Treat with furosemide and hypertonic NaCl until convulsions subside.

Asymptomatic hyponatremia

- It is almost always chronic.
- Treat with water restriction regardless of how low the serum sodium concentration is.

Symptomatic hyponatremia (chronic or unknown duration)

- Increase serum sodium promptly by 10%, i.e., approx 10 meq/L, and then restrict water intake.
- Do not exceed a correction rate of 2 meq/[L·h] at any given time.
- Do not increase serum sodium by more than 20 meq/L.

---

tion. Similarly, low-serum blood urea nitrogen concentrations have been found in SIADH. This is probably owing to an increase in total body water, where urea is normally distributed, but a decrease in protein intake could also contribute. The concentration of plasma atrial natriuretic factor has been found to be increased in patients with SIADH and to correlate with urinary sodium excretion.

10. SIGNS, SYMPTOMS, AND TREATMENT OF HYPONATREMIA

The majority of the manifestations of hyponatremia are of a neuropsychiatric nature, and include lethargy, psychosis, seizures, and coma. The elderly and young children with hyponatremia are most likely to become symptomatic. The degree of the clinical impairment is not strictly related to the absolute value of the lowered serum sodium concentration, but, rather, it relates to both the rate and the extent of the fall of ECF osmolality. Arrieff quotes a mortality rate of approx 50%. On the other hand, none of the 10 acutely hyponatremic patients reported by Sterns had permanent neurologic sequelae. Most patients who have seizures and coma have plasma sodium concentrations <120 meq/L. The signs and symptoms are most likely related to the cellular swelling and cerebral edema associated with hyponatremia.

The treatment of symptomatic hyponatremic patients has been the subject of a large-scale debate in the literature. This debate has been prompted by the description of both pontine (central pontine myelinolysis [CPM]) and extrapontine demyelinating lesions in patients whose hyponatremia has been treated. Numerous experiments have demonstrated that hyponatremia *per se* is not the underlying cause of CPM, but that the corrections of hyponatremia of greater than 24-h duration may play a central role in the development of CPM. The critical rate and the magnitude of the correction have been addressed, and a "prudent" approach to the treatment has been published (Table 7).

ACKNOWLEDGMENTS

Danielle Binette provided secretarial and computer graphics expertise. The author's work cited in this chapter is supported by the Canadian Institutes of Health Research, the Canadian Kidney Foundation; and by the Fonds de la Recherche en Santé du Québec.

REFERENCES

Antonarakis S, and the Nomenclature Working Group. Recommendations for a nomenclature system for human gene mutations. Nomenclature Working Group. *Hum Mutat* 1998;11:1–3.

Berl T, Kumar S. Disorders of water metabolism. In: Johnson RJ, Feehally J, eds. *Comprehensive Clinical Nephrology*. London, UK: Mosby, 2000:9.1–9.20.

Bichet DG, Kortas C, Mettauer B, Manzini C, Marc-Aurele J, Rouleau JL, Schrier RW. Modulation of plasma and platelet vasopressin by cardiac function in patients with heart failure. *Kidney Int* 1986;29:1188–1196.

Burbach JP, Luckman SM, Murphy D, Gainer H. Gene regulation in the magnocellular hypothalamo-neurohypophysial system. *Physiol Rev* 2001;81:1197–1267.

Czernichow P, Pomarede R, Brauner R, Rappaport R. Neurogenic diabetes insipidus in children. In: Czernichow P, Robinson AG, eds. *Frontiers of Hormone Research, Vol. 13, Diabetes Insipidus in Man*. Basel, Switzerland: S. Karger, 1985;190–209.

Deen PMT, Verdijk MAJ, Knoers NVAM, Wieringa B, Monnens LAH, van Os CH, van Oost BA. Requirement of human renal water channel aquaporin-2 for vasopressin-dependent concentration of urine. *Science* 1994;264:92–95.

Greger NG, Kirkland RT, Clayton GW, Kirkland JL. Central diabetes insipidus. 22 years' experience. *Am J Dis Child* 1986;140: 551–554.

Maghnie M, Cosi G, Genovese E, Manca-Bitti ML, Cohen A, Zecca S, Tinelli C, Gallucci M, Bernasconi S, Boscherini B, Severi F, Arico M. Central diabetes insipidus in children and young adults. *N Engl J Med* 2000;343:998–1007.

Miller M, Dalakos T, Moses AM, Fellerman H, Streeten DH. Recognition of partial defects in antidiuretic hormone secretion. *Ann Intern Med* 1970;73:721–729.

Moses AM, Blumenthal SA, Streeten DHP. Acid-base and electrolyte disorders associated with endocrine disease: pituitary and thyroid. In: Arieff AI, de Fronzo RA, eds. *Fluid, Electrolyte and Acid-Base Disorders*. New York, NY: Churchill Livingstone, 1985;851–892.

Mouillac B, Chini B, Balestre MN, Elands J, Trumpp-Kallmeyer S, Hoflack J, Hibert M, Jard S, Barberis C. The binding site of neuropeptide vasopressin V1a receptor. Evidence for a major localization within transmembrane regions. *J Biol Chem* 1995; 270:25,771–25,777.

Robertson GL. Diagnosis of diabetes insipidus. In: Czernichow P, Robinson AG, eds. *Frontiers of Hormone Research, Diabetes Insipidus in Man*, vol. 13. Basel: Karger 1985:176–189.

Robertson GL. Diseases of the posterior pituitary. In: Felig D, Baxter JD, Broadus AE, Frohman LA, eds. *Endocrinology and Metabolism*. New York, NY: McGraw-Hill, 1981:251–277.

Stern P, Valtin H. Verney was right, but . . . [editorial]. *N Engl J Med* 1981;305:1581–1582.

Valenti G, Procino G, Liebenhoff U, Frigeri A, Benedetti PA, Ahnert-Hilger G, Nurnberg B, Svelto M, Rosenthal W. A heterotrimeric G protein of the Gi family is required for cAMP-triggered trafficking of aquaporin 2 in kidney epithelial cells. *J Biol Chem* 1998;273:22,627–22,634.

Vokes T, Robertson GL. Physiology of secretion of vasopressin. In: Czernichow P, Robinson AG, eds. *Diabetes Insipidus in Man*. Basel: S. Karger 1985:127–155.

Wilson Y, Nag N, Davern P, Oldfield BJ, McKinley MJ, Greferath U, Murphy M. Visualization of functionally activated circuitry in the brain. *Proc Natl Acad Sci USA* 2002;99:3252–3257.

Zerbe RL, Robertson GL. Disorders of ADH. *Med North Am* 1984;13:1570–1574.

SELECTED READINGS

Bichet DG. Polyuria and diabetes insipidus. In: Seldin DW, Giebisch G, eds. *The Kidney: Physiology and Pathophysiology*, 3rd. Ed. Philadelphia, PA: Lippincott Williams & Wilkins 2000:1261–1285.

Bichet DG, Fujiwara TM. Nephrogenic diabetes insipidus. In: Scriver CR, Beaudet AL, Sly WS, Vallee D, Childs B, Kinzler KW, Vogelstein B, eds. *The Metabolic and Molecular Bases of Inherited Disease*, 8th Ed., Vol. 3. New York, NY: McGraw-Hill, 2001: 4181–4204.

Clapham DE. Symmetry, selectivity, and the 2003 Nobel Prize. *Cell* 2003;115:641–646.

Nielsen S, Frokiaer J, Marples D, Kwon TH, Agre P, Knepper MA. Aquaporins in the kidney: from molecules to medicine. *Physiol Rev* 2002;82:205–244.

Nilius B, Watanabe H, Vriens J. The TRPV4 channel: structure-function relationship and promiscuous gating behaviour. *Pflugers Arch* 2003;446:298–303.

Russell TA, Ito M, Yu RN, Martinson FA, Weiss J, Jameson JL. A murine model of autosomal dominant neurohypophyseal diabetes insipidus reveals progressive loss of vasopressin-producing neurons. *J Clin Invest* 2003;112:1697–1706.

Thibonnier M, Coles P, Thibonnier A, Shoham M. The basic and clinical pharmacology of nonpeptide vasopressin receptor antagonists. *Annu Rev Pharmacol Toxicol* 2001;41:175–202.

15 Endocrine Disease

Value For Understanding Hormonal Actions

Anthony P. Heaney, MD, PhD
and Glenn D. Braunstein, MD

CONTENTS

1. INTRODUCTION

Disorders involving the endocrine glands, their hormones, and the targets of the hormones may cover the full spectrum ranging from an incidentally found, insignificant abnormality that is clinically silent to a flagrant, life-threatening metabolic derangement. Some endocrine diseases such as well-differentiated thyroid carcinoma present as neoplastic growths, which rarely are associated with evidence of endocrine dysfunction. However, most clinically relevant endocrine disorders are associated with over- or underexpression of hormone action. There is a great deal of phenotypic variability in the clinical manifestations of each of the endocrine disorders, reflecting in part the severity of the derangement and the underlying pathophysiologic mechanisms. Although most of the individual clinical endocrine syndromes have multiple pathophysiologic mechanisms, the qualitative manifestations of the disease states are similar owing to the relatively limited ways in which the body responds to too much or too little hormone action.

This chapter emphasizes the diversity of pathophysiologic mechanisms responsible for endocrine diseases and illustrates the concept that despite the underlying pathophysiology, the clinical manifestations of diseases leading to over- or underexpression of hormone action are quite similar.

2. PATHOPHYSIOLOGY OF ENDOCRINE DISEASES

Endocrine diseases can occur on a congenital, often genetic, basis or can be acquired. Many of the congenital abnormalities are from mutations that result in structural abnormalities, defects in hormone biosynthesis, or abnormalities in hormone-receptor structure or postreceptor signaling mechanisms. Tables 1 and 2 provide examples of identified mutations that result in over- and underexpression of hormone action. Most endocrine diseases are acquired and fit broadly into the categories of neoplasia, destruction or impairment of function of the endocrine gland through infection, infiltrative processes, vascular disorders, trauma, or immune-mediated injury, as well as functional aberrations owing to multiorgan dysfunction, metabolic abnormalities, or drugs.

These processes may disrupt the biosynthesis of protein hormones through interference with transcription, mRNA processing, translation, posttranslational protein modifications, protein storage, degradation, or secretion. Abnormalities in steroid hormone, thyroid

From: *Endocrinology: Basic and Clinical Principles, Second Edition*
(S. Melmed and P. M. Conn, eds.) © Humana Press Inc., Totowa, NJ

Table 1
Examples of Mutations That Cause Endocrine Hyperfunction

Type of mutation	Disorder
Membrane receptor	
• TSH receptor constitutive activation	Thyroid adenoma; hyperthyroidism
• LH/hCG receptor constitutive activation	Familial male precocious puberty (testotoxicosis)
• Calcium-sensing receptor defect	Familial hypocalciuric hypocalcemia; neonatal hyperparathyroidism
Signal pathway	
• Pituitary $G_s\alpha$ activation	Acromegaly
• Thyroid $G_s\alpha$ activation	Thyroid adenoma; hyperthyroidism
• Generalized $G_s\alpha$ activation	McCune-Albright syndrome
• Temperature-sensitive $G_s\alpha$ activation	Testotoxicosis and pseudohypoparathyroidism
• Thyroid p53	Neoplasia
• *Ret* protooncogene	MEN 2a
• Cyclin D1 fusion to PTH promoter (PRAD-1) activation	Parathyroid adenoma
• (PRAD-1) activation	
• $G_1\alpha$ (gip oncogene in adrenal and ovaries)	Adrenocortical and ovarian tumors
• *MENIN* gene	MEN 1
Enzyme	
• Aldosterone synthase-11β-hydroxylase chimera	Glucocorticoid-remediable hypertension

hormone, and calcitriol production may result from loss of the orderly enzymatic conversion of precursor molecules into active hormones. Many disease states as well as medications may alter the transport and metabolism of hormones. Finally, there is a multitude of lesions that can affect hormone-receptor interaction, as well as postreceptor signal pathways. From a functional standpoint, clinical endocrine disease can be broadly classified into diseases of the endocrine glands that are not associated with hormonal dysfunction, diseases from overexpression of hormone action, and diseases characterized by underexpression of hormone action (Table 3). Occasionally, situations exist in which endocrine testing with immunoassays detects elevated hormones, but no clinical endocrine syndrome is apparent. An example of this is so-called idiopathic hyperprolactinemia, in which prolactin (PRL) is bound by a circulating immunoglobulin or the PRL protein is modified by glycation resulting in delayed degradation and excretion of often biologically inactive PRL. Endocrine diseases without hormonal aberrations are generally nonfunctional neoplasms such as thyroid carcinoma or the frequently found incidental pituitary and adrenal adenomas. These neoplasms generally cause symptoms through their anatomic effects on the surrounding structures or, in the case of some malignant neoplasms, through their metastases.

2.1. Overexpression of Hormone

Most endocrine disorders that result in overexpression of hormone action do so through excessive produc-

Table 3
Pathophysiology of Endocrine Diseases

Neoplastic growth of endocrine glands without hyper- or hypofunction.
Overexpression of hormone action
• Excessive production of hormones
  ◆ Eutopic
    ▪ Autonomous
    ▪ Excessive physiologic stimulation
    ▪ Altered regulatory feedback set point
  ◆ Ectopic
    ▪ Direct secretion by tumor
    ▪ Indirect
    ▪ Dysregulation
• Excessive activation of hormone receptors
  Constitutively activated receptors
  Hormone mimicry
  Receptor crossreactivity
• Postreceptor activation of hormone action
• Altered metabolism of hormones
Underexpression of hormone action
• Aplasia or hypoplasia of hormone source
• Acquired destruction of source of hormone
• Congenital absence of hormone
• Production of inactive forms of hormone
• Substrate insufficiency
• Destruction of target organ
• Enzyme defects in hormone production
• Antihormone antibodies
• Hormone resistance
Absent or altered receptor
• Receptor occupancy
• Downregulation of normal receptors
• Postreceptor defects
Altered metabolism of hormones

Table 2
Examples of Mutations That Cause Endocrine Hypofunction

Type of mutation	Disorder
Hormone/hormone precursor	
• GH gene deletion	Growth retardation
• TSH β-subunit gene	Hypothyroidism
• LH β-subunit gene	Hypogonadism
• Neurophysin/ADH processing	Central diabetes insipidus
• PTH processing	Hypoparathyroidism
• Proinsulin processing	Diabetes mellitus
• Insulin gene	Diabetes mellitus
• Thyroglobulin	Hypothyroidism with goiter
Membrane receptor	
• GH	Laron dwarfism
• TSH	Hypothyroidism
• LH/hCG	Resistant testes syndrome
• FSH	Resistant ovary syndrome
• ACTH	Familial glucocorticoid deficiency
• Vasopressin V2	NDI
• PTH	Pseudohypoparathyroidism
• Insulin	Insulin resistance
• β3-adrenergic	Obesity
Nuclear receptor	
• Thyroid hormone	Thyroid hormone resistance syndrome (generalized or pituitary)
• Glucocorticoid	Glucocorticoid resistance syndrome
• Androgen	Androgen insensitivity syndromes
• Estrogen	Delayed epiphyseal closure, osteoporosis
• Mineralocorticoid	Generalized pseudohypoaldosteronism
• Progesterone	Progesterone resistance
• Vitamin D	Vitamin D–resistant rickets
• DAX-1, SF-1	X-linked adrenal hypoplasia congenital
Signal pathway	
• $G_s\alpha$ inactivation	Albright hereditary osteodystrophy (pseudohypoparathyroidism with resistance to PTH, TSH, gonadotropins)
Transcription factors	
• SRY translocation	XX male
• SRY mutation	XY female
• HESX1	Variable degree of hypopituitarism
• PROP1, Pit1 mutation	Growth retardation and hypothyroidism (GH, TSH, and PRL deficiencies)
• RIEG	Occasional GH deficiency
Enzymes	
• Thyroid	
—Peroxidase	Hypothyroidism with goiter
—Iodotyrosine deiodinase	Goiter + hypothyroidism
• Adrenal and testes	
—Cholesterol side-chain cleavage	CAH with hypogonadism (20,22-desmolase)
—3β-Hydroxysteroid dehydrogenase	CAH with ambiguous genitalia
—17α-Hydroxylase	CAH with androgen deficiency and hypertension
• Adrenal	
—11β-Hydroxylase	CAH, androgen excess, hypertension
—21α-Hydroxylase	CAH with androgen excess + salt wasting
• Testes	
—17,20-Desmolase	Hypogonadism
—17-Ketosteroid reductase	Hypogonadism
• Pancreas and Liver	
—Glucokinase gene	Maturity onset diabetes of the young
• Multiple tissues	
—Aromatase	Estrogen deficiency with virilization, delayed epiphyseal closure, tall stature
—5α-Reductase	Male pseudohermaphroditism
—PC1, PC2	ACTH deficiency, hypopigmentation, diabetes mellitus
Other	
• KAL protein deficiency	Kallmann syndrome
• AQP-2 water channel	NDI

tion of hormones. Such production may be eutopic, in which the normal physiologic source of the hormone secretes excessive quantities of that hormone, or ectopic, in which a neoplasm or other pathology involving a tissue, that is not the known physiologic source of the hormone produces excessive quantities of the hormone. Eutopic hypersecretion may be due to autonomous production of the hormone with loss of normal target organ product feedback regulation. This is found in many hormone-secreting benign and malignant neoplasms.

An example would be a cortisol-secreting adrenal cortical adenoma that continues to secrete cortisol despite the suppression of endogenous adrenocorticotropic hormone (ACTH) levels. Dysfunction of endocrine glands leading to hyperplasia may be found in situations when there is excessive physiologic stimulation such as occurs in secondary hyperaldosteronism owing to cirrhosis or congestive heart failure, in which there is decreased effective vascular volume, resulting in stimulation of aldosterone secretion through the renin-angiotensin system. Alterations in the normal feedback set point also cause dysfunction of the endocrine gland, as is seen in the hypercalcemia found in patients with familial hypocalciuric hypercalcemia or in hypercalcemic patients receiving lithium. In both situations, there are alterations in the calcium-sensing mechanism in parathyroid cells, which require higher serum calcium concentrations than normal to suppress parahormone production. The concept of an altered set point for feedback regulation also forms the basis for the low- and high-dose dexamethasone suppression tests in patients with pituitary-dependent Cushing disease. In such patients, ACTH and cortisol production is not suppressed normally following low-dose dexamethasone, but generally it is suppressed following administration of to a high-dose of dexamethasone. A wide variety of hormones have been found to be secreted ectopically by tumors, especially solid tumors of the lung, kidney, liver, and head and neck region. These tumors may directly secrete excessive quantities of a prohormone or active hormone or, in some instances, may secrete releasing factors, which, in turn, stimulates the release of hormone from the normal endocrine glands. Thus, the ectopic ACTH syndrome may be found in patients with oat cell carcinoma of the lung owing to ectopic production of ACTH by the tumor, and it may also be found in patients with bronchial carcinoid tumors that secrete corticotropin-releasing factor, which, in turn, stimulates the pituitary to secrete ACTH. Another form of ectopic hormone production is found with some benign and malignant diseases in which there is dysregulation of metabolic pathways. Patients with sarcoidosis or other granulomatous processes, as well as patients with some forms of lymphoma, may develop hypercalcemia owing to excessive quantities of 1,25-$(OH)_2$-vitamin D produced from normal circulating quantities of 25-(OH)-vitamin D because of dysregulation of macrophage 1α-hydroxylase in the lesions.

A second broad mechanism responsible for overexpression of hormone action is through excessive activation of hormone receptors. Constitutive activation of thyroid-stimulating hormone (TSH) receptors owing to point mutations is found in some patients with toxic thyroid adenomas, and several families with constitutive activation of the luteinizing hormone (LH) receptor in the testes who present with familial male precocious puberty (testotoxicosis) have been described. Hormone receptors may also be activated by hormones that share close homology with the hormone for which the receptor is the primary target. Thus, human chorionic gonadotropin (hCG) when present in high concentrations, as occurs in some women with large hydatidiform moles, may stimulate the TSH receptor, resulting in hyperthyroidism. Other examples of receptor crossreaction include insulin binding to the insulin-like growth factor-1 receptor (IGF-1R) in the ovary, thereby stimulating androgen production, and growth hormone (GH) interaction with the PRL receptor, resulting in galactorrhea in some patients with acromegaly. Some nonhormonal substances can mimic hormone action through interraction with the hormone receptor. The thyroid-stimulating immunoglobulins present in the sera of patients with Graves disease and the hypoglycemia found in some patients with type B insulin resistance with insulin receptor autoantibodies are examples of this phenomenon.

On binding its receptor, a hormone induces a conformational change in the hormone/receptor complex, which, in turn, activates a variety of intracellular signaling pathways to mediate hormone action and regulate cellular function. There are several intracellular signaling pathways that regulate hormone function. Among these are the adenylyl cyclase–cyclic adenosine monophosphate (cAMP) system, tyrosine kinase, guanylyl cyclase, and activation of phospholipase C. Many of these regulatory processes involve the guanylyl nucleotide–binding proteins (G proteins). Some activating mutations of the G protein subunits "turn on" these signaling pathways, which results in the hyperfunction of an endocrine cell. In some situations, the activating G protein subunit mutation is confined to a single cell type, as in the case of ~40% of pituitary somatotroph tumors associated with acromegaly or in a minority of thyroid follicular adenomas associated with neonatal hyperthyroidism. In inherited conditions, such as McCune-

Albright syndrome, G protein subunit mutations are found in multiple tissues, resulting in polyendocrine overactivity including acromegaly and LH-releasing hormone (GnRH) –independent sexual precocity, as well as nonendocrine manifestations. In both cases, G protein subunit mutation results in constitutive activation of the G protein subunit–stimulated cAMP, regardless of the presence or absence of ligand, and the cAMP intracellular signaling pathway is permanently "turned on"This occurs in some somatotrophs associated with acromegaly or thyroid follicular cells associated neonatal hyperthyroidism.This also occurs in the endocrine target cells, which when activated through a G protein mutation function as if they were exposed to excessive quantities of the hormone. This mechanism is responsible for the precocious puberty and other clinical manifestations of the McCune-Albright syndrome (Table 1).

Hormone metabolism may be altered by disease states and medications. Hyperthyroidism, obesity, liver disease, and spironolactone increase the aromatization of testosterone and androstenedione, leading to enhanced production of estradiol and estrone, respectively, which can cause gynecomastia in affected individuals. Clinicians caring for patients with type 1 diabetes mellitus have long known that the unexpected onset of frequent hypoglycemic reactions necessitating the reduction in insulin dosages may herald the onset of renal insufficiency with loss of the ability of the kidneys to metabolize the exogenous insulin.

Multiple mechanisms also exist resulting in the underexpression of hormone action. Certainly, congenital aplasia or hypoplasia of endocrine tissue will prevent the normal synthesis or secretion of hormones by that tissue. Anencephaly, which is associated with an absence or maldevelopment of the hypothalamus, leads to a loss of hypothalamic-releasing hormones, which in turn, leads to profound panhypopituitarism. Other examples of abnormal hypothalamic development are holoprosencephaly, owing to chromosomal-mediated abnormalities of the transcription factor pituitary adenylate cyclase–activating polypeptide (PACAP) or PACAP receptor, resulting in abnormal midline forebrain development and hypothalamic insufficiency, and Kallman syndrome, owing to mutations in the *KAL* gene, which encodes the KAL adhesion protein, called anosmin, responsible for the coordinated migration of the gonadotropin-releasing hormone (GnRH)-secreting neurons from the olfactory placode into the hypothalamus.

Another example of an abnormal development of at least a portion of the hypothalamus is X-chromosome-linked Kallmann's syndrome. Loss of this normal migration results in inadequate production and secretion of

GnRH, leading to a hypogonadotropic hypogonadism. In addition to congenital structural defects, destruction of endocrine organs can occur from replacement by tumor or involvement with one of the many processes listed earlier. Congenital absence of a hormone owing to a gene deletion is rare and has been described for GH. More commonly, point mutations in the genes encoding a hormone or a hormone subunit may result in a biologically inactive form of the hormone, which may or may not retain its immunologic activity. Other mechanisms may result in hormone deficiency. Substrate required for hormone production may be limited, as occurs in individuals with vitamin D deficiency owing to inadequate intake, lack of sun exposure, or the presence of malabsorption. Without an appropriate amount of native vitamin D, insufficient quantities of 25(OH)-vitamin D and 1,25(OH)$_2$-vitamin D may be produced. Because many hormones are produced in a prohormone form,some point mutations may result in a defect that preventsthe normal processing of the biologically inactive prohormone to the biologically active hormone (Table 2).

Although antibodies that bind circulating hormone do not usually impair do not cause a major interference in hormone action, however,some antibodies may sufficiently interfere with hormone action to result in hormone deficiency.insufficiency state. Examples include the high-titer, high-affinity antibodies against insulin that occasionally cause insulin resistance, gonadotropin antibodies that occasionally form in individuals with hypogonadotropic hypogonadism receiving exogenous gonadotropins, and the extremely rare GH inactivating antibody found in some GH-deficient children receiving exogenous GH. Spontaneous antihormone antibodies are occasionally seen in patients with autoimmune diseases but rarely cause clinical manifestations. In addition,the target organ may not appropriately respond to hormonal stimulation because of structural defects in the hormone receptor; acquired disease; or in the case of thyroid hormones, steroid hormones, and vitamin D, congenital or acquired defects in the enzymes responsible for conversion of the hormone into its final active form (Table 2).

Another mechanism for the underexpression of hormone action is hormone resistance at the target organ level due to receptor or postreceptor abnormalities. A number of inactivating mutations in both membrane and nuclear hormone receptors have been described (Table 2). In addition, the receptors may be occupied by autoantibodies, which prevent the normal hormone-receptor interaction from taking place. In contrast to the stimulatory effects of thyroid-stimulating Igs in patients with Graves disease, blocking of autoantibodies to the TSH receptor is a cause of goitrous hypothyroidism. Similarly, anti-insulin receptor antibodies may block the effect of insulin in some patients, whereas in others the antibodies may mimic the effect of insulin and cause hypoglycemia. Normal receptors exposed to large quantities of its complementary hormone may be downregulated. Therapeutically, this is the mechanism by which long-largeacting analogs of GnRH lead to a loss of responsiveness by the gonadotropes to endogenous GnRH, which, in turn, leads to a lowering of LH and follicle-stimulating hormone (FSH) concentrations. Finally, hormone resistance may occur because of postreceptor defects involving the signal pathway. Albright hereditary osteodystrophy, which is manifest by resistance to parathyroid hormone (PTH), TSH, and gonadotropins, results from inactivation of $G_s\alpha a$ in a variety of tissues. Another type of postreceptor defect is homologous desensitization, which refers to the inability of a hormone to stimulate the signaling pathway after extensive interaction with its receptor at a time when other factors are able to continue to stimulate that pathway. Such homologous desensitization is seen in the corpus luteum during early pregnancy when hCG has completely occupied its receptors. Although early in pregnancy hCG is able to stimulate adenylyl cyclase activity after interaction with the hCG/LH receptor in the corpus luteum, once the receptors are occupied, adenylyl cyclase activity decreases, but it is still able to be stimulated by forskolin and phorbal esters, which act on the signaling mechanism at the postreceptor sites. Certain disease states, drugs, and medications are known to alter the metabolism of hormones and may result in overerexpression of hormone action. Alcohol enhances the A-ring metabolism of testosterone, increasing its metabolism. Phenobarbital decreases the production of 25-(OH)-vitamin D from its precursors, by stimulating the formation of more polar metabolites by the liver.

3. EXAMPLES OF CLINICAL SYNDROMES WITH MULTIPLE PATHOPHYSIOLOGIC MECHANISMS

For virtually every hormone, there exists a pathologic state of over- or underexpression of hormone action. In some instances, there may be no clinical manifestations because of physiologic compensation by normal homeostatic mechanisms or because the hormonal abnormality may have little or no relevance. Hypoprolactinemia in males is an example of the latter. In most cases, over- or underexpression of hormone action results in clinical manifestations. Although the predominant manifestations of hormone excess or deficiency will be the same no matter what the underlying pathologic lesion, there

are usually unique clinical or biochemical findings present with each type of pathology that leads the clinician to the correct diagnosis. This section illustrates these concepts as well as the array of different pathophysiologic mechanisms that may result in the consteillation of signs and symptoms that characterize some of the common endocrine syndromes.

3.1. Growth Hormone

3.1.1. ACROMEGALY/GIGANTISM

Acromegaly and gigantism are the result of excessive GH secretion. Gigantism occurs when GH is hypersecreted prior to fusion of the epiphysial plates of the long bones, resulting in excessive linear growth as well as growth of the bones of the jaw, supraorbital ridges, and spine. Once the epiphysial plates of the long bones are fused, the occurrence of excessive GH secretion results only in overgrowth of soft tissues and bones that retain cartilaginous plates such as the supraorbital ridges and the spine. Thus, these patients exhibit large, beefy hands as well as a large tongue; coarsening of the facial features; skin tags; prognathism; dorsal kyphosis; enlargement of the heart and kidneys; colonic polyps; and osteoarthritis. Symptoms include excessive perspiration; lethargy or fatigue; weight gain; and if the pathology is owing to a large intracranial neoplasm, visual abnormalities and headaches. Glucose intolerance with hyperinsulinemia is often present. These manifestations are owing to the excessive secretion of GH and its primary mediator, insulin-like growth factor-1 (IGF-1). Table 4 lists the various pathophysiologic mechanisms for acromegaly/gigantism. Excessive production of GH-releasing hormone (GHRH) occurs eutopically in some patients with hypothalamic hamartomas or gangliocytomas that secrete the releasing factor in an autonomous fashion. Autonomous ectopic production of GHRH has also been described with bronchial or pancreatic islet cell and carcinoid tumors. With both eutopic and ectopic GHRH secretion, the pituitary somatotropes are stimulated to secrete excessive quantities of GH. Somatotrope hyperplasia is seen pathologically in these conditions. The majority of patients with acromegaly or gigantism harbor a somatotrope adenoma that secretes excessive quantities of GH eutopically. Rarely, GH may be secreted ectopically by tumors such as pancreatic or lung carcinomas. In each of these situations, the clinical manifestations of acromegaly are similar, and it may be very difficult to distinguish the underlying pathology unless there are other local manifestations from the nonpituitary tumors that direct the attention to other areas. Of interest, similar clinical manifestations may be seen in a condition known as acromegaloidism, which is not owing to excessive secretion of GH but is associated with another tropic hormone that can be measured in a bone marrow stem cell assay.

Table 4
Etiologies of Acromegaly/
Gigantism

Excessive GHRH secretion
- Eutopic
- Ectopic

Excessive GH secretion
- Eutopic
- Ectopic

Acromegaloidism

Table 5
Etiologies of GHD Syndromes

Hypothalamic GHRH deficiency
- Congenital
- Acquired

Stalk lesions

GHRH receptor mutations

Pituitary

Structural defects involving somatotrophs
- Congenital *PROP*-1, *HESX*-1, *Pit*-1 mutation
- Acquired

Deletion or mutation of *GH* gene

Biologically inactive GH

GH insensitivity
- GH receptor defect (Laron dwarfism)
- Postreceptor defect in IGF-1 generation (?Pygmies)
- Resistance to IGF-1

3.1.2. GH Deficiency Syndromes

On the other end of the spectrum from acromegaly and gigantism are the clinical syndromes of GH deficiency (GHD). When present in childhood, profound growth retardation and, often, hypoglycemia are seen, and in adults weakness and deficiencies in skeletal muscle mass may be present. A variety of different conditions may give rise to similar clinical findings of underexpression of GH action (Table 5). GHRH may be deficient owing to congenital (anencephaly, holoprosencephaly) or acquired lesions of the hypothalamus (tumor, granulomatous disease). This, in turn, results in pituitary somatotrope atrophy and insufficient production of GH. A similar result can be found in lesions that destroy the hypothalamo-hypophyseal portal system through which GHRH is transported to the somatotropes. Although no defects in the *GHRH* gene have yet been reported, multiple kindreds exhibiting homozygous mutations in the *GHRH* receptor (GHRH-R) resulting in a truncated GHRH-R protein-binding site have been described. Deficient production of GH may also occur if pituitary tissue is missing, as is found in pituitary aplasia, or if somatotropes are absent through a mutation of the *Pit*-1, *PROP*1, or *HESX*1 genes. Complete deletion of the *GH* gene also results in absent GH production, and a variety of mutations and/or rearrangements of the *GH* gene that produce a partially functional GH protein and are associated with varying degrees of GHD have been described. Some of these mutations lead to biologically inactive but immunologically reactive (i.e., detectable normal GH levels) GH protein that has defects in the amino acids for GH binding to its receptor. Immunologically active but biologically inactive forms of GH, presumably due to point mutations in the *GH* gene or to post-translational processing abnormalities may alsoresulting in growth retardation, as seen in can acquired structural abnormalities of the pituitary.

3.1.2.1. GH Insensitivity

The term *GH insensitivity* describes a condition in which patients have a phenotype consistent with GHD

but have normal or elevated serum GH levels and diminished IGF-1. GH insensitivity may be caused by (1) gene deletion or missense mutation of the GH receptor (Laron dwarfism); (2) postreceptor abnormalities of GH signal transduction resulting from failed STAT, JAK1, or mitogen-actived protein kinase activation; or (3) genetic insensitivity to IGF-1 action as a consequence of abnormalities in growth hormone (GH) transport and clearance, mutated IGF receptor, or abnormal IGF-postreceptor signaling activation, although these defects are exceedingly rare. In addition, GH insensitivity may occur secondary to renal or hepatic failure, administration of pharmacologic steroids, malnutrition, or other chronic disease. The low IGF-1 in this syndrome may represent a post-receptor abnormality in IGF-1 generation. Finally, growth retardation can be seen with resistance to the biologic effects of IGF-1, which may be the mechanism through which pharmacologic doses of glucocorticoids inhibit cartilaginous growth during childhood.

3.2. Adrenal Glucocorticoids

3.2.1. Cushing Syndrome

Long-standing glucocorticoid excess, whether owing to endogenous hypersecretion from the adrenal gland or exogenous intake, results in obesity, redistribution of body fat, hypertension, proximal muscle weakness, loss of connective-tissue support with abdominal striae and easy bruisability, emotional symptoms, osteopenia, and glucose intolerance. If gluocorticoid excess is present in childhood, significant growth retardation is also seen. Glucocorticoid excess can becaused from autonomously produced from a primary adrenal gland abnormality.

Table 6
Etiologies of Cushing Syndrome

ACTH dependent	*ACTH independent*

• Excessive ectopic CRH secretion (bronchial carcinoid, medullary thyroid, or prostatic carcinoma)
• Excessive ACTH secretion
  ◆ Eutopic (pituitary corticotroph adenoma)
  ◆ Ectopic (small cell lung carcinoma, bronchial and pancreatic carcinoid)
• Macronodular adrenal hyperplasia (long-standing ACTH stimulation causing autonomous adrenal adenoma)
	• Cortisol-secreting adrenal adenoma or carcinoma
	• Primary pigmented nodular adrenal hyperplasia and Carney Complex
	• McCune-Albright syndrome
	• Macronodular adrenal and hyperplasia and aberrant receptor expression (ACTH-R, GIP-R)
	• Iatrogenic owing to exogenous glucocorticoids

Table 7
Etiologies of Adrenal Insufficiency

Hypothalamic (CRH deficiency)
• Congenital
• Structural
• Functional

Pituitary (ACTH deficiency)
• Congenital (POMC mutation, PC1 and PC2 deficiency)
• Acquired (lymphocytic hypophysitis)

Adrenal
• CAH (*DAX*-1, *SF*-1 mutation)
• CAH
• *ACTH* or *MCR*-4 receptor mutation (familial glucocorticoid deficiency)
• Adrenoleukodystrophy
• Acquired
• Structural
• Antibodies to adrenal enzymes
• ACTH receptor antibodies
• Infective (fungal, tuberculosis, AIDS)
• Drug induced

Target tissues
• Glucocorticoid resistance

Alternatively, excessive stimulation of the adrenal gland from increased quantities of ACTH from a pituitary adenoma or an ectopic tumor source, or through excessive pituitary ACTH stimulation by corticotropin-releasing hormone (CRH) from a hypothalamic lesion or nonhypothalamic tumor secreting CRH ectopically, may lead to excess adrenal steroid levels (Table 6). With all of these conditions, the patient will demonstrate clinical findings of glucocorticoid and/or mineralocorticoid excess. However, each of the causes presented in Table 6 has its own unique clinical manifestations. For instance, the onset of the clinical and metabolic abnormalities is more rapid in patients who have ectopic production of ACTH or adrenocortical carcinoma than with

the other causes. Patients with adrenocortical carcinoma tend to secrete increased quantities of mineralocorticoids and adrenal androgens in addition to the glucocorticoids, resulting in hypokalemic alkalosis and virilization in women and feminization in men. Finally, some patients have a rare familial syndrome associated with glucocorticoid resistance owing to mutations in the nuclear glucocorticoid receptor. These individuals have increased cortisol secretion but do not have the stigmata of Cushing syndrome and often exhibit precocious puberty since pituitary ACTH levels are elevated, which also stimulates adrenal androgen production.

3.2.2. ADRENAL INSUFFICIENCY

Loss of adrenal glucocorticoid production is associated with weight loss, fatigue, weakness, anorexia, and postural hypotension. Pure glucocorticoid insufficiency may be found with hypothalamic or pituitary lesions. If the adrenal gland is absent or destroyed, then mineralocorticoid and adrenal androgen deficiency also may be present, as will be hyperpigmentation from excessive secretion of pituitary-derived proopiomelanocortin (POMC)-derived peptides. Adrenal insufficiency can occur on a congenital basis or through involvement with various acquired disease processes (Table 7). Normal glucocorticoid secretion requires a coordinated production of CRH, which stimulates pituitary ACTH release, which, in turn, stimulates cortisol production and release. Thus, a congenital deficiency of CRH or a process that destroys hypothalamic CRH production will result in low ACTH and low cortisol and clinical findings of glucocorticoid insufficiency. The most common functional abnormality of the hypothalamic-pituitary-adrenal (HPA) axis is seen in patients who have received pharmacologic doses of exogenous glucocorticoids for long periods of time, and adrenal atrophy and subsequent deficiency should be anticipated in any subject who has taken more than the equivalent of 20 mg of hydrocortisone daily orally for more than 3 wk. Suppression of HPA axis following withdrawal of thesteroids may be present for up to 1 yr and during that time, patients may experience weakness, weight loss, and fatigue as well as develop acute adrenal insufficiency if physically stressed. Congenital and acquired structural lesions in the anterior pituitary cause secondary adrenal insufficiency due to inadequate adrenal stimulation and low cortisol levels, often other pituitary hormones in addition to ACTH are deficient, and patients present with partial or complete hypopituitarism. Isolated ACTH deficiency is a rare but difficult diagnosis to make; this deficiency can occur in association with lymphocytic hypophysitis, an inflammatory disorder of the hypothalamic-pituitary region. An additional rare but fascinating cause of ACTH deficiency owing to defective posttranslational POMC processing is caused by lack of the prohormone convertase (PC) enzymes PC1 and PC2. Patients may have more generalized defects in peptide processing including impaired proinsulin to insulin cleavage resulting in diabetes mellitus. Patients have also been described with mutations in the *POMC* gene. Because α-melanocyte-stimulating hormone (α-MSH), an additional cleavage POMC product, regulates appetite via the melanocortin-4 receptor, patients with *POMC*-gene mutations exhibit severe obesity and red hair, in addition to adrenal insufficiency. With both hypothalamic and pituitary adrenal insufficiency, patients do not exhibit mineralocorticoid insufficiency, because the renin-angiotensinaldosterone system generally remains intact. The other clinical manifestations of hypothalamic-pituitary diseases reflect the "neighborhood" neurologic findings.

Primary adrenocortical insufficiency is much more common than the secondary or tertiary causes; patients usually have both glucocorticord and mineralocorticoid deficiency; and it is usually owing to autoimmune destruction, either as an isolated phenomenon or as part of a polyglandular autoimmune (PGA) endocrine syndrome. Patients with PGA syndrome demonstrate antibodies to the side-chain cleavage or hydroxylase enzymes involved in steroid biosynthesis and processing. The PGA syndrome has been mapped to chromosome 21q22.3 and is associated with mutations in a transcription regulation gene called *AIRE*, or to infectious destruction, especially from tuberculosis and fungal infections. Worldwide, infectious diseases are the most common cause of adrenal insufficiency, especially from tuberculosis and fungal infections and, more recently, owing to acquired immunodeficiency syndrome (AIDS) –associated cytomegalovirus or atypical mycobacterium-induced adrenalitis. In addition, adrenal insufficiency may be precipitated in patients

with AIDS as the result of concomitant use of anti-infectives such as ketoconazole, which inhibits cortisol synthesis, and rifampicin, which increases cortisol metabolism. Congenital causes include congenital adrenal hyperplasia due to mutations in adrenal steroid biosynthesis enzymes or X-lined congenital adrenal hypoplasia, comprising adrenal insufficiency and hypogonadism, and due to mutations in the transcription factors dosage-sensitive, sex reversal, adrenal hypoplasia congenital, X chromosome gene (*DAX*1) or steroidogenic factor-1 (SF-1) resulting in failed development. Mutations in the melanocortin-2 (*MCR*-2) or *ACTH* receptor are also isassociated with familial congenital glucocorticoid deficiency, and antibodies that react to and block the *ACTH* receptor have been found in some patients with an autoimmune diathesis. Enzyme defects in the glucocorticoid pathway in the adrenal lead to a combination of glucocorticoid insufficiency with evidence of defects in the mineralocorticoid and/or adrenal androgen pathways that result in combinations of adrenal insufficiency; ambiguous genitalia; and, in some patients, precocious puberty and hypertension. In a similar fashion, drugs and some medications such as ketoconazole, metapyrone, aminoglutethimide, and trilostane also result in adrenal enzyme inhibition and, in certain circumstances, may lead to adrenal insufficiency. Finally, some patients have a rare familial syndrome associated with glucocorticoid resistance due to mutations in the nuclear glucocorticoid receptor.These individuals often exhibit precocious puberty since pituitary ACTH levels are elevated andstimulate adrenal androgen production.

3.3. Gonadal Steroid Hormones

3.3.1. PRECOCIOUS PUBERTY

Precocious puberty is the appearance of secondary sexual characteristics prior to age 9 in boys and 8 in girls. Thus, development of axillary and pubic hair and rapid bone growth in both sexes, penile (and most often testicular) enlargement in males, and breast development and menarche in females are the major clinical manifestations. Precocious puberty can be classified as occurring through gonadotropin-dependent or -independent mechanisms (Table 8). Among the former, the most common cause is premature activation of GnRH secretion either on a familial basis or owing to a structural or nonstructural (idopathic) central nervous system (CNS) disorder. One of the more common CNS disorders associated with precocious puberty is a hypothalamic hamartoma involving the tuber cinereum, which contains GnRH-secreting cells. Other CNS tumors that impinge on the neural pathways that normally inhibit the GnRH

Table 8
Etiologies of Precocious Puberty

Gonadotropin dependent
- Premature activation of GnRH secretion
  (head injury, CNS tumors, GnRH-secreting hamartoma)
- hCG-secreting tumors
- Primary hypothyroidism

Gonadotropin independent
- Constitutive activation of testicular LH/hCG receptors
  (testotoxicosis)
- Constitutive activation of gonadal adenylyl cyclase
  (McCune-Albright syndrome)
- Ovarian cysts
- Gonadal neoplasms
- CAH
- Adrenal or testicular neoplasms
- Exogenous sex steroid or endocrine disruptor exposure
  (pesticide)

pulse generator in childhood may cause precocious puberty. This problem may arise by a similar mechanism following cranial irradiation for local tumors or leukemias. The GnRH stimulates the gonadotropes to secrete LH and FSH, which, in turn, stimulate the gonads to secrete the gonadal steroid hormones. hCG-secreting neoplasms in males such as germ-cell tumors of testes or extragonadal tumors including those located in the pineal region, and hepatoblastomas, are associated with gonadotropin-dependent precocious puberty owing to direct interaction of hCG with the LH/hCG receptors present in the gonads. Another form of gonadotropin-dependent precocious puberty is seen in children with severe primary hypothyroidism, often in association with galactorrhea (Van Wyk–Grumbach syndrome). This is considered to be an example of a "hormonal-overlap" syndrome that may be associated with gonadotropin hypersecretion. Alternatively, the close similarity of TSH with the other glycoprotein hormones raises the possibility that the massively increased levels of TSH in children with primary hypothyroidism may actually interact with the LH/hCG receptors in the gonads. Gonadotropin-independent precocious puberty is found in girls who are exposed to exogenous estrogens or who develop estrogen-secreting tumors of the ovary or follicular cysts. In males, androgen-secreting neoplasms or CAH with androgen excess may result in isosexual precocious puberty, whereas in girls virilization is found. Several point mutations in the seven-transmembrane G protein–linked LH/hCG receptor present in the testicular Leydig cells that result in constitutive activation of the receptor leading to autonomous overproduction of testosterone and precocious puberty (testotoxicosis) have been

described. In males, McCune-Albright syndrome, which includes polyostotic fibrous dysplasia of the bones, café au lait spots, along with precocious puberty in both sexes, has been found to be owing to a mutation present in the $G_s\alpha$ that results in constitutive activation of gonadal adenylyl cyclase mimicking gonadotropin stimulation.

3.3.2. Hypogonadism

The manifestations of hypogonadism depend on the age at which the deficient production of sex steroid hormones occurs. In males, androgen deficiency occurring during the first 12 wk of fetal development will result in insufficient development of Wolffian duct structures, and deficient conversion of testosterone into dihydrotestosterone (DHT) in the genital ridge tissue leading to a failure to fuse the labial-scrotal folds, which normally results in the development of a scrotum and penile urethra. Androgen deficiency at this time presents with male pseudohermaphroditism.

Androgen deficiency late in gestation may only be manifest by cryptorchidism and micropenis. If androgen deficiency occurs postnatally but prepubertally, secondary sexual characteristics including hair growth in the androgen-sensitive areas of the body, deepening of the voice, and increased muscle mass fail to develop. The epiphyses of the long bones do not close and continue to grow under the influence of GH, and, therefore, the individual develops eunuchoidal proportions. If the androgen deficiency is acquired and occurs postpubertally, then there may develop testicular atrophy, muscle weakness, decreased libido, infertility, and impotence are the usual presenting features. In girls, prenatal estrogen deficiency owing to ovarian dysgenesis or lack of appropriate pituitary gonadotropin stimulation does not result in anatomic abnormalities because the female genital tract develops the same in the presence or absence of an ovary. Therefore, hypogonadism owing to congenital lesions or those acquired during childhood presents much the same way with absence of pubertal development including menarche. Postpubertal development of hypogonadism in women leads to amenorrhea, uterine atrophy, and regression of breast glandular tissue. In males, hypogonadism can be divided into two groups: hypogonadotropic hypogonadism owing to a lesion in the hypothalamic or pituitary region and hypergonadotropic hypogonadism from defects in the testes or in the androgen target tissues (Table 9).

Isolated gonadotropin deficiency with anosmia or hyposmia characterizes Kallmann syndrome. The most common form of this syndrome is X-linked and has been shown to be owing to gene deletions as well as point

Table 9
Etiologies of Male Hypogonadism

Hypogonadotropic hypogonadism	*Hypergonadotropic hypogonadism*

Hypothalamic
• Developmental defects
  • Kallmann syndrome (*KAL* gene defect)
  • Other complex genetic syndrome
• Structural defects (gliomas, astrocytomas)
• Functional defects (Langerhans cell histiocytosis)
	Testicular defects
	• Genetic (Klinefelter syndrome)
	• Gross structural lesions
	• LH/hCG receptor defect
	• Testosterone steroidogenic defects
	• Acquired (chemotherapy, gonadal radiation)

Stalk lesions Pituitary • *GnRH* receptor mutations • *LH*β mutation • Structural lesions	End organ defects • Androgen insensitivity syndromes • 5α-Reductase deficiency

mutations in the KAL gene or promoter, which, as previously noted, encodes for an adhesion protein called anosmin that resembles fibronectin. Anosmin is responsible for the migration of GnRH-secreting neurons from the olfactory placode to the hypothalamus, and lack of anosmin inhibits this migration, resulting in a GnRH deficiency. Several complex genetic syndromes associated with hypothalamic-hyppogonadism have been described, and include the Prader-Willi syndrome, comprising early onset hyperphagia, pathologic obesity and glucose intolerance, infantile central hypotonia, and mild to moderate mental retardation, and the Laurence-Moon (L-M) and Bardet Biedl (B-B) syndromes, now regarded as distinct entities. Both these autosomal recessive traits combine retinitis pigmentosa and hypogonadism but differ in that L-M is associated with spastic paraplegia, whereas B-B involves postaxial polydactyly. Hypothalamic dysfunction can also result from a variety of disease states associated with acute and chronic weight loss as well as suppression of GnRH release by several medications. Interruption of the hypothalamo-hypophyseal portal system by tumor, radiation, or infiltration, as in Langerhans cell histiocytosis, leads to hypogonadotropic hypogonadism through inadequate stimulation of thepituitary gonadotropes. Primary pituitary problems, especially large pituitary adenomas and CNS developmental defects owing to transcription factor mutations (*Prop*-1, *HESX*-1, *LHX*-3), are often associated with gonadotropin deficiency, in association with other endocrine deficiencies. An unusual congenital form of pituitary hypogonadism is owing to a mutation in the gene encoding the β-subunit of LH, resulting in a biologically inactive but immunologically active form of the hormone, and several families with mutations in the GnRH receptor have also been described.

Hypergonadotropic hypogonadism in males is often owing to acquired testicular defects. It is quite common for serum free testosterone levels to decrease with age, with a concomitant increase in LH, reflecting a mild hypogonadism. Klinefelter syndrome, resulting from the XXY genotype, is the most prevalent genetic abnormality involving the testes, and it results in hyalinization and fibrosis of the gonad at the time of puberty, hypogonadism, eunuchoidal skeletal proportions, and gynecomastia. The role of *DAX*-1 mutations in adrenal insufficiency was discussed earlier; because DAX-1 is also expressed in the testis (and weakly in the ovary), hypothalamus, and pituitary, hypogonadotropic hypogonadism can be part of the clinical picture. In addition, several inherited defects in the enzymes responsible for testosterone biosynthesis have been described (Table 2) including 17α-hydroxylase (17, 20) lyase deficiency and lack of the steroid acute regulatory protein, which enables synthesis of C21 and C19-steroids and allows conversion of cholesterol into pregnenolone. These enzyme defects and usually results in varying degrees of male pseudohermaphroditism because the defect is present during embryogenesis. Leydig cell hypoplasia is a congenital lesion associated with an absent or mutated *LH/hCG* receptor in the gonad. Activation of the receptor in the developing gonad is necessary for the mesenchymal tissue present in the developing gonad to differentiate into Leydig cells, and absent Leydig cells and undetectable testosterone. Therefore, leydig cells are neither seen nor is testosterone production from the testes presentwithcharacterize this syndrome. The androgen insensitivity syndromes are another form of hypergonadotropic hypogonadism and run the gamut from mild androgen resistance in phenotypic men who have normal male genitalia and gynecomastia to the

Table 10
Etiologies of Female Hypogonadism

Hypogonadotropic hypogonadism	*Hypergonadotropic hypogonadism*
Hypothalamic	Ovary
• Congenital	• Gonadal dysgenesis
• Acquired	• 17α-Hydroxylase deficiency
◆ Structural	• Resistant ovary syndrome
◆ Functional	• Acquired structural defects
Pituitary	Aromatase enzyme deficiency
• Congenital	
• Acquired	

complete testicular feminization syndrome characterized by complete androgen resistance with a female phenotype and the absence of pubic or axillary hair. All patients with these defects have a problem with the nuclear androgen receptor. A variety of lesions with the receptor have been characterized and include complete absence or truncation of the receptor, point mutations that cause inactivation or decreased ability of the receptor to be activated, as well as lesions that cause thermal instability of the receptor. The phenotypic manifestations of androgen resistance in these patients depends on the type of receptor lesion and severity of the lesion.

Finally, male hypogonadism can result from a deficiency of the enzyme 5α-reductase in androgen target tissues. This enzyme is responsible for the conversion of testosterone into DHT, and inwith its absence both testosterone and LH levels are both elevated. Because this defect is present during embryogenesis, there is incomplete development of male external genitalia, resulting in the appearance of a bifid scrotum and "clitoromegaly." At puberty, either through mass action resulting from an increase in testosterone or through other mechanisms such as a direct action of testosterone, virilization occurs with an increase in muscle mass, enlargement of the phallus, and deepening of the voice.

Female hypogonadism can also be divided into hypogonadotropic and hypergonadotropic forms (Table 10). The hypothalamic and pituitary abnormalities described in males may also present in women as primary amenorrhea with deficient secondary sexual characteristic development or secondary amenorrhea if a lesion develops following menarche. In the majority of patients with hypergonadotropic hypogonadism with primary amenorrhea and lack of secondary sexual development, gonadal dysgenesis including XO Turner syndrome and XX or XY pure gonadal dysgenesis is the cause. In addition to the streak ovaries and estrogen deficiency, patients with Turner syndrome

have other physical stigmata including short stature, webbed neck, lymphedema, micrognathia, low-set ears, epicanthal folds, shield like chest, and renal and vascular abnormalities. By contrast, patients with 46XX and 46XY gonadal dysgenesis only demonstrate sexual infantilism and develop eunuchoidal proportions because of the lack of estrogen-mediated epiphysial closure of the long bones. A rare form of CAH owing to 17α-hydroxylase deficiency is also associated with sexual infantilism because of a block in the conversion of pregnenolone into progesterone. Another rare conditions include the resistant ovary syndrome, which is associated with a defect in the ovarian *FSH* receptor, which, in some patients, may be overcome with pharmacologic concentrations of exogenous gonadotropins; premature ovarian failure in association with eyelid dysplasia owing to haploid insufficiency of the *FOXL2* gene; and congenital disorders of glycosylation. A variety of acquired structural defects may destroy ovarian function and lead to premature ovarian failure. Recently, an aromatase deficiency syndrome in females has been described. Because the aromatase enzyme is required to convert androstenedione into estrone and testosterone into estradiol, lack of this enzyme will result in elevated concentrations of androgens and deficient levels of estrogens. Clinically, this is manifest by estrogen deficiency with virilization from unopposed androgen effect, as well as delayed epiphysial closure resulting in tall stature.

3.4. Antidiuretic Hormone

3.4.1. SYNDROME OF INAPPROPRIATE SECRETION OF ANTIDIURETIC HORMONE

Syndrome of inappropriate secretion of antidiuretic hormone (SIADH) is manifest by signs and symptoms of water intoxication owing to enhanced reabsorption of free water by the kidney, which leads to hyponatremia, hypoosmolarity, and urine that is inappropriately concentrated with respect to the serum with continued sodium excretion despite the hyponatremia. To make a diagnosis of SIADH, there should be normal adrenal and thyroid function since glucocorticoids and thyroid hormones are required for free water clearance. In addition, kidney function should be normal, and there should be no evidence of a secondary cause of appropriate ADH secretion such as volume depletion, edema, or cardiac or hepatic disease. The signs and symptoms are owing to the degree of water intoxication and rate of fall of the sodium. When the serum sodium levels reach 115–120 meq/L, anorexia, nausea, vomiting, abdominal cramps, bloating, ileus, restlessness, confusion, withdrawal, hostility, headache, or muscle weakness may be prominent. If the serum sodium level falls below 110 meq/L, often there will be focal neurologic findings including weakness, hemiparesis, ataxia, stupor, convulsions, or coma. Both eutopic and ectopic sources of excessive ADH secretion have been identified (Table 11). Because the magnicellular vasopressin-secreting neurons receive multiple excitatory and inhibitory inputs from the brain stem cardiovascular and regulatory centers as well as osmoreceptive cells in the hypothalamus, any diffuse CNS disorder can cause vasopressin hypersecretion, in contrast to CNS causes of diabetes insipidus which are limited to lesions of the suprasellar hypothalamus.

Pulmonary disorders such as tuberculosis, pneumonia, and advanced carcinoma may cause SIADH, and this appears owing to a nonosmotic stimulation of vasopressin and possibly owing to hypercarbia. Several drugs stimulate vasopressin release including chlorpropamide and clofibrate, whereas other drugs may activate V2 renal receptors or potentiate stimulate ADH release or enhance its vasopressin activity at the renal level. Of particular recent interest are the selective serotonin reuptake inhibitors, which have been reported to cause hyponatremia by vasopressin stimulation in up to 28% of elderly patients. A similar mechanism is thought to be responsible for fatal hyponatremia following use of the recreational drug 3,4- methylenedioxymethamphetamine (Ecstasy). Some patients appear to have developed a resetting of the osmostat present in the hypothalamus. These patients begin to release ADH at a lower level of serum osmolality than in healthy individuals. In essence, the release of ADH parallels the normal curve, but the serum osmolality in the affected patients is lower than normal at any given plasma concentration of ADH. A number of tumors have been found to secrete ADH ectopically, especially oat cell carcinoma of the lung. Indeed, even in the absence of clinical SIADH, many patients with lung carcinomas will demonstrate an inadequate urinary excretion of a water load.

3.4.2. Diabetes Insipidus

Diabetes insipidus results from deficiency of ADH action leading to polyuria, polydipsia, and a urine osmolality that is low despite a high serum osmolality. From a pathophysiologic standpoint, diabetes insipidus can develop because of inadequate production of ADH from the hypothalamus and posterior pituitary (central or neurogenic diabetes insipidus), an inability of ADH to act on the kidney to enhance resorption of free water (nephrogenic diabetes insipidus [NDI]), or excessive metabolism of ADH (Table 12). Central diabetes insipidus may be present at birth from structural defects

Table 11
Etiologies of SIADH

Eutopic production of ADH
- CNS disorders
- Pulmonary disorders
- Drug induced
- Reset osmostat

Ectopic production of ADH

Table 12
Etiologies of Diabetes Insipidus

Central (neurogenic)
- Defect in neurophysin or vasopressin-processing defect
- Structural hypothalamic/stalk/posterior pituitary lesions (tumor, infiltration, trauma, surgery)
- Idiopathic (vasopressin antibody in 33%)

Nephrogenic Diabetes Insipidus
- Vasopressin *V2* receptor mutation
- *AQP*-2 water channel mutation
- Acquired

Excessive vasopressinase activity in pregnancy

involving the hypothalamus, pituitary stalk, or posterior pituitary. In addition, a point mutation interfering with the processing of the neurophysin-ADH prohormone that not only causes diabetes insipidus but may also lead to neuronal degeneration in the hypothalamic supraoptic and periventricular nuclei has been described. Other structural defects affecting the region include tumors, cysts, hypothalamic-pituitary surgery or trauma, infiltrative processes, autoimmune destruction, and lymphocytic infundibulohypophysitis, the latter may be associated with anterior pituitary dysfunction. NDI may occur congenitally from a mutation of the vasopressin V2 receptors in the renal collecting duct epithelium that disrupts receptor folding and interferes with are responsible for activation of G-proteins and the generation of cAMP. Ninety percent of cases of NDI are X-linked and occur in males, but females may exhibit a similarly severe defect in ADH action owing to inactivation of the normal X chromosome. In females, however, the likely genetic defect is a mutation of the aquaporin-2 (*AQP*-2) water channel, which mediates the renal effects of ADH and may also cause congenital NDI. When obvious causes of diabetes insipidus are not present, most cases of diabetes insipidus are termed *idiopathic*, although vasopressin antibodies have been detected in ~33% of patients, providing an alternative mechanism for the observed central diabetes insipidus. An additional genetic defect involving the aquaporin-2 water channel which represents the terminal renal effect of ADH may also cause congenital nephrogenic diabetes insipidus.

Other causes of NDI include chronic renal disease; hypercalcemia; hypokalemia;conditions which interrupt the renal medullary concentrating mechanism and drugs including lithium, demeclocycline, colchicine, and methoxyflurane anesthesia. Many of these factors have recently been shown to downregulate AQP-2 and AQP-3, thereby disrupting the renal medulla concentrating mechanism. ADH deficiency may also occur during pregnancy owing to the excessive secretion of placental vasopressinase, which destroys the circulating ADH, and may be associated with preeclampsia, coagulopathies, and rarely oligohydramnios. This disorder remits following parturition, as the vasopressinase concentrations rapidly disappear from the maternal circulation.

3.5. Thyroid Hormones

3.5.1. Hyperthyroidism

Excessive circulating quantities of thyroid hormone bind to the widely distributed nuclear thyroid hormone receptor and lead to an increase in metabolic rate and cell proliferation and increase tissue sensitivity to catecholamines. Thus, the signs and symptoms of hyperthyroidism include tachycardia, tremor, piloerection, increased perspiration, weight loss, elevation of cardiac output with a wide pulse pressure, nervousness, heat intolerance, hyperreflexia, proximal muscle weakness, and hyperdefecation.

Several different mechanisms and pathologic states have been identified that lead to similar signs and symptoms of thyrotoxicosis (Table 13). Activation of the TSH receptor or TSH receptor–coupled signal pathway is the most common endogenous cause of hyperthyroidism. The rare TSH-producing pituitary adenoma leads to the presence of hyperthyroidism and goiter because of excessive autonomous secretion of TSH by the pituitary tumor. TSH stimulates both growth of thyroid follicular cells and thyroid hormone synthesis and release. Receptor crossreaction is the mechanism by which hCG-secreting tumors account for hyperthyroidism. Although this may occasionally be seen in a patient with choriocarcinoma of the testes or ovary, most patients who have hCG-induced hyperthyroidism harbor a hydatidiform mole, which secretes enormous quantities of the placental glycoprotein hormone. Since the α-subunit of each of the glycoprotein hormones is virtually identical and the β-subunits share some degree of homology, it is not surprising that hCG has intrinsic TSH-like activity. The most common cause of endogenous hyperthyroidism is Graves disease, an autoimmune process associated with the production of thyroid-stimulating Igs. These Igs bind with the TSH receptor and mimic the action of TSH, causing growth

Table 13
Etiologies of Thyrotoxicosis

TSH receptor and signaling pathway mediated
- TSH-producing pituitary tumors
- hCG-producing tumors
- Thyroid-stimulating Ig production (Graves disease)
- Constitutive activation of TSH receptor
- Constitutive activation of $G_s\alpha$

Autonomous production
- Toxic nodule or toxic multinodular goiter
- Thyroid carcinoma

Release of preformed thyroid hormone (thyroiditis)
- Autoimmune process (Graves)

Exogenous thyroid hormone intake

Drug induced (amiodarone)

of the thyroid and synthesis and release of thyroid hormones. Constitutive activation of the TSH receptor owing to a mutation leads to continuous stimulation of its G protein and adenylyl cyclase. This type of lesion has been shown to cause congenital hyperthyroidism in neonates without a maternal history of Graves disease. The congenital form is caused by a germ-line mutation in the receptor. Activating somatic mutations in the thyrotropin receptor gene have also been noted in some patients with autonomously functioning adenomas associated with hyperthyroidism (hot nodules). Similarly, constitutive activation of the $G_s\alpha$-subunit has been found in some patients with toxic thyroid adenomas. Another mechanism of hyperthyroidism is release of preformed thyroid hormone from the thyroid gland. This is found in various inflammatory conditions involving the thyroid gland. It is perhaps most prominent in patients with subacute thyroiditis in which a viral inflammation of the thyroid gland leads to disruption of the normal follicles and release of thyroid hormone. This is a self-limited condition, and once all of the thyroid hormone is released, patients usually go through a period of hypothyroidism before the thyroid recovers and the thyroid hormone levels return to normal. Acute release of thyroid hormone can also be seen in some patients with autoimmune (Hashimoto) thyroiditis and in the postpartum state in women who develop a self-limited autoimmune thyroiditis. Thyroid hormone may be produced autonomously by toxic adenomas without a known defect in the TSH receptor or signal pathway as well as in patients with a large body burden of thyroid carcinoma. In the latter situation, although individual thyroid carcinoma cells are relatively inefficient in the production of thyroid hormone, a large mass of well-differentiated thyroid cancer may produce sufficient quantities of thyroxine and triiodothyronine (T_3)

to cause hyperthyroidism. In addition, several drugs may interfere with thyroid function, leading to thyrotoxicosis. Amiodarone is an iodine-rich drug that has become extremely popular because of its effectiveness in controlling cardiac arrythmias. The drug strikingly resembles levorotatory thyroxine (T_4) and it exerts complex effects on the thyroid by inhibition of types 1 and 2 5′-deiodinases and direct cytotoxic effects on thyroid cells resulting in increased T_4 and decreased TSH levels.

3.5.2 HYPOTHYROIDISM

The clinical manifestations of hypothyroidism depend on the age of onset. Untreated congenital hypothyroidism results in cretinism associated with diffuse puffiness, short stature, mental retardation, and neurologic abnormalities. In children and adolescents, growth retardation, decreased mental concentrating ability and school performance, as well as precocious puberty may be found. In adults, periorbital and peripheral puffiness, cold intolerance, weight gain, constipation, muscle cramps, decreased mental concentrating ability, and easy fatigability are common. Table 14 gives the etiologies of hypothyroidism according to the level of the defect. Tertiary or hypothalamic hypothyroidism may accompany multiple tropic hormone deficiencies in patients with panhypopituitarism or may occur as a monotropic deficiency in the secretion of thyrotropin-releasing hormone (TRH). It is not known whether this is owing to mutation in the TRH gene or owing to processing or secretory abnormality. Drugs, including thyroid hormones and α-adrenergic blockers, decrease hypothalamic TRH production. Secondary or pituitary hypothyroidism may be seen in patients with structural abnormalities of the thyrotrope because of replacement by tumor; infiltrative processes or vascular compromise; or congenital absence of the thyrotrope because of a mutation in the *PROP*1, *HESX*1, and *Pit*-1 genes, which is apituitary-specific intranuclear transcription factors necessary for the development and function of somatotropes, lactotropes and thyrotropes. Point mutations in the *TSH*-β-subunit gene may cause congenital hypothyroidism. A form of TSH with reduced biologic activity because of altered glycosylation has been found in some patients with hypothalamic hypothyroidism who exhibit slightly increased levels of immunoreactive TSH activity despite profound central hypothyroidism.

Congenital primary hypothyroidism is found in patients who have mutations in thyroid-specific transcription factors *PAX*8 and *TTF*2 resulting in dysgenesis of the thyroid gland, or thyroid hypoplasia owing to loss-of-function mutations in the *TSH* receptor.

Table 14
Etiologies of Hypothyroidism

Tertiary (hypothalamic) hypothyroidism
- TRH deficiency
- Drug induced

Secondary (pituitary) hypothyroidism
- Thyrotrope destruction
  - Congenital *PROP*-1, *HESX*-1, *Pit*-1 mutation
  - Acquired
- *TSH*-β-subunit mutation
- Altered glycosylation

Primary (thyroidal) hypothyroidism
- Congenital
  - Thyroid dysgenesis
  - TSH receptor defects
    - Congenital owing to receptor mutation
    - Autoimmune blocking antibodies
- TSH postreceptor $G_s\alpha$ mutation
- Iodide transport defect
- Biosynthetic enzyme defects
- Thyroglobulin mutation
- Acquired
  - Destruction
  - Iodine deficiency
  - Drug induced

End organ defects
- Thyroid hormone nuclear receptor defect (thyroid hormone resistance syndromes)

Goitrous congenital primary hypothyroidism may occur with inactivating point mutations of the *TSH* receptor or the G protein that couples the receptor to adenylyl cyclase. A more common cause of a TSH receptor problem is TSH receptor blocking antibodies produced in women with autoimmune thyroid disease that cross the placenta, enter the fetal circulation, and bind to the fetal thyroid TSH receptors. Deficiencies of thyroid peroxidase enzyme, iodotyrosine deiodinase, or of the follicular cell iodide transport (trapping mechanism) also result in hypothyroidism. Mutations in the *thyroglobulin* gene have been found to result in a thyroglobulin molecule that is incapable of functioning properly for the formation of T_4 or T_3. Iodine deficiency, the ingestion of goitrogens, and thyroiditis are additional acquired causes of primary hypothyroidism. Defects in the thyroid hormone nuclear receptors lead to resistance to the effect of thyroid hormones. The defects are due to mutations in the *thyroid hormone–receptor* β-gene, and the clinical manifestations depend on whether there is generalized resistance to thyroid hormones or selective pituitary resistance.

There is a great deal of phenotypic variability in different families with generalized resistance to thyroid hormone. Some individuals demonstrate marked hypothyroidism, whereas other have very mild degrees of hypothyroidism that are compensated for by an increased secretion of TSH resulting in thyroid growth and production of normal quantities of thyroid hormones. Patients with pituitary resistance to thyroid hormones secrete increased quantities of TSH, which results in goiter and hyperthyroidism, because the peripheral tissues are not resistant to the effects of the thyroid hormone.

3.6. Calcium Abnormalities

3.6.1. HYPERCALCEMIA

An elevation of serum calcium concentration leads to depression of CNS function, increased gastrin secretion and gastric acid production, decreased renal response to ADH, increased peripheral vascular resistance, increased ionotropic effect on the myocardium, and decreased contractility of smooth and skeletal muscles. Hence, patients with hypercalcemia often complain of weakness, anorexia, nausea, vomiting, abdominal pain, constipation, polyuria, and thirst. They may exhibit confusion, personality disturbances, obtundation, and coma.

Multiple pathophysiologic mechanisms are responsible for the development of hypercalcemia (Table 15). Overproduction of PTH from a parathyroid adenoma or hyperplastic parathyroid glands results in hyperparathyroidism, which stimulates osteoclastic bone resorption with release of calcium and phosphorus into the circulation. This may occur sporadically or as part of the multiple endocrine neoplasia (MEN) syndromes type 1 due to inactivating mutations of the tumor suppressor gene encoding the transcription factor *MENIN* or as part of the MEN 2a resulting from mutations in the *RET* tyrosine kinase receptor gene.

The elevated PTH also stimulates the renal 1α-hydroxylation of 25-(OH)-vitamin D, converting it into $1,25\text{-}(OH)_2$-vitamin D, which enhances the absorption of calcium from the gastrointestinal (GI) tract. In a similar manner, the overproduction of PTH-related protein, which binds to the PTH receptor, may also cause hypercalcemia through similar mechanisms. A number of cytokines including the interleukins IL-1β and IL-6, tumor necrosis factor-β, and RANKL, as well as prostaglandins produced locally by tumors present in the bone, may stimulate osteoclastic bone resorption, releasing calcium into the circulation. If the calcium load exceeds the ability of the kidneys to excrete it, then hypercalcemia results. Some tumors such as lymphomas cause hypercalcemia through the presence of a 25-(OH)-vitamin D-1αa-hydroxylase enzyme that converts 25-(OH)-vitamin D into $1,25\text{-}(OH)_2$-vitamin D, causing a hypervitaminosis D syndrome. A similar mechanism of hypercalcemia is found in patients with granulomatous

Table 15
Etiologies of Hypercalcemia

Hyperparathyroidism

Malignancy associated
- PTH-related protein production
- Cytokine production
- Prostaglandin secretion
- Dysregulation of 25-(OH)-Vitamin D-1α-hydroxylase

Granulomatous disease

Other endocrine disease
- Hyperthyroidism
- Hypothyroidism
- Adrenal insufficiency

Metabolic bone disease with immobilization

Drug induced

Familial hypocalciuric hypercalcemia

diseases. Mild hypercalcemia can be found in patients with hyperthyroidism presumably owing to the rapid turnover of bone during the hypermetabolic state. Hypercalcemia is also associated with hypothyroidism and adrenal insufficiency through mechanisms that are presently unclear. Patients with metabolic bone disease associated with rapid bone turnover who are immobilized lose the piezoelectric effect, which stimulates osteoblastic bone formation, and, therefore, there can be at least transient uncoupling of bone resorption and bone formation favoring resorption. A number of drugs are associated with hypercalcemia including vitamin D and vitamin A excess and lithium carbonate. Familial hypocalciuric hypercalcemia is found in patients who have a mutation in the calcium-sensing receptor. This results in an increase in the feedback regulatory set point of serum calcium on parathyroid gland PTH secretion. Thus, a higher level of serum calcium is needed to inhibit PTH secretion in patients with this syndrome. Such patients generally demonstrate mild hypercalcemia and hypocalciuria and may have parathyroid hyperplasia. The effects of PTH on the kidney increase the reabsorption of calcium; hence, for a given level of serum calcium, these patients have hypocalciuria in contrast to healthy individuals or those with non-PTH-mediated hypercalcemia.

3.6.2. HYPOCALCEMIA

A decrease in the serum ionized calcium concentration results in CNS depression and muscular irritability. Patients usually complain of lethargy, confusion, irritability, dry skin, and muscle cramps and often demonstrate emotional lability and confusion. Neuromuscular irritability can be demonstrated on physical examination.

Since calcium is regulated by both PTH and vitamin D, disorders of these hormonal systems may result in hypocalcemia (Table 16). Decreased PTH secretion can be found in patients born with structural defects in the parathyroid gland as well as in individuals who have mutations involving parathyroid hormone processing. Structural defects of the parathyroid gland can occasionally occur with infiltrative disorders, but the most common acquired structural problem results from thyroid or parathyroid surgery with extirpation of the parathyroid glands or compromise of their vascular supply. A functional defect in the secretion of PTH is found in patients who have magnesium deficiency, which also results in decreased responsiveness of the bone to PTH. Other causes of PTH resistance are defective PTH receptors owing to a mutation to the receptor itself (pseudohypoparathyroidism type IB) or to an inactivating $G_{s\alpha}$ mutation in the *PTH receptor*–signaling pathway (Albright hereditary osteodystrophy, pseudohypoparathyroidism type 1A). PTH resistance is also found in patients who have renal insufficiency.

Abnormalities in vitamin D production, absorption, or metabolism result in a decrease in absorption of calcium and phosphorus from the GI tract. Mutations of the *vitamin D* nuclear receptor also result in decreased absorption of calcium and phosphorus from the diet and are responsible for the syndrome of $1,25\text{-}(OH)_2$-vitamin D–resistant rickets. Hypocalcemia may also occur from chelation with phosphate, which leads to deposition of calcium phosphate in soft tissues, and from saponification of fat in patients with fulminant acute hemorrhagic pancreatitis. Rarely osteoblastic metastases may be so extensive that hypocalcemia is found. Finally, a variety of drugs may bring about hypocalcemia through inhibition of osteoclastic bone resorption, chelation, or alterations in vitamin D metabolism.

3.7. Glucose Abnormalities

3.7.1. HYPOGLYCEMIA

Hypoglycemia results in two types of symptoms: those caused by a rapid rate of fall of the blood glucose resulting in stimulation of the sympathoadrenal system and those reflecting the low level of blood sugar on CNS function (neuroglycopenic systems). When the sympathetic nervous system and adrenal medulla are activated, patients develop tachycardia, piloerection, anxiety, tremulousness, diaphoresis, and hunger. Levels of plasma glucose below 36 mg/L lead to difficulties with concentration, fatigue, headache, confusion, seizures, and coma. Table 17 presents a simple classification scheme of the causes of hypoglycemia based on pathophysiology. Excessive stimulation of the insulin receptor can occur when the pancreatic islet of Langerhans

Table 16
Etiologies of Hypocalcemia

Decreased PTH secretion
- Congenital structural defects of parathyroids
- PTH-processing defect
- Acquired structural defects
- Acquired functional defects

PTH resistance
- Defective PTH receptor (pseudohypoparathyroidism type IB)
- PTH $G_{s\alpha}$ mutation (pseudohypoparathyroidism type IA)
- Renal insufficiency
- Magnesium deficiency

Active vitamin D production abnormalities
- Deficient intake or sunlight
- Vitamin D malabsorption
- Abnormal metabolism
- Congenital renal 1α-hydroxylase deficiency (Vitamin D–dependent rickets type I)

Vitamin D receptor abnormalities
- $1,25\text{-}(OH)_2$-Vitamin D–resistant rickets
- Renal insufficiency

Excessive tissue deposition
- Hyperphosphatemia
- Acute hemorrhagic pancreatitis
- Osteoblastic metastases

Drug induced

secretes excessive quantities of insulin. Islet cell hyperplasia from adenomatosis or nesidioblastosis, as well as autonomously functioning benign or malignant islet cell neoplasms, secretes insulin regardless of the blood sugar concentration. Hyperstimulation of the insulin receptor leads to increased glucose uptake by a multitude of tissues while inhibiting hepatic glucose production. Similarly, increased insulin secretion is found in patients who have an alimentary form of hypoglycemia following gastric surgery. The rapid transit and absorption of carbohydrate leads to stimulation of insulin secretion and elevation of insulin levels at a time when the plasma glucose has decreased. The hyperinsulinemia reduces the glucose further, leading to hypoglycemic symptoms. IGF-2 is produced ectopically by nonislet cell tumors associated with hypoglycemia. Many of these tumors are derived from mesenchymal tissues such as retroperitoneal fibrosarcomas and mesotheliomas. The hypoglycemia associated with ectopic IGF-2 production may be the result of IGF-2 acting through the insulin receptor or the IGF-1 receptor. Although the majority of patients with the Kahn type B insulin resistance syndrome associated with anti–insulin receptor antibodies have hyperglycemia, some will develop intermittent hypoglycemia. The syndrome occurs in individuals with

Table 17
Etiologies of Hypoglycemia

Excessive insulin receptor stimulation
- Increased insulin secretion
  - Islet cell tumor
  - Islet hyperplasia
  - Alimentary
- Ectopic IGF-2 production
- Anti–insulin receptor antibodies
- Anti–insulin antibodies

Deficiency of glucose contraregulatory hormones
- GH
- ACTH
- Cortisol
- Thyroid hormone
- Catecholamines
- Glucagon

Defective hepatic glucose production
- Liver disease
- Gluconeogenic substrate deficiency

Drug induced

Table 18
Etiologies of Hyperglycemia

Inadequate insulin production
- Type 1 and 2 diabetes mellitus
- Mutation of proinsulin/insulin gene
  - Proinsulin-processing defect
  - Insulin gene point mutations
- Pancreatic disease
- Drug induced

Insulin receptor defect
- Mutation of insulin receptor gene
- Receptor downregulation
- Antireceptor antibody

Excessive production of glucose contraregulatory hormones
- GH
- Cortisol
- Catecholamines
- Glucagon

other abnormalities of the immune system including elevated levels of antinuclear and and anti-DNA antibodies; elevated IgG, IgM, and IgA concentrations; leukopenia; decreased serum complement levels; proteinuria; alopecia; and vitiligo. This condition has also been found in patients with systemic lupus erythematosus, thrombocytopenia, primary biliary cirrhosis, and scleroderma. Another rare immune-mediated cause of hypoglycemia is the appearance of antiinsulin antibodies in individuals who have not been exposed to exogenous insulin. These antibodies bind endogenous insulin

and, at times, the insulin will disassociate from the antibody, resulting in hypoglycemia. This phenomenon has been found in patients with Graves disease and conditions such as multiple myeloma and lymphoma.

GH, ACTH, cortisol, thyroid hormones, catecholamines, and glucagon are all required for glucose homeostasis. Congenital or acquired deficiencies of one or more of these hormones may be associated with hypoglycemia. In the absence of food intake, plasma glucose concentrations are maintained initially through glycogenolysis and then gluconeogenesis. Patients who have liver disease or are unable to generate sufficient quantities of gluconeogenic amino acids develop hypoglycemia. Finally, several drugs are associated with hypoglycemia either through induction of hyperinsulinemia (sulfonylureas, pentamidine) or without hyperinsulinemia (alcohol).

3.7.2. HYPERGLYCEMIA

Hyperglycemia, whether owing to insulin-dependent type 1 or non-insulin-dependent type 2 diabetes mellitus or to secondary diabetes, results in osmotic diuresis with loss of water and electrolytes. Patients therefore develop polyuria, polydipsia, polyphagia, weight loss, weakness, and fatigue. If the serum hyperosmolality is very high and the degree of dehydration severe, then obtundation and coma may be present. With severe insulin deficiency, ketoacidosis may develop, resulting in dehydration; rapid, deep respirations; stupor; and coma. Patients with long-standing, poorly controlled diabetes may also exhibit retinopathy, neuropathy, and nephropathy.

From a pathophysiologic standpoint, hyperglycemia may be caused by inadequate insulin production, insulin receptor defects, or excessive production of glucose contraregulatory hormones (Table 18). Both type 1 and 2 diabetes mellitus are associated with inadequate insulin production, with type 1 showing a more profound defect. Inadequate biologically active insulin production is also seen with point mutations of the *proinsulin/insulin* gene resulting in either a proinsulin-processing defect with hyperproinsulinemia or an abnormal circulating insulin.

Pancreatic diseases such as acute pancreatitis or pentamidine-induced β-cell destruction are associated with inadequate insulin production, as is also seen with a variety of drugs such as diazoxide, thiazide diuretics, or phenytoin, which reduce the release of insulin from the pancreas.

Several different mutations affecting the *insulin receptor* gene have been found. Some of these mutations are associated with decreased insulin binding to the receptor, whereas others result in impaired transport of insulin to the cell surface; a decrease in the receptor-associated tyrosine kinase activity; or, in some instances, accelerated receptor degradation. Occupation of the insulin receptor by anti–insulin receptor antibodies is associated with insulin resistance in Kahn type B insulin resistance. Patients who exhibit marked insulin resistance because of mutations or antireceptor antibodies also may have acanthosis nigricans. In women with this syndrome, polycystic ovaries are often present and are associated with increased ovarian production of testosterone, hirsutism, and virilization. Several conditions that are associated with hyperinsulinemia also lead to downregulation of insulin receptor. This is commonly seen in patients with type 2 diabetes as well as obesity. Excessive production of the glucose contraregulatory hormones—GH, cortisol, catecholamines, or glucagon—is also associated with hyperglycemia, generally through a postreceptor antagonism of insulin action.

3.8. Abnormalities of Adipocytes (Table 19)

3.8.1. OBESITY

It is estimated that approx 60% of individuals in the United States are obese, and the consequences account for almost 300,000 deaths/yr. Obese persons, particularly those with excess abdominal fat, are at increased risk of diabetes, hypertension, dyslipidemia, and ischemic heart disease. Clearly body size depends on a complex interaction between genetic background and environmental factor. In humans, genetic background explains only approx 40% of the variance in body mass, whereas eating large serving sizes and having a sedentary lifestyle account in large part for the recent dramatic increase in obesity. Striking examples of the powerful effect of environment on obesity and diabetes include the Pima Indians who live in Arizona and now derive 50% of their energy from fat, as opposed to 15% in their traditional diet, and the aborigines of Northern Australia, where urbanized populations are much heavier than their usually lean (body mass index [BMI] <20 kg/m^2) hunter-gatherer kindred.

Traditionally, adipocytes have been viewed as energy depots that store triglycerides during feeding, but, increasingly, the role of adipocyte factors, "adipokines," in a complex variety of physiologic functions has emerged and has important implications for understanding the relationship between obesity and other diseases including diabetes, and lipid abnormalities. For example, adipocytes produce leptin, which mediates pleiotrophic effects on food intake, hypothalamic neuroendocrine regulation, reproductive function, and energy expenditure. Leptin deficiency due to frameshift or single-base mutations in the *leptin* gene and transmembranal and

Table 19
Etiologies of Obesity and Lipodystropyhy

Obesity

Hypothalamic
- Congenital (Prader-Willi)
- Structural (hypothalamic tumor)

Pituitary
- Congenital (*POMC, MCR*-4, *PC*1, *PC*2 mutation)

Adipocyte
- *Leptin* receptor
- *PPAR*-γ

Lipodystrophy
- Familial or genetic types
- Congenital generalized lipodystrophy (Berardinelli-Seip syndrome)
- Familial partial lipodystrophies (Dunnigan, Kobberling, and mandibuloacral dysplasia varieties)
- Acquired
  - Generalized (Lawrence syndrome)
  - Partial (Barraquer-Simons syndrome)
  - HIV associated
- Localized (drug or pressure induced, panniculitis variety, idiopathic)

intracellular mutations in the *leptin receptor* are rare and have only been described in several extremely obese individuals. Indeed, leptin levels are generally proportionate to adipose mass, and the vast majority of obese humans may be considered to manifest a leptin-resistant rather than a leptin-deficient state. One potential mechanism underlying the development of leptin resistance in humans is thought to be suboptimal transport of leptin through the blood-brain barrier. Although clinical studies have demonstrated that leptin treatment is safe, well tolerated, and effective in individuals with congenital leptin deficiency, only modest weight reduction and loss of fat mass were seen following high-dose leptin treatment (0.3 mg/kg) in two short-term studies of obese individuals, indicating that exogenously administered leptin is unlikely to overcome leptin resistance and cause effective weight reduction in obese humans.

A mutation in the prohormone convertase 1 (*PC*1) gene that cleaves POMC and proinsulin among other peptides led to reduced melanocortins in a single patient, and, interestingly, haploinsufficiency of the MCR-4 appears to be the most common monogenic cause of human obesity, responsible for up to 5% of severe pediatric obesity. A null mutation in the *POMC* gene has also been described in two children with hyperphagia; in addition to ACTH insufficiency, these children had red hair, presumably owing to lack of α-MSH (another POMC cleavage product)-stimulated melanin.

The nuclear receptor peroxisome proliferator–activated receptor-γ (PPAR-γ) plays a key role in adipogenesis and is essential for adipocyte development. Recently, a gain-of-function mutation in the N-terminal domain of *PPAR-γ* resulting in a receptor with constitutive transcriptional function has been described in four morbidly obese subjects (BMI >38 kg/m^2). PPAR-γ exists as two isoforms, PPAR-γ-1 and -2, derived by alternate promoter usage, and much interest has focused on a polymorphism in the *PPAR-γ-2* gene that is exclusively expressed in the adipocyte and occurs in almost 15% of some Caucasian populations. However, although in some functional assays the PPAR-γ variant exhibited reduced DNA binding and modest impairment of transcriptional activation, and these properties correlated with reduced BMI, subsequent studies have been inconclusive.

3.8.2. LIPODYSTROPHY

The lipodystrophies are a heterogeneous group of adipose tissue disorders characterized by loss of fat that can be limited, resulting in well-demarcated SC depressed areas or indentations (localized forms), or extensive, with nearly complete loss of body fat, as seen in generalized forms. The extent of fat loss determines the severity of metabolic complications, such that patients with localized lipodystrophy may have cosmetic problems, whereas those with generalized lipodystrophy have severe insulin resistance, hypertriglyceridemia, diabetes mellitus at an early age, and fatty liver. As in some forms of obesity-associated insulin resistance, acanthosis nigricans may be a feature. In recent years, the pathogenesis of some of these extremely rare conditions has been elucidated. For example, loss-of-function mutations in the ligand-binding domain of *PPAR-γ* have been described in several adults. Intriguingly, these subjects all exhibit a stereotyped form of partial lipodystrophy, in which SC fat is lost from the limbs and gluteal region, but preserved in both the SC and visceral abdominal fat deposits. In addition, mutations in 1-acylglycerol-3-phosphate *O*-acyltransferase (*AGPAT*2), an enzyme that catalyzes the acylation of lysophosphatidic acid to form phosphatidic acid, and a key intermediate in the biosynthesis of triacylglycerol and glycerophospholipids, and BSCL2, which encodes seipin, a protein of unknown function, have also been described. Furthermore, the molecular characterization of lipodystrophy has led to further subclassification. For example, patients with typical features of mandibuloacral dysplasia and exhibiting marked loss of fat from the extremities but normal or increased truncal fat harbor mutations in the *LMNA* (lamin A/C gene), whereas patients with mandibuloacral dysplasia but generalized fat loss appear to have mutations in other as-yet unidentified

genes. Some patients with acquired generalized and localized lipodystrophy have clinical or serologic evidence of other autoimmune diseases such as Hashimoto thyroiditis or chronic active hepatitis, and autoantibodies to adipocyte membranes have recently been described in some individuals, raising the possibility that acquired generalized lipodystrophy may itself be an autoimmune disease. Combination antiretroviral therapy that includes human immunodeficiency virus-1 (HIV-1) protease inhibitors has been reported to cause lipodystrophy in many HIV-infected patients, and localized lipodystrophy was a frequent complication of insulin therapy before the availability of purified or human recombinant insulins. The presence of a high titer of insulin antibodies and response to local steroid injections again suggest an autoimmune mechanism. Occasionally, patients with lipodystrophy present a diagnostic dilemma, because the phenotype can resemble that seen in Cushing syndrome or following rapid weight loss in other conditions.

4. CONCLUSIONS

The study of each of the endocrine disorders presented in Tables 4–19 nicely illustrates the progression of clinicians' knowledge from bedside to bench and back to the patient. The initial descriptions of diseases such as precocious puberty, hypogonadism, hyperthyroidism, and hypothyroidism were confined to clinical and then biochemical observations of patients presenting with the disorders. As more patients were studied, it became clear that although the predominant clinical findings were similar, subtle differences existed with some of the clinical manifestations existed. For instance, boys who have central, gonadotropin-dependent precocious puberty exhibit enlargement of the testicles, whereas those who develop precocious puberty because of an androgen-secreting adrenal neoplasm retain small testicles. In a similar fashion, a patient presenting with secondary hypothyroidism will have a small thyroid gland, whereas an individual with primary hypothyroidism may have a goiter. As bioassays and immunoassays became available to measure the hormones involved, patients presenting with similar signs and symptoms could be subclassified and different pathophysiologic mechanisms to explain the findings formulated. The explosion of knowledge in cellular and molecular biology has allowed clinicians to understand further the diversity of mechanisms that give rise to endocrine diseases and to understand the differences in clinical manifestations of their patients. Just as advances in the understanding of endocrine diseases provides insight into the target tissue response to hormonal action, the advances in understanding of hormonal action provide insight into the mechanisms of endocrine disease. One of the lessons that clinicians have learned from clinical medicine, which is being reinforced by advances in understanding the molecular mechanisms for the various disease states, is that although a patient may present with signs and symptoms of a certain endocrine disease, the therapies used to treat one patient with the disease may not be appropriate for another patient presenting with a similar disease, because of a different hormonal or molecular pathologic abnormality. Thus, using methimazole or propylthiouracil to treat a patient with hyperthyroidism from Graves disease is appropriate because the hyperthyroxinemia in that disease results from enhanced synthesis and release of thyroid hormones. However, those drugs are inappropriate for a patient who has hyperthyroidism from subacute thyroiditis, because the hyperthyroxinemia in that situation results from disruption of the normal integrity of the thyroid with release of preformed thyroid hormones into the circulation. Clinicians' increased understanding of the unique pathophysiology of endocrine disease through molecular and cellular biology will ultimately lead to development and application of disease mechanism–specific subcellular therapies for patients.Once we are able to understand the specific pathophysiology for an endocrine disease presenting in aparticular patient, we should be able to design more specific therapies for treating that patient.

SELECTED READINGS

Bell GI, Froguel P, Nishi S, et al. Mutations of the human glucokinase gene and diabetes mellitus. *Trends Endocrinol Metab* 1993; 4:86.

Braunstein GD. Ectopic hormone production. In: Felig P, Baxter JD, Frohman LA, eds. *Endocrinology and Metabolism*, 3rd Ed. New York, NY: McGraw-Hill 1995:1733–1783.

Brent GA. The molecular basis of thyroid hormone action. *N Engl J Med* 1994;331:847.

Cohen L, Radovik S. Molecular basis of combined pituitary hormone deficiencies. *Endocr Rev* 2002; 23:431–442.

Garg A. Lipodystrophies. *Am J Med* 2000;108:143–152.

Gershenghorn M, Osman R. Insights into G protein–coupled receptor function using molecular models. *Endocrinology* 2001;142: 2–10.

Gurnell M, Savage DB, Chatterjee KK, O'Rahilly S. The metabolic syndrome: peroxisome proliferator-activated receptor γ and its therapeutic modulation. *J Clin Endocrinol Metab* 2003;88:2412–2421.

Haavisto A-M, Pettersson K, Bergendahl M, Virkamaki A, Huhtaniemi I. Occurrence and biological properties of a common genetic variant of luteinizing hormone. *J Clin Endocrinol Metab* 1995;80:1257.

Heaney AP, Melmed S. Molecular pathogenesis of pituitary tumors. In: Wass JAH, Shalet SM, eds. *Oxford Textbook of Endocrinology*. Oxford, UK: Oxford University Press 2002;109–120.

Jameson JL. Applications of molecular biology in endocrinology. In: DeGroot LT, et al., eds. *Endocrinology*, 3rd Ed. Philadelphia, PA: W.B. Saunders 1995:119–147.

Kopp R, van Sande J, Parma J, et al. Brief report: congenital hyperthyroidism caused by a mutation in the thyrotropin-receptor gene. *N Engl J Med* 1995;332:150.

Leo CP, Hsu SY, Hsueh AJW. Hormonal genomics. *Endocr Rev* 2003;23:369–381.

Ludgate ME, Vassart G. The thyrotropin receptor as a model to illustrate receptor and receptor antibody diseases. *Clin Endocrinol Metab* 1995;9:95.

Moreno JC, de Vijlder JJM, Vulsma T, Ris-Staplers C. Genetic basis of hypothyroidism: recent advances, gaps and strategies for future research. *Pediatr Endocrinol* 2003;14:318–326.

Nielsen S, Frokiaer J, Marples D, Kwon TH, Agre P, Knepper MA. Aquaporins in the kidney: from molecules to medicine. *Physiol Rev* 2002; 82:205–244.

Oral EA. Lipoatrophic diabetes and other related syndromes. *Rev Endocr Metab Disord* 2003;4:61–77.

Schwindinger WF, Levine MA. McCune-Albright syndrome. *Trends Endocrinol Metab* 1993;4:238.

Shenker A, Laue L, Kosugi S, Merendine JJ, Minegishi T, Cutler GB. A constitutively activating mutation of the luteinizing hormone receptor in familial male precocious puberty. *Nature* 1993; 365:652.

Silveira LFG, MacColl GS, Bouloux PMG. Hypogonadotropic hypogonadism. *Semin Reprod Med* 2002;20:327–338.

Smith EP, Boyd J, Frank GR, et al. Estrogen resistance caused by a mutation in the estrogen-receptor gene in a man. *N Engl J Med* 1994;331:1056.

Stewart PM. The adrenal cortex. In: Larsen PR, Kronenberg HM, Melmed S, Polonsky KS, eds. *Williams Textbook of Endocrinology*, 10th Ed. Philadelphia, PA: Saunders 2003:491–551.

Sunthornthepvarakul T, Gottschalk ME, Hayashi Y, Refetoff S. Brief report: resistance to thyrotropin caused by mutations in the thyrotropin-receptor gene. *N Engl J Med* 1995;332:155.

Taylor SI, Cama A, Kadowaki H, Kadowaki T, Accili D. Mutations of the human insulin receptor gene. *Trends Endocrinol Metab* 1990;1:134.

Vaisse C, Clement K, Durand E, et al. Melanocortin-4 receptor mutations are a frequent and heterogenous cause for morbid obesity. *J Clin Invest* 2000;106:185–187.

Veniant MM, LeBel CP. Leptin: from animals to humans. *Curr Pharm Des* 2003;9:811–818.

16 The Pineal Hormone (Melatonin)

Irina V. Zhdanova, MD, PhD
and Richard J. Wurtman, MD

1. INTRODUCTION

The pineal gland, or epiphysis cerebri (Fig. 1), a neuroendocrine organ, is one of the major parts of the circadian system, which also includes the eyes and the suprachiasmatic nuclei of the hypothalamus. The pineal gland exerts important regulatory influences by secreting its hormone, melatonin (Fig. 2), in variable amounts, depending on the time of day; the animal's age; and, in some species, the time of year. The daily rhythm in circulating melatonin is characterized by very low concentrations during the day and high levels at night (Fig. 3). This rhythm persists in constant darkness but can be altered by nighttime light exposure, because light can acutely suppress melatonin production. Normal daily variations in melatonin secretion synchronize numerous body rhythms and, in diurnal species, probably are important for nighttime sleep initiation and maintenance. Since the onset and offset of melatonin production by the pineal gland occur at dusk and dawn, respectively, the length of time per 24-h period that plasma melatonin levels are elevated can synchronize physiologic processes to seasonal changes and, in seasonal animals, can affect season-dependent functions

such as body temperature, locomotor activity, and reproductive behavior.

Lerner and colleagues first identified melatonin in 1958, as the constituent of bovine pineal glands that lightens isolated frog skin (by causing the melanin granules within the dermal melanophores to aggregate around the cell's nucleus). Initial studies on possible physiologic roles of melatonin focused on its effects on pigmentation (a phenomenon that is not observed in mammals) and on gonadal maturation. Kitay and Altschule had demonstrated that pinealectomy accelerated gonadal maturation in rats, and that administration of pineal extracts had the opposite effect. We then showed that melatonin was the constituent of bovine pineal extracts that was responsible for their antigonadal activity and suggested that melatonin thus is a hormone in mammals. On the basis of evidence that either removing a rat's pineal gland or exposing the maturing animal to continuous illumination caused equivalent—but not additive—increases in gonadal weight, we further proposed that light exposure suppressed the formation of the pineal gland's antigonadal hormone. Later results confirmed that light indeed suppresses melatonin synthesis, and that the rhythm in melatonin synthesis parallels the natural diurnal rhythm in environmental

From: *Endocrinology: Basic and Clinical Principles, Second Edition*
(S. Melmed and P. M. Conn, eds.) © Humana Press Inc., Totowa, NJ

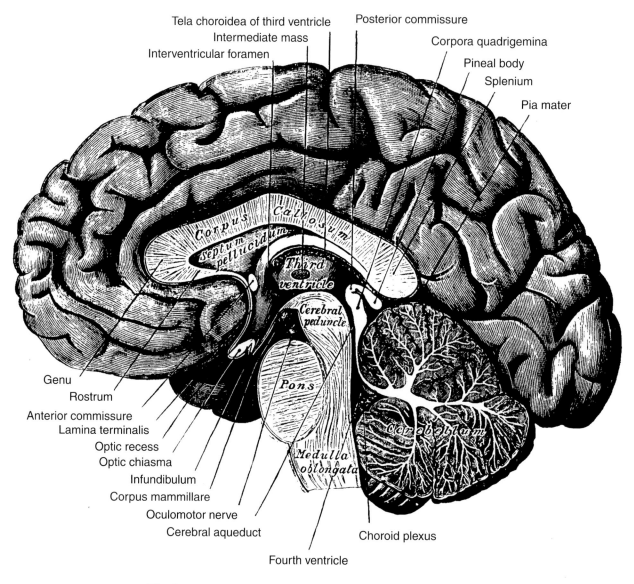

Tela choroidea of third ventricle
Intermediate mass
Interventricular foramen
Posterior commissure
Corpora quadrigemina
Pineal body
Splenium
Pia mater

Genu
Rostrum
Anterior commissure
Lamina terminalis
Optic recess
Optic chiasma
Infundibulum
Corpus mammillare
Oculomotor nerve
Cerebral aqueduct
Choroid plexus
Fourth ventricle

Fig. 1. Median sagittal section of brain. (Reproduced from Gray, 1985.)

illumination. Our laboratory also observed that serum melatonin levels in humans exhibit a characteristic daily pattern; levels are very low during the day (0.5–3 pg/mL), and can be as high as 200 pg/mL at night, with typical nighttime levels in adults of about 100 pg/mL. (Fig. 3).

The pineal gland and its hormone melatonin apparently are important components of the systems that organize rhythmic biochemical, physiologic and behavioral processes in living organisms. This chapter explores some of the fundamental mechanisms that control pineal function and that mediate melatonin's effects. It also considers possible clinical implications of impaired pineal function.

2. THE PINEAL GLAND

The pineal gland is a small unpaired organ located near the geometric center of the brain (Fig. 1). Its function has puzzled researchers for centuries. Postulates regarding this function have ranged from it being a mere vestigial appendage of the brain to Descartes' designation of the pineal gland as the "seat of the rational soul." Experimental investigation over the last half century has revealed that the pineal gland is indeed a biologically significant organ that has undergone profound changes in both form and cytologic differentiation during the course of evolution while retaining a functional role in the temporal organization of animal life.

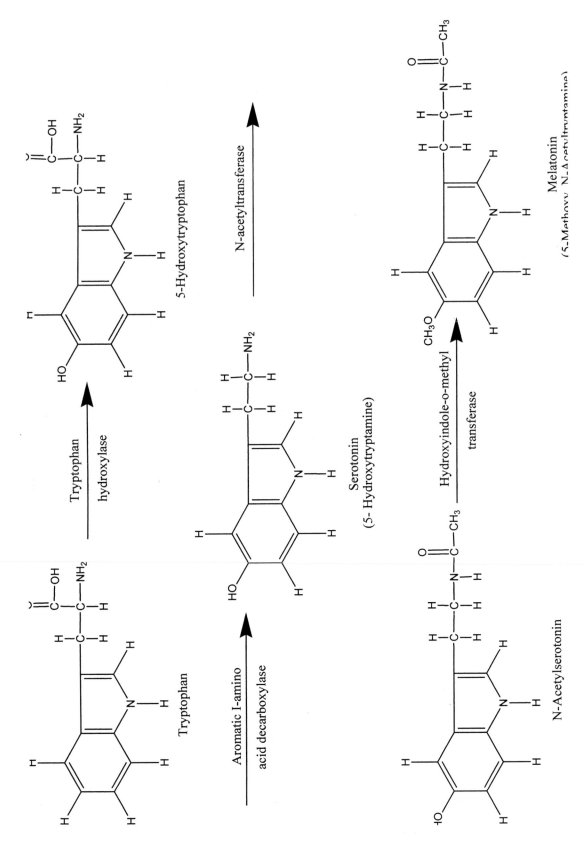

Fig. 2. Metabolism of tryptophan to melatonin in pineal gland.

257

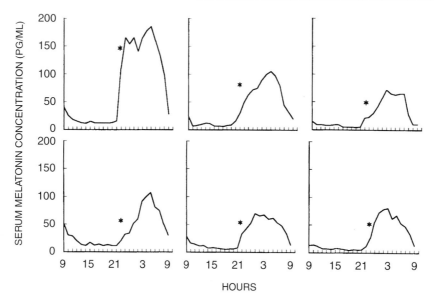

Fig. 3. Twenty-four-hour serum melatonin profiles measured from 9 ᴀᴍ to 9 ᴀᴍ in group of six young healthy males; *time of onset of habitual evening sleepiness.

Embryologically, the pineal organ arises as an evagination of the roof of the diencephalon. The diencephalon also gives rise to the lateral eyes and to the hypothalamus. This common embryologic origin is reflected in a common physiologic property—the capacity to respond to cyclic changes in environmental illumination. A fixed temporal pattern of photic input is an ubiquitous phenomenon, generated by Earth's daily rotation in reference to the sun. Viewed from an evolutionary perspective, the pineal origin is part of a sophisticated photoneuroendocrine system with photoreceptors represented both in the lateral eyes and, in some species (but not mammals), in the pineal organ itself. With development, this organ-system has acquired a unique feature: an endogenous, circadian (*circa* = around, *dian* = day) rhythmic pattern in its metabolic and/or neural activity. In mammals, a neuronal component of this neuroendocrine complex, the suprachiasmatic nuclei of the hypothalamus, displays a regular pattern of spontaneous neuronal discharges, entrained to the cyclic photic input, with a higher frequency during the daylight hours; this pattern persists in the absence of a day-night cycle. In vertebrate classes whose pineal organ possesses true photoreceptors (e.g., birds and reptiles), the pineal organ itself manifests a sustained circadian oscillation in melatonin biosynthesis. In the mammalian pineal organ, the absence of true photoreceptors is accompanied by the loss of this endogenous pace-setting capacity. Mammals thus rely on the suprachiasmatic nuclei for auto-

nomous circadian stimulation. Under natural conditions, the environmental light-dark cycle and the suprachiasmatic nuclei's endogenous oscillator act in concert to produce the daily rhythm in melatonin production. A complex neural pathway has evolved that relays information regarding environmental illumination from the ganglion layer of the retina to pinealocytes via the optic nerve, the suprachiasmatic nuclei, the lateral hypothalamus, and through the spinal cord by preganglionic fibers synapsing in the superior cervical ganglion. Postganglionic fibers reaching the pineal organ via the nervi conarii release norepinephrine at night. This neurotransmitter then activates adenylate cyclase, stimulating production of the second messenger cyclic adenosine monophosphate (cAMP), which accelerates melatonin synthesis. Exposure to sufficiently bright light qiuckly suppresses melatonin synthesis; however, under conditions of constant darkness a circadian rhythm in melatonin production persists, generated by the cyclic suprachiasmatic nuclei output.

3. MELATONIN SYNTHESIS AND SECRETION

The circulating amino acid L-tryptophan is the precursor of melatonin. Within pineal cells, it is converted to serotonin by a two-step process, catalyzed by the enzymes tryptophan hydroxylase and 5-hydroxytryptophan decarboxylase. Pineal serotonin concentrations in mammals are high during the daily light phase and decrease during the dark phase, when much of this indoleamine is converted into melatonin. This process, which occurs principally but not exclusively in the pineal gland (e.g., also in retina), involves serotonin's N-acetylation, catalyzed by an *N*-acetyltransferase enzyme, and its subsequent methylation by hydroxy-indole-*O*-methyltransferase gland (Fig. 2).

There is no evidence that melatonin is stored in the pineal gland; rather, the hormone is thought to be released directly into the bloodstream and the cerebrospinal fluid as it is synthesized. The pattern of melatonin secretion in humans is characterized by a gradual nocturnal increase, starting about 2 h prior to habitual bedtime, and a morning decrease in serum concentrations of the hormone (Fig. 3). About 50–70% of circulating melatonin is reportedly bound to plasma albumin; the physiologic significance of this binding remains unknown. Inactivation of melatonin occurs in the liver, where it is converted into 6-hydroxymelatonin by the P-450-dependent microsomal mixed-function oxidase enzyme system. Most of the 6-hydroxymelatonin is excreted into the urine and feces as a sulfate conjugate (6-sulfatoxymelatonin), and a much smaller amount as a glucuronide. Some melatonin may be converted into *N*-acetyl-5-methoxykynurenamine in the central nervous system. About 2 to 3% of the melatonin produced is excreted unchanged in the urine.

4. ONTOGENY OF MELATONIN SECRETION

Lower vertebrates start secreting melatonin at an early embryonic age. However, in mammals, including humans, the fetus and the newborn infant do not produce their own melatonin but rely on the hormone supplied via the placental blood and, postnatally, via the mother's milk. The few studies of the development of circadian functions in full-term human infants, including the melatonin secretory rhythm, the sleep-wake rhythm, and the body temperature rhythm, reveal an absence of circadian variation neonatally until 9–12 wk. Preterm babies display a substantial delay in the appearance of rhythmic melatonin production. Total melatonin production rapidly increases during the first year of life, with highest nighttime melatonin levels observed in children ages 1–3 yr. These high levels start to fall around the time of onset of puberty, decreasing substantially with physiologic aging (Fig. 4). Marked, unexplained interindividual variations in "normal" melatonin levels are observed in all age groups, so some elderly people do still exhibit relatively high serum melatonin levels. Several factors may explain the decline in melatonin concentration during the life-span, such as the increase in body mass from infancy to adulthood (which

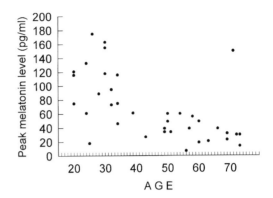

Fig. 4. Nighttime peak serum melatonin levels in subjects of different age (years).

results in a greater volume of distribution and, therefore, a decline in the melatonin concentration in body fluids even if melatonin production is almost constant); the calcification of the pineal gland with advancing age (which may suppress melatonin production); or a reduction in the sympathetic innervation of the pineal gland, which is essential for melatonin's nocturnal secretion (which may result in diminished melatonin production). High variability in melatonin production among individuals of the same age group could reflect, among other things, genetic predisposition, general health, and particular environmental lighting conditions. Determining the sources of this variability requires further investigation.

5. EFFECTS OF MELATONIN ON CELLULAR METABOLISM

Melatonin is a highly lipophilic hormone, permitting its ready penetration of biologic membranes and its ability to reach each cell in the body. The effects of melatonin appear to be mediated via specific melatonin receptors, two of which (MT1 and MT2) have been cloned and characterized in mammals. These G protein–coupled receptors are present in various body tissues, such as brain, retina, gonads, spleen, liver, thymus, and gastrointestinal tract, and inhibit the formation of two second messengers, cAMP (both MT1 and MT2) or cyclic guanosine 5′-monophosphate (MT2). In mammals, high-affinity melatonin receptors are consistently found in the pars tuberalis of the pituitary gland; such labeling is especially intensive in seasonal breeders and is believed to mediate the seasonal reproductive effects of melatonin. The suprachiasmatic nucleus (SCN) is another brain region rich in melatonin receptors. Animal-based studies suggest that its receptors allow melatonin to inhibit SCN neuronal firing and metabolism at nighttime. This effect, presumably mediated via MT1

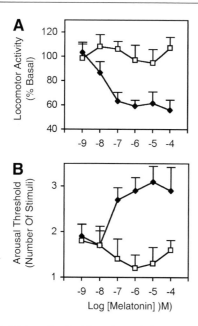

Fig. 5. Melatonin significantly and dose dependently reduces zebrafish locomotor activity (**A**) and increases arousal threshold (**B**) in larval zebrafish. Each data point represents the mean ± SEM group changes in a 2-h locomotor activity relative to basal activity, measured in each treatment or control group for 2 h prior to administration of treatment. Arousal threshold data are expressed as the mean ± SEM group number of stimuli necessary to initiate locomotion in a resting fish. (◆) treatment; (□) – vehicle control (*n* = 20 for each group). (Reproduced from Zhdanova et al., 2002.)

receptors, may contribute to the sleep-promoting effects of melatonin in diurnal species. On the other hand, MT2 receptors in the SCN can affect the circadian phase of SCN activity, either advancing or delaying it, depending on when in the cycle the melatonin is administered. These effects of melatonin might be important among lower vertebrates, in which the pineal gland responds directly to light.

Melatonin receptors are saturated at close-to-physiologic nocturnal melatonin concentrations; thus, their capacity to exhibit dose dependency is limited. One example of limited dose dependency, documented in both humans and diurnally active animals, is melatonin's sleep-promoting and activity-inhibiting effects. These behavioral effects in humans are initiated at melatonin levels close to those normally observed at the beginning of the night (about 50 pg/mL in blood plasma) but are not significantly enhanced when circulating levels are increased to substantially higher values (about 150 pg/mL). We found similar melatonin dose dependencies in macaques and zebrafish (Fig. 5). Furthermore, melatonin's effects depend on diurnal variations in the sensitivity of the melatonin receptors. Typically,

melatonin receptors are more sensitive during the daytime—i.e., at the time endogenous melatonin is not secreted—perhaps reflecting receptor upregulation in the absence of endogenous ligand. Augmented sensitivity to melatonin in the morning or in the evening hours may facilitate circadian phase shifts in response to small increases in melatonin secretion.

6. MELATONIN AND PHYSIOLOGIC FUNCTIONS

Diversity in the adaptive strategies employed by particular mammalian species may dictate how each species responds to the circadian signal provided by the release of melatonin. In both laboratory animals and humans, the effects of melatonin on behavioral rhythmicity, sleep, reproduction, and thermoregulation have been studied most extensively and are discussed in the following sections. Some investigators have also proposed that melatonin might affect immune function, intracellular antioxidative processes, aging, tumor growth, and certain psychiatric disorders.

6.1. Homeostatic and Circadian Regulation of Sleep

The concurrence of melatonin release from the pineal gland and the habitual hours of sleep in humans had led to the hypothesis that the former might be causally related to the latter. The effects of the administration of melatonin made it clear that melatonin can affect both homeostatic and circadian sleep regulation (i.e., the need to sleep after having been awake for a sufficient number of hours, and the desire to sleep at certain times of day or night), and that it does so at normal plasma melatonin levels. Although the acute sleep-promoting effect of doses of physiologic melatonin has been documented only in diurnal species (e.g., humans, fish, birds, monkeys), the circadian effects of melatonin appear to be similar in both nocturnal and diurnal species.

This phenomenon can be explained by temporal organization of the circadian system in diurnal and nocturnal species and its relation to habitual hours of sleep. Activation of the SCN and synthesis of melatonin in the pineal gland vary inversely in both nocturnal and diurnal species, with the metabolic and neuronal activity of the SCN high during the day, and the production of pineal melatonin low. This pattern is reversed during the night, when the SCN is relatively inactive and melatonin production is substantially increased. Acute exposure to light stimulation, mediated through the lateral eyes, produces an excitatory response in SCN neurons and inhibits melatonin production. On the other hand, melatonin itself exerts an acute inhibitory effect on SCN neuronal activity (Fig. 6). When environmental light

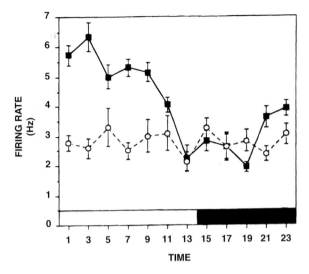

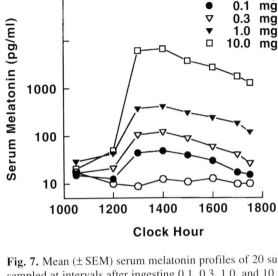

Fig. 6. Mean (± SEM) firing rates of SCN cells recorded in 2-h bins throughout daily cycle in slices from hamsters housed in a lighting cycle (■) or transferred to constant light for ~48 h before slice preparation (○). The lighting cycle for light:dark (LD) animals is illustrated at the bottom. (Reproduced from Guang-Di et al., 1993.)

Fig. 7. Mean (± SEM) serum melatonin profiles of 20 subjects sampled at intervals after ingesting 0.1, 0.3, 1.0, and 10 mg of melatonin or placebo at 11:45 AM. (Reproduced from Dollins et al., 1994.)

or melatonin is applied at an unusual time of day, such as bright light at the beginning of the night or melatonin in the afternoon, the phase of the circadian activity of the SCN shifts and, thus, advances or delays other circadian rhythms. Such circadian effects are similar in nocturnal and diurnal species. By contrast, the temporal relationship between sleep and activation of the circadian system is different in diurnal and nocturnal species. Nocturnal melatonin secretion is concurrent with habitual hours of sleep in diurnal animals and with peak activity levels in nocturnal animals. As a result, melatonin is linked to sleep initiation and maintenance in diurnal but not nocturnal species. Indeed, physiologic melatonin levels promote sleep in humans, diurnal primates, birds and fish, but not in rats or mice.

Initial human studies regarding the acute effects of melatonin treatment utilized pharmacologic doses of the hormone (1 mg to 6 g, orally), which tended to induce sleepiness and sleep. These effects of the pineal hormone were commonly considered to be "side effects" of the pharmacologic concentrations of melatonin induced. We then showed that low melatonin doses (0.1–0.3 mg), which elevate daytime serum melatonin concentrations to those normally occurring nocturnally (50–120 pg/mL) (Fig. 7), also facilitate sleep induction in young healthy adults when administered at the time of low sleep propensity (Fig. 8). The response occurs within 1 h of administration of the hormone and is independent of the time of day that the treatment is administered.

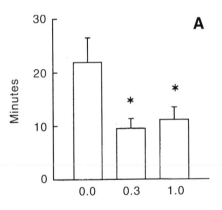

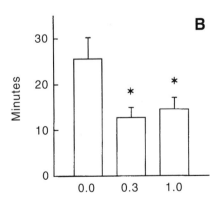

Fig. 8. Effects of melatonin (0.3 or 1.0 mg, orally) on average (± SEM) latency to (**A**) sleep onset and (**B**) stage 2 sleep relative to placebo (*n* = 11). Treatment was administered at the time of low sleep propensity, 2–4 h before habitual bedtime (*p < 0.005). (Reproduced from Zhdanova et al., 1996.)

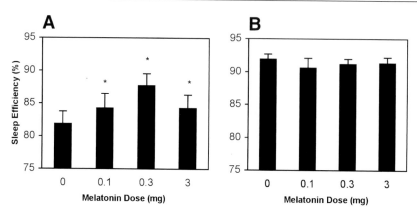

Fig. 9. Sleep efficiency in subjects with age-related insomnia (**A**) and normal sleep (**B**) following melatonin or placebo treatment ($^*p < 0.05$). (Reproduced from Zhdanova et al., 2001.)

Elevation of circulating melatonin level within the physiologic range, although improving sleep in people who have insomnia, does not cause significant changes in nocturnal sleep structure in people who experience normal sleep, and it is without untoward side effects (i.e., drowsiness) on the morning following treatment.

These results support the idea that in humans melatonin secretion is physiologically related to normal sleep. This relationship would explain the high correlation between the onset of evening sleepiness or habitual bedtime in people and the onset of their melatonin release late in the evening. It might also partially explain the high incidence of insomnia in the elderly, whose circulating melatonin levels are, in general, significantly lower than those in young adults. This hypothesis is further supported by the fact that the sleep of aged people with insomnia was significantly improved by doses of both physiologic (e.g., 0.1–0.3 mg) and pharmacologic (e.g., 3 mg) oral melatonin administered 30 min before habitual bedtime (Fig. 9A). Such treatments increased overnight sleep efficiency, principally by increasing it during the middle portion of the nocturnal sleep period and, to a lesser extent, during the latter third of the night (Fig. 10). By contrast, bedtime melatonin treatment did not modify sleep efficiency in older people in whom sleep already was normal (Fig. 9B), affirming melatonin's physiologic mode of action. Furthermore, melatonin had no discernible effect on sleep architecture, such as latency to rapid eye movement sleep or percentage of time spent in any of the five sleep stages, among healthy individuals or aged individuals with insomnia. Such disturbances are common complications encountered with many of the existing hypnotics.

Desynchronization of daily rhythms of sleep and melatonin secretion could occur as a result of: (1) complete blindness, when the melatonin rhythm free-runs

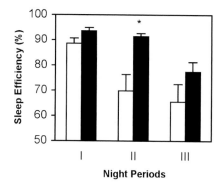

Fig. 10. Sleep efficiency in individuals with insomnia during three consecutive parts (I, II, III) of the night following placebo (□) or melatonin (0.3 mg, ■) treatment ($^*p < 0.05$). (Reproduced from Zhdanova et al., 2001.)

with a period either longer or shorter than 24 h; (2) pinealectomy or functional destruction of the pineal, resulting in a lack of melatonin production; (3) temporal displacement of the daylight period, as in transmeridian flight (the jet-lag syndrome) or shift work; or (4) the administration of drugs that block the release of norepinephrine from pineal sympathetic nerves, or the postsynaptic effects of the neurotransmitter. Such desynchronization might diminish the quantity and quality of sleep, a condition that then might be ameliorated by the timely administration of exogenous melatonin. If the goal is to entrain the circadian system to a specific time schedule (e.g., 24-h periodicity), it is critical to administer physiologic melatonin doses (0.1–0.3 mg, orally) at the same time, typically about 30 min prior to habitual bedtime. However, if the goal is to reentrain the circadian system to a new schedule (e.g., after a jet lag), the timing of melatonin treatment has to be carefully calculated in order to facilitate a phase shift, rather than oppose it. Administration of the hormone in the morning causes a phase delay, whereas evening treatment results in a phase advance. In this case, it is also important not to exceed physiological melatonin levels. The reason is that the residual circulating melatonin left, e.g., after evening melatonin treatment (Fig. 11) designed to advance the circadian rhythms, would produce a phase delay if still acting during the morning hours, thus dampening the overall efficacy of melatonin.

Because sleep is under control of the circadian clock, changes in the circadian phase will either cause a delay in the onset of evening sleepiness or advance it to an earlier hour. This property of melatonin found a useful application in the treatment of blindness-related sleep disorders; sleep alterations related to jet lag after transmeridian flight; and sleep disruption experienced by workers on rotating shifts, whose endogenous circadian rhythms are not synchronized with their rest-activity cycle.

6.2. Reproductive Physiology

The idea that pineal gland function in some way relates to gonadal expression originated with Heubner's 1898 description of a 4-yr-old boy who exhibited both precocious puberty and a nonparenchymal tumor that destroyed his pineal gland. The efficacy of the pineal hormone, melatonin, in modifying reproductive functions has been found to vary markedly, depending on the species and age of the animal tested, and the time of administration of melatonin relative to the prevailing light-dark schedule. Animal studies show that in seasonal breeders melatonin mediates the effects of changes in the photoperiod and, thus, the season of reproductive activity. Interestingly, the effects of exogenous melatonin on animals in which reproductive activity is inhibited during fall–winter (e.g.,

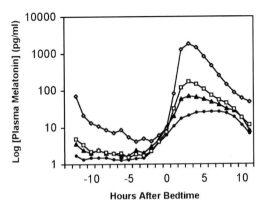

Fig. 11. Mean group ($n = 30$) plasma melatonin profiles during repeated melatonin or placebo treatment administered 30 min before bedtime. Daytime melatonin levels (i.e. before bedtime) reflect those after the previous night's treatment. (●) placebo; (▲) 0.1 mg; (□) 0.3 mg; (◆) 3 mg. (Reproduced from Zhdanova et al., 2001.)

hamsters) are opposite from its effects on animals that are reproductively passive during spring–summer (e.g., sheep) (Fig. 12).

Whether pineal melatonin secretion influences reproductive activity in nonseasonal mammals such as humans is still unclear. Melatonin could normally affect sexual maturation; however, observations regarding the relation between circulating melatonin levels and the onset of puberty in humans are inconsistent. There also are conflicting observations regarding serum melatonin levels during normal menstrual cycles in women. Some investigators report a transient decrease in nocturnal melatonin levels during the preovulatory phase; others fail to document any association between circulating

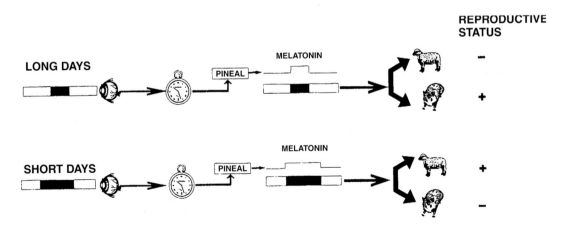

Fig. 12. Opposite effects of seasonal variation in day length and melatonin secretion period on reproductive status in different species. (Reproduced from Goldman, 2001.)

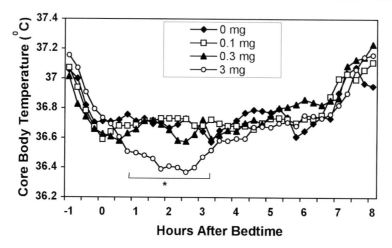

Fig. 13. Core body temperature profiles in adults over 50 yr of age following melatonin or placebo treatment ($^*p < 0.05$). (Reproduced from Zhdanova et al., 2001.)

melatonin and the phase of the menstrual cycle. Some patients with tumors involving pinealocytes, which result in an increased secretion of melatonin, reportedly displayed delayed puberty; nonparenchymal tumors, which presumably destroy pinealocytes and suppress melatonin production, have been associated with precocious puberty.

In women with amenorrhea whose estrogen levels are extremely low, serum melatonin concentrations are often substantially elevated. Exogenous estrogen also reportedly suppresses nocturnal melatonin secretion in women with secondary amenorrhea. Long-term suppression of estrogen synthesis in healthy women may lead to elevations in their circulating melatonin. Interestingly, in women with normal menstrual cycles and initially normal estrogen levels, treatment with conjugated estrogen did not suppress circulating melatonin levels. These findings suggest that there is an inhibitory feedback control of pineal function by estrogen, and that responses depend on the initial status of the organism. Other dysfunctions of the reproductive system may also be associated with abnormal melatonin levels: girls with central idiopathic precocious puberty may show diminished levels of circulating melatonin, and some cases of male primary hypogonadism are reportedly associated with elevated serum melatonin.

6.3. Thermoregulation

The daily decline in body temperature occurs 1 to 2 h prior to the onset of increased melatonin release from the pineal gland, and peak plasma melatonin concentrations precede the temperature minimum by about 2 h. Thus, although these two circadian rhythms have an inverse relationship, their extremes do not coincide and the decline in daytime temperature normally precedes the increase in melatonin production.

Animal studies reveal a hyperthermic effect of pinealectomy in some species (sparrows, chickens, rabbits, sheep), and an absence of effect or hypothermia in others (rats and hamsters). Exposure to bright light or administration of a β-adrenergic antagonist at night, which blocks sympathetic input to the pineal gland, suppresses melatonin production and increases core body temperature. Both pharmacologic and physiologic doses of melatonin are reported to be effective in reestablishing such experimentally modified temperature levels. By contrast, the administration of a physiologic melatonin dose (0.1–0.3 mg, orally) to human subjects whose core body temperature was not experimentally altered left temperature values unchanged, whereas a hypothermic effect of melatonin powerfully manifested after a pharmacologic dose (3 mg) of the hormone had been administered (Fig. 13). Indeed, human studies consistently show that pharmacologic doses of the hormone suppress daytime and nighttime core body temperature. It has been suggested, for some time, that sleep-promoting effects of melatonin in humans might be related to its hypothermic effects. Although a substantial reduction in body temperature following administration of high pharmacologic doses of melatonin might contribute to overall sedation, the clear dissociation between the doses required to produce hypnotic and hypothermic effects (compare the data in Figs. 9 and 13, collected in the same group of subjects) suggests that these two phenomena may not be related. Studies in fish and in birds showing dissociation between sleep and temperature-related effects of melatonin further confirm this notion.

7. CLINICAL IMPLICATIONS

The pineal gland, through the rhythmic secretion of its hormone, melatonin, is part of a complex neuroendocrine mechanism that controls the temporal organization of physiologic, biochemical, and behavioral processes within the organism and synchronizes the patterns of their activities to that of environmental cycles. The characteristic time course of nocturnal melatonin secretion, together with the somnogenic effect of exogenous melatonin in physiologic doses, underlies its involvement in processes that generate normal sleep and its potential use as a treatment for insomnias, including difficulty falling or remaining asleep.

A sleep-promoting effect of exogenous melatonin might be particularly important in elderly people with insomnia whose nocturnal serum melatonin levels tend to be diminished. The ability of "physiologic" doses of melatonin to shorten latency to sleep onset, or to improve sleep efficiency in elderly people with insomnia, suggests the potential use of melatonin as a hypnotic agent, with—at physiologic doses—an extremely low probability of untoward side effects. Administration of pharmacologic melatonin doses can lead to increased daytime melatonin levels (Fig. 11) and reduced nighttime core body temperature (Fig. 13).

Studies in children with various neurologic disorders, associated with severe insomnia, showed that administration of melatonin could substantially improve their sleep patterns and increase sleep duration. Similarly, our study of children with Angelman syndrome, a rare genetic disorder characterized by severe mental retardation, hyperactivity, and disturbed sleep, found that administration of low oral melatonin doses (0.3 mg) at bedtime both promoted sleep onset and increased the duration of nighttime sleep. In some patients—those with documented delays in the circadian rhythm of melatonin secretion—treatment with melatonin at bedtime advanced the circadian rhythm and synchronized it with the environmental light-dark cycle. Furthermore, some children with Angelman syndrome showed a reduction in daytime hyperactivity and enhanced attention. Whether these are consequences of improved nighttime sleep or represent additional results of melatonin treatment that could be beneficial to other populations suffering from attention deficits needs further investigation.

The phase shift–inducing effects of melatonin treatment on the activity pattern of the SCN can entrain sleep and other rhythmic functions to an altered time schedule. Thus, prudent administration of the pineal hormone can help ameliorate blindness-induced insomnia and jet-lag symptoms, and to assist shift workers in coping with their changing rest-activity schedule.

Manipulation of circulating melatonin levels may also prove useful in the clinical management of pathologic conditions of the reproductive system, such as amenorrhea in women or hypogonadism in men. The results of clinical and experimental investigations indicate that, with further study, melatonin may become a useful therapeutic tool for these disorders.

SELECTED READINGS

Goldman BD, Nelson RJ. Melatonin and seasonality in mammals. In: Yu H-S, Reiter RJ, eds. *Melatonin: Biosynthesis, Physiological Effects, and Clinical Applications.* Boca Raton, FL:CRC Press 1993:225–231.

Lewy AJ, Sack RL. Circadian rhythm sleep disorders: lessons from the blind. *Sleep Med Rev* 2001;5:189–206.

Reppert SM. Melatonin receptors: molecular biology of a new family of G protein–coupled receptors. *J Biol Rhythms* 1997;12:528–531.

Zhdanova IV, Wurtman RJ, Lynch HJ, et al. Sleep-inducing effects of low doses of melatonin ingested in the evening. *Clin Pharmacol Ther* 1995;57:552–558.

REFERENCES

Dollins AB, et al. Effect of inducing nocturnal serum melatonin concentrations in daytime on sleep, mood, body temperature, and performance. *Proc Natl Acad Sci USA* 1994;91:1824–1828.

Goldman BD. Mammalian photopenidic time measurement. *J Biol Rhythms* 2000;16:283–301.

Gray H. In: Clemente CD, ed. *Anatomy of the Human Body.* Philadelphia, Pa: Lea & Febiger 1985:989.

Yu, G-D, et al. Regulation of melatonin-sensitivity and firing-rate rhythms of hamster suprachiasmatic nucleus neurons: constant light effects. *Brain Res* 1993;602:191–199.

Zhdanova IV, Wurtman RJ, Morabito C, Piotrovska V, Lynch HL. Effects of low doses of melatonin, given 2–4 hours before habitual bedtime, on sleep in normal young humans. *Sleep* 1996;19:423–431.

Zhdanova IV, Wurtman RJ, Regan MM, Taylor JA, Shi JP, Leclair OU. Melatonin treatment for age-related insomnia. *J Clin Endocrinol Metab* 2001;86:4727–4730

17 Thyroid Hormones (T$_4$, T$_3$)

Takahiko Kogai, MD, PhD and Gregory A. Brent, MD

1. INTRODUCTION

Thyroid hormone is produced by all vertebrates. In mammals, the thyroid gland is derived embryologically from endoderm at the base of the tongue and develops into a bilobed structure lying anterior to the trachea. The structure and arrangement of thyroid tissue, however, vary significantly among species. Several key transcription factors, thyroid transcription factors 1 and 2 (TTF 1 and 2) and Pax8, are required for normal thyroid gland development and regulate gene expression in the adult thyroid gland. The thyroid gland receives a rich blood supply, as well as sympathetic innervation, and is specialized to synthesize and secrete thyroxine (T$_4$) and triiodothyronine (T$_3$) into the circulation (Fig. 1). This process is regulated by thyroid-stimulating hormone ([TSH], or thyrotropin) secreted from the pituitary, which is, in turn, stimulated by thyrotropin-releasing hormone (TRH) from the hypothalamus. Both TSH and TRH are regulated in a negative-feedback loop by circulating T$_4$ and T$_3$. Iodine and the trace element selenium are essential for normal thyroid hormone metabolism. Regulatory mechanisms within the thyroid gland allow continuous production of thyroid hormone despite variation in the supply of dietary iodine. Thyroid hormone influences a wide range of processes, including amphibian metamorphosis, development, reproduction, growth, and metabolism. The specific processes that are influenced differ among species, tissues, and developmental phase.

2. THYROID HORMONE SYNTHESIS

The synthesis of thyroid hormones requires iodide, thyroid peroxidase (TPO), thyroglobulin, and hydrogen peroxide (H$_2$O$_2$). Iodine is transported into the thyroid in the inorganic form by the sodium/iodide symporter (NIS), oxidized by the TPO-H$_2$O$_2$ system, and then utilized to iodinate tyrosyl residues in thyroglobulin. Coupling of iodinated tyrosyl intermediates in the TPO-H$_2$O$_2$ system produces T$_4$ and T$_3$, which are hydrolyzed and then secreted into the circulation. These processes are closely linked, and defects in any of the components can lead to impairment of thyroid hormone production or secretion.

2.1. Structure of Thyroid Follicle

The functional unit for thyroid hormone synthesis and storage, common to all species, is the thyroid fol-

From: *Endocrinology: Basic and Clinical Principles, Second Edition*
(S. Melmed and P. M. Conn, eds.) © Humana Press Inc., Totowa, NJ

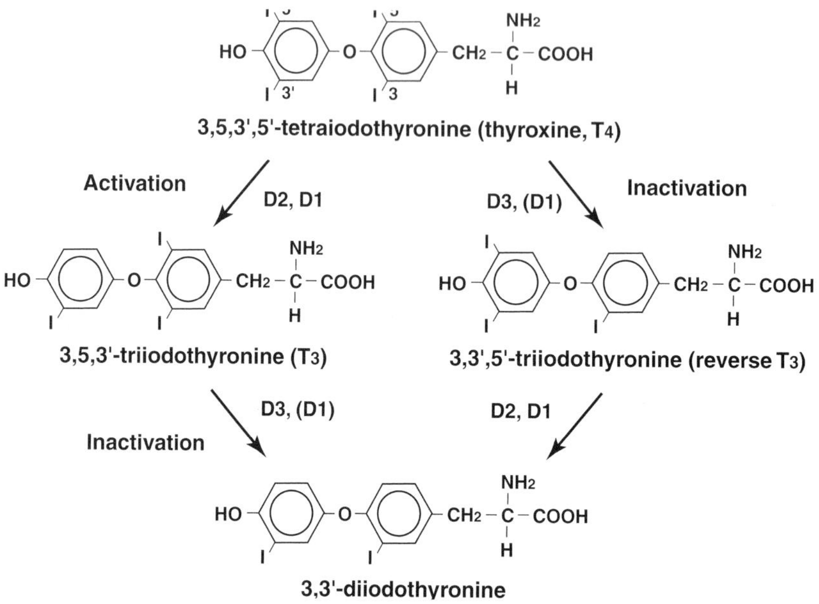

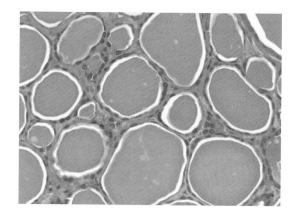

Fig. 1. Structure of L-thyroxine (T$_4$) and its major metabolites, T$_3$ and reverse T$_3$ (rT$_3$). The enzymes include type I 5′-deiodinase (D1), type II 5′-deiodinase (D2), and type III 5-deiodinase (D3).

Fig. 2. Photomicrograph of thyroid follicles of varying sizes. Each follicle consists of a ring of cells filled with colloid.

licle (Fig. 2). The follicle consists of cells arranged in a spherical structure. The thyroid cell synthesizes thyroglobulin, which is secreted through the apical membrane into the follicle lumen. The secreted substance containing thyroglobulin, colloid, serves as a storage form of iodine and is resorbed to provide substrate for T$_4$ and T$_3$ synthesis. The amount of stored colloid varies as a result of a number of conditions, including the level of TSH stimulation and availability of iodine. With TSH stimulation, colloid is resorbed to synthesize thyroid hormone, and with chronic stimulation, the size of the follicular lumen decreases. TSH also stimulates expression of elements of the cytoskeleton, which mediate changes in follicular cell shape that favor thyroid hormone production. The organization of thyroid cells in culture from monolayer to follicles stimulates NIS gene expression and iodide uptake. Defects in thyroid hormone synthesis or release can result in increased colloid stores.

2.2. Thyroglobulin

Thyroglobulin is the major iodoprotein of the thyroid gland. It is a large dimeric glycoprotein (660 kDa) that serves as a substrate for efficient coupling of mono-iodotyrosine (MIT) and diiodotyrosine (DIT) by the TPO-H$_2$O$_2$ system, to produce T$_4$ and T$_3$, as well as provides a storage form of easily accessible thyroid hormone (Fig. 3). Because of this storage capacity, the

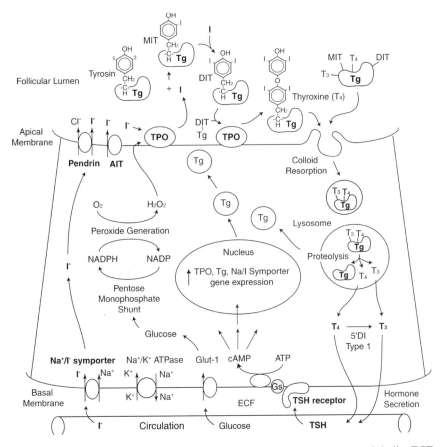

Fig. 3. Diagram of major steps involved in thyroid hormone synthesis and secretion. Tg = thyroglobulin; ECF = extracellular fluid; 5′ D Type I = 5′-iodothyronine deiodinase type I; Na/I symporter = sodium iodide symporter; ATP = adenosine triphosphate; DIT = diiodityrosine; MIT = monoiodotyrosine.

thyroid gland can continue to secrete thyroid hormone despite transient deficiencies in environmental iodine. The amount of stored thyroglobulin varies among species, with rodents having limited stores and humans very large stores, sufficient for up to 1 mo of thyroid hormone production. Thyroglobulin synthesized on the endoplasmic reticulum is transported to the Golgi apparatus, where carbohydrate moieties are added. The thyroglobulin is then localized at the apical membrane, where internal tyrosyl residues are iodinated by TPO and H$_2$O$_2$. Because iodide is bound to an organic compound, this process is known as "organification" of iodide.

The intracellular generation of H$_2$O$_2$ is essential for thyroglobulin iodination and coupling and is generated by the thyroid follicular cell (Fig. 3). TSH stimulates uptake of glucose, which is metabolized by the pentose monophosphate shunt, generating NADPH from NADP. The reduced adenosine nucleotide, NADPH, and NADPH oxidase are considered the major mechanisms for the reduction of molecular oxygen to H$_2$O$_2$.

Coupling between two DIT moieties forms T$_4$, and coupling of MIT and DIT produces T$_3$ (Fig. 3). The coupling reaction is catalyzed by TPO and involves the cleavage of a tyrosyl phenolic ring, which is joined to an iodinated tyrosine by an ether linkage. The structural integrity of the thyroglobulin protein matrix is essential for efficient coupling. The usual thyroidal secretion contains about 80% T$_4$ and 20% T$_3$, however, the ratio of secreted T$_4$:T$_3$ can be altered. Hyperstimulation of the TSH receptor is associated with an increase in the relative fraction of T$_3$ secretion. TSH receptor stimulation can be owing to IgG in Graves disease or a constitutive activating TSH receptor mutation found in many hyperfunctioning autonomous nodules. The excess in T$_3$ is owing to preferential MIT/DIT coupling as well as increased activity of the intrathyroidal type I (D1) and type II (D2) 5′-deiodinase that converts T$_4$ into T$_3$ (*see* Section 3). Repletion of iodine after a period of iodine deficiency also results in an increase in the fraction of T$_3$ in the thyroidal secretion.

The process of thyroid hormone release and secretion begins with TSH-stimulated resorption of colloid (Fig. 3). Pseudopods and microvilli are formed at the apical membrane, and pinocytosis of colloid produces multiple colloid droplet vesicles. Lysosomes move from the basal to apical region of the cell and fuse with colloid droplets to form phagolysosomes. Proteolysis of thyroglobulin releases iodothyronines, free iodotyrosines, and free amino acids. T_4 and T_3 then diffuse across the cell and into the circulation.

2.3. Iodine Transport

The thyroid contains 70–80% of the total iodine in the body (15–20 mg). The thyroid gland must trap about 60 µg of iodine/d from the circulation to maintain adequate thyroid hormone production. The urinary excretion of iodine generally matches intake, and low levels indicate inadequate iodine intake. NIS is a membrane-bound protein located in the basolateral portion of the thyroid follicular cell that passively transports two Na^+ and one I^- down the Na^+ ion gradient, resulting in an iodine concentration gradient from the thyroid cell to extracellular fluid of 100:1 (Fig. 3). The iodide gradient can be increased to as high as 400:1 in conditions of iodine deficiency. Iodine transport is driven by the Na^+ gradient generated from Na^+/K^+ adenosine triphosphatase (ATPase). Ouabain, which inhibits the Na^+/K^+ ATPase, blocks thyroidal iodide uptake. Iodide uptake by NIS, therefore, is a passive, but efficient, transport process that occurs against an iodide electrochemical gradient. The process is stimulated by TSH via cyclic adenosine monophosphate (cAMP). TSH induces NIS gene expression through the thyroid-selective enhancer located far upstream of the gene with cAMP-regulated transcription factors, such as Pax-8 and cAMP-response element–binding protein (CREB). Trapped iodide in the follicular cells is further transferred to the lumen by other iodide transporters at the apical membrane, pendrin or the apical iodide transporter (AIT), and "organified" with thyroglobulin for subsequent thyroid hormone synthesis. Iodine transport by NIS is seen in other tissues, including the salivary gland, gastric mucosa, lactating mammary gland, ciliary body of the eye, and the choroid plexus. A low level of iodide uptake has been demonstrated in breast cancer. Iodine is not organified in these tissues, other than lactating mammary glands, and NIS gene expression is unresponsive to TSH.

Endemic goiter is the presence of thyroid enlargement in >10% of a population, a higher fraction than that owing to intrinsic thyroid disease alone, and indicates that the etiology is likely to be owing to dietary and/or environmental factors. Most endemic goiters are the result of reduced thyroidal iodine resulting from deficient dietary iodine. Mountainous areas, including the Andes and Himalayas, as well as central Africa and portions of Europe, remain relatively iodine deficient. Reduced thyroidal iodine may also be the result of factors that inhibit NIS. Inhibitors can be natural dietary "goitrogens," such as the cyanogenic glucosides found in cassava, a staple in parts of Africa and Asia. Cyanogenic glucosides are hydrolyzed in the gut by glucosidases to free cyanide, which is then converted into thiocyanate. Thiocyanate inhibits thyroid iodide transport and at high concentrations interferes with organification. Other inhibitors include perchlorate, chlorate, periodate, and even high concentrations of iodide, which cause transient inhibition of thyroid hormone synthesis (Wolff-Chaikoff effect). This has been shown to be primarily owing to reduced NIS expression. Perchlorate causes release of nonorganified iodine and is used diagnostically, after radioiodine tracer uptake, to distinguish defects of iodine uptake from organification (radioiodine transported but not organified will be released after administration of perchlorate). Perchlorate is used in the aircraft and rocket industry and has been detected in various concentrations in water supplies worldwide. The impact of various levels of perchlorate on thyroid function in adults and children is being studied. A wide range of heritable defects also result in impaired iodide transport or organification, including genetic mutations of iodide transporters, NIS and *PDS*, which encodes pendrin. Mutation of *PDS* in patients with Pendred syndrome leads to inefficient iodide transport to the follicular lumen and brings about a "partial" organification defect in the thyroid. In this case, trapped radioiodine in the thyroid can be discharged by perchlorate faster than normal.

NIS is utilized clinically for both diagnostic and therapeutic applications. Radioisotopes of iodine can be given orally and are taken up into thyroid tissue with high efficiency. Nonincorporated iodine is rapidly excreted by the kidneys. Short-half-life, low-energy isotopes, such as I^{123}, are used to make images of functional thyroid tissue. Longer-half-life, high-energy isotopes, such as I^{131}, are used therapeutically to destroy thyroid tissue in both hyperthyroidism and thyroid cancer. Thyroid cancer requires a high level of TSH stimulation, either endogenous after thyroidectomy and cessation of thyroid supplementation, or exogenous administration of recombinant TSH. Less-differentiated thyroid cancers, however, either do not have or lose the ability to transport iodine. Agents that target stimulation of NIS expression or augmentation of its function in these situations are being developed as therapeutic tools.

2.4. Thyroid Peroxidase

TPO is a membrane-bound glycoprotein with a central role in thyroid hormone synthesis catalyzing iodine oxidation, iodination of tyrosine residues, and iodothyronine coupling. The human cDNA codes for a 933-amino-acid protein with transmembrane domains at the carboxy terminus. The extracellular region contains five potential glycosylation sites. The human thyroid peroxidase gene is found on chromosome 2 and spans approx 150 kb with 17 exons. The 5′-flanking sequence contains binding sites for a number of thyroid-specific transcription factors, including TTF 1 and 2. TSH stimulates TPO gene expression by an increase in intracellular cAMP, although the level of regulation (transcriptional vs posttranscriptional) varies by species.

IgG autoantibodies to TPO are pathogenic in several thyroid diseases. The predisposition to forming TPO autoantibodies is inherited as an autosomal-dominant trait in women but has incomplete penetrance in men. This pattern of inheritance is consistent with the female preponderance of autoimmune thyroid disease. In addition to the diagnosis of autoimmune thyroid disease, the magnitude of elevation of these antibodies correlates with disease activity. TPO antibodies are known to damage cells directly by activating the complement cascade. A number of epitopes for TPO autoantibodies have been defined. Several animal models with thyroid autoantibodies have demonstrated that a second insult, such as injection of interferon or other cytokine, is required for thyroid destruction and hypothyroidism. Clinically, thyroid destruction can be transient, with temporary phases of increased and then decreased thyroid hormone levels (lymphocytic thyroiditis) or permanent hypothyroidism (Hashimoto disease). Lymphocytic thyroiditis is often seen in the postpartum period.

2.5. Influence of Thyrotropin on Thyroid Hormone Synthesis

The major stimulus to thyroid hormone production and thyroid growth is stimulation of the TSH receptor. Other factors that modify this response include neurotransmitters, cytokines, and growth factors. In addition to physiologic regulation via TSH, there are a number of clinical disorders of excess and reduced thyroid hormone production mediated by the TSH receptor.

The human TSH receptor gene is on the long arm of chromosome 14 and consists of 10 exons spread over 60 kb. Analysis of the regulatory region of the gene has identified binding sites for TTF 1 and 2, as well as cAMP response elements. TSH is a G protein–coupled receptor with a classic seven-transmembrane domain structure. The primary structure contains leucine-rich motifs and six potential *N*-glycosylation sites. Such motifs are similar to those that form amphipathic α-helices and may be involved in protein-protein interactions. A number of recent studies have demonstrated that full function of the TSH receptor results from cleavage of a portion of the extracellular domain. This appears to be a unique feature of the TSH receptor, and antibodies to the cleaved portion may play an important role in the pathogenesis of Graves disease and especially extrathyroidal manifestations. The receptors for the pituitary glycoprotein hormones—TSH, follicle-stimulating hormone (FSH), and leutinizing hormone (LH)/chorionic gonadotropin (CG)—are very similar in the transmembrane domain containing the carboxy-terminal portion (70%) but have less similarity in the extracellular domain (about 40%). The similarity is clinically relevant in glycoprotein hormone "spillover" syndromes, in which marked elevations in these hormones stimulate related receptors. Excess CG from trophoblastic disease can stimulate thyroid hormone production via the TSH receptor, and excess TSH in prepubertal children with primary hypothyroidism can stimulate precocious puberty via stimulation of the FSH and/or LH/CG receptors. A TSH receptor mutation that retained normal TSH affinity, but a marked augmentation of hCG affinity has been reported. Affected individuals were thyrotoxic only during pregnancy. Gain-of-function mutations have been identified in the TSH receptor, resulting in constitutive activation (TSH independent) of thyroid hormone production. These mutations are manifest in the heterozygous state, produce thyroid growth as well as an increase in thyroid function, and have been found in the majority of hyperfunctioning thyroid nodules. Similar constitutive mutations in the germ line produce diffuse thyroid hyperfunction and growth. Inactivating TSH receptor gene mutations have also been reported. Characterization of these mutations has helped to map functional domains of the TSH receptor.

TSH stimulation of thyroid follicular cells promotes protein iodination, thyroid hormone synthesis, and secretion. These effects can be reproduced by agents that enhance cAMP accumulation (theophylline, cholera toxin, forskolin, cAMP analogs). At high concentrations of TSH, there is activation of the Ca^{2+} phosphatidylinositol-4,5-bisphosphate (PIP$_2$) cascade. The relative influence of the cAMP and PIP$_2$ pathways appears to differ by species; for example, dog have only the cAMP pathway and humans have both. TSH acting via cAMP generation stimulates the expression of a number of genes involved in thyroid hormone synthesis and secretion, including NIS, thyroglobulin, and TPO. In many species (e.g., human, rat, and dog), TSH is mitogenic and promotes thyroid growth.

Table 1
Properties of Iodothyronine Deiodinases

	D1	*D2*	*D3*
Developmental expression	Expressed in later development	Expressed in early development	Expressed first in development
Tissue distribution	Thyroid, liver, kidney	Brain, pituitary, brown adipose tissue	Placenta, uterus, developing brain, skin
Preferred substrate	$rT_3 >> T_4 > T_3$	$T_4 > rT_3$	T_3 (sulfate) $> T_4$
Target	Outer ring	Outer ring	Inner ring
Response to hypothyroidism	Decrease	Increase	Decrease
Inhibition by propylthiouracil	Yes	No	No
Inhibition by ipodate	Yes	Yes	Yes
Physiologic role	Extracellular T_3 production	Intracellular and rapid T_3 production	Inactivation of T_4 and T_3

T_4 = thyroxine; T_3 = triiodothyronine; rT_3 = reverse T3.

2.6. Interference of Antithyroid Drugs With Thyroid Hormone Synthesis

In the 1940s, the thionamides were first observed to produce goiters in laboratory animals. Propylthiouracil and methimazole are the most commonly used of these compounds, and both have intrathyroidal and extrathyroidal actions. They reduce thyroid hormone production by interfering with the actions of TPO, which include the oxidation and organification of iodine, and the coupling of MIT and DIT to form T_4 and T_3. The thionamides compete with thyroglobulin tyrosyl residues for oxidized iodine. These medications are primarily used in patients with hyperthyroidism resulting from Graves disease but are effective in any form of hyperthyroidism owing to overproduction of thyroid hormone. Propylthiouracil has an additional effect at high serum T_4 concentrations of reducing peripheral T_4 to T_3 conversion by inhibiting the D1. Both agents are thought to have additional immunosuppresive actions that may help in the treatment of autoimmune hyperthyroidism.

3. THYROID HORMONE METABOLISM

The thyroid gland secretes primarily T_4, which must be converted into the active form, T_3, by D1 (Fig. 1). The various pathways of thyroid hormone metabolism allow regulation of hormone activation at the target tissue level as well as adaptation for times of reduced thyroid hormone production. A large number of iodothyronine metabolites are degradation products of T_4, in addition to T_3, including rT_3 (3,3′,5′-triiodothyronine), T_{2S}, 3′-T_1, and T_0. The levels of these products vary in a number of thyroid states and, in some situations, have been used diagnostically. Reverse T_3 e.g., is metabolically inactive but is elevated in illness and fasting. The liver solubilizes T_4 metabolites by sulfation or glucuronide formation for excretion by the kidney or in the bile. The process allows the conservation of body iodine stores.

Deiodinase enzymes have distinctive characteristics based on developmental expression; tissue distribution; substrate preference; kinetics; and sensitivity to inhibitors, such as propylthiouracil and iopanoic acid. Deiodinases can be separated into phenolic (outer ring) 5′-deiodinases or tyrosyl (inner ring) 5-deiodinases (Table 1, Fig. 1).

3.1. Type I 5′-Deiodinase (D1)

The primary source of T_3 in the peripheral tissues is D1, although rodents and humans differ in the contribution of D1 (Fig. 4). This enzyme is found predominantly in thyroid, liver, and kidney. T_3, TSH, and cAMP all increase expression of D1 in FRTL5 thyroid cell cultures. Consistent with this observation are the in vivo findings of increased D1 activity in hyperthyroidism and reduced activity in hypothyroidism. The biochemical properties of D1 include a preference for rT_3 as a substrate over T_4. D1 requires reduced thiol as a cofactor and is sensitive to inhibition by propylthiouracil and gold. Other inhibitors of D1 include illness, starvation, glucocorticoids, and propranolol.

3.2. Type II 5′-Deiodinase (D2)

D2 is a related 5′-deiodinase with distinct tissue distribution, biochemical properties, and physiologic function. D2 is found primarily in the pituitary, brain, muscle, and brown fat. This enzyme functions to regulate intracellular T_3 levels in tissue, where an adequate concentration is critical. In humans, D2 may be the major contributor to T_3 production (Fig. 4). The biochemical properties include a preference for T_4 over rT_3 as a substrate and insensitivity to inhibition by propylthiouracil. The activity of D2 increases in hypothyroidism, appar-

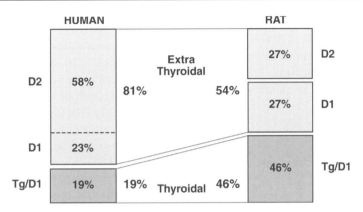

Fig. 4. Comparison of relative source of circulating T$_3$ in humans and rodents as a result of activity of Type 1 (D1) and Type II (D2) 5′-deiodinase enzymes. Tg = thyroglobulin (Data from Bianco et al., 2002.)

ently to sustain intracellular T$_3$ levels despite falling levels of T$_4$, especially in the brain. The mechanism of D2 regulation has been found to involve ubiquitination by specific enzymes that then lead to proteasomal degradation. De-ubiquitination prolongs D2 activity, and the system allows rapid up- and downregulation in specific tissues, such as brown adipose tissue. Both D1 and D2 activity are inhibited by the iodine contrast agent iopanoic acid.

3.3. Type III 5-Deiodinase (D3)

D3 is found in the developing brain, placenta, uterus, and skin and inactivates T$_3$ by removal of a tyrosyl ring iodide. The activity of the enzyme, like D1, is regulated by thyroid hormone, with less enzyme activity when thyroid hormone levels are low. This deiodinase may play a role in regulating T$_4$/T$_3$ availability across the placenta and uterus, especially during development. This is supported by the finding that D3 gene knockout mice have excess neonatal mortality, indicating an essential role of this enzyme in early development. Overexpression of D3 in an infantile hemangioma was associated with "consumptive" hypothyroidism in a patient requiring massive amounts of thyroid hormone replacement. A young woman with a large hepatic vascular tumor was also found to have consumptive hypothyroidism that reversed after treatment of the tumor. D3 overexpression in the failing heart and in severe non thyroidal illness may be responsible for reduced serum T$_3$ concentration and reduced thyroid hormone action.

3.4. Selenium and Deiodination

The role of selenium in thyroid hormone metabolism was suggested by studies of rats fed a selenium-deficient diet. Compared with control animals, those with selenium deficiency had elevated serum T$_4$ and reduced serum T$_3$ concentrations associated with reduced hepatic D1 activity. Analysis of the D1 cDNA identified a TGA codon, usually indicating a stop codon, which codes for the amino acid selenocysteine (an analog of cysteine with selenium in place of sulfur). Substitution of cysteine for selenocysteine completely reduced enzyme activity. A number of other glutathione-requiring enzymes contain a selenocysteine and share properties with the deiodinase. A common stem loop structure that is present in the 3′-untranslated region of the D1 mRNA directs insertion of a selenocysteine, rather than terminates translation at the TGA codon.

Epidemiologic studies have also demonstrated the importance of selenium for thyroid hormone metabolism. Groups in Africa and China with selenium-deficient diets have been studied and have a high incidence of goiter and reduced serum T$_3$ concentrations. In some areas of these countries, selenium deficiency coexists with iodine deficiency. In these situations, it is harmful to replace selenium without iodine, because this activates D1 and accelerates degradation of T$_4$, the primary source of T$_3$ to the brain. The slowed metabolism of T$_4$ from selenium deficiency may be partially protective for the reduced T$_4$ production in iodine deficiency.

4. THYROID HORMONE–BINDING PROTEINS AND MEASUREMENT OF THYROID HORMONE LEVELS

4.1. Serum Proteins That Bind Thyroid Hormones

The thyroid hormones are hydrophobic and circulate predominantly bound to serum proteins. The free fraction, which represents the metabolically active form of hormone, comprises only 0.02% of the total T$_4$ concentration and 0.30% of the total T$_3$ concentration. The predominant serum protein that binds thyroid hormone is thyroxine-binding globulin (TBG), which carries approx 70% of serum T_4 and T_3. TBG is synthesized in the liver and is a 54-kDa glycoprotein with approx 20% of its weight from carbohydrates. The extent of sialylation directly influences the clearance of TBG from the serum. Desialylated TBG has a circulating half-life of only 15 min, whereas fully sialylated TBG has a circulating half-life as long as 3 d. The variation in the carbohydrate component is likely to be responsible for microheterogeneity on isoelectric focusing. However, it causes little effect on ligand affinity or immunogenic properties. The remainder of thyroid hormone is bound to transthyretin (previously called thyroid-binding prealbumin) and albumin. Transthyretin is a 55-kDa protein consisting of four identical subunits of 127 amino acids each and is synthesized in the liver and choroid plexus. In addition to binding thyroid hormone, transthyretin transports retinol by forming a complex with retinol-binding protein.

Owing to the large fraction of circulating thyroid hormone bound to protein, alterations in binding significantly change total hormone measurements. Mutations of the TBG gene, located on the X chromosome, produce abnormalities that range from partial or complete deficiency to excess. Abnormalities of T_4 binding have also been reported as a result of transthyretin and albumin mutations. The most common thyroid hormone–binding disorder, dysalbuminemic hyperthyroxenemia, is the result of a mutation in the albumin gene, which produces a mutant albumin with increased affinity for T_4, but not T_3. Affected individuals have elevated total T_4, normal total T_3, and normal TSH.

In addition to inherited defects in thyroid hormone–binding proteins, there are a number of conditions and medicines that can alter serum-binding protein concentrations and thyroid hormone–binding affinity. The most common cause of excess TBG is estrogen, either exogenous (oral contraceptives or postmenopausal replacement) or from pregnancy. Rather than increased TBG synthesis, this is the result of estrogen-stimulated increase in sialylation, prolonging the circulating half-life. TBG is also increased in acute hepatitis and by medications, including methadone, 5-fluorouracil, perphenazine, and clofibrate. Reduced TBG has been reported in cirrhosis of the liver; from excess urinary loss in nephrotic syndrome; and from medications, including androgens, glucocorticoids, and L-asparaginase.

In the majority of cases, individuals with abnormalities of binding proteins have normal serum concentrations of thyrotropin and free T_4 and free T_3. Total T_4 and T_3 levels are abnormal but are rarely measured in the clinical setting.

4.2. Measurement of T_4, T_3, and TSH

Total serum T_4 and T_3 are measured by radioimmunoassay (RIA). The free fraction, however, is relatively small, and changes in binding proteins can significantly affect total hormone levels, even when the free fraction is normal. The free fraction can be measured directly by RIA or ultrafiltration. Most available free T_4 assays are automated and utilize the analog method. The concentration of TBG can also be measured directly by RIA.

TSH is measured by a double-antibody "sandwich" method, which allows precise measurement of very low levels of hormone. Previous assay techniques could determine only abnormally elevated levels associated with an underactive thyroid, not the abnormally low levels associated with hyperthyroidism. Because TSH, in most cases, is regulated based on the concentration of free hormone, this is the most useful way to assess thyroid hormone action, as long as the pituitary is functioning normally.

4.3. Conditions That Alter Thyroid Hormone Measurements

Measurement of thyroid hormones can be influenced by a variety of factors, including illness and medications. Severe illnesses are associated with an elevation in the free fraction measured relative to the total hormone concentrations. Medications, such as salicylates, diphenylhydantoin, and furosemide, may impair thyroid hormone binding and artificially elevate measurements of free hormone concentration. Serum TSH can be reduced in severe illness or by medications, such as dopamine and glucocorticoids. TSH can remain suppressed below normal levels for several months after treatment of long-standing hyperthyroidism, even when circulating thyroid hormone levels are normal or low, presumably owing to impairment of TSH synthesis.

5. MOLECULAR ACTION OF THYROID HORMONE

5.1. Thyroid Hormone Receptor α and β Genes

Thyroid hormone receptor (TR) is a member of the superfamily of nuclear receptors that are ligand-modulated transcription factors. Within the superfamily, TR is most closely related to the *trans*-retinoic acid receptor (RAR) and the retinoid X receptor (RXR), whose ligand is 9-*cis* retinoic acid, the isomer of *trans*-retinoic acid. The DNA-binding domain (DBD) is the most highly conserved region among the members of the family and consists of a pair of "zinc fingers," which interact with target DNA sequences. The DNA sequence that these nuclear receptors recognize is determined by a few amino acid residues at the base of the first zinc finger, termed the *P box*. Sequences in the amino terminus have been shown to influence DNA-binding site recognition. A unique carboxy-terminal domain mediates ligand binding.

There are two TR genes, α and β, which are cellular homologs of the viral oncogene v-*erb*A, one of the two oncogenes carried by avian erythroblastosis virus. TRα and TRβ are coded on chromosomes 17 and 3, respectively, and each gene has at least two alternative mRNA and protein products. The TRβ isoforms, TRβ1 and TRβ2, contain identical DBDs and ligand-binding domains (LBDs) but differ in their amino termini. The β-2-specific exon is regulated separately from the β-1-specific exon, leading to differential expression of TRβ1 and TRβ2. By contrast, the TRα variants have identical transcription initiation sites but diverge after the DBD. TRα2 differs from TRα1 at the 3′ end and has a unique carboxy terminus that does not bind T$_3$. TRα2 antagonizes T$_3$ action in a transient transfection assay.

5.2. Tissue-Specific Expression and Function of TR Isoforms

TR isoforms have both developmental and tissue-specific patterns of expression, suggesting unique functions of the different isoforms. Expression of TRβ2 was originally thought to be restricted to the pituitary but has subsequently been shown in a number of other brain areas and the retina. A recent study using a variety of TRβ2-specific antibodies concluded that TRβ2 represents as much as 10–20% of T$_3$-binding capacity in the adult brain, liver, kidney, and heart. The other TR isoforms are found in virtually all other cells, although the proportion varies among tissues and cell types. In the heart, levels of TRα1 and TRβ1 are nearly equal, whereas in liver TRβ1 is the predominant species. In brain, TRα1 and TRα2 are predominantly expressed. The finding that TRβ1 and TRβ2 are expressed in rat embryonic cochlear tissue supports the hypothesis that TRβ has a specific function in the development of hearing. Several investigators have studied the spatial and temporal expression of TR isoforms during development. TRα2 is the first isoform to be expressed during central nervous system development and is expressed at high levels throughout all locations in the developing brain. TRβ1 is expressed later, predominantly in regions of cortical proliferation, whereas TRα1 is found predominantly in regions of cortical differentiation. Several genes expressed in the brain have been shown to be preferentially regulated by the TRβ isoform, including a Purkinje cell gene (PCP-2), thyrotropin-releasing hormone, and myelin basic protein. Within the pituitary,

Table 2
TR Isoform–Specific Actions

Thyroid hormone target	Mediating receptor
TSH suppression	TRβ2 > TRα
Ligand-independent TSH elevation	TRα > TRβ
Bone development	TRα > TRβ
Cochlear development	TRβ
Retinal development	TRβ2
Small intestine maturation	TRα
Cardiac gene expression	TRα > TRβ
Heart rate	TRα
Somatic growth	TRα > TRβ
Hepatic gene expression	TRβ > TRα
Catecholamine potentiation	TRα
UCP1 stimulation[a]	TRβ

[a] UCP1 = uncoupling protein 1.

TRβ2 is expressed at the highest level in thyrotropes and somatotropes. Expression increases further in hypothyroidism.

A wide variety of TR gene "knockout" and "knockin" point mutations have been utilized in mouse models to determine TR isoform–specific function. Mice with deletion or mutation of the TRβ gene display the clinical syndrome resistance to thyroid hormone (RTH) with increased serum thyroid hormone levels and TSH, goiter, and impaired action of thyroid hormone in the pituitary and liver. In one model of a TRβ gene dominant-negative mutation, mice had impaired brain development. The phenotype of the TRα gene deletions has been variable, depending on the site of disruption. In general, the thyroid levels are only modestly elevated or in some models reduced. In most TRα mutant models, the homozygous condition is an embryonic or neonatal lethal. Dominant-negative mutations of the TRα gene are also an embryonic or neonatal lethal in the homozygotes. Heterozygotes have impaired thyroid hormone action, bradycardia, and reduced thermogenic response to cold. These results suggest that the early expression of TRα is likely required for normal development. A summary of TR isoform–specific actions in various tissues is based on these various models (Table 2).

A number of TR isoform–specific agonists and antagonists have been designed based on the TR crystal structure. The primary focus has been on TRβ agonists that reduce cholesterol and produce weight loss with limited cardiac actions. TR antagonists will be useful in identifying key stages of thyroid hormone action in development and have already been utilized to identify steps in amphibian metamorphosis.

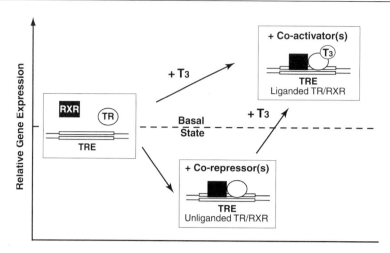

Fig. 5. Schematic of the action of complexes of TR RXR with and without T_3 ligand bound to DNA TREs in basal promoter of T_3-regulated target genes.

5.3. Mechanism of Gene Regulation by Thyroid Hormone

A number of recent observations are changing the view of the mechanism of thyroid hormone action. Although a number of investigators have suggested the presence of a membrane thyroid transporter, mono-carboxylate transporter 8 (MCT8) has been identified as a specific transporter of T_4 and T_3. Of even greater significance is the identification of several kindreds with MCT8 gene mutations associated with abnormal thyroid function tests and neurologic abnormalities including developmental delay and central hypotonia. The thyroid function tests show a marked elevation of serum TSH and T_3 concentration, but normal T_4. The MCT8 gene is located on the X chromosomes, and only males are affected with neurologic abnormalities; heterozygous females have a milder thyroid phenotype and no detectable neurologic deficit.

TR interacts with specific DNA sequences, T_3 response elements (TREs), that positively or negatively regulate gene expression. Mutational analysis of TREs from a number of T_3-regulated genes has identified a consensus hexamer-binding nucleotide sequence, A/G GGT C/A A. Most elements that confer positive regulation consist of two such elements arranged as a direct repeat with a 4-bp gap. A number of other arrangements are seen, including inverted repeats and palindromes. Flanking sequences are important, with a marked increase in affinity by the addition of AT to the 5′ end of the hexamer. Elements that confer negative regulation are often single hexamers and are located adjacent to the transcriptional start site. Although receptor monomers and homodimers can bind to a TRE

and transactivate a gene, TR heterodimers (with such partners as RXR) bind DNA with higher affinity to most elements. A number of potential functional TR complexes confer T_3 regulation. Receptor dimers can consist of homodimers (α/α, α/β, or β/β), and also heterodimers with RXR, RAR, or other nuclear receptor partners. Regions of the TR LBD that are highly conserved among members of the nuclear receptor superfamily are important for TR dimerization. There is polarity to the heterodimer-DNA interactions with RXR occupying the upstream hexamer. T_3 action is further complicated by observations that unliganded TR reduces expression from positively regulated genes and that T_3 disrupts TR homodimers bound to DNA, but not TR-RXR heterodimers. The complexity of the ligand-receptor-DNA interaction suggests that the specific TRE, as well as tissue level concentrations of ligand, TR, and nuclear cofactors, dictates the functional complex.

Unliganded TR represses gene expression of positively regulated genes, and this is now known to be mediated, at least in part, by binding to various corepressor proteins (Fig. 5). Ligand disrupts TR corepressor binding and promotes coactivator binding. Histone deacetylation promotes gene repression and is linked to the corepressors (Fig. 6). Coactivators bind to the liganded receptor and promote transcription through a variety of mechanisms including histone acetyltransferase and complexing with p300/CBP. Negative regulation of genes by TR is even more complex but appears to involve enhancement of expression in the presence of corepressor. A wide range of proteins complex with TR to promote or inhibit transcription (Fig. 6).

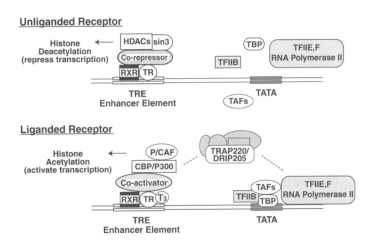

Fig. 6. Schematic of relative gene expression mediated by TR/RXR complex with and without ligand. Binding of unliganded receptor to the TRE promotes corepressor binding and reduces gene expression. Binding of ligand disrupts corepressor binding, promotes coactivator binding, and enhances gene expression.

5.4. Specific Genes Positively Regulated by Thyroid Hormone

Transcriptional regulation by T_3 has been shown for a number of genes. In the liver, these include α-glycerol phosphate dehydrogenase, malic dehydrogenase, and the lipogenic enzyme "spot 14." T_3 stimulates α-myosin heavy-chain expression in cardiac muscle, as well as cardiac and skeletal muscle forms of sarcoplasmic reticulum CaATPase. A complex response element that confers T_3 responsiveness has been identified in the 5′-flanking region of the D1 gene. Growth hormone expression in rats is transcriptionally regulated by T_3. Growth and thermogenesis are highly dependent on the presence of thyroid hormone. In rodent brown fat, thyroid hormone is required for facultative thermogenesis. T_3 stimulates heat production by increasing expression of the uncoupling protein (which generates heat by uncoupling oxidative phosphorylation), and by augmenting of the adrenergic system signal.

Thyroid hormone is an absolute requirement for amphibian metamorphosis. TRα is expressed at the earliest developmental phase, before thyroid hormone is available, and then stimulates expression of the TRβ gene. Unliganded TR may function to modulate retinoic acid action. Thyroid hormone acts initially to increase the expression of TR in all tissues, which corresponds to the onset of metamorphosis. Prolactin antagonizes the action of thyroid hormone, and if administered at the time of metamorphosis, it can completely halt the process. A number of thyroid hormone-responsive genes that may mediate this process have been identified and are being characterized.

5.5. Specific Genes Negatively Regulated by Thyroid Hormone

The most potent examples of negative regulation of gene expression by thyroid hormone are the TSH β- and α-subunit genes and the TRH gene. These are transcriptionally regulated by T_3, mediated by specific TR-binding elements identified within the gene. Interactions with *Fos* and *Jun* as well as the cAMP-stimulated CREB may be important for negative gene regulation. The importance of accessory factors is demonstrated by the observation that negative regulation of TRH gene expression by T_3 varies by tissue (e.g., regulated in paraventricular nucleus of the hypothalamus and prostate, but not in other brain areas or gut), despite the presence of nuclear TR in all of these tissues.

5.6. Extranuclear Effects of Thyroid Hormone

Both T_3 and T_4 have documented extranuclear actions, including stimulation of ion pumps, CaATPase, and Na⁺/K⁺ ATPase, mediated by specific membrane-binding sites. Cellular uptake of amino acids and 2-deoxyglucose is rapidly stimulated by T_3. A direct effect of thyroid hormone on relaxation of vascular smooth muscle has been shown. Thyroid hormone regulates polymerization of the actin cytoskeleton in astrocytes by extranuclear action. Thyroid hormone stimulates adenosine 5′-diphosphate uptake and oxygen consumption by mitochondria. These actions of thyroid hormone are rapid (within seconds) and are not blocked by inhibitors of transcription or translation.

6. CLINICAL MANIFESTATIONS OF REDUCED THYROID HORMONE LEVELS

6.1. Clinical Settings in Which Thyroid Hormone Levels Are Reduced

The most common causes of primary thyroid failure are autoimmune destruction caused by Hashimoto thyroiditis or as a sequela of radioiodine or surgical ablation for hyperthyroidism (Table 3). Hypothyroidism as a result of pituitary/hypothalamic dysfunction is rare. Congenital hypothyroidism affects about 1 in 4500 live births, and thyroid testing is part of routine neonatal screening in most countries. A variety of defects of thyroid growth and function have been identified as causes. When adequate amounts of thyroxine replacement are administered to hypothyroid infants within the first few weeks after delivery, growth and neurologic function are normal. Maternal hypothyroidism, even mild disease, has been associated with a number of complications of pregnancy and fetal development. These include preterm delivery; pregnancy-induced hypertension; and intellectual deficit in children of hypothyroid mothers as demonstrated in IQ tests conducted at ages 5 to 8. Maternal hypothyroidism from iodine deficiency, however, results in maternal and fetal hypothyroidism. Some offspring of severely iodine-deficient mothers have permanent and severe neurologic deficiencies, including mental deficiency, deafness/mutism, and motor rigidity. This condition, neurologic cretinism, is part of the spectrum of endemic cretinism in iodine-deficient areas. Iodine supplementation in the first trimester, but not later in pregnancy, largely prevents these abnormalities. Maternal TSH receptor–blocking antibodies can produce hypothyroidism in the mother and transient hypothyroidism in the fetus and infant. Rare but informative cases of hypothyroidism have been reported from defects in the Pit 1 pituitary-specific transcription factor reducing TSH expression, from defects in TTF1 associated with deficient thyroglobulin expression, and from germ-line TSH receptor gene-inactivating mutations. Genetic mutations of iodide transporters, the NIS and pendrin, have been reported in some case of hypothyroidism. Iodide transport defects cause reduced thyroid hormone synthesis, elevated serum TSH, and goiter. Pendrin is important for inner-ear development as well as iodide transport into the follicular lumen. Genetic mutation of *PDS*, which encodes pendrin, therefore leads to Pendred syndrome (iodide organification defect, goiter, and congenital sensory deafness).

6.2. Clinical Findings

Mild hypothyroidism is associated with relatively nonspecific symptoms, including weight gain, low energy level, amenorrhea, and mood disorders (especially depression). More severe hypothyroidism is associated with hypothermia, hypoventilation, hyponatremia, and eventually coma. Other findings include constipation, hair loss, and dry skin. The characteristic puffy facial appearance and nonpitting edema of arms and legs are the result of increased glycosaminoglycans, such as hyaluronic acid. This deposition is the result of reduced degradation by hyaluronidase. Changes in serum chemistries include elevations in cholesterol, creatine kinase from skeletal muscle, and carotene.

6.3. Treatment

Thyroid hormone deficiency can, in most cases, be easily treated with oral supplementation of T_4. Historically, thyroid extracts were used to replace patients with hypothyroidism. Such combinations of T_4 and T_3 were either animal thyroid extracts or synthetic combinations and were used because they simulated normal thyroidal secretion. The disadvantages, however, include the rapid absorption and short half-life of T_3 as well as variation in tablet content. The observation was convincingly made that the majority of circulating T_3 (80%) was generated from peripheral conversion of T_4. T_4 alone could, therefore, replicate the normal function of the thyroid gland and is recommended for thyroid hormone replacement. Several studies have suggested an advantage of adding T_3 to T_4 in selected patients for improvement of mood, cognition, and energy level. T_4 has a long half-life of 7–10 d, which means that once steady-state levels are achieved, levels are quite stable despite variation in timing of doses and so on. The adequacy of replacement is primarily determined by the measurement of the serum concentration of TSH. Owing to the availability of the sensitive TSH assay, it is possible to determine when the T_4 dose is too large or small. Even moderate excessive replacement has been associated with cardiac complications of left ventricular enlargement and an increased risk of atrial fibrillation in the elderly. Postmenopausal women taking excessive doses of T_4, according to some studies, are at risk of accelerated reduction in bone density.

7. CLINICAL MANIFESTATIONS OF EXCESS THYROID HORMONE LEVELS

7.1. Clinical Settings in Which Thyroid Hormone Levels Are Increased

The most common etiology of excess thyroid hormone production is Graves disease, associated with circulating autoantibodies that stimulate TSH receptors (Table 4). Stimulation of these receptors results in thyroid growth and an increase in thyroid hormone produc-

Table 3
Conditions Associated With Reduced Serum Concentrations of T_4/T_3

Diagnosis	Etiology	Thyroid gland	Serum TSH concentration	Antibodies	Outcome/treatment
Hashimoto thyroiditis	Mediated by IgG to TPO	Modestly enlarged, ultimately becomes atrophic	Elevated	TPO antibodies positive	Usually permanent, small subset (<5%) possibly owing to TSH receptor blocking antibodies and may be reversible
Postablative therapy	After radioiodine or surgical treatment for hyperthyroidism	Absent or atrophic	Elevated	Negative	Permanent
Congenital hypothyroidism	Thyroid agenesis, defect in thyroglobulin synthesis, iodine transport, or organification	Absent or ectopic	Elevated	Negative	Most cases permanent, reversible when owing to maternal TSH receptor blocking antibodies, sequelae reversible if treatment begun promptly
Central hypothyroidism	Pituitary or hypothalamic dysfunction, genetic defects in PROP1 or Pit 1 genes	Normal to atrophic	Reduced bioactivity, can be normal or low, but inappropriate for reduced T_4 concentration	Negative	Generally permanent, can be reversible if underlying pituitary or hypothalamic condition treated
Subacute thyroiditis	Painless immune mediated and often seen postpartum, painful usually sequelae of viral illness	Often slightly enlarged	Elevated during hypothyroid phase, can be transiently low during hyperthyroid phase	Painless often TPO antibody positive	Usually resolves without treatment, can evolve to permanent hypothyroidism, usually recurrence postpartum in subsequent pregnancies
TSH resistance	Reduced sensitivity of TSH receptor	Atrophic	Elevated	Negative	Permanent

TPO = thyroid peroxidase.

Table 4
Conditions Associated With Elevated Serum Concentrations of T_4/T_3[a]

Diagnosis	Etiology	Thyroid gland	Serum TSH concentration	Antibodies	Outcome/treatment
Graves disease	Circulating antibodies that stimulate TSH receptor	Usually symmetrically enlarged	Suppressed	TSI positive	Usually characterized by exacerbations and remissions
Neonatal Graves disease	Owing to transplacental transfer of maternal TSI	Enlarged	Suppressed	Maternal TSI	Self-limited, although may require temporary antithyroid drug treatment
Toxic nodule	Independent/autonomous production owing to activating mutation of TSH receptor	Focal enlargement	Suppressed	Negative	Hormone production proportional to size; treated with medicine, radioiodine, or surgery
Toxic goiter	Areas of autonomy throughout thyroid	Diffuse irregular enlargement	Suppressed	Negative	Usually progresses slowly; treated with medicine, radioiodine, or surgery
TSH-secreting pituitary adenoma	Excess TSH unresponsive to negative feedback from T_4/T_3	Diffusely enlarged	Inappropriately "normal" for high T_4/T_3 or elevated	Negative	Requires resection of pituitary adenoma
RTH	Genetic defect in TRβ gene, some with no identified defect	Enlarged	Inappropriately "normal" for high T_4/T_3 or elevated	Negative	Not progressive, thyroxine treatment recommended by some

[a] TSI = thyroid-stimulating immunoglobulin; TSH = thyrotropin.

tion. The relative concentration of T_3 in the thyroidal secretion increases and is, in general, proportional to the severity of the disease. Cloning of the TSH receptor has allowed mapping of the specific epitopes for Graves-associated antibody. The manifestations of Graves disease in the eye include periorbital swelling, infiltration of the extraocular muscles, and protrusion of the eye globe outside of the orbit and are mediated by the same or related antibodies.

The thyroid gland can make thyroid hormone autonomously independent of the usual regulation by TSH. The underlying pathology can be an autonomously functioning nodule or a diffusely hyperfunctioning goiter. A large fraction of autonomous nodules studied have a somatic mutation of the TSH receptor gene, which results in constitutive activation of the TSH receptor and, therefore, thyroid hormone production and thyroid cell growth. Approximately 1 in 100 infants born to mothers with Graves disease will have transient (several weeks to months) hyperthyroidism owing to transplacental passage of maternal IgG. An infant with a germ-line TSH receptor–activating mutation has been identified with severe neonatal hyperthyroidism.

7.2. Tissue-Specific Manifestations

A large fraction of hyperthyroid symptoms—nervousness, tachycardia, excess perspiration, and tremulousness—are a manifestation of increased sensitivity to stimulation from the adrenergic nervous system. The molecular basis of this sensitivity is not known, but the effect is thought to be augmentation of adrenergic signaling, including augmentation of receptor number, affinity, and signaling. Longer-term effects of thyroid hormone include weakness, muscle wasting, and weight loss owing to acceleration of the basal metabolic rate.

7.3. Treatment

The treatments available for hyperthyroidism include antithyroid drugs, radioiodine, and surgery. The choice of treatment varies by the clinical situation and even geographically. For example, radioiodine is used to a much greater extent in the United States compared with Asia or Europe, where antithyroid drugs are more commonly used.

8. THYROID HORMONE RESISTANCE

8.1. Clinical Presentation

RTH is a syndrome characterized by the presence of a diffuse goiter; elevated serum T_4 and T_3 concentrations; inappropriately "normal" (given elevated serum T_4 and T_3 concentrations) or elevated serum TSH concentration; and varying manifestations of hypothyroidism, including growth retardation, mental retardation, dysmorphisms, and deafness. Although most manifestations are consistent with reduced thyroid hormone action, an elevated heart rate in many patients indicates retained sensitivity to thyroid hormone effects on the heart. Attention deficit disorder is a frequent finding, seen in as many as 60% of RTH patients. Most patients are identified based on the findings of a goiter and elevated thyroid hormone levels, or as a result of family screening after an affected individual is identified.

8.2. Associated TR Mutations

All reported cases of RTH in which a genetic defect has been found have been associated with mutations in the TRβ gene. As many as 15% of patients with a clinical diagnosis of RTH will not have TRβ mutations and may have mutations in TR coactivator partners. Mutations have been described in three "hot spots" in the carboxy-terminal regions of the TRβ gene. Reduced affinity for T_3 is seen in all of the mutant receptors, and they function as dominant-negative inhibitors of wild-type receptor. In most kindreds, RTH is inherited as an autosomal-dominant trait. In the original kindred described, however, the trait was autosomal recessive, and individuals heterozygous for the defect had no abnormal phenotype. The affected individuals from this kindred were later found to have complete deletion of the coding region of the TRβ gene. Only one patient, the product of consanguineous parents, has been described who was homozygous for a dominant-negative TRβ mutation. This child was severely affected with very high serum thyroid hormone concentrations and profound neurologic abnormalities and died after a few years of life. TRα mutations have not been identified in patients with RTH, although analogous TRα mutants studied in vitro can function as a dominant-negative receptor. Mouse knockout models indicate that the TRα is very important for early development.

8.3. Mechanisms of Mutant Receptor Inhibition of Thyroid Hormone Action

The heterogeneity of clinical manifestations of RTH support the hypothesis that tissues differ in their ability to compensate for an absent or mutant TR isoform. There are a number of proposed mechanisms for inhibition of T_3 action by mutant TRβ receptors. It is known that there is a correlation between mutations or deletions that interfere with T_3 binding and inhibition of wild-type receptor. Examples of naturally occurring mutants that have this property include the oncogene *verb* A and the α2 variant of TRα. Several studies have demonstrated the importance of an intact DBD for inhibition. Mutant receptors can heterodimerize with the wild-type receptor and may form inactive complexes. The mutant receptor may compete with wild-type receptor for some limiting cofactor that is required for a response. Mutant receptors vary in their ability to have normal function restored by high concentrations of T$_3$. Furthermore, this normalization of function varies by the specific response element used, implying that a specific gene may be differentially affected. This may explain why tissues vary in their response to thyroid hormone; for example, some kindreds have primarily RTH action in the pituitary.

REFERENCE

Bianco AC, Salvatore D, Gereben B, Berry MJ, Larsen PR. Biochemistry, cellular and molecular biology, and physiological roles of the iodothyronine selenodeiodinases. *Endocr Rev* 2002; 23:38–89.

SELECTED READING

Brent GA. The molecular basis of thyroid hormone action. *N Engl J Med* 1994;331:847–853.

Brent GA. Tissue-specific actions of thyroid hormone: insights from animal models. *Rev Endocr Metab Disord* 2000;1/2:27–34.

Dohan O, De la Vieja A, Paroder V, Riedel C, Artani M, Reed M, Ginter CS, Carrasco N. The sodium/iodide symporter (NIS): characterization, regulation, and medical significance. *Endocr Rev* 2003;24:48–77.

Glinoer D. The regulation of thyroid function in pregnancy: pathways of endocrine adaptation from physiology to pathology. *Endocr Rev* 1997;18:404–433.

Knobel M, Medeiros-Neto G. An outline of inherited disorders of the thyroid hormone generating system. *Thyroid* 2003;13:771–801.

Lee H, Yen PM. Recent advances in understanding thyroid hormone receptor coregulators. *J Biomed Sci* 1999;6:71–78.

McLachlan SM, Rapoport B. The molecular biology of thyroid peroxidase: cloning, expression and role as autoantigen in autoimmune thyroid disease. *Endocr Rev* 1992;13:192–206.

Motomura K, Brent GA. Mechanism of thyroid hormone action: implications for the clinical manifestations of thyrotoxicosis. *Endocrinol Metab Clin North Am* 1998;27:1–23.

Paschke R, Ludgate M. The thyrotropin receptor in thyroid diseases *New Eng J Med* 1997;337:1675–1681.

Refetoff S. Resistance to thyrotropin. *J Endocrinol Invest* 2003;26: 770–779.

Weiss RE, Refetoff S. Resistance to thyroid hormone. *Rev Endocr Metab Disord* 2000;1:97–108.

18 Calcium-Regulating Hormones

Vitamin D and Parathyroid Hormone

Geoffrey N. Hendy, PhD

Contents

1. INTRODUCTION

This chapter describes the structure and actions of vitamin D, which is essential for maintaining a positive calcium balance and skeletal integrity, and the parathyroid hormone (PTH), responsible for minute-to-minute maintenance of calcium homeostasis, which is critical for neuromuscular activity.

2. VITAMIN D

Vitamin D originally attracted attention because of its antirachitic properties. It is now appreciated to be a natural product of the body and is the precursor of the calcium-regulating hormone, 1,25-dihydroxyvitamin D (1,25[OH]$_2$D). This is produced in the kidney; is released into the circulation, and exerts its effects on mineral homeostasis by acting on intestine, bone, kidney, and the parathyroid gland. The hormone acts like a steroid hormone in the nuclei of target cells, and its production is subject to feedback regulation. Vitamin D and its metabolites form the basis of an endocrine system that interacts with the parathyroid glands and is of fundamental importance in the hormonal control of mineral metabolism.

2.1. Production and Metabolism of Vitamin D

2.1.1. Chemical Structure

Vitamin D is a 9-10 secosterol with the A-ring rotated into the *cis* configuration. Although it is related to a C$_{21}$

From: *Endocrinology: Basic and Clinical Principles, Second Edition*
(S. Melmed and P. M. Conn, eds.) © Humana Press Inc., Totowa, NJ

steroid, it differs in structure by disruption of the bond between C-9 and C-10, opening the B-ring, and thus forms a conjugated triene structure. It also has an elongated side chain (Fig. 1). Cholecalciferol (vitamin D$_3$) is the natural form of the vitamin. This C$_{27}$ compound is produced by irradiation of the precursor 7-dehydrocholesterol. Ergocalciferol (vitamin D$_2$) is a synthetic C$_{28}$ compound originally produced by irradiation of the plant sterol, ergosterol. The side chain of vitamin D$_2$ differs from that of vitamin D$_3$ by having a double bond between C-22 and C-23 and a methyl group at C-24. Vitamins D$_2$ and D$_3$ are metabolized along similar pathways, and vitamin D written without a subscript can refer to either form of the vitamin.

2.1.2. Photoproduction

Normally, synthesis of vitamin D$_3$ in the skin can provide the body's full requirement unless exposure to sunlight is restricted. Production of vitamin D$_3$ occurs by nonenzymatic photolysis of 7-dehydrocholesterol (provitamin D) in the epidermis (Fig. 2). Near-ultraviolet (UV) light with a wavelength of 290–315 nm opens the B-ring by cleaving the bond between C-9 and C-10 of 7-dehydrocholesterol, forming previtamin D$_3$, and rearrangement of the molecule, which is temperature dependent and favored at body temperature, yields vitamin D$_3$. Two other biologically inert products, lumisterol and tachysterol, are produced by photolysis of previtamin D. The skin pigment melanin can

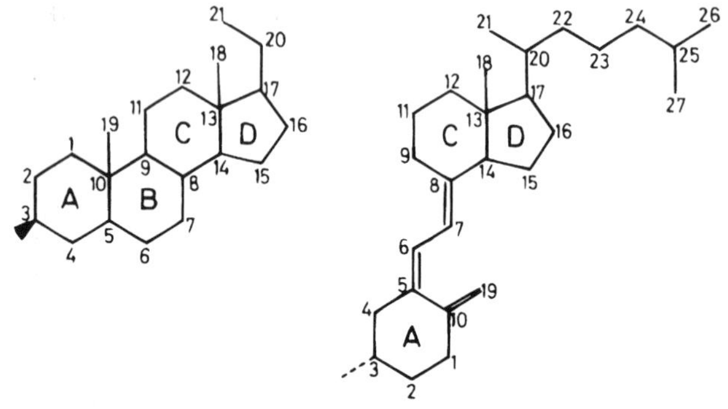

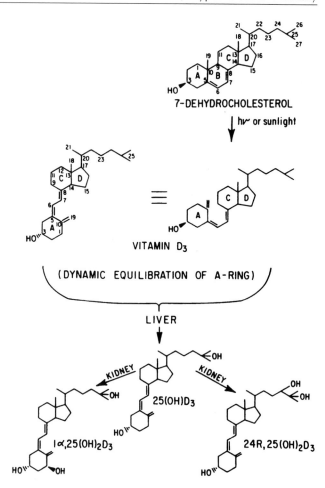

Fig. 1. Structure of a C_{21} steroid (**left**) compared with a C_{27} secosterol (**right**), such as vitamin D_3.

also absorb UV light and when present in large amounts competes with 7-dehydrocholesterol for this energy source. Given the same UV exposure, heavily pigmented individuals produce less vitamin D_3 than lightly pigmented individuals.

Vitamin D can also be obtained from the diet either as vitamin D_3 from foods that contain it naturally (e.g., liver of fatty fish) or from milk and dairy products, which are frequently fortified with either vitamin D_2 or D_3.

2.1.3. METABOLIC ACTIVATION OF VITAMIN D

Biologic responses to vitamin D_3 after its administration to animals are apparent only after a significant time lag. Vitamin D must undergo two hydroxylation steps before it assumes the physiologically active form, $1,25(OH)_2D$. This allows it to bind to intracellular receptors in target tissues.

2.1.3.1. 25-Hydroxylation in Liver. Vitamin D_3
either produced in the skin or absorbed from the small intestine rapidly accumulates in the liver, where it is hydroxylated at C-25 of the side chain to form 25-hydroxycholecalciferol ($25[OH]D_3$), the most abundant form of the vitamin (Fig. 2). Vitamin D_2 is similarly metabolized to 25-hydroxyergocalciferol ($25[OH]D_2$). This step is obligatory for further metabolism of the sterol. The liver is the principal site of production in vivo, and total hepatectomy causes the virtual disappearance of $25(OH)D$ from the circulation. Hepatic 25-hydroxylase activity is associated with mitochondrial and microsomal fractions, and both activities are the result of cytochrome P-450 enzymes. The mitochondrial enzyme is CYP27A1 sterol 27-hydroxylase. Loss-of-function mutations in humans and mice manifest in markedly altered cholesterol metabolism as this enzyme catalyzes an essential step in bile acid synthesis. By contrast, vitamin D metabolism is normal, indicating that the microsomal vitamin

Fig. 2. Metabolic pathway of vitamin D_3 production and activation beginning with synthesis of previtamin D_3 by UV irradiation of 7-dehydrocholesterol in skin. Rearrangement of previtamin D_3 yields vitamin D_3, which is metabolized to $25(OH)D_3$ in the liver. In the kidney, $25(OH)D_3$ is either metabolized to the hormonally-active $1,25(OH)_2D_3$ or catabolized to $24,25(OH)_2D_3$. (Adapted from Minghetti and Norman, 1988.)

D–hydroxylase compensates for loss of the mitochondrial activity. An enzyme, CYP2R1, having the appropriate biochemical properties and tissue and subcellular distribution has been identified. In contrast to CYP27A1, a low-affinity, high-capacity enzyme that activates cholecalciferol but not ergocalciferol, CYP2R1 is a high-affinity, low-capacity enzyme that catalyzes hydroxylation of both vitamins D_2 and D_3.

$25(OH)D_3$ is more effective than vitamin D_3 in curing rickets and acts more rapidly in stimulating both intestinal calcium absorption and calcium mobilization from bone. At one time, it was believed to be the final active metabolite of vitamin D_3. However, although it is not biologically active at physiologic concentrations in vivo, it is active in binding the intestinal vitamin D receptor (VDR) and stimulating calcium transport at high concentrations. The hypercalcemia produced by vitamin D intoxication is mediated by 25(OH)D.

2.1.3.2. 1α-Hydroxylation in Kidney. Further metabolism of 25(OH)D occurs in mitochondria of renal proximal tubules to the most biologically active metabolite of vitamin D known, 1,25(OH)$_2$D (Fig. 2). Although other tissues and cultured cells can produce 1,25(OH)$_2$D, these sources do not normally contribute significantly to the circulating 1,25(OH)$_2$D concentration. 1,25(OH)$_2$D is absent from the serum of anephric animals and humans. In pregnancy, additional hormone is supplied to the circulation by placental production of 1,25(OH)$_2$D. Hypercalcemia associated with granulomatous diseases, such as sarcoidosis and tuberculosis, and certain lymphomas, is also the result of extrarenal synthesis of 1,25(OH)$_2$D.

The renal 1α-hydroxylase, CYP27B1, is of the P-450 mixed-function type, and requires a ferrodoxin and NADPH, which is generated in the mitochondria by an energy-dependent transhydrogenase.

2.1.3.3. 24-Hydroxylation. Hydroxylation of 25(OH)D at C-24 produces 24,25(OH)$_2$D (Fig. 2), the second most abundant circulating metabolite of vitamin D. It circulates at concentrations 10-fold lower than those of 25(OH)D. Most circulating 24,25(OH)$_2$D is derived from the kidney, but many other tissues can also produce this metabolite. The renal tubular 24-hydroxylase enzyme is located in mitochondria but is distinct from the renal 1α-hydroxylase. The P-450 component of this enzyme, CYP24A1, has been cloned and characterized in the human and other species. Its main substrate is 25(OH)D, but the enzyme also hydroxylates 1,25(OH)$_2$D to form 1,24,25(OH)$_3$D. 24,25(OH)$_2$D is far less active than 1,25(OH)$_2$D in bioassays, and a clear physiologic role has been difficult to ascribe. 24-Hydroxylation renders the vitamin D molecule susceptible to side-chain cleavage and oxidation, and 24,25(OH)$_2$D represents the first metabolic step in hormonal inactivation.

2.1.3.4. Further Metabolism of Vitamin D. Other forms of vitamin D have been identified in the circulation. 25,26-Dihydroxyvitamin D (25,26[OH$_2$]D), which is produced in the kidney and liver, circulates at a concentration slightly lower than that of 24,25(OH)$_2$D. 1,25(OH)D can be catabolized by two pathways to either the C$_{23}$ calcitroic acid (1[OH]-24,25,26,27-tetranor-23-COOH-D) or 1,25(OH)$_2$D-26,23-lactone. 24,25(OH)$_2$D can also be metabolized by two pathways leading to either 25,26,27-trinor-24-COOH-D or 24,25,26,27-tetranor-23-COOH-D.

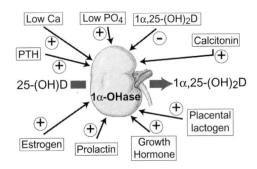

Fig. 3. 1,25(OH)$_2$D is produced in the kidney by metabolism of 25(OH)D. The renal 1α-hydroxylase is modulated both positively (+) and negatively (−) by several regulators (shown in boxes) including mineral ions, hormones, and 1,25(OH)$_2$D itself.

2.1.4. REGULATION OF VITAMIN D METABOLISM

Dietary intake and endogenous synthesis of vitamin D are variable, and there is a need for regulation of the production of the more active metabolites. Potentially, this is feasible at the stages of hepatic and renal hydroxylation. Hepatic 25-hydroxylation is not regulated by serum calcium or phosphate. Although it is more efficient at low levels of substrate, it is not tightly regulated, because suppression of the enzyme can be overcome by large amounts of vitamin D. This has practical application in the clinical administration of a synthetic form of vitamin D$_3$, 1α-hydroxycholecalciferol (1α[OH]D$_3$), which requires hepatic hydroxylation at C-25 to become active. This might give a safety factor if there was product inhibition of 25-hydroxylase, but, in fact, hypercalcemia can be produced with 1α(OH)D$_3$ even in microgram doses, and careful monitoring of treatment with this drug is necessary.

More important is the control of 1α- and 24-hydroxylases in the kidney. There is a switching mechanism that determines the relative activity of these two enzymes. Normally, serum concentrations of 1,25(OH)$_2$D change little in response to administration of vitamin D. Several circulating factors modulate the fine control of the 1α-hydroxylase, the most important being parathyroid hormone (PTH), calcium, phosphate, and 1,25(OH)$_2$D (Fig. 3).

2.1.4.1. Calcium and PTH. In hypocalcemia, 25(OH)D is preferentially converted into 1,25(OH)$_2$D, whereas in normo- and hypercalcemia, it is mainly metabolized to 24,25(OH)$_2$D. This effect is achieved largely by hypocalcemia stimulating the parathyroid gland to secrete PTH, which enhances renal proximal tubular 1α-hydroxylase activity and raises serum 1,25(OH)$_2$D. This enhances intestinal calcium absorp-

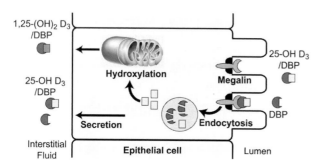

Fig. 4. Renal uptake and activation of 25(OH)D. Complexes of 25(OH)D and DBP undergo glomerular filtration and are taken up from the lumen into proximal tubular cells by the endocytic receptor megalin. The complexes go to lysosomes, DBP is degraded; and 25(OH)D is released and taken up by mitochondria, where it is 1α-hydroxylated. The active vitamin D metabolite is secreted into the interstitial fluid.

tion, and the increased serum calcium concentration inhibits PTH secretion, closing the feedback loop. The circulating calcium concentration acting via the calcium-sensing receptor (CASR) can also directly modulate the renal 1α-hydroxylase (Fig. 3).

2.1.4.2. Phosphate . Low serum phosphate concentrations stimulate and high-phosphate concentrations inhibit renal 1α-hydroxylase activity (Fig. 3). These effects are independent of PTH.

2.1.4.3. 1,25(OH)₂D . 1,25(OH)$_2$D controls its own synthesis (Fig. 3) by decreasing 1α-hydroxylase activity and stimulating 24-hydroxylase activity. When large doses of 1,25(OH)$_2$D$_3$ are given to vitamin D–deficient chicks, the switch in enzyme activity occurs rapidly, and this can be prevented by actinomycin D. This suggests that 1,25(OH)$_2$D regulates its own production by the synthesis of new protein. Indirect regulation may also occur via the effect of 1,25(OH)$_2$D on the parathyroid glands, and the consequent changes in serum calcium and phosphate.

2.1.4.4. Other Regulators . Calcium requirements are increased in physiological states, such as growth, pregnancy, lactation, and egg laying, and hormonal changes occurring during these conditions influence vitamin D metabolism. In mammals, prolactin, insulin, growth hormone (GH), and calcitonin all stimulate 1α-hydroxylase (Fig. 3). In birds, enhanced estrogen and progesterone secretion during egg laying enhance 1α-hydroxylation and increase serum 1,25(OH)$_2$D levels.

2.2. Absorption, Transport, and Excretion

After absorption from the duodenum and distal ileum, vitamin D is incorporated into chylomicrons. Disrup-

tion of this process, as in steatorrhea, can lead to vitamin D malabsorption. Normally, as much as half of the absorbed vitamin is stored in body fats.

Vitamin D derived from either diet or epidermis is bound in the circulation by the vitamin D–binding protein (DBP), an α-globulin of 55,000 Daltons, previously known as group-specific component. This has a single high-affinity binding site that binds vitamin D and all its metabolites, although it has higher affinity for 25(OH)D, 24,25(OH)$_2$D, and 25,26(OH)$_2$D than for vitamin D or 1,25(OH)$_2$D. This facilitates partitioning of vitamin D in lipid stores and favors entry of 1,25(OH)$_2$D into target cells. The serum DBP concentration greatly exceeds the concentration of all vitamin D metabolites, such that only 3–5% of available binding sites are occupied. Hepatic synthesis of the protein is increased in pregnancy and decreased in chronic liver disease, and serum concentrations are also reduced in the nephrotic syndrome. DBP concentrations are not influenced by vitamin D status; they are unaltered in disorders of mineral homeostasis. Mice null for DBP and fed a vitamin D–deficient diet exhibit osteopathy and resistance to vitamin D toxicity. The latter may reflect more rapid urinary excretion of 25(OH)D, and a more rapid conversion into inactive polar metabolites.

Megalin and cubulin are large, membrane-associated endocytic receptor proteins on the luminal surface of the kidney proximal tubule that recognize and bind DBP. Together, they constitute part of a functional unit for delivery of 25(OH)D to the 1α-hydroxylase enzyme (Fig. 4). Filtered 25(OH)D-DBP is endocytosed and delivered to lysosomes, where DBP is degraded and 25(OH)D is released to the cytosol. 25(OH)D is either secreted or hydroxylated in the mitochondria to 1,25(OH)$_2$D before release into the interstitial fluid and complex formation with DBP. Intracellular DBPs that are members of the heat-shock protein family promote the uptake and preferential 1α-hydroxylation of 25-hydroxylated vitamin D metabolites. After 1,25(OH)$_2$D has performed its function in target tissues, it is converted into inactive metabolites, such as calcitroic acid, via a 24-oxidation pathway and excreted in bile. Administration of anticonvulsant drugs increase the biliary excretion of vitamin D metabolites.

2.3. Biologic Actions of Vitamin D
2.3.1. Intestine

In the small intestine, 1,25(OH)$_2$D actively stimulates calcium transport, and this is accompanied by passive movement of phosphate. In addition, an independent active phosphate transport system is stimulated throughout the small and large bowels. The calcium transport response to a dose of 1,25(OH)$_2$D is biphasic, with the first phase peaking at 6 h and the second phase maintaining elevated calcium transport for several days. In vitro both $1,25(OH)_2D$ and $25(OH)D$ can increase calcium absorption by a direct action on the gut, whereas vitamin D cannot.

The synthesis of several intestinal epithelial cell proteins that may function in the calcium transport process, including apical calcium transport protein 1 and the epithelial calcium channel, is induced by $1,25(OH)_2D$. Additionally, production of a calcium-binding protein (calbindinD28K in chick and calbindinD9K in mammals) is dependent on vitamin D in the intestine, and its appearance in villus enterocytes is induced within a few hours of administration of $1,25(OH)_2D_3$.

$1,25(OH)_2D$ induces changes in plasma membrane phospholipase activity in intestinal epithelial cells with a similar time course to that of $1,25(OH)_2D$-stimulated uptake of calcium into brush border membrane vesicles. It has been suggested that $1,25(OH)_2D$-induced alteration in membrane lipids initiates the calcium transport process.

2.3.2. SKELETON

The antirachitic effects of vitamin D are mainly indirect, relying more on increasing serum calcium and phosphate through its actions on intestinal absorption than a direct action on bone formation. Intravenous infusion of calcium and phosphate in vitamin D–deficient rats or feeding mutant mice lacking either the VDR or the $1\alpha(OH)$ase gene a "rescue diet" rich in lactose, calcium, and phosphate can cure rickets in the absence of circulating $1,25(OH)_2D$. However, $1,25(OH)_2D$ does act directly on bone-forming cells. In cultured osteoblasts, $1,25(OH)_2D_3$ stimulates matrix deposition and terminal differentiation. Conversely, when dietary sources are inadequate to maintain normocalcemia, $1,25(OH)_2D$ may stimulate calcium mobilization from the bone by promoting the action of PTH to differentiate mononuclear precursor cells into mature, multinuclear bone-resorbing osteoclasts. Overall, $1,25(OH)_2D$ facilitates bone remodeling.

2.3.3. KIDNEY

As it does in other tissues, $1,25(OH)_2D$ induces the transcriptional activity of the 24-hydroxylase gene in the kidney. $1,25(OH)_2D$ causes a decrease in both calcium and phosphate excretion by increasing renal proximal tubular reabsorption, although the phosphate-conserving action may in part be indirect via PTH.

2.3.4. OTHER TISSUES

$1,25(OH)_2D$ inhibits PTH synthesis and secretion as part of an important feedback loop in regulating mineral ion homeostasis. This has led to the use of iv $1,25(OH)_2D_3$ and its analogs in the treatment of secondary hyperparathyroidism of chronic renal failure.

In addition to the classic actions of vitamin D on mineral metabolism, $1,25(OH)_2D$ has pleiotropic actions in many tissues that are not necessarily related to its role as a calcium-regulating hormone. These often involve the sterol acting as an antiproliferative, prodifferentiation agent in both normal and cancer cells. For example, $1,25(OH)_2D_3$ induces maturation of basal epidermal skin cells into keratinocytes and stimulates mouse myeloid leukemic cells to differentiate into macrophages.

The VDR also functions as a receptor for the bile acid, lithocholic acid (LCA). LCA activates the VDR and induces expression of the enzyme, CYP3A, that detoxifies the growth-promoting LCA in the liver and intestine. In the digestive tract, the VDR could function as a part of a protective mechanism to inhibit enhanced cellular proliferation leading to colon carcinoma.

2.3.4.1. Nonhypercalcemic Vitamin D Analogs. Because of its antiproliferative effects, $1,25(OH)_2D_3$ is potentially useful clinically in the control of secondary hyperparathyroidism and various cancers, and in the treatment of the common, benign hyperproliferative skin disorder psoriasis. However, hypercalcemia results from $1,25(OH)_2D_3$ treatment. Recently, synthetic $1,25(OH)_2D_3$ analogs have been developed that display reduced calcemic activity (Fig. 5). Many of these carry side-chain modifications that reduce affinity for the serum DBP, alter tissue distribution, and accelerate metabolic degradation. Several of these derivatives have been shown to be highly effective in controlling cellular differentiation and maintain a high affinity for the VDR. One of these compounds, Calcipotriol (MC903), is currently available for the treatment of psoriasis.

2.4. Biochemical Mechanism of Action

2.4.1. GENOMIC ACTIONS

Tissues responsive to vitamin D contain a specific, high-affinity intracellular receptor, the VDR, that mediates the ability of $1,25(OH)_2D$ to regulate gene expression by binding vitamin D–responsive elements (VDREs). The present understanding is that free $1,25(OH)_2D$ (that fraction of circulating $1,25[OH]_2D$ not bound to the serum DBP) diffuses across the cell membrane. It is not known if a specific endocytic receptor is involved in this process. In the cell, $1,25(OH)_2D$ binds the VDR in the cytoplasm followed by ligand-bound VDR translocation to the nucleus. The VDR is closely related structurally to the thyroid hormone and retinoic acid receptors, which all function as ligand-activated transcription factors.

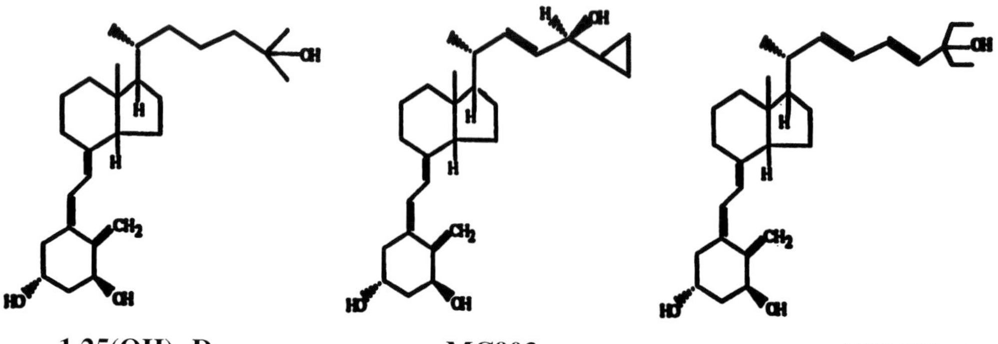

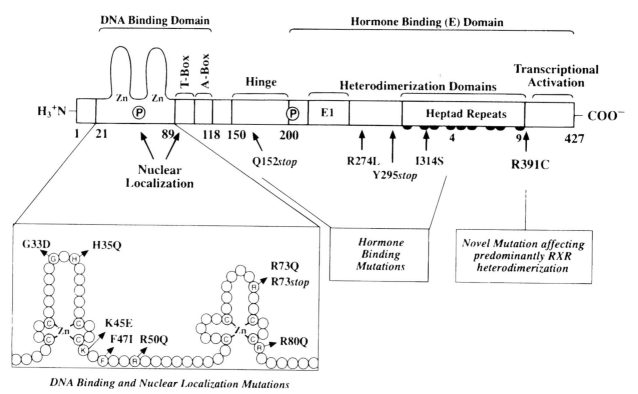

Fig. 5. Structure of 1,25(OH)$_2$D$_3$ and its "noncalcemic" analogs, MC903 and EB1089. MC903 and EB1089 differ only in the side chain compared to 1,25(OH)$_2$D$_3$ and demonstrate reduced calcemic activity but are equipotent or more potent than 1,25(OH)$_2$D$_3$ in inhibiting cell proliferation (Yu et al., 1995).

Fig. 6. Structure/function map of human VDR showing naturally occurring mutations causing hereditary vitamin D–dependent rickets type II. P indicates a phosphorylation site (Haussler et al., 1995).

The VDREs in positively controlled genes are direct hexanucleotide repeats with a spacer of 3 nucleotides. The VDR associates with the VDRE as a heterodimer with a retinoid X receptor (RXR). The VDR has several functional domains: an NH$_2$-terminal zinc finger DNA-binding domain, a hinge region, and a COOH-terminal hormone-binding domain that also contains regions responsible for heterodimerization with the RXR (Fig. 6). Binding of 1,25(OH)$_2$D to the VDR

alters the conformation of the VDR, facilitating dimerization with RXR and enhancing association with the VDRE. RXR binds the 5′-VDRE repeat, and the VDR binds the 3′-VDRE repeat. After heterodimerization with RXR, the VDR binds several coregulatory proteins (coactivators or corepressors) that couple to the basal RNA polymerase II transcription machinery. Positive VDREs have been identified in several genes, including those for osteocalcin, osteopontin, 24-

hydroxylase, β_3 integrin, and the CASR. Negative VDREs have been described in the *PTH* and bone sialoprotein genes, although it remains less clear how 1,25(OH)$_2$D negatively modulates gene transcription. Coregulatory proteins other than RXR are likely to interact with the VDR and modulate its effect on gene transcription.

The cells of a patient resistant to vitamin D action but with normal VDR expression were demonstrated to have increased expression of a VDRE-interacting protein that blocks binding of the VDR-RXR heterodimer to DNA. The mechanism underlying the increased expression of this heterogeneous nuclear ribonucleoprotein is not known.

2.4.2. NONGENOMIC ACTIONS

1,25(OH)$_2$D can also act on target cells via nongenomic mechanisms. Unlike genomic events, which take several hours or days to be apparent, nongenomic effects take place in minutes or less after hormonal treatment. The nongenomic effects include stimulation of Ca^{2+} influx, release of Ca^{2+} from intracellular stores, protein phosphorylation, and phospholipid turnover. An important finding is that genomic and nongenomic effects are pharmacologically separable. Thus, it has been speculated that a distinct membrane VDR exists, possibly coupled to a phospholipase, that mediates these nongenomic actions. It should be emphasized, however, that such a receptor has yet to be identified. Some of the nonhypercalcemic analogs discussed in Section 1.3.4.1. retain the genomic activities of 1,25(OH)$_2$D and decrease cellular proliferation and promote differentiation but lack the nongenomic effects that stimulate calcium mobilization. These compounds have the greatest therapeutic potential for the treatment of hyperproliferative disorders while minimizing hypercalcemic side effects.

2.5. Pathophysiology of Hypervitaminosis D and Hypovitaminosis D, Receptor Defects

2.5.1. ASSESSMENT OF VITAMIN D STATUS

Assays for vitamin D and its metabolites in serum use radioligand-binding techniques—radioreceptor or radioimmunoassay—most of which require prior chromatography to separate the metabolite to be measured. The circulating concentration of 25(OH)D is the best index of overall vitamin D status. There is a seasonal fluctuation in serum 25(OH)D concentrations, with highest values occurring in late summer and lowest values in late winter. The physiologic status of an individual should be considered in interpreting serum 1,25(OH)$_2$D levels, which may be increased during growth, pregnancy, or lactation. Table 1 provides the

frequently encountered clinical conditions that may present with an abnormal serum concentration of 25(OH)D or 1,25(OH)$_2$D. Insufficient dietary intake or cutaneous synthesis of vitamin D can lead to inadequate production of 25(OH)D substrate for conversion into 1,25(OH)$_2$D. Disturbances in vitamin D metabolism at the level of liver or kidney can cause reduced production of 1,25(OH)$_2$D. In renal failure, a decline in functional renal mass, with increased phosphate retention, reduces or eliminates 1α-hydroxylase activity. Hypoparathyroidism and pseudohypoparathyroidism are associated with low circulating 1,25(OH)$_2$D concentrations. In vitamin D–dependent rickets type I, serum 1,25(OH)$_2$D levels are low because of an inherited defect in the renal 1α-hydroxylase enzyme. By contrast, in vitamin D–dependent rickets type II, resulting from an inherited defect in the VDR, the end-organ resistance can lead to grossly elevated serum 1,25(OH)$_2$D concentrations.

Clinical deficiency of vitamin D can result from perturbations at several different levels—synthesis, metabolism, or action. Consequently, for accurate assessment of the pathophysiology, it may be necessary to consider both 25(OH)D and 1,25(OH)$_2$D concentrations. For example, low 1,25(OH)$_2$D levels need not necessarily indicate defective renal production of the metabolite. They could result from insufficient vitamin D intake, and this would be indicated by a low serum 25(OH)$_2$D concentration. However, if 1,25(OH)$_2$D values are low in the presence of a normal 25(OH)D value, decreased renal synthesis of 1,25(OH)$_2$D is likely.

2.5.2. RECEPTOR DEFECTS

Vitamin D–dependent rickets type II is a rare, autosomal-recessive disorder in which severe hypocalcemia and rickets develop in early childhood. The disease is unresponsive to all forms of vitamin D, including high doses of 1,25(OH)$_2$D$_3$. In affected individuals, a number of naturally occurring mutations in the VDR gene have been identified (Fig. 6), which disrupt DNA binding and/or nuclear localization, ligand binding, or RXR heterodimerization.

2.6. Summary

The crystal structures of the DBP and the ligand-binding domain of the VDR are now known. This will aid in understanding how vitamin D metabolites circulate and how 1,25(OH)$_2$D and its pharmacologically important analogs transactivate its target genes. Novel 1,25(OH)$_2$D target genes that have been identified include the epithelial calcium channels in proximal intestine and distal nephron and the *CASR* in parathy-

Table 1
Concentrations of Vitamin D Metabolite in Patients
With Disordered Calcium Homeostasis [a]

	25(OH)D	1,25(OH)$_2$D
Hypocalcemia		
• Vitamin D deficiency	↓	↓ or ↑ or →
• Severe hepatocellular disease	↓	↓ or →
• Nephrotic syndrome	↓	↓ or →
• Renal failure	→	↓
• Hyperphosphatemia	→	↓
• Hypoparathyroidism	→	↓ or →
• Pseudohypoparathyroidism	→	↓ or →
• Hypomagnesemia	→	↓ or →
• Vitamin D–dependent rickets type I	→ or ↑	↓
• Vitamin D–dependent rickets type II	→ or ↑	↑
Hypercalcemia/hypercalciuria		
• Vitamin D, 25(OH)D intoxication	↑	↓ or →
• 1,25(OH)$_2$D intoxication	→	↑
• Granuloma-forming diseases	→	↑
• Lymphoma	→	↓ or ↑
• Hyperparathyroidism	→	↓ or ↑
• Williams syndrome	→	↑
• Idiopathic hypercalciuria	→	↑
• Idiopathic osteoporosis	→	↑ or →
• PTHrP associated	→	↓

[a] ↓ = decreased; ↑ = increased; → = normal. (Adapted from Clemens and Adams, 1996.)

roid and kidney tubule. It is suggested that the *VDR* gene, as marked by allelic variants, is a predictor of bone mass in some populations. 1,25(OH)$_2$D exhibits pleiotropic actions, not only playing a key role in mineral metabolism but also influencing cell differentiation. These effects are achieved through genomic mechanisms involving the widely expressed VDR and nongenomic mechanisms. The essential roles of vitamin D metabolites in vivo have been revealed by murine knockout models of the VDR as well as the key metabolic enzymes involved.

3. PARATHYROID HORMONE

PTH is essential for the maintenance of calcium homeostasis, and an excess or deficiency can cause severe and potential fatal illness. PTH is synthesized in the parathyroid glands in the neck, and after secretion, PTH exerts its effects directly on the skeleton and kidneys.

3.1. Hormone Gene

3.1.1. STRUCTURE

PTH is the product of a single-copy gene and in mammals has 84 amino acids. The gene, which encodes a larger precursor molecule of 115 amino acids,

preproPTH, is organized into three exons. Exon I encodes the 5′ untranslated region (UTR) of the messenger RNA; exon II encodes the NH$_2$-terminal pre- or signal peptide and part of the short propeptide; and exon III encodes the Lys^{-2}-Arg^{-1} of the prohormone cleavage site, the 84 amino acids of the mature hormone, and the 3′-UTR of the mRNA (Fig. 7).

This general organization is shared by the PTH-related peptide (PTHrP) gene, in which the same functional domains—the untranslated region, preprosequence of the precursor peptide, and the prohormone cleavage site and most or all of the mature peptide—are encoded by single exons (Fig. 7). For the *PTHrP* gene, exons encoding alternative 5′ UTRs, carboxyl-terminal peptides, and 3′ UTRs may also be present, depending on the species.

The *PTH* and *PTHrP* genes map to chromosome 11p15 and chromosome 12p12.1-11.2, respectively. These two human chromosomes are thought to have been derived by an ancient duplication of a single chromosome, and the *PTH* and *PTHrP* genes and their respective gene clusters have been maintained as syntenic groups in the human, rat, and mouse genomes. Because of the similarity in NH$_2$-terminal sequence of their mature peptides, their gene organization, and chro-

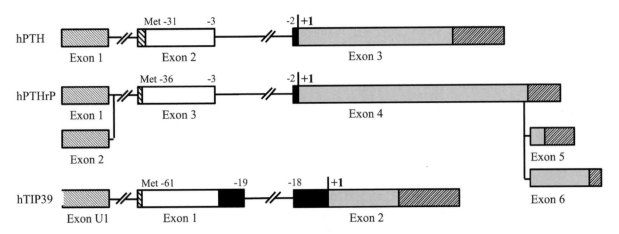

Fig. 7. Comparison of structural organization of the human PTH, PTHrP, and TIP39 genes. Exons are boxed: from left to right, stippled and hatched boxes denote 5′UTRs, white boxes denote presequences, black boxes denote prosequences, light gray stippled boxes denote mature polypeptide sequences, and dark gray stippled boxes denote 3′UTRs. +1 denotes the beginning of the mature polypeptide. (Adapted from John et al, 2002.)

mosomal locations, it is likely that the *PTH* and *PTHrP* genes evolved from a single ancestral gene and form part of a single gene family.

The gene for tuberoinfundibular peptide of 39 residues (TIP39), a more distantly related member of the gene family, resides on chromosome 19q13.33. The *TIP39* gene shares organizational features with the *PTH* and *PTHrP* genes having one exon encoding the 5′UTR, one encoding the precursor leader sequence, and one encoding the prohormone cleavage site and the mature peptide (Fig. 7).

3.1.2. REGULATION

Transcription of the *PTH* gene occurs almost exclusively in the endocrine cells of the parathyroid gland and is subject to strong repressor activity in all other cells. Ectopic PTH synthesis (i.e., synthesis outside parathyroid tissue) has been documented in only a very few cases of malignancies associated with hypercalcemia. In the majority of instances of hypercalcemia associated with malignancies, PTHrP is the responsible causal factor.

Activation of genes in particular tissues is often related to demethylation of cytosine residues, and the *PTH* gene in parathyroid cells is hypomethylated at CpG residues relative to other tissues. The human *PTH* gene has two functional TATA transcriptional start sites, a cyclic adenosine monophosphate (cAMP) response element, and a VDRE in its proximal promoter. Distally, several kilobase pairs upstream of the transcription start site sequences that function to repress transcription in nonparathyroid cells are present. *PTH* gene transcription is negatively regulated by the hormonally active metabolite of vitamin D, 1,25(OH)$_2$D.

3.1.3. COMPARISON OF SPECIES

The primary structure of the major glandular form of PTH, PTH(1-84), has been determined in several mammalian species, including human, bovine, porcine, and rat (Fig. 8). In the chicken, the PTH polypeptide contains 88 rather than 84 amino acids. The NH$_2$-terminal 34 amino acids are the most well-conserved portion of the molecule, and structure and function studies have emphasized the importance of the NH$_2$-terminal region to bioactivity in all species. Considerable deletion of the middle and COOH-terminal region of the intact polypeptide can be tolerated without apparent loss of important biologic activity.

3.1.4. ULTRASTRUCTURE

In aqueous solution, PTH(1-34) and PTHrP(1-34) have little secondary structure. In the presence of organic solvents or lipids, there is a dramatic increase in the α-helical content of the peptides. A common three-dimensional model was proposed for both PTH(1-34) and PTHrP(1-34) in which amino- and carboxy-terminal α-helical domains align side by side in antiparallel fashion with inwardly facing hydrophobic residues forming a core. Hydrophilic residues comprise a loop connecting the helices and also line their outer surfaces. By contrast, the crystal structure of PTH(1-34) reveals it to be in a slightly bent, extended helical conformation. While the NH$_2$-terminal PTH could be in a flexible conformation in solution (in the extracellular fluid), an extended helical conformation may be induced as the peptide approaches the hydrophobic plasma membrane before receptor binding.

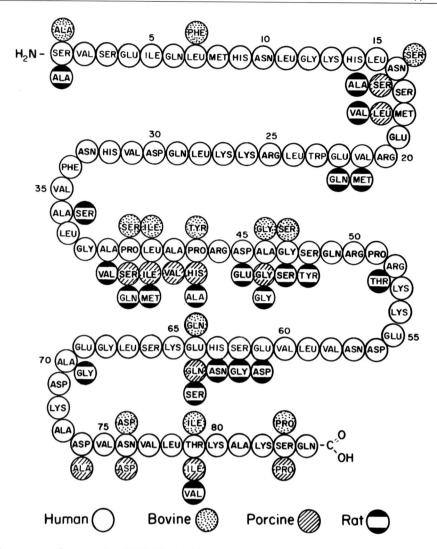

Fig. 8. Amino acid sequence of mammalian PTH. The backbone is that of the human sequence, and substitutions in the bovine, porcine, and rat hormones are shown (Goltzman and Hendy, 2001).

3.2. PTH Receptor Gene

Like other peptide hormones, PTH and PTHrP bind receptors on the plasma membrane of target cells. The PTH/PTHrP receptor belongs to a new subgroup (B or II) of the G protein–coupled seven-transmembrane-spanning receptor superfamily that, by virtue of their structural similarities, also includes the receptors binding secretin, calcitonin, vasoactive intestinal peptide, glucagon, glucagon-like peptide-1, and GH-releasing hormone.

3.2.1. STRUCTURE

The rat, mouse, and human *PTH/PTHrP receptor* genes have a similar complex organization and possess at least 17 exons. The first three exons encode two different 5′ UTRs of the mRNA, and the remaining 14 exons encode the receptor. This has 585–593 amino acids depending on species. Four exons encode portions of the extracellular domain, and eight exons encode the seven predicted transmembrane domains. This arrangement is not only well conserved within species but is also very similar to that of related subgroup family members, such as the GH-releasing factor receptor, calcitonin receptor, and glucagon receptor genes. This suggests that these receptor genes evolved from a common precursor.

Both promoters in the human *PTH/PTHrP receptor* gene (on chromosome 3p21.1-p22) lack a consensus TATA element, and the downstream promoter is (G + C) rich, containing several Sp-1 sites. By contrast, the upstream promoter is not (G + C) rich but does possess a CCAAT box. Whereas transcripts derived from the downstream promoter are widely expressed in many tissues, the upstream promoter is highly tissue specific, being strongly active in kidney and weakly active in liver, but not expressed at all in other tissues. $1,25(OH)_2D$ via the downstream promoter downregulates the *PTH/PTHrP receptor* gene in osteoblasts but not chondrocytes.

A related receptor, PTHR2, has been identified and appears to be the natural receptor for the neuromodulator TIP39.

3.2.2. REGULATION

Homologous downregulation of PTH/PTHrP receptors by PTH is observed in bone and kidney cells. This may explain, in part, the well-recognized resistance to PTH action in primary and secondary hyperparathyroidism. Posttranscriptional mechanisms, such as receptor-ligand recycling and membrane reinsertion, are involved since the steady-state levels of PTH/PTHrP receptor mRNA are unaltered by PTH exposure. Heterologous regulation of the PTH receptor also occurs. For example, glucocorticoids increase and decrease PTH/PTHrP receptors in bone cells and kidney cells, respectively. $1,25(OH)_2D$ and retinoic acid decrease PTH receptors in bone cells. In these cases of heterologous regulation, parallel changes in the steady-state receptor mRNA levels have been observed implicating direct effects on gene transcription and/or mRNA stability.

3.2.3. COMPARISON OF SPECIES

The primary structure of the PTH/PTHrP receptor has been elucidated for several mammalian species including human, rat, mouse, and opossum. There is a high degree of conservation with the greatest divergence between rat and opossum, whose sequences are 78% identical. The most striking differences in sequence are in parts of the amino-terminal extracellular regions, and the first intracellular loop and the intracellular carboxy-terminal domain. Other parts of the amino-terminal extracellular region and the membrane-spanning regions are especially well conserved. Cysteine residues in the amino-terminal extension and in each of the first two putative extracellular loops, as well as potential asparagine-linked glycosylation sites in the extracellular domain, are highly conserved not only in the PTH/PTHrP receptor among species, but also in other members of the subgroup of G protein–coupled receptors described in Section 3.2.1.

3.3. Embryology and Cytogenesis

Humans have two pairs of parathyroid glands lying in the anterior cervical region, which are of endodermal origin, being derived from the third and fourth pharyngeal pouches. Rats have a single pair of glands embedded in the cranial part of the thyroid. The chief cell is the predominant cell type in human with some oxyphil cells, which have an acidophilic cytoplasm and mitochondria, also present. Only, the chief cell is present in rat. Parathyroid cells have limited numbers of secretory granules containing PTH, indicating that relatively little hormone is stored in the gland. Parathyroid cells normally divide at an extremely slow rate; mitoses are rarely observed.

3.4. PTH Secretion

The NH_2-terminal 25-residue portion of preproPTH, characterized by its hydrophobicity, is called the signal sequence or presequence, and facilitates entry of the nascent hormone into the cisternae of the endoplasmic reticulum to begin its journey through the regulated secretory pathway. After removal of the signal sequence, the resultant proPTH molecule—extended at the NH_2-terminus of PTH(1-84) by six amino acids—is transported to the Golgi apparatus. In the *trans*-Golgi, proPTH is converted into PTH by the action of furin and proprotein convertase 7, mammalian proprotein convertases that are related to bacterial subtilisins. Little proPTH is stored within the gland, and the mature 84-amino-acid form of the hormone is packaged in secretory granules. The hormone is released by exocytosis in response to the principal stimulus to secretion, hypocalcemia.

3.4.1. CALCIUM

Calcium regulates the amount of PTH available for secretion in different ways (Fig. 9). In hypocalcemia, there is increased binding of regulatory proteins to the 3′ UTR of the PTH mRNA, thereby stabilizing PTH transcripts, allowing enhanced preproPTH synthesis. Also in the absence of a stimulus for release, intraglandular metabolism of PTH occurs, causing complete degradation to its constituent amino acids or partial degradation to fragments through a calcium-regulated enzymatic mechanism. In the case of hypercalcemia, the predominant hormonal entities released from the gland are biologically inactive fragments composed of midregion and COOH-terminal sequences. In response to hypocalcemia, degradation of PTH within the parathyroid cell is minimized, and the major hormonal entity released is the bioactive PTH(1-84) molecule. Thus, in the presence of hypocalcemia, increased amounts of bioactive PTH are secreted even in the absence of immediate additional synthesis of hormone. In the presence of a sustained severe hypocalcemic stimulus, additional PTH synthesis and secretion depends on an increase in the number of parathyroid cells. Such an increase may also be stimulated by the

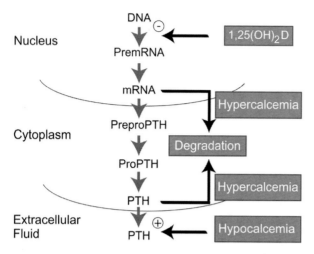

Fig. 9. Sites of regulation for PTH biosynthesis, intraglandular metabolism, and secretion. PTH gene transcription is downregulated by $1,25(OH)_2D$. Elevations in the level of extracellular fluid calcium reduce the stability of preproPTH mRNA and increase the production and release of biologically inactive COOH-terminal fragments. Reduction in the concentration of extracellular fluid calcium maximize stability of the preproPTH mRNA, minimize the breakdown of preformed PTH, and increase secretion of the biologically active mature form of PTH.

reduction in circulating $1,25(OH)_2D$ that often accompanies hypocalcemia. Normally, the sterol inhibits parathyroid cell proliferation by inhibiting expression of early immediate response genes, such as the *MYC* protooncogene.

There is an inverse relationship between ambient calcium levels and PTH release that is curvilinear rather than proportional. This relationship between PTH and extracellular calcium is in stark contrast to the influence of the calcium ion as a secretagogue in most other secretory systems in which elevations in this ion enhance release of the secretory product. This distinction between the parathyroid cell and other secretory cells is maintained intracellularly, where elevations rather than decreases in cytosol calcium correlate with decreased PTH release. Alterations in extracellular fluid calcium levels are transmitted through the parathyroid plasma membrane CASR that couples through G_i and $G_{q/11}$ proteins to inhibit adenylyl cyclase or stimulate phospholipase C (PLC), respectively. Potentially, the CASR can signal through several pathways. The activated CASR appears to signal the inhibition of PTH release via a mitogen-activated protein kinase pathway.

3.4.2. 1,25-Dihydroxyvitamin D

Vitamin D metabolites modulate PTH release. There is a feedback loop between PTH-induced increase in

$1,25(OH)_2D$ and vitamin D metabolite–induced decrease in PTH levels. $1,25(OH)_2D$ modulates hormone synthesis within the gland, by direct action on preproPTH gene transcription, thus altering the quantities of hormone available for immediate release by secretagogues (Fig. 9). In addition, the secosterol upregulates CASR expression, enhancing responsiveness of the gland to extracellular calcium and further reducing PTH synthesis and secretion, and inhibiting parathyroid cell proliferation.

3.4.3. Other Factors

In addition to calcium and vitamin D metabolites, several other factors influence the release of PTH from parathyroid glands. The cation magnesium affects PTH release like calcium, although with reduced efficacy. High concentrations of aluminum also suppress PTH release. Hyperphosphatemia is associated with increased circulating levels of PTH. This effect is often a result of the hypocalcemia that accompanies the rise in serum phosphate. However, high serum phosphate levels also increase PTH levels independently, although it is not known how the chief cells sense changes in extracellular phosphate concentrations. In the longer term, hyperphosphatemia promotes binding of *trans* factors to PTH mRNA and stabilizes it. Parathyroid cell proliferation is increased by chronic hyperphosphatemia. Glucocorticoids increase PTH secretion. Such agents as biogenic amines, which increase parathyroid gland cAMP levels, induce PTH secretion, and those that lower cAMP levels within the parathyroid gland decrease PTH secretion. Peptides derived from chromogranin A, inhibit low-calcium-stimulated PTH release from parathyroid cells in culture. The physiologic significance of these observations is unclear.

3.5. PTH Action

The major function of PTH is the maintenance of a normal level of extracellular fluid calcium. The hormone exerts direct effects on bone and kidney and indirectly influences the gastrointestinal (GI) tract. In response to a fall in the concentration of extracellular fluid ionized calcium, PTH is released from the parathyroid cell and acts on the kidney to enhance renal calcium reabsorption and promote the conversion of 25(OH)D into $1,25(OH)_2D$. This active metabolite increases GI absorption of calcium and with PTH induces skeletal resorption, causing restoration of extracellular fluid calcium and neutralization of the signal initiating PTH release. PTH also perturbs the extracellular concentration of other ions, the most important of which is phosphate. As a consequence of PTH-enhanced $1,25(OH)_2D$

production, the GI absorption of phosphate is increased to some extent, and with PTH-induced skeletal lysis, extracellular phosphate as well as calcium levels are increased. PTH acts to inhibit renal phosphate reabsorption, producing phosphaturia and a net decrease in extracellular fluid phosphate concentration. The phosphaturic action of PTH is a classic manifestation of renal PTH responsiveness.

In target tissues, the result of interaction of PTH with the plasma membrane PTH/PTHrP receptor has classically been appreciated to be stimulation of the enzyme adenylyl cyclase on the inner surface of the plasma membrane, although the same receptor can couple to phosphatidylinositol turnover as well (Fig. 10). The product of this adenylyl cyclase activity, cellular cAMP, and the products of phospholipase activity, isositol triphosphate (IP$_3$), diacylglycerol (DAG), and intracellular Ca^{2+}, initiate a cascade of events leading to the final cellular response to the hormone. The PTH/PTHrP receptor may not activate both these intracellular signaling pathways equivalently in all target tissues but act preferentially by means of one or another pathway in different cells.

3.5.1. BONE

The best-documented effect of PTH is a catabolic one, which results in the breakdown of mineral constituents and bone matrix, as manifested by the release of calcium and phosphate, by increases in plasma and urinary hydroxyproline, and other indices of bone resorption. This process is mediated by osteoclastic osteolysis, but the mechanism is indirect, since PTH does not bind directly to multinucleated osteoclasts. However, the PTH/PTHrP receptor is expressed on osteoblasts, and PTH stimulates second-messenger accumulation in osteoblast-enriched populations of cells from skeletal tissues and in osteosarcoma cells of the osteoblast lineage. PTH-induced stimulation of multinucleated osteoclasts occurs through the action of PTH-stimulated osteoblast activity via intermediary factors.

One of the key intermediary factors is receptor activator of nuclear factor-κB ligand (RANKL), which is expressed in the bone-lining cells or osteoblast precursors that support osteoclast recruitment. RANKL is a member of the tumor necrosis factor (TNF) family and is important for lymphocyte development and lymph node organogenesis, as well as osteoclastogenesis. Several bone resorbing factors such as PTH, PTHrP, prostaglandin E$_2$, some of the interleukins, and 1,25(OH)$_2$D upregulate RANKL gene expression in osteoblasts and bone stromal cells. Interaction of RANKL with its receptor (RANK) on osteoclast progenitors and osteoclasts then stimulates their recruit-

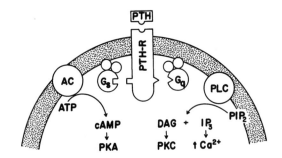

Fig. 10. PTH/PTHrP receptors can activate two intracellular signaling pathways. G$_s$ couples to adenylyl cyclase (AC) and stimulates production of cAMP, which activates protein kinase A (PKA). G$_q$ couples to PLC to form IP$_3$ and DAG from phosphatidylinositol-4,5-bisphosphate (PIP$_2$). IP$_3$ releases calcium (Ca^{2+}) from intracellular stores, and DAG stimulates PKC activity. Each heterotrimeric G protein comprises a unique α-subunit and βγ-dimer (Levine et al., 1994). ATP = adenosine triphosphate.

ment and activation and delays their degradation. Osteoprotegerin (OPG), although a soluble factor, is a member of the TNF receptor family, and it inhibits recruitment, activation, and survival of osteoclasts. OPG acts as a natural decoy receptor that disrupts the interaction of RANKL, released by osteoblast-related cells, and its receptor on osteoclast progenitors.

The consequences of the effects of PTH on osteoblast activity are complex. Examination of bone after in vivo administration of PTH has demonstrated an increase in osteoblasts and new bone formation, indicating that PTH may also play an anabolic role under some circumstances. In mice, daily injections of PTH attenuate osteoblast apoptosis, increasing osteoblast number, bone formation rate, and bone mass. Osteoclast number is not affected. By contrast, sustained elevation of PTH does not affect osteoblast apoptosis but increases osteoclast number. The antiapoptotic effect of PTH depends on the key osteoblastic transcriptional factor, Runx2, which upregulates survival genes such as Bcl-2. However, PTH increases proteosomal proteolysis of Runx2, thus contributing to the self-limiting nature of the PTH-induced anabolic actions.

PTH (and PTHrP) regulate bone cell differentiation, proliferation, and skeletal development and are now considered to be anabolic skeletal agents when made available periodically rather than continuously in vivo. Low and intermittent doses of PTH(1-34) and PTHrP (1-34) and related analogs promote bone formation. In clinical studies, daily PTH(1-34) injections increased hip and spinal bone mineral density and the NH$_2$-terminal PTH peptide has been approved for treatment of osteoporosis in the United States and Europe.

3.5.2. KIDNEY

PTH has diverse actions on the renal tubule, most of which can be mimicked by infusion of cAMP onto the luminal aspect of tubular cells. This is consistent with cAMP's postulated role as a second messenger for many renal responses. Nevertheless, it is evident that inositol phosphates and intracellular calcium also play an important role in the renal action of PTH. In some cells the PTH/PTHrP receptor binds to Na^+/H^+ exchanger regulatory factor1 (NHERF1) and NHERF2 via a PDZ domain at the COOH-terminus of the PTH/PTHrP receptor. In the kidney proximal tubule, whereas the PTH/PTHrP receptor is expressed on both brush-border and basolateral membranes, NHERF1 is expressed only at the brush border, where it interacts with the PTH/PTHrP receptor and the type IIa sodium phosphate cotransporter and regulates PTH-mediated phosphate reabsorption. NHERF-2 markedly activates PLCβ and inhibits adenylyl cyclase through stimulation of inhibitory G proteins.

PTH-induced inhibition of phosphate reabsorption is localized to the proximal convoluted tubule and the pars recta. The proximal tubule is the major site of action of PTH in stimulating 1α-hydroxylase and increasing the production of $1,25(OH)_2D$. The important site of PTH action to increase calcium and magnesium transport is the thick ascending limb of the loop of Henle, and the distal convoluted tubule and earliest portion of the cortical collecting duct.

3.5.3. OTHER TARGET TISSUES

Hepatocyte binding of PTH has been associated with adenylyl cyclase stimulation and may reflect PTH-enhanced gluconeogenesis. Other actions of PTH include effects on vascular tone, stimulation or inhibition of mitosis of various cells in vitro, promotion of increased concentrations of calcium in mammary and salivary glands, and enhancement of lipolysis in isolated fat cells. The widespread expression of the *PTHrP* gene and the equally broad expression of the *PTH/PTHrP receptor* gene suggest that many of the noncalcemic actions ascribed to PTH may be carried out by PTHrP acting in an autocrine or paracrine manner.

3.6. Pathophysiology of Hypersecretion/Hyposecretion/Receptor Defects

3.6.1. HYPERPARATHYROIDISM

Abnormally increased parathyroid gland activity may be primary or secondary. Primary hyperparathyroidism is associated with hyperplasia and neoplasia, with the latter predominantly the result of adenomas, parathyroid carcinoma is extremely rare. Parathyroid adenomas are monoclonal, involving molecular genetic derangements,

such as loss of the multiple endocrine neoplasia (MEN) type 1 gene on chromosome 11q13, which encodes a tumor suppressor called menin, loss of another putative tumor suppressor gene on chromosome 1p; or overexpression of the cyclin D1 gene on chromosome 11q. Hyperparathyroidism may occur as part of rare familial syndromes, which include MEN 1, MEN 2A, familial hypocalciuric hypercalcemia (FHH), and neonatal severe hyperparathyroidism (NSHPT). Parafibromin, the product of the tumor suppressor gene associated with the hyperparathyroid–jaw tumor syndrome and some cases of familial isolated hyperparathyroidism, is implicated in several cases of sporadic parathyroid carcinoma.

Inactivating mutations throughout the parathyroid *CASR* located on chromosome 3q13.3-21 have been described in FHH and NSHPT. These might disrupt biosynthesis of the protein or its targeting to the plasma membrane. Mutations within the extracellular domain could modify the ligand-binding properties of the receptor, and those within transmembrane and cytoplasmic domains could disrupt coupling with G proteins and subsequent activation of signal transduction pathways. Mutations in the *CASR* gene itself do not contribute to sporadic parathyroid tumorigenesis. However, CASR expression levels (as well as those for the VDR) are often reduced in parathyroid tumors, contributing to the altered calcium set point.

Mice heterozygous for deletion of the *CASR* gene demonstrate a phenotype analogous to that of humans with FHH, and homozygous animals, like humans with NSHPT, demonstrate more markedly elevated serum calcium and PTH levels, parathyroid hyperplasia, bone abnormalities, and premature death.

Excess circulating PTH leads to altered function of bone cells, renal tubules, and GI mucosa. This may result in kidney stones and calcium deposits in renal tubules, and decalcification of bone, resulting in bone pain and tenderness and spontaneous fractures. The hypercalcemia may also lead to muscle weakness and GI symptoms.

Secondary hyperparathyroidism occurs when the levels of extracellular fluid calcium and/or $1,25(OH)_2D$ fall below normal, as in chronic renal disease or vitamin D deficiency. Tertiary hyperparathyroidism refers to the condition that ensues when a parathyroid adenoma arises from the secondary hyperplasia caused by chronic renal failure.

3.6.2. HYPOPARATHYROIDISM

There are a variety of causes of hypoparathyroidism in which the deficiency of PTH secretion results in hypocalcemia and hyperphosphatemia. Isolated or idiopathic hypoparathyroidism develops as a solitary endocrinopathy: familial forms occur with either autosomal-dominant, autosomal-recessive, or X-linked recessive modes of inheritance. In some cases of familial autosomal hypoparathyroidism, inactivating mutations in the *PTH* gene have been identified, and in other cases, activating mutations in the parathyroid CASR have been documented. A patient with neonatal hypoparathyroidism was homozygous for a partial deletion of the glial cell missing-2 gene. This gene encodes a transcription factor that is critical for the development of PTH-secreting cells of the parathyroid gland. Hypoparathyroidism may also occur as a part of a pluriglandular autoimmune disorder or as a complex congenital defect, including the DiGeorge, Kenny-Caffey, or Barakat syndromes, among others. For the DiGeorge syndrome, the Tbx1 transcription factor has been implicated although the full expression of the syndrome may involve loss of other contiguous genes. The autosomal–recessive Kenny-Caffey or Sanjad-Sakati syndrome is owing to mutations in the tubulin-specific chaperone E gene that encodes a protein critical for the tubulin assembly pathway important for development of the parathyroid. Haploinsufficiency of the transcription factor GATA3 has been implicated by the finding of heterozygous loss-of-function mutations in patients suffering from the Barakat or HDR (hypoparathyroidism, nerve deafness, and renal dysplasia) syndrome. Thus, GATA3 appears essential for normal embryonic development of the parathyroids, auditory system, and kidney.

3.6.3. Pseudohypoparathyroidism

Pseudohypoparathyroidism (PHP) describes a heterogeneous collection of conditions characterized by biochemical hypoparathyroidism—hypocalcemia and hyperphosphatemia—but increased circulating PTH levels and target tissue unresponsiveness to PTH. Patients with PHP type 1a exhibit a distinctive physical appearance, referred to as Albright hereditary osteodystrophy (AHO), characterized by skeletal and developmental defects. The urinary cAMP and phosphorous response to PTH is defective and serum calcium levels are low. There is evidence of target organ resistance to other hormones. However, within families, some affected members may show all the aforementioned features, whereas others manifest only the features of AHO with no evidence of biochemical abnormalities—so-called pseudo-pseudohypoparathyroidism (pseudo-PHP). The trait is inherited in an autosomal-dominant fashion, and affected individuals demonstrate reduced $G_s\alpha$ activity and carry heterozygous mutations in the $G_s\alpha$ gene. In addition, the PHP type 1a trait (AHO + hormone resistance) is inherited maternally whereas the pseudo-PHP trait (only AHO) is paternally transmitted.

PHP type 1b patients have a normal appearance, no mutations in the $G_s\alpha$-coding exons, and hormone resistance almost exclusively limited to the PTH-responsive proximal renal tubules. However, the PHP type 1b trait is inherited maternally and maps to the *GNAS* locus (chromosome 20q13.3) close to the region containing the $G_s\alpha$ gene exons. The *GNAS* locus has several additional upstream exons that are genetically imprinted. Just upstream of $G_s\alpha$ exon 1 is exon 1A (also known as A/B), which is paternally expressed. In PHP type 1b patients, the maternal imprinting of exon 1A is lost. This appears to be owing to the heterozygous deletion of a putative imprinting control region in PHP type 1b patients some 220 kb centromeric to the $G_s\alpha$ exons. How this genetic defect causes the PTH resistance in this type of PHP is not known.

3.6.4. Receptor Defects

Ablation of the *PTHrP* gene in mice is lethal, with death occurring in the perinatal period. Likewise, knockout of the *PTH/PTHrP receptor* gene leads to an even more severe phenotype, with few fetuses surviving to term. These animals manifest extensive skeletal abnormalities owing to impaired endochondral ossification, which is the highly organized process responsible for longitudinal growth of bones during embryogenesis and early postnatal life. Both PTHrP and the PTH/PTHrP receptor are expressed in proliferating chondrocytes, but not by terminally differentiated chondrocytes. In PTHrP-less mice, the chondroplastic phenotype results from disruption of multiple stages of chondrogenesis, from reduced cellular proliferation to premature terminal differentiation and programmed cell death. This results in premature ossification of the developing skeleton. Thus, PTHrP normally maintains chondrocytic cells in a dedifferentiated state and protects them from apoptosis. The latter property may be the result in part of PTHrP's ability to localize to the nucleolus, which is mediated by a functional nucleolar targeting signal sequence located in the midregion of the molecule.

In humans, inactivating mutations in the PTH/PTHrP receptor have been implicated in the molecular pathogenesis of Blomstrand lethal chrondrodysplasia. This rare autosomal-recessive disease is characterized by advanced endochondral bone maturation, short-limbed dwarfism, and fetal death, thus mimicking the phenotype of PTH/PTHrP receptor–less mice.

In contrast to the PTHrP-less and PTH/PTHrP receptor–less mice, patients with Jansen-Type metaphyseal chondrodysplasia (JMC) with short-limbed dwarfism demonstrate little ossification at the chondroosseous junctions of their long bones. They also manifest features of hyperparathyroidism, such as severe hypercal-

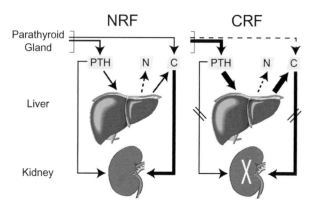

Fig. 11. Model of PTH metabolism in presence of normal renal function (NRF) and chronic renal failure (CRF). In the presence of NRF, PTH(1-84) released from the parathyroid gland is cleared by the kidney or metabolized in the liver, where amino (N:NH$_2$) and carboxyl (C:COOH) fragments are generated. COOH, but generally not NH$_2$, fragments are released into the circulation; the pool of COOH fragments, which includes a contribution from the parathyroid gland, is cleared by the kidney. In CRF, PTH secretion is increased, in part by a tendency toward hypocalcemia, and fewer COOH fragments are released from the parathyroid glands. Failure of the kidney to clear PTH results in increased hepatic metabolism. Under these conditions, COOH-terminal fragments reach high circulating concentrations because of increased production and reduced renal clearance.

cemia and hypophosphatemia, despite normal or undetectable levels of circulating PTH and PTHrP. JMC patients are heterozygous for activating missense mutations in the PTH/PTHrP receptor. Patients with enchondromas, benign cartilage tumors of bone, having either germ-line or somatic heterozygous activating mutations in the PTH/PTHrP receptor, have been identified. Collectively, these genetic disorders provide evidence that the PTH/PTHrP receptor does indeed mediate both the endocrine actions of PTH and the autocrine or paracrine actions of PTHrP necessary for orderly endochondral bone formation.

3.7. Measurement of PTH

Circulating PTH is heterogeneous. The major circulating bioactive moiety is similar or identical to intact PTH(1-84). This is metabolized by the liver, which releases midregion and COOH-terminal fragments into the circulation for subsequent clearance by the kidney (Fig. 11).

The circulating biologically inert moieties generated by metabolism and secretion from the parathyroid gland are cleared more slowly than intact PTH and comprise the majority of the circulating immunoreactive PTH. Circulating bioactive PTH is best measured by sensitive immunometric assays that simultaneously recognize

NH$_2$ and COOH epitopes on the PTH molecule and detect only intact PTH(1-84). This is the method of choice for the accurate diagnosis of patients with hypercalcemia, especially in distinguishing patients with primary hyperparathyroidism from those with hypercalcemia of malignancy in whom PTHrP levels are increased and intact PTH levels are suppressed but those of midregion and carboxyl-terminal PTH fragments are not suppressed.

3.8. Summary

PTH is the key polypeptide hormone responsible for minute-to-minute maintenance of calcium homeostasis. PTHrP plays a critical role in development, especially skeletogenesis, but is not involved in normal calcium homeostatic control in the adult. Both factors act through the PTH/PTHrP receptor, which is widely expressed and signals through multiple second-messenger pathways. Calcimimetics are small, orally active, organic molecules that allosterically increase the sensitivity of the CASR to circulating calcium, reducing PTH secretion and serum calcium concentration. The calcimimetic cinacalcet normalizes serum calcium levels in patients with primary hyperparathyroidism and lowers PTH levels in patients with secondary hyperparathyroidism on hemodialysis, pointing the way to future medical management of hyperparathyroidism.

REFERENCES

Clemens TL, Adams JS. Vitamin D and metabolites. In: Favus MJ, ed. *Primer on the Metabolic Bone Diseases and Disorders of Mineral Metabolism*. 3rd Ed. New York, NY: Raven 1996: 109–114.

Goltzman D, Hendy GN. Parathyroid hormone. In: Becker KL, ed. *Principles and Practice of Endocrinology and Metabolism*, 3rd Ed. Philadelphia, PA: JB Lippincott, 2001:497–512.

Haussler MR, Jurutka PW, Hsieh J-C, Thompson PD, Selznick SH, Haussler Ca, Whitfield GK. New understanding of the molecular mechanism of receptor-mediated genomic actions of the vitamin D hormone. *Bone* 1995;17(Suppl):33S–38S.

John MR, Arai M, Rubin DA, Jonsson KB, Juppner H. Identification and characterization of the murine and human gene encoding the tuberoinfundibular peptide of 39 residues. *Endocrinology* 2002;143:1047–1057.

Levine MA, Schwindinger WF, Downs RW Jr, Moses AM. Pseudohypoparathyroidism: clinical, biochemical, and molecular features. In: Bilezikian JP, Marcus R, Levine MA, eds. *The Parathyroids. Basic and Clinical Concepts*. New York, NY: Raven 1994: 781–800.

Minghetti PP, Norman AW. 1,25(OH)$_2$-Vitamin D$_3$ receptors: gene regulation and genetic circuitry. *FASEB J* 1988;2:3043–3053.

Yu J, Papavasiliou V, Rhim J, Goltzman D, Kremer R. Vitamin D analogs: new therapeutic agents for the treatment of squamous cancer and its associated hypercalcemia. *Anti-Cancer Drugs* 1995;6:101–108.

SELECTED READINGS

Bilezikian JP, Marcus R, Levine MA, eds. *The Parathyroids: Basic and Clinical Concepts*. New York, NY: Raven 2001.

Brown EM, Macleod J. Extracellular calcium sensing and extracellular calcium signaling. *Physiol Rev* 2001;81:239–297.

Christakos S, Dhawan P, Liu Y, Peng X, Porta A. New insights into the mechanisms of vitamin D action. *J Cell Biochem* 2003;88: 695–705.

Cole DEC, Hendy GN. Hypoparathyroidism and pseudohypoparathyroidism. In: Arnold A, ed. *Endotext.com. Bone/Mineral Metabolism section*. Website: www.endotext.org/index.htm, 2002.

Favus MF, ed. *Primer on Metabolic Bone Diseases and Disorders of Mineral Metabolism*, 5th Ed. New York, NY: Raven 2003.

Hendy GN, Arnold A. Molecular basis of PTH overexpression. In: Bilezikian JP, Raisz LG, Rodan GA, eds. *Principles of Bone Biology*. San Diego, CA: Academic 2002:1017–1030.

Hendy GN, Cole DEC. Parathyroid disorders. In: Emery AEH, Rimoin DL, eds. *Principles and Practice of Medical Genetics*, 4th Ed., vol. 2. Edinburgh: Churchill Livingstone 2002:2203–2230.

Holick MF. Vitamin D: importance in the prevention of cancers, type 1 diabetes, heart disease, and osteoporosis. *Am J Clin Nutr* 2004;79:362–371.

Juppner H, Potts JT Jr. Immunoassays for the detection of parathyroid hormone. *J Bone Miner Res* 2002;17(Suppl 1):N81–N86.

Karaplis AC, Goltzman D. PTH and PTHrP effects on the skeleton. *Rev Endocr Metab Disord* 2000;1:331–341.

Sutton ALM, MacDonald PN. Vitamin D: more than a "bone-a-fide" hormone. *Mol Endocrinol* 2003;17:777–791.

19 Oncogenes and Tumor Suppressor Genes in Tumorigenesis of the Endocrine System

Anthony P. Heaney, MD, PhD and Shlomo Melmed, MD

1. INTRODUCTION

Tumor formation is a multistep process that involves uncoupling of the interdependent mechanisms of cell proliferation and differentiation. Mutations of either protooncogenes or tumor suppressor genes may confer a growth advantage to mutant cells, enabling them to proliferate more rapidly than normal cells, and to alter their interaction with their surroundings, resulting in local invasion and or distant metastases. Studies of cellular protooncogenes and tumor suppressor genes during the past decade have yielded major advances in the understanding of the molecular basis of tumorigenesis. This chapter focuses on the role of these genes in development of tumors of the endocrine system.

2. ONCOGENES

Studies of tumor viruses capable of infecting normal cells and transforming them into tumor cells led to the initial discovery of oncogenes. The discovery that the Rous sarcoma virus–associated oncogene, *Src*, originated from the genome of normal chicken cells sug-

gested the existence of a cellular gene (protooncogene) with oncogenic potential that could be activated by a virus. The compelling evidence that genetic alterations of cellular protooncogenes are involved in human tumor formation came from DNA transfection experiments. DNA from tumor cells was extracted and introduced into normal fibroblast cells. Some transfected cells grew in culture with similar characteristics to transformed cells and when injected into nude mice formed rapidly growing tumor masses. Subsequent isolation and molecular cloning of several oncogenes from transfected cells showed that they are structurally very similar to genes present in DNA of normal cells but contain one or more somatic mutations that occurred during tumor pathogenesis. A subtle change in gene structure even at the single base pair level appeared sufficient to convert a normal cellular protooncogene into a transforming oncogene.

Protooncogenes play important roles in regulating normal cell growth and differentiation, and, to date, more than 200 have been identified. The cellular functions of protooncogenes fall into several groups, includ-

From: *Endocrinology: Basic and Clinical Principles, Second Edition*
(S. Melmed and P. M. Conn, eds.) © Humana Press Inc., Totowa, NJ

Table 1
Representative Oncogenes in Human Tumors [a]

Oncogene	Tumor	Mechanism of activation	Properties of gene product
erb-B	Mammary cacinoma glioblastoma	Amplification	Growth factor receptor
ret	Papillary thyroid carcinoma	Rearrangement	Cell-surface receptor
raf	Stomach carcinoma	Rearrangement	Cytoplasmic serine/threonine kinase
H-ras	Stomach carcinoma	Point mutation	GDP/GTP binding
K-ras	Bladder carcinoma	Point mutation	Signal transducer
N-ras	Leukemia	Point mutation	Signal transducer
myc	Lymphomas, carcinomas	Amplification, chromosome translocation	Nuclear transcription factor
bcl-2	Follicular and undifferentiated lymphomas	Chromosome translocation	Cytoplasmic membrane protein
gsp	Pituitary tumors	Point mutation	GDP/GTP signal transducer
PTTG	Pituitary tumors	Unclear	Securin protein, regulates bFGF

[a]Adapted from Weinberg (1994).

ing membrane-associated receptors (e.g., *Erb2* and epidermal growth factor receptor), their extracellular ligands (e.g., *v-sis* and platelet-derived growth factor), cytoplasmic signal transduction molecules (e.g., *Src*, *ras*, and *raf*) or nuclear mitogen-inducible transcription factors (e.g., *Jun*, *fos*, *myc*), and nuclear transcription factors (e.g., estrogen receptor-α, peroxisome proliferators–activated receptor-γ [PPAR-γ]). Table 1 provides representative protooncogenes of these different groups associated with human tumors.

Activation of protooncogenes can result from either a point mutation in the structural region, which encodes for amino acids of a protein, or changes in the regulatory region, which modulates gene expression in response to developmental or physiologic stimuli. Point mutations that activate the ras oncogene are the best characterized mutations found in the former category. These mutations occur most frequently at codons 12, 13, and 61. The ras protein is a guanine nucleotide–binding protein, which acts as a proximal membrane-associated signal transducer resulting in a complex cascade transmitting growth stimulatory signals. Binding to guanosine 5′-triphosphate (GTP) results in ras activation and signal transduction, whereas hydrolysis of bound GTP to guanosine 5′-diphosphate (GDP) by guanosine 5′-triphosphatase (GTPase) leads to inactivation of ras and termination of signal transduction. The three-dimensional structure of ras has revealed that the amino acid residues most commonly mutated in the ras protein are directly involved in GTP binding and hydrolysis. Thus, mutations in these residues abolished the ability of the ras protein to hydrolyze GTP to GDP, resulting in constitutively activated ras protein, which leads to overexpression of growth stimulatory signals.

Oncogenic conversion of the nuclear protein, myc, results from aberrant expression of the protein rather than a point mutation. A variety of genetic changes can increase the level of *myc* expression. In Burkitt lymphoma, e.g., a chromosome translocation occurs whereby the *myc* protooncogene is placed under the control of a regulatory sequence derived from an immunoglobulin gene, uncoupling *myc* from its normal physiologic modulator and leading to continuous *myc* expression. In other types of tumor cells, the *myc* gene is amplified to multiple copies, resulting in a proportional increase in the level of myc protein. In both of these cases, deregulation of myc gene expression results in uncontrolled cell proliferation.

3. TUMOR SUPPRESSOR GENES

The notion that neoplastic transformation may involve alterations in genes whose products negatively regulate cell proliferation was originally derived from evidence obtained from cell hybrid experiments, studies of familial neoplasms, and observed loss of allelic heterozygosity in tumors. These genes are termed *tumor suppressor genes*. In contrast to protooncogenes, which induce tumors when converted into oncogenes, tumor suppressor genes are present in tumor cells as an inactive or null allele. Since tumor suppressor genes act in normal cells to suppress proliferation, tumor cells lacking these genes exhibit unconstrained growth associated with malignancy.

Evidence from somatic cell hybrid experiments first suggested that genetic alterations underlying neoplastic transformation might result from the loss of function of normal alleles. Hybrid cells generated between tumorigenic and normal cells did not always give rise to tumors

Table 2
Representative Tumor suppressor Genes in Human Tumors [a]

Chromosomal localization	Name of locus	Tumors involved	Properties of gene product
5p	APC	Familial adenomatous polyposis, colotectal carcinoma	Cytoplasmic protein
10q	—	MEN 2, astrocytoma	—
11p	WT-1	Wilms tumor, rhabdomyo- sarcoma, hepato-blastoma, bladder and lung carcinoma	DNA-binding protein
11q	Menin	MEN 1	Transcription factor
13q	Rb-1	Retinoblastoma, osteosarcoma, breast and bladder carcinoma	DNA-binding protein
17p	p53	Small-cell and squamous cell lung carcinoma, breast carcinoma, colorectal carcinoma, and other	DNA-binding protein
17q	NF-1	Neurofibromatosis type 1	Induces GTP hydrolysis of ras protein
18q	DCC	Colorectal carcinoma	Cell-surface receptor

[a]Adapted from Weinberg (1994).

when injected into suitable hosts, unless specific chromosomes were lost from the hybrids. This phenomenon of tumor suppression suggested that recessive genetic changes were responsible for the tumorigenic phenotype. Although cell hybrid studies of tumor suppression provided very useful information on chromosomal assignment, this method could not lead to gene identification, and, to date, no suppressor gene thus has been isolated.

The identification of tumor suppressor genes has been greatly facilitated through studies of familial cancers. This is best illustrated in the identification and isolation of the retinoblastoma susceptibility gene (*Rb*). The essential features of retinoblastoma are that, in the familial forms of the tumor, the affected individual inherits a mutant, "loss-of-function" allele from an affected parent and a second somatic mutation inactivates the normal allele derived from the unaffected parent. By contrast, the sporadic forms of the tumor involve two somatic mutational events. According to this recessive mutation model, homozygous deletion of the *Rb* gene would be expected in some tumors, and *Rb* gene expression could be altered in retinoblastoma compared to normal tissue. Homozygous deletion of chromosome 13q14 was in fact detected in retinoblastomas, and using chromosomal walking to identify sequences conserved in evolution that were expressed in retinoblasts but were absent or altered in retinoblastomas, the candidate gene for Rb was isolated.

Another powerful strategy for discovering new tumor suppressor genes in human tumors is to identify specific genetic markers that are repeatedly reduced to homozygosity in many tumors of a given type. Loss of heterozygosity (LOH) for this specific marker suggests the presence of a closely linked suppressor gene whose second allele has been eliminated from tumor cells during tumor pathogenesis. For example, losses of allele on the long arm of chromosome 18 are a frequent occurrence in colorectal carcinomas but not in adenomas, suggesting the presence of a suppressor gene on this chromosome whose loss frequently accompanies the conversion of benign adenomas to carcinomas. Based on this evidence, the responsible gene, termed *DCC* for "deleted in colorectal carcinoma," was identified and a transmembrane protein with a sequence similarity to the neural cell-adhesion family of molecules isolated. Similar methodology was used to identify other tumor suppressor genes such as p53 and *WT-1* (Table 2).

4. PROTOONCOGENES AND TUMOR SUPPRESSOR GENES IN ENDOCRINE TUMORS

Like tumors in other tissues, tumors in the endocrine system arise as monoclonal expansions of a signal-mutated cell. For most tumor types, multiple genes are involved and different combinations of gene mutations may result in similar phenotypes. Some genes contribute to tumors of only one cell type whereas other genes are involved in different types of tumors. The role of protooncogenes and tumor suppressor genes in tumorigenesis of the endocrine system is presently being actively studied. Table 3 summarizes the oncogenes and tumor suppressor genes that have been implicated in endocrine tumor formation, and some of these genes are discussed in detail.

Table 3
Oncogenes and Tumor Suppressor Genes in Endocrine Tumors

Gene	Defect	Tumor phenotype
H-*ras*	Point mutation	Thyroid adenomas and carcinomas, pituitary carcinoma metastases
K-*ras*	Point mutation	Thyroid tumors
N-*ras*	Point mutation	Thyroid tumors
Ret	Chromosomal rearrangement, point mutations	Papillary thyroid carcinoma, MEN 2
trk	chromosomal rearrangement	Papillary thyroid carcinoma
$G_s\alpha$	Point mutation	Pituitary tumors, thyroid adenomas
PTTG	Unclear	Various cancers including pituitary and thyroid tumors
Menin	Mutation	MEN 1, parathyroid tumors
11q	LOH	Pituitary tumors
13q	LOH	Parathyroid and pituitary carcinomas
p53	Point mutation	anaplastic thyroid carcinoma
PRAD1	Chromosomal rearrangement	Parathyroid adenoma
c-*myc*	Overexpression	Thyroid carcinoma
c-*fos*	Over expression	Thyroid carcinoma
GADD45	Unclear	Melanoma, pituitary tumors
PPAR-γ/PAX-8	Chromosomal translocation	Follicular thyroid carcinoma

4.1. Multiple Endocrine Neoplasia Type 1

Multiple endocrine neoplasia type 1 (MEN 1) is an autosomal dominant disorder characterized by tumors of the parathyroid gland, pancreatic islet, and anterior pituitary. Based on the assumption that tumorigenesis involves loss of function for a tumor suppressor gene (see above), and by utilizing restriction fragment length polymorphisms, the MEN 1 locus was mapped to chromosome 11q13. Extensive characterization of the 11q13 region in a panel of MEN 1–associated tumors identified a gene, called *menin*, that functions as a nuclear protein that interacts specifically with the activator protein-1 transcription factor JunD. Mutations in *menin*, resulting in failed menin binding to JunD, have been identified in tumors derived from MEN 1 kindreds, supporting the hypothesis that MEN 1 encodes a tumor suppressor gene. The clinical phenotype can also be largely recapitulated in transgenic mice in which the menin gene is inactivated. It is now possible to test MEN 1 kindreds for *menin* mutations at an early age, allowing affected individuals to be monitored for the development of endocrine tumors (Table 4).

4.2. Multiple Endocrine Neoplasia Type 2

Multiple endocrine neoplasia type 2 (MEN 2) consists of three clinically distinct, dominantly inherited cancer syndromes. MEN 2A is the most common, and patients develop familial medullary thyroid carcinoma (FMTC), pheochromocytoma, and primary hyperparathyroidism. Those with MEN 2B have FMTC, pheo-

Table 4
Chromosome 11 Deletions in Sporadic Endocrine Tumors

Adenoma[a]	Deletion present (%)
Nonfunctioning	20
GH cell	16
PRL cell	12
ACTH cell	28
Parathyroid	25

[a] PRL, prolactin; ACTH, adrenocorticotrophic hormone

chromocytoma, mucosal neuromas of the tongue, hyperplasia of neuronal Schwann cells in the cornea, ganglioneuromatosis of the gastrointestinal tract, and an asthenic marfanoid habitus. In familial MTC, only the thyroid is affected. All three syndromes result from one of several different germline mutations of the receptor tyrosine kinase *RET* protooncogene, located on chromosome 10q11.

The *RET* gene was identified and cloned through rearrangements that occur in papillary thyroid carcinomas and in vitro during transfection studies. It consists of 21 exons and encodes a receptor kinase. *RET* mRNA is expressed in developing central and peripheral nervous system and during renogenesis in the mouse embryo. Mice homozygous for mutant *RET* fail to develop kidneys and enteric neurons and die within 16–24 h after birth.

RET protooncogene missense mutations have been detected in 95% of patients with MEN 2A and MEN 2B, and in about 88% of families with FMTC. Families with MEN 2A have a *RET* mutation in exon 10 or 11, involving five conserved cysteine residues (609, 611, 618, 620, and 634) in the cysteine-rich region of the cadherin-like ligand-binding domain. These mutations probably interfere with ligand binding. Missense mutations of *RET* in the same cysteine residues were also identified in families with FMTC, although additional mutations in exons 13, 14, and 15 have been identified in a small number of families. Germ-line mutations in the *RET* protooncogene, at exon 16, were found in >95% of MEN 2B cases. Almost all cases have the same missense change (918T), resulting in a methionine-to-threonine change in the substrate-recognition pocket of the tyrosine kinase domain, although recently a methionine-to-valine substitution, involving exon 15, has been identified. The same (918T) mutation was also detected in about 30–40% of sporadically occurring MTCs and pheochromocytomas. It has been suggested that this mutation is a dominant tyrosine kinase–activating mutation, perhaps altering target specificity, which would explain the tissue hyperplasia leading to both tumors and ganglioneuromas. In papillary thyroid cancer, the genetic defect in the *RET* gene results from rearrangements, rather than a point mutation. The exons that encode the tyrosine kinase domain of *RET* are fused to 5′-regulatory sequences of other genes, leading to constitutive activation in this malignancy.

5. PITUITARY TUMORS

Tumors of the pituitary gland are mostly benign adenomas that are either hormonally functional or nonfunctional. Functional tumors are characterized by autonomous hormone secretion, leading to clinical hormone excess syndromes such as acromegaly or Cushing disease, whereas nonfunctioning pituitary adenomas often secrete clinically inactive glycoprotein hormones or their free subunits. Pituitary carcinomas are extremely rare, and, to date, only about 40 cases have been documented.

5.1 Oncogenes

The first point mutations detected in pituitary tumors were localized in the G protein α-subunit. Signal transduction of many peptide hormones and their cell-surface receptors are coupled with G proteins, which consist of three polypeptides: an α-chain that binds to guanine nucleotide, a β-chain, and a γ-chain. Activation of receptor accelerates the binding of GTP, which induces a conformational change in G protein, releases α-subunit from β and γ, and allows it to interact with target proteins. Hydrolysis of bound GTP to GDP by the intrinsic

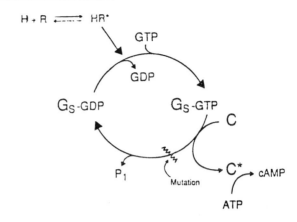

Fig. 1. Activation of G protein on hormone stimulation. Hormone binding to its cell-surface receptor results in GTP binding to the $G_s\alpha$ subunit, which activates adenylyl cyclase to increase intracellular cAMP levels. Hydrolysis of bound GTP to GDP by intrinsic GTPase activity of $G_s\alpha$ results in inactivation of $G_s\alpha$ and termination of signal transduction. Mutations in $G_s\alpha$ result in inhibition of GTP hydrolysis leading to constitutive activation of $G_s\alpha$. H = hormones, R = receptor, C = catalytic subunit of the G protein; ATP = adenosine triphosphate.

GTPase acivity of the α-subunit terminates signal transduction (Fig. 1). Growth hormone–releasing hormone (GHRH) utilizes cyclic adenosine monophosphate (cAMP) as a second messenger to stimulate growth hormone (GH) secretion and somatotrope proliferation. The GHRH receptor contains seven transmembrane domains and is coupled to a G protein. Characterization of GH-secreting pituitary adenomas revealed that a subgroup of these tumors has elevated basal cAMP and GH secretion and is no longer responsive to GHRH stimulation. Subsequently, point mutations of $G_s\alpha$ were identified in approx 40% of GH-secreting and 10% of nonfunctioning pituitary tumors derived from Caucasian and Korean patients, although $G_s\alpha$ mutations appear less frequently (approx 10%) in GH-secreting pituitary tumors derived from Japanese patients. These missense mutations, Arg201Cys or His and Gln227 Arg or Leu, occur at two sites critical for GTPase activity and result in a permanently activated adenylate cyclase system, by preventing GTP hydrolysis. Subsequent studies have not identified significant differences in the biologic and clinical phenotypes between GH-secreting tumors harboring the *gsp* mutant or nonmutant proteins. Moreover, the increased cAMP levels exert a positive feedback on the cAMP phosphodiesterase (PDE4), leading to enhanced degradation of cAMP, potentially limiting the activating effects of *gsp* mutation. Accordingly, the true oncogenic potential of these mutations is as yet unclear. $G_s\alpha$ point mutations have also been found in other types of endocrine tumor (*see* Section 6).

Because the pituitary gland is under the control of multiple hormones and growth factors, signal transduction of these factors utilizes pathways other than those coupled to G protein. For example, mutations of the tyrosine kinase receptor, RET, are implicated in the pathogenesis of a subset of pituitary tumors, and a truncated fibroblast growth factor (FGF) receptor-4 isoform (ptd-FGFR4) has been reported in approx 40 % of pituitary adenomas. However, no single, causatory factor for sporadic pituitary tumorigenesis has been isolated. The product of protooncogene *ras* plays an important role in growth factor signal transduction. There are three functional *ras* genes—H-, N-, and K-*ras*—that encode for a 21-kDa protein, P^{21ras}. P^{21ras} is a guanine nucleotide–binding protein that possesses intrinsic GTPase activity and is associated with the plasma membrane. The similarities between P^{21ras} and G proteins suggest that *ras* protein is involved in signal transduction pathways regulating growth and differentiation. Recent evidence indicates that *ras* is brought into close contact with tyrosine kinase receptors through interaction with other proteins. Signaling downstream of *ras* involves a cascade of protein kinases that transmit the incoming signal to the nucleus. Point mutations of the *ras* gene can convert *ras* into a constitutively active oncogene (*see* Section 2). *ras* oncogenes have been implicated in the development of a variety of tumors and represent one of the most common mutations detected in human neoplasia. However, *ras* gene mutations appear to be a rare event in pituitary tumors. To date, only one invasive prolactinoma was found to harbor a missense mutation of *ras*. Mutations of *ras* were also detected in metastatic deposits of pituitary carcinomas, but not in the primary pituitary tumors. These findings suggest that activation of *ras* oncogene is not the initial event in pituitary tumorigenesis, however, point mutations of *ras* may be important in the formation or growth of metastases originating from the rarely occurring pituitary carcinomas.

Since its initial isolation, from rat pituitary tumor cells, pituitary tumor–derived transforming gene (PTTG) has been identified as the index mammalian securin protein, which functions to ensure faithful chromosomal separation during mitosis. The nucleotide sequence of the human homolog of this transforming gene shares 89% identity with rat PTTG. PTTG exhibits potent in vitro and in vivo transforming actions, and higher basic FGF (bFGF) levels were detected in conditioned medium derived from stable PTTG transfectants. PTTG expression is low in most normal adult tissues, and abundant in the testis. By contrast, abundant PTTG expression is observed in a variety of solid and hemopoietic neoplasms including pituitary, thyroid, endometrial, and colorectal tumors. Inappropriately high cellular

PTTG expression promotes uneven sister chromatid separation, leading to aneuploidy, a frequent occurrence in endocrine tumors, and this chromosomal gain or loss may render the cell more prone to protooncogene activation or loss of heterozygosity of tumor suppressors. PTTG abundance may therefore be a key early determinant of tumorigenesis, and PTTG is the first human transforming gene found to be expressed at increased levels in the majority of pituitary tumors tested.

5.2. Tumor Suppressor Genes

Because pituitary tumors comprise part of the MEN 1 syndrome, the *menin* gene region has been the focus of intense research in sporadic pituitary tumors. LOH of chromosome 11q13 (where *menin* is located) was found in up to 20% of sporadic pituitary tumors; no inactivating menin mutation has been demonstrated, indicating the existence of a still unidentified tumor suppressor gene in this region.

The retinoblastoma susceptibility gene (*Rb*), a well-characterized tumor suppressor gene, is inactivated on both alleles in a variety of human tumors. Individuals with germ-line mutations on one *Rb* allele have a >90% chance of developing retinoblastoma during childhood. The *Rb* gene maps to chromosome 13q14, and loss of LOH at this locus was demonstrated in retinoblastoma cells. The *Rb* gene product, pRB, is a major determinant of cell-cycle control and acts as a signal transducer interfacing the cell-cycle apparatus with the transcriptional machinery. pRb is phosphorylated in a cell-cycle-dependent manner, being maximal at the start of the S phase and low after mitosis and entry into G1, and its state of phosphorylation regulates its activity. pRb interacts with a variety of viral and cellular proteins, and through this interaction, pRb allows the cell-cycle "clock" to control genes that mediate the advance through a critical phase of the cell growth cycle. Thus, loss of pRb function deprives the cell of an important mechanism for controlling cell proliferation through regulation of gene expression.

The role of the *Rb* gene in pituitary tumor formation was initially suggested by studies in transgenic mice, in which one allele of the *Rb* gene was disrupted. Embryos homozygous for the *Rb* mutation die between 14 and 15 d of gestation and exhibit neuronal cell death and defective erythropoiesis. Mice heterozygous for the *Rb* gene mutation are not predisposed to retinoblastoma but, interestingly, develop pituitary tumors at a high frequency. These tumors originate from the intermediate lobe of the pituitary and are classified histopathologically as proopicmelanocortin immunoreactive adenocarcinomas. DNA derived from these tumors shows the absence of the wild-type *Rb* allele, and retention of the mutant allele. Pituitary tumor tissue in the mouse also displays expression of a dysfunctional Rb protein. In 13 invasive pituitary adenomas and in pituitary carcinomas, allelic deletion of *Rb* was observed, whereas no LOH at the *Rb* locus was detected in four noninvasive pituitary tumors, although all these tumors showed normal expression of Rb protein. It is therefore likely that another tumor suppressor gene on chromosome 13 located in close proximity to the *Rb* locus might be involved in the formation of pituitary tumor. Interestingly, although *p53* tumor suppressor gene mutations have been detected in a wide variety of human tumors, no such mutation has been found in pituitary tumors that were comprehensively screened.

A recent study examining *GADD45γ* expression, a member of a growth arrest and DNA damage-inducible gene family, demonstrated that although *GADD45γ* was abundant in normal human pituitary tissues, it was detectable in only 1 of 18 clinically nonfunctioning pituitary tumors and was not expressed in most GH- or prolactin-secreting pituitary tumors. Transfection of *GADD45γ* cDNA into pituitary tumor cells inhibited tumor cell colony formation, indicating growth-suppressive actions of *GADD45γ*.

6. THYROID TUMORS

Thyroid neoplasia comprises benign follicular adenomas, differentiated carcinomas (follicular carcinoma and papillary carcinoma), and anaplastic or undifferentiated carcinomas, and many distinct molecular events occur in thyroid neoplasia. The most common mutations found in thyroid tumors are point mutations of the *ras* protooncogene. Mutations of all three *ras* genes have been identified in follicular adenomas and in thyroid carcinomas. Besides activating point mutations of *ras*, some thyroid tumors exhibit *ras* gene amplifications.

Thyrotropin (thyroid-stimulating hormone [TSH]) not only regulates differentiated function of thyroid cells, but also acts as a growth factor for thyrocytes. The growth-inducing function of TSH on thyrocyte growth is mediated by cAMP, which is induced after adenylyl cyclase activation by $G_s\alpha$ protein. As in GH-secreting pituitary tumors, point mutations that inhibit the intrinsic GTPase activities of $G_s\alpha$ have been detected in 25% of hyperfunctioning thyroid adenomas. Some hyperfunctioning adenomas have mutations in the third intracellular loop of the TSH receptor, resulting in a constitutively active receptor and inappropriate activation of adenylyl cyclase.

A novel oncogene, *PTC-RET*, is unique to papillary thyroid carcinomas. *PTC-RET* arises as the result of an intrachromosome inversion that juxtaposes unrelated gene sequences to the tyrosine kinase domain of the *RET* protooncogene (*see* Section 4.2). Other activating gene rearrangements found in this group of thyroid carcinomas include the nerve growth factor receptor (trk). Recently, a translocation t(2;3)(q13;p25) involving the fusion of the thyroid transcription factor, PAX8, and PPAR-γ was suggested to arise in follicular thyroid carcinomas, and this rearrangement may be a useful diagnostic marker to differentiate follicular thyroid carcinoma and adenoma. Anaplastic carcinoma is the most aggressive form of thyroid cancer and displays complete loss of thyroid differentiation. These tumors exhibit a high prevalence of *p53* tumor suppressor gene missense mutations that are not present in differentiated thyroid carcinomas. p53 is a sequence-specific DNA-binding protein that binds to DNA as a tetramer and regulates transcription of genes that negatively control cell growth and invasion. p53 induces differentiation and acts as a checkpoint protein that arrests the cell cycle in response to DNA damage, allowing DNA repair to take place, or to activate pathways for apoptosis. The *p53* gene is the most frequently mutated locus in human neoplasia, involved in 50% of human cancers. Typically, one allele of the *p53* gene is lost and point mutations occur in the remaining allele, resulting in production of a mutant protein. The majority of missense mutations occur within the evolutionarily conserved regions of the gene. Some mutants lose the ability either to bind to DNA or to transactivate target genes. Other mutations seem to affect p53 function by changing the global conformation of the protein. All mutant p53 proteins have lost the ability to suppress transformation, and some mutants can also act as dominant oncogenes in cooperation with *ras* in transformation of primary cells. The presence of p53 point mutations in anaplastic carcinomas but not in differentiated thyroid tumors suggests that inactivation of the *p53* tumor suppressor gene may play a role in transition to the more malignant phenotype of thyroid carcinomas.

7. PARATHYROID NEOPLASIA

Parathyroid adenomas arise either sporadically or in association with MEN 1. Multiple chromosomal regions, 1p-pter (40% of adenomas), 6q (32%), 15q (30%), and 11q (25–30%), are missing in individual parathyroid adenomas, probably reflecting the deletion of tumor suppressor genes, some of which have been characterized. For example, the majority of MEN 1–associated and about 25% of sporadic parathyroid adenomas exhibit 11q deletions that are associated with mutations in the *menin* gene (located on the undeleted 11q). A subgroup of parathyroid adenomas contains a chromosome 11 inversion in which the 5′-regulatory region of the parathyroid hormone is fused to the coding

Table 5
Clinical Impact of Genetic
Screening in Endocrine Tumors

1.   Allows early prediction of tumor behavior
2.   Portends a response to therapeutic interventions
3.   Provides genetic screening for tumor prediction
4.   Allows design of novel subcellular therapies

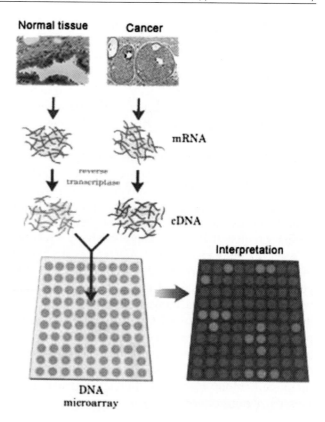

Fig. 2. Schematic representation of microarray. Any known DNA sequence, generated by chemical synthesis or polymerase chain reaction, is positioned on specifically treated glass slides with the aid of a robotic device capable of depositing very small drops (nanoliters) in precise patterns. Ultraviolet light is then used to crosslink the DNA to the glass slides, and the microarry can then be probed with fluorescently labeled nucleic acids. For example, mRNA samples are collected from normal and cancer cells (representing all the genes being expressed in these cells), cDNA probes for each sample are made with nucleotides that fluoresce in different colors, and a mixture of the cDNAs is used to probe the microarray. Spots that fluoresce green represent mRNAs more abundant in the cancer, whereas spots that fluoresce red represent sequences more abundant in normal tissue. The molecular phenotype of the tumor is thereby interrogated and characterized by computer modeling to identify potential drug targets and "tailor design" appropriate treatment.

region of the *PRAD1* gene. This gene rearrangement leads to overexpression of the *PRAD1* gene in tumor cells. Cloning of PRAD1 cDNA revealed that it is structurally related to the cyclins, and it is now termed *cyclin D1*. Cyclins are a group of proteins that play important roles in controlling cell-cycle progression. Cell-cycle progression is regulated at two critical checkpoints: the G2/M border and the G1/S transition. Cyclin D1 is a "G1 cyclin" and functions to propel cells through the G1/S transition checkpoint. Cyclin D1 forms complexes with cyclin-dependent kinases, and also interacts directly with the product of *Rb* gene to participate in cell-cycle regulation. Overexpression of cyclin D1 could lead to excessive cell proliferation. The implication of cyclin D1 as a parathyroid oncogene indicates the important role that the cell-cycle machinery can play in inducing parathyroid tumors, by regulating the biochemical pathways that control parathyroid cell proliferation. Most parathyroid carcinomas show LOH at the *Rb* allele. As in pituitary tumors, inactivation of *Rb* is only found in more aggressive tumors, not in benign parathyroid adenomas, suggesting that *Rb* gene assessment could be used as a diagnostic or prognostic molecular marker for parathyroid carcinoma. A subset of parathyroid tumors harbors amplification of regions on chromosomes 16p and 19p that contain as yet uncharacterized protooncogenes.

8. CLINICAL IMPLICATIONS

Genetic changes in protooncogenes and tumor suppressor genes play important roles in the development and progression of endocrine tumors. The identification and characterization of new tumor suppressor genes and oncogenes will not only provide important insights into normal growth regulation of endocrine cells and elucidate the genetic alterations that lead to tumor formation, but may also provide diagnostic or prognostic tools for these lesions (Table 5).

For example, *ras* protooncogene point mutations have been found in all types of thyroid tumors but rarely in pituitary tumors. The advent of rapid throughput and powerful molecular biologic techniques, such as DNA microarray (Fig. 2) and proteomic analyses, that will ultimately enable characterization of individual tumors at the mechanistic level, as well as the parallel development of specific receptor and signal transduction cascade targeted therapies, potentially will identify tumors that exhibit an aggressive phenotype, and guide clinicians in determining the need for more aggressive postoperative management and follow-up. As these tools increase the understanding of key underlying molecular mechanisms of endocrine tumor development, in tandem they will pave the way to designing subcellular therapeutic modalities for managing endocrine neoplasia in the future (Table 6).

Table 6
Potential Endocrine Tumor–Targeted Gene Therapy

Replacing functions of tumor suppressor gene	13q, 11q, 17p
Interrupting self-stimulatory autocrine loops	gsp, hypothalamic hormone receptor antagonists
Interrupting aberrant signal responsiveness	RET
Using specific immunotherapy	Mutant receptors, growth factors

SELECTED READING

Agarwal SK, Guru SC, Heppner C, et al. Menin interacts with the AP1 transcription factor JunD and represses JunD activated transcription. *Cell* 1999;96:143–152.

Bos J L. Ras genes in human cancer: a review. *Cancer Res* 1989;49: 4682.

Chandrasekharappak SC, Guru SC, Manickam P, et al. Positional cloning of the gene for multiple endocrine neoplasia-type 1. *Science* 1997;276: 404–406.

Evan GI, Littlewood TD. The role of myc in cell growth. *Curr Opin Genet Dev* 1993;3:44.

Ezzat S, Zheng L, Zhu XF, Wu GE, Asa SL. Targeted expression of a human pituitary tumor-derived isoform of FGF receptor-4 recapitulates pituitary tumorigenesis. *J Clin Invest* 2002;109: 69–78.

Fagin JA. Minireveiw: branded from the start-distinct oncogenic initiating events may determine tumor fate in the thyroid. *Mol Endocrinol* 2002:16:903–911.

Hahn WC, Weinberg RA. Rules for making human tumor cells. *N Engl Med* 2002;347:1593–1603.

Heaney AP, Horwitz GA, Wang Z, Singson R, Melmed S. Early involvement of estrogen-induced pituitary tumor transforming gene and fibroblast growth factor expression in prolactinoma pathogenesis. *Nat Med* 1999;5:1317–1321.

Hoff AO, Cote GJ, Gagel RF. Genetic screening of endocrine disease. In: Baxter JD, Melmed S, New MI, eds. *Genetics in Endocrinology*. Philadelphia, PA: Lippincott Williams & Wilkins 2002:189–221.

Knudson AD. All in the (cancer) family. *Nature Genet* 1993;5:103.

Kroll TG, Saraff P, Pecciarini L, Chen CJ, Mueller E, Spiegelman BM, Fletcher JA. PAX8-PPARgamma1 fusion oncogene in human thyroid carcinoma [corrected]. *Science* 2000;289:1357–1360.

Motokura T, Arnold A. Cyclins and oncogenesis. *Biochem Biophys Acta* 1993;1155:63.

Santoro M, et al. Activation of RET as a dominant transforming gene by germline mutations in MEN2A and MEN2B. *Science* 1995; 267:381.

Weinberg RA. Molecular mechanisms of carcinogenesis. In: Philip Leder, David A. Clayton, Edward Rubenstein, eds. *Scientific American Introdtuction to Molecular Medicine*, New York, NY: Scientific American, 1994.

20 Insulin Secretion and Action

Run Yu, MD, PhD, Hongxiang Hui, MD, PhD, and Shlomo Melmed, MD

1. INTRODUCTION

Because glucose is the primary energy source of most cells in the body, control of constant circulating glucose levels is of utmost importance. Too little serum glucose (hypoglycemia) suppresses central nervous system functions and prolonged hypoglycemia leads to death. Too much serum glucose (hyperglycemia) as seen in diabetes mellitus, results in grave consequences such as kidney, nerve, eye, muscle, and immune system damage. The body has an elaborate system to control circulating glucose levels in a narrow range (72–126 mg/dL) to prevent untoward fluctuations. For populations in Western societies, the predominant problem in glucose metabolism is diabetes mellitus although other derangements are significant but not often encountered. Of all the humoral and neuronal regulatory mechanisms for glucose metabolism, insulin is the hormone that lowers serum glucose whereas most other mechanisms function to increase serum glucose.

Insulin is a peptide hormone secreted by β-cells in the pancreatic islets of Langerhans. The main function of insulin is to lower serum glucose. Insulin is a major anabolic hormone that is critical in lipid and protein synthesis, and insulin is also an essential growth factor

required for normal development. Intact insulin function requires four components: islet β-cell mass; insulin synthesis; glucose-dependent insulin secretion; and, ultimately, insulin signaling at the target cells. Although theoretically any of these components can go awry and cause disease, abnormal insulin signaling is the most common problem, followed by decreased islet cell mass. Abnormal insulin synthesis or secretion rarely causes diseases. Understanding the physiology of all four components, however, is important to prevent and treat diabetes and related diseases.

2. DEVELOPMENT OF ENDOCRINE PANCREAS AND REGULATION OF ISLET β-CELL MASS

The islet β-cell mass is dynamic and regulated. Maintaining an appropriate β-cell mass in response to metabolic demand is critical for maintaining glucose homeostasis. Decreased β-cell mass underlies several types of diabetes. In type 1 diabetes, β-cells are destroyed by an autoimmune mechanism. In late-stage type 2 diabetes, β-cells undergo excessive apoptosis owing to glucose toxicity. Intrinsic genetic defects play a central role in causing decreased β-cell mass in maturity-onset diabetes of the young (MODY), diabe-

From: *Endocrinology: Basic and Clinical Principles, Second Edition*
(S. Melmed and P. M. Conn, eds.) © Humana Press Inc., Totowa, NJ

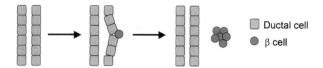

Fig. 1. Schematic illustration of pancreatic β-cell neogenesis from ductal cells.

tes associated with genetic syndromes, and diabetes encountered in genetically modified animal models. Unlimited growth of transformed β-cells comprising insulinoma tumor causes hypoglycemic coma. The net β-cell mass results from the difference between β-cell proliferation and cell death. β-Cell proliferation is achieved in two ways: (1) neogenesis (formation of β–cells from precursor pancreatic ductal cells) and (2) replication of differentiated β-cells. β-Cell death can be due to either apoptosis (programmed and controlled) or necrosis (associated with inflammation). It has recently been realized that β-cells continue to proliferate throughout adult life. The average islet size is more than 10-fold larger in adult mice than in younger animals. The most robust islet growth occurs in the intrauterine and neonatal period. β-Cell proliferation is also prominent during pregnancy.

An islet of Langerhans comprises three main cell types: (1) glucagon-secreting α-cells at the periphery (15–20% of islet cells), (2) insulin-secreting β-cells at the inside (60–80%), and (3) peripheral somatostatin-secreting δ-cells (5–10%). Glucagon functions to increase serum glucose levels and somatostatin suppresses insulin secretion. During embryonic pancreatic development, primordial islet cell clumps are derived from nascent pancreatic ducts and detach from the ducts to expand and coalesce with other clumps (Fig. 1). β-Cells are first detected at the wk 13 of gestation and begin to secrete insulin at the wk 17. β-Cell proliferation and differentiation are under tight control of a number of transcription factors. Pancreatic duodenal homeobox gene-1 (PDX-1), hepatocyte nuclear factor-1α (HNF-1α), HNF-1β, HNF-4α, insulin promoter factor-1 (IPF-1), and β-cell E-box transactivator 2 (BETA2) are some that have clinical implications since their respective mutations result in neonatal diabetes or MODY. PDX-1 is required for normal pancreatic development. A patient with deficient PDX-1 expression has failed pancreatic development. In adults, PDX-1 is also important for normal islet function because it regulates insulin gene expression. HNF-1α gene mutations are found in MODY3 and HNF-4α gene mutations in MODY1; mutations in HNF-1β, IPF-1, and BETA2 cause MODY5, MODY4, and

MODY6, respectively. All those MODY subtypes (1, 3–6) are characterized by insufficient β-cell mass. Genetic defects are also responsible for several clinical diabetes syndromes and diabetes in some animal models. Defective expression of β-cell mitochondrial protein frataxin, a gene that is deficient in Friedreich ataxia, results in decreased β-cell proliferation and increased apoptosis in experimental mice, suggesting that the diabetes associated with Friedreich ataxia may be owing to decreased β-cell mass. Wolframin, an endoplasmic protein that is defective in Wolfram syndrome (diabetes, blindness, and deafness at early childhood), appears to protect β-cells from apoptosis, thus explaining the decreased β_cell mass observed in this syndrome. Diabetes is found in a number of knockout mice deficient in various genes. In many cases, the experimentally disrupted gene is expressed in many cell types, but the β-cells seem to be particularly vulnerable to the disruption. Securin (also called PTTG), a regulatory protein critical for progression of mitosis, is expressed in all proliferative cells. Disruption of murine securin results in defective proliferation of β-cells, a cell type not known for rapid division, while sparing more proliferative cells such as hemopoietic and spermatogenic cells. Another intriguing feature of diabetes owing to genetic defects is that in most cases, they do not immediately manifest themselves but occur after a considerable latent period in childhood or young adulthood, suggesting that other insults during postnatal growth must cooperate with the genetic defects to result in the clinical phenotype.

Besides genetic determinants, β-cell mass is regulated by nutrients, growth factors, and hormones. Glucose is a major stimulator of β-cell proliferation, and in rodents, infusion of glucose for 24 h results in a rapid increase in β-cell mass, mostly owing to neogenesis. Ironically, glucose also induces β-cell apoptosis, as seen in prolonged type 2 diabetes. Amino acids and free fatty acids are also potent stimulators of β-cell proliferation. Several growth factors such as epidermal growth factor, fibroblast growth factor, and vascular endothelial growth factor stimulate β-cell proliferation. Many hormones including insulin, insulin-like growth factor-1 (IGF-1), IGF-2, glucagon, gastroinhibitory peptide, gastrin, cholecystokinin, growth hormone (GH), prolactin (PRL), placental lactogen, leptin, and glucagon-like peptide-1 (GLP-1) stimulate β-cell proliferation. Most of the hormones have significant systemic effects and therefore are not good candidates for potential therapeutic agents, whereas GLP-1 is rather specific in increasing β-cell mass. GLP-1, a gastrointestinal peptide hormone secreted by enteroendocrine L-cells, stimulates β-cell mass growth in animal models and in

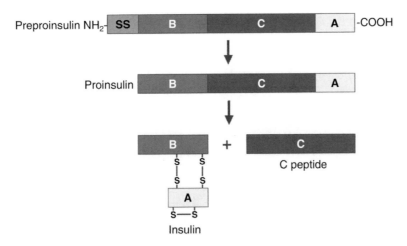

Fig. 2. Insulin synthesis and processing. SS = signal sequence.

human islet cultures through three potential pathways: (1) promotion of β-cell proliferation, (2) stimulation of β-cell neogenesis from ductal epithelium, and (3) inhibition of β-cell apoptosis. In rodents, GLP-1 treatment results in an increase in β-cell proliferation. Multiple signaling pathways including phosphatidylinositol 3- kinase (PI3K), Akt, mitogen-activated protein kinase (MAPK) and protein kinase C (PKC) mediate the proliferative effects. Islet neogenesis may also be stimulated, because the number of small islets increases after chronic administration of GLP-1 analogs. PDX-1 appears important in mediating the GLP-1 stimulation of islet neogenesis. GLP-1 prevents apoptosis in immortalized rodent β-cell lines treated with apoptosis-promoting agents including peroxide, streptozotocin, fatty acids, and cytokines. GLP-1 also prevents apoptosis in human islet cultures. PI3K, Akt, and MAPK are the likely mediators for the antiapoptotic effects.

3. INSULIN SYNTHESIS

Insulin synthesis appears to be very error proof because defects are extremely rare. The only known defects are rare mutations in the insulin gene producing defective proinsulin. Understanding insulin synthesis, however, is important, because pharmacologic interventions can be designed to manipulate insulin synthesis. The human insulin gene is located on chromosome 11p15.5 and contains three exons and two introns. The final spliced mRNA transcript is 446 bp long and encodes preproinsulin peptide (with a B-chain, a C-chain, and an A-chain). The structure of the insulin gene has been remarkably conserved throughout evolution. Most animals have a single copy of the insulin gene, with the exception of rat and mouse, which carry a duplicate. The mammalian insulin gene is exclusively

expressed in β-cells of the islet of Langerhans. Intensive physiologic and biochemical studies have led to identification of regulatory sequence motifs along the insulin promoter and the binding proteins, such as islet-restricted proteins (BETA2, PDX-1, RIP3b1-Act/C1) and ubiquitous proteins (E2A, HEB). Their DNA-binding activity and transactivating potency can be modified in response to nutrients (glucose, free fatty acids) or hormonal stimuli (insulin, leptin, GLP-1, GH, PRL) through kinase-dependent signaling pathways (PI3K, p38MAPK, PKA, calmodulin kinase). It is notable that transcriptional regulation results not only from specific combinations of these activators through DNA-protein and protein-protein interactions, but also from their relative nuclear concentrations, generating cooperativity and transcriptional synergism unique to the insulin gene.

As in the case of many other peptide hormones, insulin mRNA encodes preproinsulin peptide. A signal sequence is removed from preproinsulin while preproinsulin is inserted into the endoplasmic reticulum, which results in proinsulin. Proinsulin is further processed to form insulin and a byproduct, C peptide, both of which are packaged into secretory vesicles. The mature insulin molecule comprises two peptide chains (A and B) linked together by two disulfide bonds, and an additional disulfide bond is formed within the A chain (Fig. 2). In most species, the A chain consists of 21 amino acids and the B chain, 30 amino acids. Although the amino acid sequence of insulin varies among species, key structural features (including the positions of the three disulfide bonds, both ends of the A chain, and the carboxyl-terminal residues of the B chain) are highly conserved, and the three-dimensional conformation is quite similar. Insulin from one species is usually readily active in

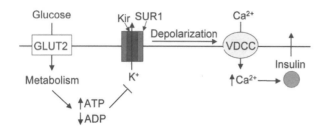

Fig. 3. Schematic illustration of glucose-stimulated insulin release from a pancreatic β-cell.

another one. Insulin exists primarily as a monomer at low concentrations ($\sim 10^{-6}$ M) and forms a dimer at higher concentrations at neutral pH. At high concentrations and in the presence of zinc ions, insulin aggregates further to form hexameric complexes. Monomers and dimers readily diffuse into blood, whereas hexamers diffuse poorly. Hence, absorption of insulin preparations containing a high proportion of hexamers is delayed and slow. By preparing different insulin analogs bearing amino acid substitutions and deletions, and comparing their ability to activate the insulin receptor, several regions of insulin have been determined to be linked to receptor binding. The three conserved regions in insulin—amino terminal A-chain (GlyA1-IleA2-ValA3-GluA4 or AspA4), carboxyl terminal A-chain (TyrA19-CysA20-AsnA21), and carboxyl terminal B-chain (GlyB23-PheB24-PheB25-TyrB26)—are located at or near the surface of insulin and therefore may interact with the insulin receptor. Understanding insulin structure has stimulated development of a number of insulin analogs, and recombinant DNA technology allows their production.

4. INSULIN SECRETION

β-cells are excitable endocrine cells that secrete insulin. The essential secretory machinery is analogous to that for other peptide hormones such as GH and PRL, as described elsewhere in this book. Although abnormalities in insulin secretion are not common, insulin secretion is of pharmacologic interest because oral hypoglycemic agents act by increasing insulin secretion. Multiple mechanisms mediate insulin secretion, the most important being glucose-stimulated, K_{ATP} channel dependent. Other pathways either augment or complement that pathway.

Glucose-stimulated, K_{ATP} channel-dependent pathway starts with intracellular transport of extracellular glucose by a glucose transporter (GLUT2) (Fig. 3). Intracellular glucose undergoes cytosolic glycolysis catalyzed by glucokinase (glucokinase gene mutations

cause MODY2). Pyruvate, a product of glycolysis, is shuttled into mitochondria as a substrate of the tricarboxylic acid cycle with production of adenosine triphosphate (ATP). As a result, cytosolic ATP levels are elevated and adenosine 5′-diphosphate (ADP) levels reduced. Increased cytosolic ATP/ADP ratio closes an ATP-sensitive K⁺ channel, K_{ATP}, which results in discontinued K⁺ outflow, thus depolarizing the β-cell membrane. Voltage-dependent calcium channels (VDCCs) on the cell membrane are opened by depolarization, and calcium influx increases intracellular calcium (phase 1), which, in turn, activates calcium-dependent calcium release from the endoplasmic reticulum (phase 2). The resultant biphasic increase in intracellular calcium triggers fusion of secretory vesicles with the plasma membrane and insulin is released.

The K_{ATP} channel plays the crucial role of converting metabolic to electric signals. All components of glucose-stimulated, K_{ATP} channel-dependent insulin secretion are found in several other cell types, except for the K_{ATP} channel, which is unique for β_cells (a similar channel is also found in muscle and brain). Each β-cell posseses thousands of K_{ATP} channels, which is a high density considering the small size of β-cells. This channel has eight subunits; four identical smaller subunits, called Kir6.2 ("ir" stands for "inward rectifier"), which form the inner pore for K⁺ passage; and four identical larger subunits, termed the sulfonylurea receptors (SUR1), which form the outer regulatory structure. ATP regulates K_{ATP} channel by binding to Kir6.2, and oral sulfonylurea hypoglycemic medications bind to SUR1 and close the K_{ATP} channel, thus stimulating insulin secretion. Not surprisingly, mutations in the K_{ATP} channel cause either hyperglycemia or hypoglycemia. Mutations in SUR1 and Kir6.2 that render the K_{ATP} channel less open cause insulin hypersecretion with neonatal hypoglycemia (nesidioblastosis). Conversely, other mutations in Kir6.2 that maintain the K_{ATP} channel in an open state result in neonatal diabetes. K_{ATP} channel mutations are also found in some patients with type 2 diabetes.

Mitochondria produce ATP, the signal for the K_{ATP} channel, and they are implicated in a subtype of diabetes termed *mitochondrial diabetes* (1% of all diabetes). The most common is a mutation in the mitochondrial gene encoding transfer RNA for leucine, which decreases production of some mitochondrial proteins. Interestingly, this mutation causes two distinct syndromes: (1) maternally inherited mitochondrial diabetes and deafness, and (2) mitochondrial encephalomyopathy, lactic acidosis, and strokelike episodes (MELAS syndrome), the latter often associated with diabetes. Uncoupling protein 2 (UCP2) is an anion carrier located on the mitochondrial inner membrane that uncouples proton gradient and ATP synthesis, thus decreasing ATP production and increasing heat generation. Mice deficient in β-cell UCP2 have increased ATP production and insulin hypersecretion. UCP2 is upregulated in obesity and may contribute to diabetes associated with obesity. Certain UCP2 gene polymorphisms are weakly associated with body mass index (measure of obesity) and type 2 diabetes.

Three other pathways are also known to stimulate insulin secretion. The augmentation pathway may facilitate the K_{ATP} channel–dependent pathway but is controversial. The second pathway is also calcium dependent and works through Gq-coupled receptors that produce inositol triphosphate (IP_3), which releases calcium from the endoplasmic reticulum through IP_3 receptors. Acetylcholine releases insulin through this mechanism. GLP-1 and vasoactive intestinal peptide act through binding to Gs-coupled receptors that produce cyclic adenosine monophosphate, which activates PKA. PKA stimulates insulin secretion through a calcium-independent mechanism. GLP-1 is an ideal hormone candidate for diabetic treatment. Besides the stimulatory effects on β-cell mass growth, GLP-1-stimulated insulin release is regulated by serum glucose and is suppressed by hypoglycemia. In clinical trials, GLP-1 normalizes serum glucose in patients with type 2 diabetes without development of hypoglycemia.

5. INSULIN SIGNALING
5.1. Insulin Receptor

Insulin is released from the islet into the bloodstream and its actions are mediated by the insulin receptor (IR) on the surface of target cells. The most common etiology in diabetes, insulin resistance, results from defects in insulin signaling. Native IR is a large cylindrical tetrameric protein with a relative mobility (*Mr*) of 3,000,000, consisting of two α- and two β-polypeptide chains linked by disulfide bonds. IR is expressed in most mammalian tissues; adipose and liver have the highest IR density (>300,000 receptors/cell). High IR density is necessary for more rapid binding kinetics since normal plasma insulin levels range from 10^{-10} to 10^{-9} *M*, which are lower than the insulin-binding affinity. IR gene is located on the short arm of chromosome 19 and is approx 150 kb long with 22 exons and 21 introns. Most cell types have multiple RNA transcripts ranging from 5.7 to 9.5 kb in size, and all appear to code for the complete proreceptor. Exons 1–12 encode the α-subunit, and exons 13–22 encode the β-subunit. Two IR isoforms exist: IR-A is more abundant in fetal tissues, whereas IR-B is more abundant in adult tissues except brain. The difference between the two isoforms is that the IR-A

transcript does not include exon 11, whereas the IR-B transcript does, and, consequently, IR-A misses 12 amino acids near the carboxyl terminus of the α-subunit. Both isoforms have similar affinities for insulin.

IR as a whole is an allosteric enzyme. The β-subunit has tyrosine kinase activity, and the α-subunit regulates the β-subunit in an insulin-binding-dependent manner. The extracellular IR α-subunit is responsible for ligand binding. It has two insulin-binding pockets that interact with corresponding regions of insulin molecule. The carboxyl-terminal domain of α-subunit interacs with the β-subunit and transmits signal from insulin binding to activation of the IR kinase. The β-subunit has a short extracellular domain interacting with the α-subunit, a transmembrane domain, and a large intracellular domain with an intrinsic tyrosine (Tyr) kinase activity that undergoes tyrosine autophosphorylation on insulin binding to α-subunit and starts the insulin signaling network. Insulin-induced IR β-subunit autophosphorylation further increases the tyrosine kinase activity, and β-subunit autophosphorylation also forms recruitment sites for bringing substrate proteins to the IR. Tyrosine residues 1146, 1150, and 1151 are essential for tyrosine kinase activity. NPEY motif (Asn-Pro-Glu-Tyr) at the juxtamembrane region is important for substrate recruitment. Insulin receptor substrate-1 (IRS-1) and Shc, both IR substrates, interact with the NPEY motif. Mutations of autophosphorylation sites demonstrate that both increased kinase activity and recruitment of target proteins are critical for insulin signaling. Autophosphorylation is achieved within seconds after insulin binding. Seconds to minutes later, substrate protein phosphorylation occurs.

IR signaling is regulated in a variety of ways. Two protein tyrosine phosphatases (PTPases) dephosphorylate the IR, terminating insulin action without degrading the IR. One of the PTPases, leukocyte common antigen-related phosphatase, is membrane bound; the other, PTPase1B, is intracellular. Cell-surface IR density is regulated by addition from the Golgi apparatus and insulin-stimulated IR endocytosis. IR serine phosphorylation also contributes to the negative regulation of IR signaling.

5.2. Insulin Signal Network

The major substrates of IR tyrosine kinase are adapter protein Src-homology-collagen-like protein (SHC) and multifunctional docking proteins IRS-1 and IRS-2 (Fig. 4). Tyrosine-phosphorylated SHC recruits the small adapter protein growth factor receptor–binding protein 2 (Grb2), which, in turn, recruits and activates the ras-guanosine 5′-diphosphate exchange

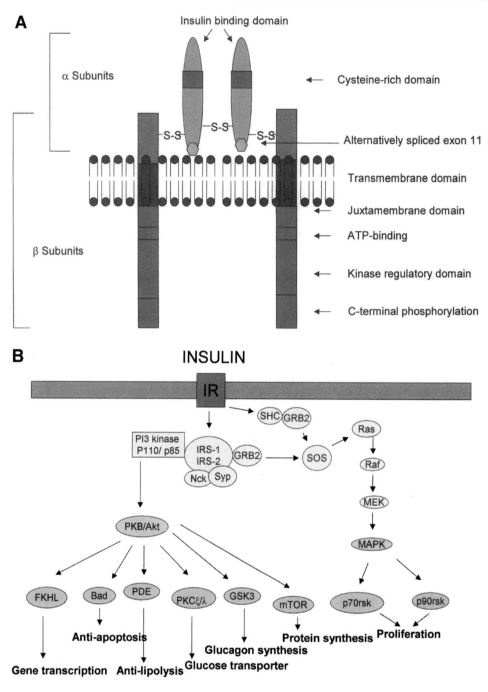

Fig. 4. (**A**) Insulin receptor structure; (**B**) signal transduction for IR.

factor mammalian son-of-sevenless protein (m-sos). The addition of m-sos into the receptor tyrosine kinase–induced complex at the plasma membrane activates ras small guanosine 5´-triphosphate–binding protein, which leads to eventual activation of the MAPK cascade involved in stimulating mitogenesis. A number of other hormones and growth factors also regulate MAPK cascade, and IR-stimulated MAPK activation mostly does not take part in insulin regulation of metabolic events. IRS-1 and IRS-2 are the major mediators for insulin metabolic action. Phosphorylation of specific tyrosine residues on IRS-1 and IRS-2 by activated IR allows recruitment of a number of signaling molecules through their Src homology 2 (SH2) domains. These include Grb2, the small adapter protein Nck, the tyrosine phosphatase Syp, and PI3K.

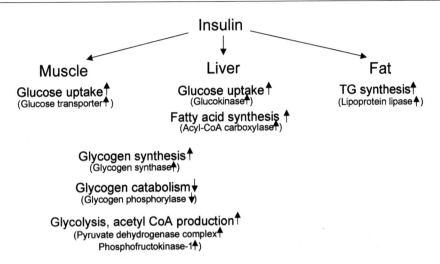

Fig. 5. Insulin-regulated metabolic activities in muscle, liver, and fat.

PI3K plays a central role in insulin signaling, leading to metabolic consequences. PI3K has two subunits. The p85 subunit acts as an adapter and targets the p110 catalytic subunit to the appropriate signaling complex. p85 contains two SH2 domains, which bind to tyrosine-phosphorylated motifs on IRS-1, IRS-2, and growth factor receptors. An inter-SH2 domain in p85 interacts with the p110 catalytic subunit. The p110 subunit is a kinase that phosphorylates phosphoinositides at the 3-position to form phosphatidylinositol-3-phosphates. Signaling proteins containing pleckstrin homology domains bind to the membrane-bound phosphaotidylinositol-3-phosphate, and their activity or localization is altered by the binding. p110 also has some serine kinase activity that appears to be largely directed toward the p85 subunit and IRS-1. PI3K recruitment increases PI3K activity because p85 interaction with specific phosphotyrosine motifs increases the p110 kinase activity and recruitment brings PI3K closer to its substrate near plasma membranes. PI3K activates phosphatidylinositol-3,4-biphosphate/phosphatidylinositol-3,4,5-triphosphate-dependent kinase 1, which activates PKB/Akt, a serine kinase. PKB in turn deactivates glycogen synthase kinase-3 (GSK-3), leading to glycogen synthase activation and thus glycogen synthesis. PKB activation also results in translocation of glucose transporter GLUT4 from intracellular vesicles to the plasma membrane, where they transport glucose into the cell. Another target of PKB is mTOR-mediated activation of protein synthesis by PHAS/elf4 and p70s6k.

5.3. Physiologic Actions of Insulin

Insulin has profound, diverse, and indispensible physiologic functions in growth and metabolism (Fig. 5).

Insulin can act very rapidly, within minutes (e.g., increased glucose uptake in muscle and fat cells); or in minutes to hours (e.g., regulation of gene expression and protein degradation); or slowly, in days (e.g., cell differentiation and organ development). Insulin is one of the few quintessential growth factors required for cell survival, proliferation, and differentiation. Indeed, most synthetic growth media (serum-free "defined media") for cell culture must contain insulin. It is not entirely clear how insulin signals as a growth factor but the MAPK pathway contributes at least partially. The metabolic activities of insulin, however, are more important clinically because metabolic derangements are the most common problems encountered in abnormal insulin signaling. Insulin regulates the metabolism of glucose, fat, and proteins and the general effects are anabolic. The metabolic activities of insulin are mediated through modulating the expression and activity of key enzymes in metabolism via the PI3K pathway.

Insulin stimulates glucose uptake, utilization, and storage in various tissues. Glucose cannot diffuse passively into the cells; the only way for a cell to take up glucose is through facilitated diffusion with hexose transporters (GLUTs). Four types of GLUT exist: GLUT1 is present in most tissues; GLUT2 is in liver and pancreatic β-cells, and GLUT2 in β-cells is important for regulating insulin secretion, as discussed earlier; GLUT3 is in brain; GLUT4 is in skeletal muscle, heart, and adipose tissue and is closely regulated by insulin through the PI3K-Akt pathway. In the absence of insulin, GLUT4 is on the membrane of intracellular vesicles, unable to transport glucose. Increased insulin levels, as seen in the postprandial state, result in binding of insulin to IR, which leads rapidly to fusion of those vesicles with the plasma membrane and insertion of GLUT4 onto the plasma membrane, thus allowing glucose uptake into the cell. When serum insulin levels decrease, as in fasting, and IR is no longer occupied, GLUT4 is recycled back into the cytoplasmic vesicles. Decreased glucose uptake into skeletal muscle has important implications in insulin resistance. The brain and liver do not require insulin for glucose uptake because these organs have an insulin-independent transporter. Insulin stimulates glycogen synthesis through the PI3K-Akt-GSK-3 pathway in muscle and liver to store glucose and inhibits gluconeogenesis.

Insulin promotes lipid synthesis and inhibits lipid degradation. Before insulin became available for treatment of type 1 diabetes, patients with this disease were invariably thin, reflecting the importance of insulin in lipid metabolism. Insulin increases fatty acid synthesis in the liver. When the liver is saturated with glycogen (roughly 5% of liver mass), glucose is diverted into synthesis of fatty acids and lipoproteins. The lipoproteins are released from the liver and undergo lipolysis in the circulation, providing free fatty acids for use in other tissues including the adipose tissue. Insulin also facilitates glucose uptake into adipocytes and glucose can be used to synthesize glycerol in these cells. Adipocytes use fatty acids produced in the liver and from food and glycerol produced in adipocytes to synthesize triglyceride. Insulin inhibits triglyceride breakdown in adipose tissue by inhibiting an intracellular lipase that hydrolyzes triglycerides. Thus insulin promotes lipid anabolism and has a fat-sparing effect so that insulin drive most cells to preferentially utilize carbohydrates instead of fatty acids for energy expenditure. Insulin also has profound effects on activity of lipoprotein lipase, fatty acid synthase, and acetylCoA carboxylase.

Insulin stimulates the intracellular uptake of amino acids through the PI3K-Akt-p70^{rsk} pathway and promotes protein synthesis. Insulin also increases the permeability of many cells to potassium, magnesium, and phosphate ions.

5.4. Insulin Resistance

The most important and readily measurable physiologic effect of insulin is on serum glucose. In a given person, serum insulin levels correspond to serum glucose levels. The relationship is inverse: the higher the insulin, the lower the glucose level. The concept of insulin resistance developed after it was found that in patients with early type 2 diabetes, both insulin and glucose levels are high, suggesting that glucose is "resistant" to insulin in these patients. Insulin resistance is defined as a clinical state of decreased insulin biologic responses to a normal or higher insulin level.

Although all biologic responses to insulin can be resistant to insulin, clinical insulin resistance refers to decreased glucose uptake, utilization, and storage at normal or higher circulating insulin levels, ultimately resulting in glucose intolerance and hyperglycemia. Insulin resistance is the most common cause of diabetes in Western societies and is the most common clinical problem encountered that involves glucose metabolism. More than 90% of type 2 diabetes is insulin resistant, and at least 25% of subjects with normal glucose tolerance may be insulin resistant but secrete sufficient insulin to overcome resistance. Insulin resistance is a key feature of the prediabetic "metabolic syndrome" (central obesity, hypertension, insulin resistance, and dyslipidemia).

Mechanisms for insulin resistance are not clear but are likely multiple. About 50% of insulin resistance can be attributed to genetic factors and another 50% to lifestyle factors. The molecular abnormality underlying insulin resistance may involve any of the multiple steps required for insulin signaling and can be classified as prereceptor or postreceptor defects. Prereceptor insulin resistance is extremely rare in humans and includes insulin mutants defective in binding with IR and antibodies to circulating insulin. Most clinical insulin resistance is owing to postreceptor defects.

Type A severe insulin resistance is an extremely rare clinical syndrome owing to IR mutations. In mice models, *Drosophila melanogaster*, and *Caenorhabditis elegans*, IR mutations have been identified that alter insulin binding and tyrosine kinase activity. Some mutations decreased mRNA stability with reduced IR expression at the cell surface. Because PI3K is critical for insulin metabolic functions, defects in PI3K could result in insulin resistance. A single mutation (326met-ile) was found in the coding sequence of p85. Mice lacking IRS-1 or IRS-2 are insulin resistant and defective in PI3K stimulation in muscle and adipocytes. These observations suggest that mutations in the insulin-signaling machinery are rare, which may not be surprising considering the critical importance of insulin signaling for survival.

IR serine/threonine phosphorylation contributes to insulin resistance. In muscle preparations derived from patients with type 2 diabetes, IR phosphorylation on serine or threonine residues is accompanied by decreased IR tyrosine phosphorylation. Serine phosphorylation of IRS molecules is elevated in the tissues of insulin-resistant or diabetic subjects with concomitant decrease in IRS tyrosine phosphorylation. Increased serine phosphorylation in insulin resistance of obesity may be due to elevated serum lipids and/or increased tumor necrosis factor-α (TNF-α). Furthermore, down-

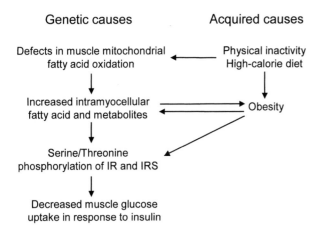

Fig. 6. A hypothesis on mechanism for insulin resistance.

stream enzymes such as PKC isoenzymes are serine/ threonine kinases and phosphorylate both IR and IRS. IR serine phosphorylation is also elevated in tissues derived from patients with polycystic ovary syndrome, who often have insulin resistance.

Because the skeletal muscles take up the majority of glucose, and muscle glycogen synthesis is about 50% lower in type 2 diabetic patients than in healthy subjects, impaired insulin-stimulated muscle glycogen synthesis is important in insulin resistance. Glucose transport (by GLUT4), phosphorylation (by hexokinase), and storage (by glycogen synthase) are three rate-limiting steps for muscle glycogen synthesis, and their defects have been suggested to be responsible for insulin resistance. In muscle of patients with type 2 diabetes, intracellular glucose and glucose-6-phosphate levels are both decreased, suggesting that glucose transport by GLUT4 is decreased, which causes impaired muscle glycogen synthesis.

Although decreased muscle glucose transport is a common theme in insulin resistance, the underlying mechanism is not clear. An interesting hypothesis based on nuclear magnetic resonance spectroscopy studies of intracellular muscle metabolites suggests that impaired mitochondrial fatty acid oxidation may be a primary lesion for insulin resistance. Compared with matched healthy control subjects, healthy, young lean but insulin-resistant offspring of patients with type 2 diabetes have an 80% increase in intracellular muscle lipid content with a 30% decrease in mitochondrial phosphorylation. The increase in intracellular fatty acids results in increased fatty acid metabolites such as diacylglycerol, fatty acid CoA, and ceramide, which may activate PKC

isoenzymes, leading to serine/threonine phosphorylation of IR and IRS molecules. A decrease in muscle glucose transport ensues.

This hypothesis explains most features of insulin resistance and type 2 diabetes (Fig. 6). A genetic primary defect in mitochondrial fatty acid oxidation leads to an increase in intramyocellular fatty acid levels, which leads to insulin resistance and an increase in triglyceride synthesis. A sedentary lifestyle and high-calorie diet further increase triglyceride synthesis and result in obesity. Central or abdominal obesity worsens insulin resistance and eventually diabetes develops. The mechanisms by which obesity promotes clinical manifestation of diabetes are poorly understood. Currently, it is thought that molecules released from adipose tissue are involved in insulin resistance, including metabolic products (e.g., free fatty acids), hormones (e.g., leptin, resistin, and adiponectin), and cytokines (e.g. TNF-α, interleukin-6, and acylation-stimulating protein). In animal models, some adipose hormones (e.g., resistin) are necessary and sufficient to cause insulin resistance. In humans, however, none has been shown to be consistently important in linking obesity to insulin resistance. The difference between mice and humans may be that adipose hormones may cause insulin resistance only in a selected genetic background. A class of drugs referred to as thiazolidinediones, including troglitazone, rosiglitazone, and pioglitazone, are insulin sensitizers and enhance insulin-stimulated glucose disposal in muscle by interacting with peroxisome proliferator–activated receptor γ, a nuclear receptor regulating adipogenesis.

SELECTED READING

Bonner-Weir S. Perspective: postnatal pancreatic beta cell growth. *Endocrinology* 2000;141:1926–1929.

Bratanova-Tochkova TK, Cheng H, Daniel S, Gunawardana S, Liu YJ, Mulvaney-Musa J, Schermerhorn T, Straub SG, Yajima H, Sharp GW. Triggering and augmentation mechanisms, granule pools, and biphasic insulin secretion. *Diabetes* 2002;51(Suppl 1): S83–S90.

Edlund H. Factors controlling pancreatic cell differentiation and function. *Diabetologia* 2001;44:1071–1079.

Le Roith D, Zick Y. Recent advances in our understanding of insulin action and insulin resistance. *Diabetes Care* 2001;24:588–597, 2001

Mauvais-Jarvis F, Kulkarni RN, Kahn CR. Knockout models are useful tools to dissect the pathophysiology and genetics of insulin resistance. *Clin Endocrinol* 2002;57:1–9.

Saltiel AR, Kahn CR. Insulin signalling and the regulation of glucose and lipid metabolism. *Nature* 2001;414:799–806.

Saudek CD. Presidential address: a tide in the affairs of medicine. *Diabetes Care* 2003;26:520–525.

Shulman GI. Cellular mechanisms of insulin resistance. *J Clin Invest* 2000;106:171–176.

21 Cardiovascular Hormones

Willis K. Samson, PhD and Meghan M. Taylor, PhD

CONTENTS

1. VASOACTIVE HORMONE FAMILIES

1.1. The Heart as an Endocrine Organ

Although the heart had long been considered merely a muscular pump that performed the physical labor of the circulation, it has been recognized for more than six decades that in addition to the contractile ultrastructure, a secretory function was evidenced by dense-core granules in the myocytes. Over the past two decades, the endocrine nature of the heart has been established, and the physiology and pathophysiology of the cardiac hormones have been extensively characterized. In both a constitutive and regulated fashion, myocytes produce two members of a family of hormones designated natriuretic peptides based on their abilities to stimulate salt and water excretion by direct renal actions and by actions in other tissues, including endocrine organs, responsible for the control of fluid and electrolyte homeostasis. Two members of the natriuretic peptide family, atrial natriuretic peptide (ANP) and brain natriuretic peptide (BNP, actually a misnomer since very little if any of this peptide is produced in the central nervous system) are produced in the heart and released in response to a variety of cues, many typical of plasma volume overload or hyperosmolality. Although numerous biologic actions have been char-

acterized, their hallmark effects are to unload the vascular tree via a combination of CNS, pituitary, adrenal, vascular, and renal actions (Fig. 1). This results in decreased venous return to the pump as a consequence of increased renal excretion of water and solute, vasorelaxation in certain vascular beds, increased capillary permeability, and decreased cardiac output. The third member of this family of hormones, although exerting many of the same actions as ANP and BNP, is unique in that it is predominantly produced in the vascular endothelium, not in the heart, and is thought to act more in a paracrine or an autocrine fashion, regulating primarily vascular tone and growth. Additionally, this hormone, designated C-type natriuretic peptide (CNP), exerts several CNS actions that oppose those of ANP and BNP.

For years the central focus of vascular endocrinology was the renin–angiotensin system (see Chapter 23); however, with the discovery of the cardiac hormones and the realization that at least some of their actions were expressed by a functional antagonism of the actions of angiotensin, a broader view of the importance of circulating hormones controlling vascular and renal function took shape. Then this doctrine of endocrine regulation of cardiovascular and renal function was challenged and expanded by the realization that

From: *Endocrinology: Basic and Clinical Principles, Second Edition*
(S. Melmed and P. M. Conn, eds.) © Humana Press Inc., Totowa, NJ

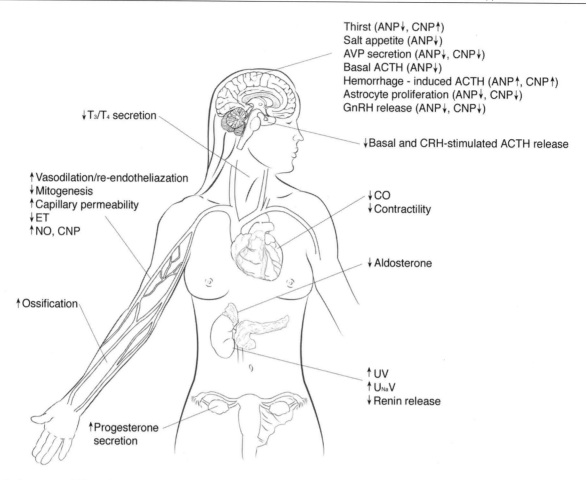

Thirst (ANP↓, CNP↑)
Salt appetite (ANP↓)
AVP secretion (ANP↓, CNP↓)
Basal ACTH (ANP↓)
Hemorrhage - induced ACTH (ANP↑, CNP↑)
Astrocyte proliferation (ANP↓, CNP↓)
GnRH release (ANP↓, CNP↓)

↓Basal and CRH-stimulated ACTH release

↓T₃/T₄ secretion

↑ Vasodilation/re-endotheliazation
↓ Mitogenesis
↑ Capillary permeability
↓ ET
↑ NO, CNP

↓CO
↓Contractility

↓ Aldosterone

↑Ossification

↑ UV
↑ U_NaV
↓ Renin release

↑Progesterone
secretion

Fig. 1. Summary of biologic actions of ANP and CNP. AVP = vasopressin; ACTH = adrenocorticotropin; GnRH = gonadotropin-releasing hormone; CRH = corticotropin-releasing hormone; CO = cardiac output; UV = urine volume; $U_{Na}V$ = urinary sodium excretion; NO = nitric oxide; ET = endothelin; T_3/T_4 = thyroid hormones.

perhaps the largest endocrine organ in the body, by virtue of its enormous surface area and ubiquitous presence, was the vasculature itself, mainly the endothelium. Not only was one member of the natriuretic peptide family produced in and released from this tissue, but it became apparent that numerous peptidergic, as well as nonpeptidergic, factors originating in the endothelium controlled vascular tone and proliferation.

1.2. Hormones of the Endothelium

The vascular endothelium controls access of blood-borne factors not only to the interstitium, but also to the contractile and proliferative elements of the vascular tree, the vascular smooth muscle cells (VSMCs). Additionally, the endothelial cells are positioned optimally to respond themselves to circulating factors and to transduce those messages to the VSMCs. Many hormonal messages are in fact delivered to the contractile ele-

ments via factors produced in the endothelium. Much attention has been focused on the ability of the endothelium to cause vasorelaxation via the generation of a soluble gas, nitric oxide (NO); however, peptidergic factors originating in the endothelial cells control VSMC function as well. Here the role of CNP as a paracrine factor has been established, and the endothelial cell–VSMC interface was the setting for the discovery and characterization of two additional, potent vasoactive hormones, endothelin (ET) and adrenomedullin (AM). The ETs are potent hypertensive agents that exert their effects directly on the VSMCs. AM, on the other hand, is a potent hypotensive agent, acting in a paracrine or an autocrine fashion in the vasculature. Thus, both circulating and locally produced vasoactive hormones can control regional blood flow, and this cellular interface has provided a model for the paracrine and autocrine effects of these peptides in other tissues as well. Agonists and antagonists selective for these peptides have been successfully tested in models of cardiovascular disease and some have even been approved for clinical use in humans.

2. NATRIURETIC PEPTIDE FAMILY

2.1. Gene Structure and Regulation

The members of the natriuretic peptide family share structural homology but are products of unique genes. Expression of separate genes and posttranslational processing of the nascent hormones is very similar. The genes for ANP and BNP have been localized to the same chromosome, whereas that for CNP resides on a separate chromosome, further suggesting the similar actions of ANP and BNP and disparate effects of CNP. Cloning of the cDNA complementarity to ANP mRNA revealed the presence of three exons in the ANP gene and the transcription of a prepro-ANP mRNA that encoded a 151- to 152-amino-acid preprohormone, depending on species. Removal of the N-terminal signal peptide results in a prohormone of 126 amino acids, which demonstrates extensive homology across species. This 126-amino-acid prohormone is the major form of the peptide stored in secretory granules in the heart. Stored pro-ANP is processed at secretion to a variety of smaller, biologically active forms, primarily the mature 28-amino-acid, C-terminal fragment. In brain, on the other hand, the prohormone is further processed to the mature peptide before packaging in secretory granules. An additional form of ANP is produced in kidney, this form being 33 amino acids of the C-terminus by posttranslational processing that includes four more amino acids on the N-terminus. This isoform, designated urodilatin, is thought to act as a paracrine regulator of tubular function. Expression of the BNP gene differs in that the resultant mRNA is less stable and the final posttranslational product is 32 amino acids long. Finally, CNP processing is quite similar to that of ANP, with the exception that the final posttranslational product lacks the C-terminal extension distal to the shared (within the natriuretic family) 17-membered disulfide loop, consisting, thus, of only 22 amino acids. In humans, owing to the presence of an arginine in the prohormone at position 73, a second form of CNP is present, which is N-terminally extended, consisting of 53 amino acids. CNP-22 and CNP-53 exert similar actions in many biologic systems. Note that in all three isoforms, the integrity of the internal disulfide loop is necessary for biologic activity.

Although little is known about the regulation of CNP gene transcription, mechanisms for activation of ANP and BNP gene transcription have been extensively studied. Gene transcription is induced by glucocorticoids, α-adrenergic agents, growth factors, calcium, and physical factors. There is a regional mismatch in the adult in gene expression of the two peptides, with ANP expressed primarily in the atria and BNP in the ventricles under basal conditions. Physical factors such as cardiac overload induce transcription of both genes, with the appearance of ANP expression in the ventricles as well. Most striking, however, is the level of induction of the BNP gene in the ventricles, resulting in a remarkable increase in circulating hormone levels. At the molecular level, ANP gene transcription is regulated by numerous members of the activating protein-1 complex, being induced by c-*jun* and in most cases suppressed by c-*fos*. A close relative of c-*fos*, fra-1, exerts biphasic effects, reducing the magnitude of c-*jun* activation of ANP gene expression in atriocytes, while amplifying the induction of expression by c-*jun* in ventriculocytes. Thus, the response of the ANP promotor to these early response elements may vary under unique physiologic conditions, permitting a wider repertoire of control of gene expression.

2.2. Hormone Secretion

2.2.1. PHYSIOLOGIC RELEASE

Plasma levels of ANP and BNP are extremely low (5–10 and 0.5–1.0 fmol/mL, respectively) and rise in response to any interventions that increase venous return and, therefore, atrial pressure and stretch. Pressor agents can release ANP in vivo and some even act in isolated tissue in vitro, suggesting direct cellular effects independent from increased venous return. The natriuretic effects of ANP and BNP are mirrored by the ability of hyperosmolality to stimulate directly, and indirectly via volume expansion, hormone secretion. In addition to secretion from the heart, these peptides are produced in and secreted from or into a variety of other tissues where distinct biologic actions have been characterized. The absolute contribution of those release sites to circulating levels of the hormones is in all likelihood minor; however, the potential importance of paracrine effects of the natriuretic peptides in those other tissues makes the study of the regulation of release in noncardiac sites extremely important. Indeed, renal, CNS, gonadal, and thymic production sites suggest a diversity of function for the peptides, and the mechanisms responsible for the regulation of secretion first must be elucidated before the physiologic or pathologic significance of those production sites is fully understood. Within the CNS, some of the same circulating factors that can stimulate ANP release from the myocytes (i.e., vasopressin and ET) similarly stimulate neuronal production and release of the peptide.

Endothelial cell production of CNP has been clearly established and the control of peptide secretion partially characterized. A variety of cytokines and growth factors (including interleukin-1α [IL-α] and IL-β, tumor necrosis factor-α [TNF-α], and transforming growth factor [TGF-β], as well as ANP and BNP) can stimulate CNP release from endothelial cells. Shear stress and hypoxia stimulate CNP release in the vasculature, as they do for ANP and BNP in the heart. Thus, the endothelial cell can, via CNP secretion, both transduce the antimitogenic effects of circulating ANP and BNP and buffer the proliferative effects of circulating cytokines and growth factors.

2.2.2. STATE OF HYPERSECRETION

Elevations in circulating natriuretic peptides have been reported in a variety of pathophysiologic states. CNP is remarkably elevated in septic shock, but not in hypertension or congestive heart failure (CHF). This again points to the more likely paracrine actions of CNP within the endothelial cell interface with VSMCs. CHF, myocardial ischemia, and hypertension all result in increased ANP and BNP secretion, reflecting possible compensatory mechanisms called into play during those conditions. Plasma BNP levels in cardiac overload states exceed those of ANP and are used clinically as diagnostic and prognostic tools to assess the progression and degree of heart failure. Although elevated during those overload states, the bioactivity of ANP and BNP appears to be reduced owing to a possible combination of effects, including reduced renal perfusion, receptor downregulation, or the counterregulatory effects of simultaneous activation of the renin-angiotensin-aldosterone system. Of these three possible explanations, the best case can be made for the latter. The increased circulating levels of ANP in critically ill trauma patients is thought to be a potential cause of suppressed adrenocorticotropic hormone levels frequently observed, because ANP can act at both the hypothalamic and pituitary levels to inhibit corticotropin release.

2.3. Sites of Action

Three natriuretic peptide receptor subtypes have been identified (Fig. 2). Two of these proteins contain intracellular kinase homology domains (adenosine triphosphate binding sites) and C-terminal guanylyl cyclase (GC) domains. Activation of these receptors results, therefore, in elevated cellular cyclic guanosine 5´-monophosphate (cGMP) levels. Their extracellular domains share 44% homology, whereas the intracellular domains share 63% homology in the kinase homology domain and 88% homology in the GC domains. These two receptors have been designated the GC-A and GC-B receptors and are alternatively called natri-

uretic peptide receptor-A (NPR-A) and NPR-B. A third receptor subtype, called the clearance receptor or NPR-C, shares approx 30% homology with NPR-A and NPR-B in the extracellular ligand-binding domain; however, this receptor lacks the intracellular C-terminal extension (i.e., it is missing the kinase and GC domains). This receptor was originally thought to have no biologic activity other than to sequester or clear natriuretic peptides from the extracellular fluid; however, it is now recognized that NPR-C plays important biologic roles and signals via a reduction in cyclic adenosine monophosphate (cAMP) levels and possibly a stimulation of polyinositol phosphate turnover (increased phospholipase C [PLC] activity). This receptor appears to mediate the antimitogenic actions of the natriuretic peptides in the CNS. A distinct hierarchy of binding affinities characterizes these receptors with all three forms of natriuretic peptides binding with equal affinity to NPR-C. NPR-A prefers ANP as a ligand (ANP > BNP >> CNP), whereas NPR-B recognizes more readily CNP (CNP >> ANP = BNP). Thus, the sites of action of the natriuretic peptides are determined by the relative distributions of the three receptors, with NPR-B predominating in the brain (e.g., the hypothalamo-hypophyseal system) and muscular component of the vasculature, whereas NPR-A is more abundant in the kidney, adrenal gland, and endothelium. The clearance (NPR-C) receptor is present throughout the body.

2.4. Biologic Actions

Originally CNP was thought to act only in a paracrine fashion to regulate vascular tone and growth; however, CNP can also exert cardiovascular, renal, and adrenal actions when infused intravenously. This may simply be a reflection of the fact that CNP is produced in a variety of tissues, and, therefore, multiple paracrine actions may occur. CNP levels are elevated in chronic renal failure, and the peptide is produced in kidney, where it exerts diuretic and natriuretic effects. One can recognize the sites of action of the natriuretic peptides by locating receptors, but the assignment of biologic activity is not as simple. Two reagents that have clarified the receptor subtype responsible for a variety of natriuretic peptide actions are the clearance receptor ligand C-ANF$_{4-23}$, which binds preferentially to NPR-C, and the GC antagonist HS-142-1, which blocks the ability of the natriuretic peptides to signal via activation of GC. By using a combination of methodologic approaches, it has been realized that although the NPR-C controls the antimitogenic effects of the natriuretic peptides centrally, NPR-B performs a similar function in the vascular compartment. Within the kidney, multiple receptors are found, explaining the ability of both

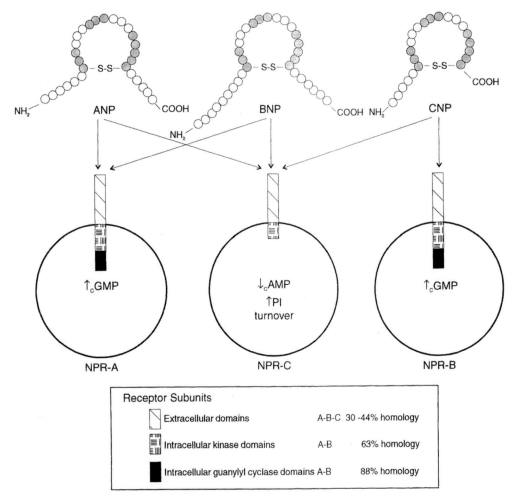

Fig. 2. Three members of the natriuretic peptide family, ANP, BNP, and CNP, share 65% homology (indicated by shaded circles) in the biologically active ring structure formed by the disulfide links and vary in amino acid composition and lengths of their N- and C-terminal extensions. All three peptides are recognized by the natriuretic peptide C (clearance) receptor (NPR-C); however, the A receptor (NPR-A) prefers ANP and BNP. The B receptor (NPR-B) recognizes with relative preference CNP. Activation of the three receptors has been reported to generate the indicated changes in intracellular levels of cGMP or cAMP and/or phosphoinositol (PI) turnover.

ANP and CNP to act as diuretic and natriuretic agents. The multiple peripheral effects of the natriuretic peptides are summarized in Fig. 1. Although not all of these actions seem related to fluid and electrolyte homeostasis, some may instead be related to the antiproliferative effects of the peptides.

Within the CNS, similar and diverging actions of ANP and CNP have been described. In most species, more CNP is produced within the brain than ANP or BNP and, for the most part, NPR-B and NPR-C predominate within the brain interstitium. It should be recognized that ANP may therefore exert its biologic actions in the brain by displacing CNP from NPR-C (clearance receptor). This has been demonstrated to be the case in the neuroendocrine hypothalamus. There are

other examples where interactive effects via the shared NPR-C cannot underlie the effects observed. Thus, the ability of ANP to inhibit the behavioral (water drinking) and endocrine (prolactin [PRL] secretion) aspects of fluid and electrolyte homeostasis is opposed by the stimulatory effects of CNP. Certainly in these cases, activation of NPR-A must underlie the effects of ANP, whereas NPR-B must be responsible for the stimulatory effects of CNP. In the absence of antagonists that can distinguish between these two GC receptor subtypes, other methodologies had to be created to make these distinctions. One such approach is receptor-specific cytotoxin cell targeting using the plant lectin ricin. With this approach, evidence for the involvement of the NPR-A in the physiologic regulation of salt appetite has been obtained, and the importance of NPR-B in the hypothalamic mechanisms controlling neuroendocrine function has been established.

Which of the pharmacologic actions of the natriuretic peptides are physiologically relevant? A combination of experimental approaches has provided evidence for the role of the peptides in a variety of tissues. Use of the selective clearance receptor ligand C-ANF$_{4-23}$ established the importance of ligand binding to the NPR-C on astrocyte proliferation (i.e., antimitogenic effects). The GC receptor antagonist HS-142-1 was employed to demonstrate that the natriuretic peptides play important roles in the maintenance of glomerular filtration and sodium excretion under basal conditions. Ricin cytotoxin adminstration studies demonstrated the role of endogenous brain-derived CNP in the neuroendocrine regulation of PRL and luteinizing hormone secretion, and the importance of central ANP to the control of sodium homeostasis (i.e., appetite). Passive immunoneutralization was employed to demonstrate the physiologic relevance of the action of ANP to inhibit thirst.

Recently two molecular techniques have provided additional insight into the physiology of the natriuretic peptides. Transgenic mouse models of overexpression of natriuretic peptide have been created. In the case of the ANP transgene, homozygotes displayed significantly lower blood pressure under basal conditions than nontransgenic littermates; however, sodium excretion was not different. Transgene-induced overexpression of BNP led to increased endochondral ossification and bony overgrowth. These studies uncovered an action of BNP that was not revealed in pharmacologic studies, probably due to the chronic effect of BNP overexpression, something not possible to accomplish in classic pharmacologic application studies. Transgene-induced overexpression of CNP or BNP improved postischemic insult neovascularization by stimulating reendothelialization and suppressing neointimal formation. These studies strongly suggest a therapeutic option for the natriuretic peptides in patients with tissue ischemia.

The second molecular approach to the study of the physiologic relevance of the pharmacologic effects of the natriuretic peptides is the generation of null mutations (knockouts), which results in the absence of a given peptide. ANP-null mice are more susceptible to the hypertensive consequences of high salt ingestion. This model reveals two important things. First, ANP is not essential for normal embryonic and postnatal development. Second, endogenous ANP must play some role in the physiologic mechanisms that protect against the development of high blood pressure. CNP knockouts are dwarfs, displaying impaired endochondral ossifica-

tion, but the condition can be rescued by simultaneous targeted overexpression of a CNP transgene. These data complement the results (just discussed) in the CNP overexpression system alone and further support a significant role of CNP in normal bone development and turnover. The CNP knockout animals display early mortality; thus, other important roles of CNP must be present and are certainly awaiting discovery.

2.5. Potential Therapeutic Uses

Although the action of the natriuretic peptides appears to be blunted in edematous states, such as CHF, cirrhosis, and the nephrotic syndrome, therapeutic use of the peptides in these states may prove at least acutely advantageous. Certainly, if the mechanism by which the biologic activity of the peptides has been reduced in these states can be elucidated, strategies might be employed that overcome those deficits. In particular, it has already been demonstrated that in CHF, administration of high doses of ANP and urodilatin can lower preload and increase diuresis and natriuresis, providing significant benefit in this life-threatening situation. Even though plasma ANP levels are elevated in CHF, further elevation by exogenous administration has provided salutary therapy. Like conventional diuretics, ANP increases urine volume and urinary sodium excretion, at least in part by inhibiting sodium reabsorption in the collecting duct by an action on the sodium/chloride transporter. However, unlike current diuretic agents, ANP inhibits the renin-angiotensin-aldosterone system by directly inhibiting renin secretion and thereby lowering aldosterone levels in plasma. In addition, administration of ANP lowers sympathetic tone, and the combined reduction in plasma renin activity and sympathetic tone effectively lowers sodium reabsorption in the proximal tubule. ANP also inhibits tubuloglomerular feedback, and the maintenance of glomerular filtration even in the face of decreased renal blood flow may be an important reason for the peptide's protective effect on renal function even in low perfusion states such as heart failure. Finally, ANP not only inhibits arginine vasopressin (AVP) release, but it blocks AVP's ability to stimulate water reabsorption in the collecting duct. ANP therapy in acute heart failure was approved in Japan almost 10 yr ago, and recently a synthetic BNP, nesiritide, was approved for use in the United States.

Because a role of endogenous ANP in the phenomenon has been suggested, perhaps a similar strategy can be used to induce mineralocorticoid escape. Interest in the postoperative use of ANP and urodilatin to prevent acute renal failure has been stimulated by early studies demonstrating the ability of high pharmacologic doses

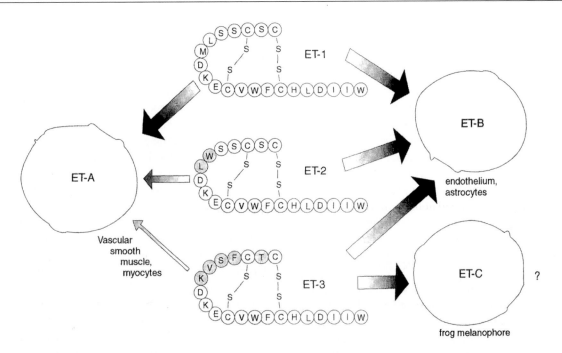

Fig. 3. Three members of the mammalian ET peptide family have been identified, each sharing remarkable homology in amino acid composition. Shaded circles indicate differing amino acids. Three receptor subtypes have been characterized. The ET-A receptor binds ET with a relative preference indicated by the thickness of the arrows (ET-1 ≥ ET-2 > ET-3). The ET-B receptor recognizes equally all three forms of ET. The third receptor, ET-C, found thus far only in nonmammals, prefers ET-3. Sites of receptor expression are indicated.

of the peptide to reduce the need for hemodialysis/ hemofiltration in these patients.

Most promising in a therapeutic sense is the potential use of the natriuretic peptides as antiproliferative agents. In a rabbit model of vascular lesions caused by balloon catheter injury, administration of CNP significantly lowered the resultant intima-to-media ratios, providing direct evidence for a paracrine action of the peptide to suppress intimal thickening. Furthermore, local CNP antagonizes the growth-promoting effects of angiotensin II (Ang II) and the vascular consequences of cyclosporine A induction of ET release and subsequent mitogenesis, again predicting a significant avenue for the prevention of vascular lesions.

3. ENDOTHELINS
3.1. Gene Structure

In addition to the production of endothelial-derived relaxing factors in the vasculature, it had been known for some time that the cells lining the blood vessels produce potent vasoconstrictive substances as well. In 1988, the sequence of a powerful, endogenous vasoconstrictor substance produced by endothelial cells was identified. This 21-amino-acid peptide was named ET. It is now recognized that there are at least three forms

of the ETs (ET-1, ET-2, and ET-3), all 21 amino acid peptides differing by only 2–5 amino acids in the 15-membered ring structure formed by two internal disulfide bonds (Fig. 3). Each are products of unique genes and are first processed similarly into a prohormone form of 203 amino acids, in the case of ET-1, and then posttranslationally modified into the 39-amino-acid prohormone intermediate, big ET. In states of hypersecretion, the prohormone forms appears in plasma; however, under normal conditions, the mature 21-amino-acid form is the major secretory product. The final cleavage of the prohormone is thought to occur at secretion and to be catalyzed by a phosphoramidon-sensitive metalloproteinase designated ET-converting enzyme (EC 3.4.24.11). Knowledge of this important conversion enzyme's presence has led to potential therapeutic intervention strategies for interruption of ET action in states of hypersecretion, because the prohormone big ET has limited biologic activity.

The human ET-1 gene has five exons and four introns, with the peptide coded in the second exon. The gene is transcriptionally regulated via *cis* elements, including a GATA-2 protein-binding site and an AP-1 site that is activated by thrombin, angiotensin II, epidermal growth factor (EGF), basic fibroblast growth factor (bFGF), insulin-like growth factor, and TGF-β. Other transcriptional regulators include vasopressin, the ILs, TNF-α, and NO, which apparently mediates the ability of heparin to stimulate ET production. Physical factors also activate transcription, including pressure and anoxia. Translational regulation is exerted by a variety of factors that also regulate secretion, since little hormone is stored intracellularly. High-density lipoproteins stimulate production and secretion, whereas insulin not only stimulates production and secretion, but also augments ET binding and action. Negative regulation of production and secretion is exerted at the transcriptional level by NO, and at the translational event by prostaglandins, prostacyclin, AM, and ANP.

3.2. Hormone Secretion

Fortunately, the majority of the ET produced is secreted abluminally, away from the vessel lumen, to act in a paracrine or autocrine fashion. Although levels of the hormone do rise in certain pathologic conditions, in general, reflecting tissue damage in most cases, this peptide should be kept out of the circulation because of its potent vasoconstrictive properties and because in experimental animals, elevation in circulating ET results in respiratory failure and/or cerebral vasospasms and aneurysms. Again, knowledge of the production sites predicts biologic activities. The major site of ET-1 production is the endothelium, where on release it causes vasoconstriction. Additional production sites include the brain, uterus, kidney mesangial cells, Sertoli cells, and breast epithelial cells. ET-3 production occurs mainly within the CNS, where a role for the peptide in neuronal and astroglial development and proliferation has been suggested. What little ET-2 is produced in the body is found in kidney, intestine (hence, the alternative name vasoactive intestinal constrictor), myocardium, and uterus. The ETs have a relatively short half-life in plasma, about 4–7 min, and are released primarily in response to hypoxia, ischemia, and shear stress.

3.3. Site and Mechanisms of Action

Two mammalian ET receptor subtypes have been cloned, and they are members of the G protein–linked, seven-transmembrane-spanning domain superfamily of biologic receptors (Fig. 3). The ET-A receptor displays a rank order of binding affinity with ET-1 being the preferred ligand (ET-1 $\geq$ ET-2 >> ET-3). This receptor predominates in VSMCs and cardiac myocytes. Activation of the receptor results, depending on tissue site, in the activation of a variety of signaling cascades, including in the lung the production of prostanoids via stimulation of PLD and PLA$_2$ activities resulting in bronchoconstriction and in the scenario of hypersecretion, pulmonary hypertension (Fig. 4). In VSMCs, ET stimulates contraction and mitogenesis via multiple signaling pathways, including activation of PLC with the resultant formation of diacylglycerol (DAG) and inositol triphosphate (IP$_3$). The DAG formed activates the kinase cascade via protein kinase C (PKC), and IP$_3$ mobilizes intracellular calcium, initiating the contractile event. ET-A receptor activation also in these cells has been reported to open potassium channels and to activate adenylyl cyclase. In the myocardium, the ET-A receptor is thought to be activated by endogenous ET released in response to ischemia following myocardial infarction. The resultant opening of potassium channels causes a decrease in the electrical activity of the myocyte and closes the chloride channel, resulting in a suppression of catecholamine activation of contractile function.

The ET-B receptor predominates in the endothelium itself and in the CNS. This receptor binds all three isoforms equally and is responsible for the activity of circulating ET to stimulate a transient vasodilatory response in the periphery, via acute release of vasodilators such as NO and CNP. The signaling cascade that follows activation of the ET-B receptor is multifaceted. G protein–coupled activation of PLC results in PKC activation and mobilization of intracellular calcium. NO synthase activity is stimulated with the resultant production of the potent vasodilator NO, which can act within the endothelial cell to activate GC or diffuse across to the smooth muscle cells to perform the same function. Additionally, ET-B activation results in opening of the sodium-hydrogen antiporter and inhibition of adenylyl cyclase. The mitogenic effects of ET are thought to be transduced via PKC activation and tyrosine phosporylation–intiated activation of the mitogen-activated protein kinase (MAPK) system. In mesangial cells, the mitogenic effect of ET is mediated via transcriptional activation of immediate early genes. Activation of *Ras* proteins and downstream induction of the kinase activity of *Raf*-1 result in transcriptional induction of the c-*fos* serum response element, perhaps providing a mechanism for the mitogenic effect of ET. One hallmark characteristic of the biologic effects of the ETs is their profound tachyphylaxis. Although some data indicate this to be the result of chronic membrane effects or overloading of the cytosolic calcium pool, evidence also exists for rapid internalization of the ligand-receptor complex and continued signaling from the internalized aggregate.

3.4. Biologic Actions

Although multiple pharmacologic effects of the ETs have been reported, there is a need to establish which of

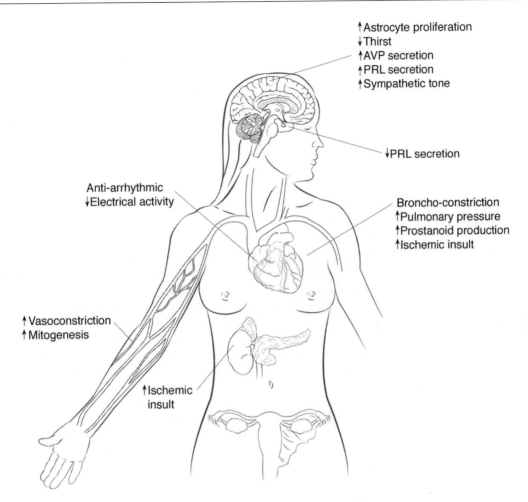

↑Astrocyte proliferation
↓Thirst
↑AVP secretion
↑PRL secretion
↑Sympathetic tone

↓PRL secretion

Broncho-constriction
↑Pulmonary pressure
↑Prostanoid production
↑Ischemic insult

Anti-arrhythmic
↓Electrical activity

↑Vasoconstriction
↑Mitogenesis

↑Ischemic insult

Fig. 4. Summary of biologic actions of ETs.

those have biologic significance and physiologic relevance. In this case, multiple pharmacologic tools are available, such that selective antagonism of the ET-A receptor is possible and isoform-specific activation of the ET-B receptor can now be accomplished. Also available are antagonists that affect both the ET-A and ET-B receptor, and a new generation of relatively specific ET-B antagonists. Much interest continues regarding the possible existence of a unique, ET-3-selective ET-C receptor in mammals similar to that found in frog melanophores, and it is hoped that eventual cloning of that protein will permit generation of similarly selective antagonists.

Surprising results from molecular approaches have provided new insight into the biology of the ETs. As discussed below, it was anticipated that these potent vasoconstrictive peptides would be found to play an important role in the development of hypertension; however, gene knockout homozygotes have, if anything, slightly elevated blood pressure, not the expected

hypotension. Unexpected results accrued from these null mutation strategies. Mice lacking expression of the normal ET-1 gene are born with severe craniofacial malformations, suggesting a developmental role of the peptide in pharyngeal arch structures. Additionally, these animals succumb to respiratory failure, suggesting an important embryonic role of the peptide in the preparation of respiratory structures for postnatal life. Knockouts of the genes encoding the ET-B receptor or ET-3 itself result in a postnatal phenotype similar to that observed in Hirschsprung disease (congenital megacolon), suggesting the importance of ET in the development of the intrinsic nervous system of the gut and the regulation of gastrointestinal smooth muscle function. Multiple CNS actions of the ETs have been reported, ranging from mitogenic effects on astrocytes mediated via the ET-B receptor to effects on descending sympathetic activity. The presence of the ET peptide and ET receptors during fetal development indicates a potential embryonic role in CNS structures, which may mirror the situation uncovered by the ET-3 and ET-B receptor knockouts in the intrinsic nervous system of the gut. Loss of the neurotropic effects of the ETs may be responsible in part for the respiratory failure seen in the immediate postpartum interval. Regarding neuromodulatory effects of the ETs, antagonist studies have revealed the physiologic relevance of the antidipsogenic effects of ET; however, the day-to-day significance of the neuroendocrine actions of the peptide (including activation of the hypothalamic mechanisms controlling anterior pituitary function and vasopressin secretion) and the effects of the peptides on sympathetic function have yet to be established.

A final CNS consequence of the administration of ET is potentially disastrous. In some species, ET infusion results in rupture of the basal artery on the ventral surface of the Pons, and a role for endogenous ET in vasospasm subsequent to subarachinoid hemorrhage has been established by the observation that pretreatment with an ET antagonist can prevent this event. This has led to the hypothesis that ET antagonists may prove therapeutically advantageous to prevent or lessen ischemic damage downstream from damaged, hypoxic endothelium of the cerebral vessels after thrombosis or infarct.

3.5. Pathophysiology of the ETs

Because of the multiple pharmacologic activities of the ETs, their involvement in numerous pathologic states has been hypothesized. These hypotheses were based largely on elevated circulating ET levels or responses seen in these conditions and, under many circumstances, it remains unclear whether the associations are causal or coincidental. The most predicted role for the ETs in pathophysiology was that in hypertensive states. Indeed, plasma levels are not consistently found to correlate with blood pressure, and although they may be elevated in some animal models of hypertension, null mutant mice actually have elevated blood pressures. Similarly controversial is the potential role for ET in reperfusion injury; one group using an isolated perfused rat heart model argued against a causative role and another utilizing isolated ventricular myocytes argued in favor. In vivo evidence favoring a role for endogenous ET in reperfusion injury comes from studies in pig in which both myocardial ischemia and infarction resulted in significantly elevated ET production and release. In rats receiving infusion of an antiserum directed against ET-1 prior to coronary artery ligation, damage distal to the ligation was markedly reduced. Similar results were obtained with an ET-A receptor antagonist in a canine myocardial infarction model. These data provide the best evidence for a role for ET in reperfusion injury and ischemia.

ET antagonists improve renal function in a genetic model of hypertension, the spontaneously hypertensive rat, and ET has been invoked in the pathogenesis of acute renal failure (postischemia renal failure). Cyclosporine A–induced nephrotoxicity has been identified to be owing at least in part to ET-induced vasoconstriction of the afferent arteriole, since the renal toxicity of immunosuppressant therapy was blocked by ET antagonist pretreatment. The mitogenic actions of ET are thought to underlie the development of graft arteriosclerosis in cardiac allografts, the establishment of atherosclerotic plaques, and the development of diabetes-related vascular lesions. Its role in vasospasm secondary to subarachnoid hemorrhage has been established in animal models. Within the lung, roles for ET in asthma and pulmonary hypertension have been proposed. The current literature favors the therapeutic use of ET antagonists in a variety of pathologic situations. However, clinical trials have not always been successful in establishing their clinical value.

Several patient trials were conducted to determine the efficacy of ET antagonists in the setting of pulmonary arterial hypertension (PAH). The rational for these trials was that lung levels of ET mRNA are increased in PAH, and a positive correlation between serum ET levels and measured pulmonary vascular resistance had been described. Although the nonselective ET antagonist, bosentan, was effective in reducing pulmonary artery pressure and pulmonary vascular resistance in one study when administered with another agent (a prostaglandin included to increase pulmonary blood flow), deaths occurred in the treatment group. In another trial, bosentan did improve exercise tolerance in patients with severe PAH. This led to the approval by the Food and Drug Administration of the use of low-dose bosentan in PAH; however, liver function tests were abnormal in a significant portion of the treatment group, and, thus, the possible negative side effect of hepatotoxicity must be weighed against the benefit obtained. Hepatotoxicity was also a problem in trials employing the selective ET-A antagonist sitaxsentan.

Again in human trials, this time in the setting of CHF, bosentan treatment resulted in a significant incidence of liver abnormalities. On the other hand, tezosentan, a nonselective ET antagonist, showed some benefit in acute heart failure patients in one trial but failed to provide protection in others. The selective ET-A antagonist darusentan improved cardiac index in patients with New York Heart Association stage III heart failure, but there were more adverse events in the treatment group than in placebo control subjects. Thus, in heart failure trials, ET antagonists have not been proven to be safe alternatives to conventional therapies. The same can be said of trials

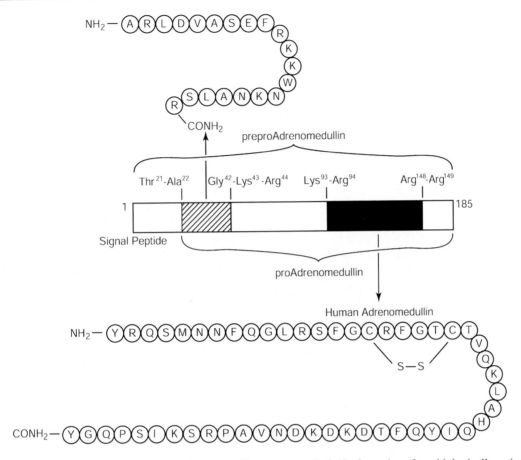

Fig. 5. Posttranslational processing of the preproadrenomedullin protein results in the formation of two biologically active peptides, AM and PAMP.

examining the efficacy of the ET antagonist in essential hypertension. Only recent, preliminary trials in patients with coronary artery disease are promising. Because ET is a vasoconstrictor and stimulates smooth muscle proliferation, neutrophil adhesion, and platelet aggregation, it was hypothesized that ET antagonists would be effective in the treatment of coronary artery disease. Indeed, ET antagonists increased coronary artery diameter and prevented vasoconstriction after percutaneous coronary angiography. However, these trials need to be repeated and extended with a careful examination of liver function in patients before any conclusions can be made.

4. ADRENOMEDULLIN GENE PRODUCTS
4.1. Gene Structure and Regulation

Utilizing a bioassay system that monitored accumulation of cAMP in platelets, Japanese investigators identified in 1993 a novel vasoactive hormone in extracts of a human pheochromocytoma. The peptide (Fig. 5) is produced in normal chromaffin cells of the adrenal gland, as well as a variety of other tissues, including

brain, kidney, endothelial cells, and VSMCs. Posttranslational processing of the 185-amino-acid prohormone results in the production and secretion of the mature 52-amino-acid form, designated AM, and a 20-amino-acid fragment from the N-terminus designated proadrenomedullin N-terminal 20 peptide (PAMP), a peptide that shares some, but not all, of the biologic activities of AM. Although activation of adenylyl cyclase was used as a screening bioassay in the initial phases of discovery, the hallmark bioassay for AM is the potent hypotensive action when infused intravenously (Fig. 6).

AM production in VSMCs and endothelial cells is regulated at the transcriptional level by a variety of cytokines, including IL-1α, IL-1β, TNF-α, and TNF-β. Production of AM in these cells is also stimulated by thrombin, aldosterone, cortisol, retinoic acid, and thyroid hormones. To a lesser degree, stimulation of production in VSMCs was reported also in response to Ang II, epinephrine, platelet-derived growth factor, EGF, and FGF. TGF-β and cAMP inhibit production.

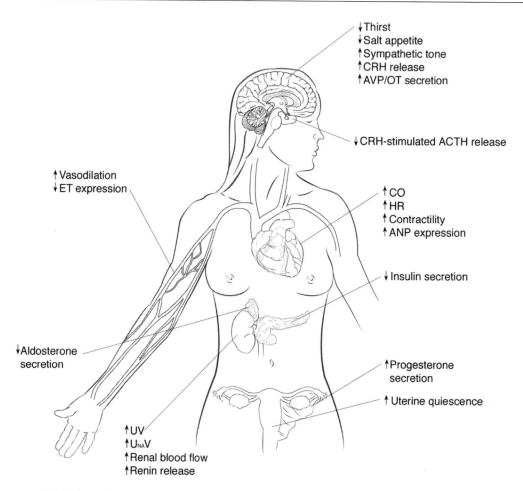

↓Thirst
↓Salt appetite
↑Sympathetic tone
↑CRH release
↑AVP/OT secretion

↓CRH-stimulated ACTH release

↑Vasodilation
↓ET expression

↑CO
↑HR
↑Contractility
↑ANP expression

↓Insulin secretion

↓Aldosterone
secretion

↑Progesterone
secretion

↑Uterine quiescence

↑UV
↑U$_{Na}$V
↑Renal blood flow
↑Renin release

Fig. 6. Summary of biologic actions of AM. CRH = corticotropin-releasing hormone; ACTH = adrenocorticotropin; AVP = vasopressin; OT = oxytocin; CO = cardiac output; HR = heart rate; ANP = atrial natriuretic peptide; UV = urine volume; U$_{Na}$V = urinary sodium excretion; ET = endothelin.

4.2. Hormone Secretion

Many of the factors that stimulate hormone production also stimulate secretion in isolated cell systems, leading to the hypothesis that AM may be responsible for the hypotension of inflammation, septic shock, and atherosclerosis. Circulating levels in humans are similar to those of other vasoactive hormones (about 3 fmol/mL of plasma), suggesting that like other vasoactive substances, the actions of AM may be predominantly autocrine or paracrine in nature. One group failed to observe elevations in plasma AM concentrations during hypertensive attacks in patients with pheochromocytomas; however, cosecretion of AM and catecholamines has been observed from cultured, bovine adrenal medullary cells. In fact, the cosecretion of PAMP and catecholamines from these cells is calcium dependent and induced by carbachol activation of nicotinic receptors. Those studies also pointed to an autocrine or paracrine

action of the peptide, since PAMP acted as an anticholinergic inhibiting sodium influx and reducing the magnitude of catecholamine response to carbachol.

4.3. Sites of Action

Some of the pharmacologic actions of AM can be blocked by the calcitonin gene–related peptide (CGRP) receptor blocker CGRP$_{8-37}$, which is not surprising because AM and CGRP share considerable structural homology. Both activate adenylyl cyclase in a variety of tissues and can displace each other in binding assays. Mesenteric vasodilatory responses to AM are blocked by CGRP$_{8-37}$ in vitro, but the in vivo vasodilatory responses are not. Additionally, the increase in cAMP levels observed in response to AM in endothelial cells in culture is not blocked by CGRP$_{8-37}$. Both AM and CGRP bind the calcitonin receptor–like receptor (CRLR), which is a unique G protein–coupled receptor. When

CRLR associates with an accessory protein (receptor activity modifying protein-1 [RAMP-1]), it functions as a selective CGRP receptor, one that can be blocked by $CGRP_{8-37}$. On the other hand, when CRLR associates with the homologous RAMP-2 and RAMP-3, the complex is more selective for AM binding. This may explain the apparent similarity in action of CGRP and AM in some systems. Not all of the biologic activities of AM can be explained by the presence of the CRLR/RAMP-2 or RAMP-3 receptor complexes; thus, additional yet-to-be described receptors may exist. In bovine aortic endothelial cells, AM binding leads to activation of adenylyl cyclase via a cholera toxin–sensitive G protein mechanism, with concomitant stimulation of PLC activity. As a result, cyctosolic calcium levels increase and NO is generated. In mesangial cells, AM inhibits MAPK, an effect that may underlie the peptide's antimitogenic actions. In VSMCs, AM activates a proline-rich tyrosine kinase. Very little is understood about the identity of the PAMP receptor. PAMP inhibits catecholamine release induced by periarterial nerve stimulation, possibly by a direct membrane action mediated via a pertussis toxin–sensitive G protein. Pertussis toxin also blocks the ability of PAMP to inhibit opening of voltage-gated (N-type) calcium channels in pheochromocytoma cells (PC-12 cells), a cell line in which PAMP also opens inwardly rectifying potassium channels. A potassium channel also appears to mediate the ability of PAMP to inhibit corticotropin-releasing hormone–stimulated adrenocorticotropin release from cultured anterior pituitary cells in vitro.

4.4. Biologic Actions

AM and PAMP exert profound effects on cardiovascular function and fluid and electrolyte homeostasis by actions in a variety of tissues (Fig. 6). The hallmark action of AM is vasodilation by an action on endothelial cells to generate NO and by direct activation of adenylyl cyclase in VSMCs. PAMP, on the other hand, exerts its hypotensive action not by an action on the endothelial cells or VSMCs, but, instead, by presynaptic inhibition of electrical activity in the sympathetic fibers that innervate the blood vessels. These vascular effects appear to be physiologically relevant because heterozygote AM gene knockout mice (missing one copy of the AM gene) display only 50% of the normal circulating levels of AM and are hypertensive compared with wild-type (normal two-gene copy) mice. The vasodilatory effect of AM is even more pronounced in circumstances of high levels of Ang II, such as in preconstricted vessels in vitro or human hypertensives in vivo. This has led to the hypothesis that the physiologic action of AM is to act as a coun-

terbalance to the renin-angiotensin-aldosterone system. Indeed, this may be the case because both AM and PAMP inhibit Ang II–stimulated aldosterone secretion in vivo and block activation of the hypothalamic-pituitary-adrenal axis at the level of the anterior pituitary gland. AM is produced in cardiomyocytes and acts locally to inhibit fibrosis stimulated by increased Ang II and aldosterone levels. It acts to increase coronary blood flow, a function that is thought to have clinical relevance in recovery of the ischemic myocardium following infarction. This is one area where a therapeutic action of AM may hold promise. Additionally, AM exerts positive inotropic and chronotropic actions in the heart, effects that may be beneficial in patients in CHF. Finally, AM upregulates expression of the vasodilatory peptide ANP in the heart, while downregulating ET expression in the vasculature.

The AM gene is expressed abundantly in kidney, where the peptide exerts numerous effects. It exerts direct natriuretic and diuretic actions (prostacyclin mediated) in renal tubule and is an important determinant of renal perfusion pressure. Even when administered intravenously, AM maintains renal blood flow in the face of profound decreases in mean arterial pressure. AM accomplishes this paradox by exerting a vasodilatory effect (NO dependent) on the afferent arteriole, thus maintaining glomerular filtration and urine flow. Although in pharmacologic studies the threshold dose in humans for the renal effects exceeded that required to observe the cardiovascular actions, it is unlikely that circulating AM explains the observed in vitro or in vivo actions of AM. Locally produced peptide instead appears to act in an autocrine/paracrine fashion to control sodium and water handling by the tubule and perhaps even glomerular filtration. The same pharmacologic administration of AM in patients displaying already high levels of plasma AM (renal failure) did improve renal function in one study, and it appears that administration of exogenous AM can improve survival in septic crisis (a hypotensive state in which endogenous AM levels are already elevated).

The AM gene is highly expressed in the CNS, and significant effects of the peptide in brain have been demonstrated, many related to the regulation of fluid and electrolyte homeostasis. The natriuretic and diuretic actions of AM in kidney appear to be mirrored by CNS effects to inhibit thirst and sodium appetite. Both of these CNS actions have been demonstrated to be physiologically relevant. AM also acts in brain to stimulate sympathetic tone and to stimulate the release of vasopressin and oxytocin. Although the actions to elevate peripheral blood pressure and circulating levels of AVP may seem counter to the peptide's renal and vascular effects (natriurestis, diuresis, and vasodilation), they may reflect brain actions that are cardioprotective in nature, just as those exerted by AM in the heart may have evolved to protect against cardiovascular collapse.

Other actions of AM include a stimulatory effect on progesterone secretion and a quiescent effect in uterus. The fact that the knockout of the AM gene resulted in embryonic death at approx d 14 of mouse gestation points to significant effects of the peptide during embryogeneis as well. Indeed, the cause of embryo demise appeared to be a constriction of the umbilical arteries and veins. The knockout also provided insight into the physiologic relevance of another pharmacologic effect of AM. Heterozygote (one gene copy) animals develop a late-onset diabetic phenotype, suggesting that the ability of AM to inhibit insulin secretion has physiologic relevance.

4.5. Pathophysiology of AM

The multiple pharmacologic effects of AM have predicted that the peptide or its analogs would be beneficial in a variety of disease states. The ability of AM to inhibit Ang II–mediated cardiomyocyte hypertrophy and fibroblast proliferation predicted a role for the peptide in protection against hypertension-induced ventricular hypertrophy and interstitial fibrosis of the heart. In addition, AM exerts antimigratory and antiproliferative effects in VSMCs, promising a possible role in the prevention of atherosclerosis and angiogenesis. This is supported by observations in heterozygote knockout animals in which perivascular fibrosis and intimal hyperplasia were exaggerated compared with wild-type controls following salt loading or chronic administration of Ang II. The protective effect of AM is also supported by results from transgenic mice in which overexpression of AM has been engineered. Much less interstitial fibrosis and a milder form of hypertrophy were observed in these animals compared with controls in several models of hypertension. In experimental animals, overexpression of AM reduces the magnitude of arterial thickening and promotes reendothelialization following balloon angioplasty. In one study, administration of AM immediately following myocardial infarction enhanced ejection fraction and improved coronary sinus blood flow. Thus, administration of AM may provide both acute and chronic benefit in this patient population.

Plasma AM levels are elevated in CHF. Because of the peptide's vasodilatory and renotropic effects, it was thought that exogenous administration might provide some benefit in these patients. Initial results were disappointing. Increases in forearm blood flow to iv administration of AM were attenuated in CHF patients compared with control subjects, as were the blood pressure–lowering effects. Later it was determined that the failure of AM in these models was owing to an impairment in NO generation in these patients. However, more promising were the observations that administration of AM decreased pulmonary capillary wedge pressure as well as pulmonary arterial pressure in patients with CHF. Furthermore, AM infusion increased heart rate, stroke volume, ejection fraction, and cardiac index in patients with CHF and in another study increased urine volume and sodium excretion. These were short-term infusion protocols; longer-term clinical studies are needed. However, chronic infusion studies in experimental animals have demonstrated the ability of AM to reduce renin levels in models of renovascular hypertension and to decrease renal injury in hypertensive animals. Similarly, animal models have demonstrated that administration of AM improves blood pressure in spontaneously hypertensive (SHR) rats, exerting a more profound effect in those animals than in their normotensive (Wistar-Kyoto) control counterparts. This should not be surprising because the vasodilatory effect of AM is more pronounced in preconstricted vessels. In one clinical trial in patients with essential hypertension, administration of AM reduced both systolic and diastolic blood pressure and also reduced total peripheral resistance.

Therapeutically, AM is already being employed for the treatment of septic crisis. It had been observed that plasma AM levels correlate positively with the severity of sepsis, which initially suggested that AM was the causative agent for the observed hypotension, since proinflammatory cytokines stimulate AM production and release. However, it was subsequently reported that there was also a direct, positive correlation between absolute levels of plasma AM and survival, in that patients with highest AM levels in circulation had a greater chance of surviving the septic event. This was observed to be owing to a preservation of renal function in the high AM group, mirroring the ability of exogenous AM to maintain renal perfusion even in the face of profound hypotension.

5. CARDIOVASCULAR HORMONES AS DIAGNOSTIC AND THERAPEUTIC TOOLS

The three families of cardiovascular hormones discussed in this chapter have proven to be potent regulators of cardiovascular and renal function. Acting as either true endocrine or autocrine/paracrine hormones, they exert a wide variety of physiologically and pathologically relevant actions. Although the effects of the ETs are predominantly pathologic in nature, this still provides promise for the use of antagonists to block those deleterious actions in a variety of disease states characterized by overproduction or secretion of the peptides. Results from the initial trials with these antagonists are discussed above. More promising are the beneficial effects of long-term administration of the natriuretic peptides or AM because their actions in general appear organ specific and protective. In addition, pathologic secretion of these two classes of peptides may reflect the recruitment of compensatory mechanisms within the body that can hallmark the onset of disease and therefore provide diagnostic advantage. Just as important are the basic biomedical lessons learned from the discovery and characterization of the actions of these peptide hormones. Emerging now is an integrated view of how these hormones can coordinate endocrine, cardiovascular, and renal mechanisms that protect against postischemia proliferative disease and tissue damage caused by volume over- or underload. The roles played by these peptides in inflammatory disease are now being recognized and their importance in normal glucose metabolism and bone health is better understood.

In summary, the roles played by these potent cardiovascular hormones in the maintenance of cardiovascular function and fluid and electrolyte homeostasis have taught investigators a great deal about integrative, systems biology. These peptides promise to open new avenues into cellular and molecular control mechanisms underlying other normal and pathologic systems as well.

SELECTED READINGS

Ando K, Fujita T. Lessons from the adrenomedullin knockout mouse. *Regul Pept* 2003;112:185–188.

Charles CJ, Lainchbury JG, Nicholls MG, Rademaker MT, Richards AM, Troughton RW. Adrenomedullin and the renin-angiotensin-aldosterone system. *Regul Pept* 2003;112:41–49.

Costello-Borrigter LC, Boerrigter G, Burnett JC. Revisting salt and water retention: new diuretics, aquaretics, and natriuretics. *Med Clin North Am* 2003;87:475–491.

Eto T, Kato J, Kitamura K. Regulation of production and secretion of adrenomedullin in the cardiovascular system. *Regul Pept* 2003;112:61–69.

Moreau P, Schiffrin EL. Role of endothelins in animal models of hypertension: focus on cardiovascular protection. *Can J Physiol Pharmacol* 2003;81:511–521.

Rich S, McLaughlin VV. Endothelin receptor blockers in cardiovascular disease. *Circulation* 2003;108:2184–2190.

Stoupakis G, Klapholz M. Natriuretic peptides: biochemistry, physiology, and therapeutic role in heart failure. *Heart Dis* 2003;5:215–223.

Taylor MM, Samson WK. Adrenomedullin and the integrative physiology of fluid and electrolyte balance. *Microsc Res Tech* 2002;57:105–109.

Taylor MM, Shimosawa T, Samson WK. Endocrine and metabolic actions of adrenomedullin. *The Endocrinologist* 2001;11:171–177.

22 Adrenal Medulla (Catecholamines and Peptides)

William J. Raum, MD, PhD

CONTENTS

1. DEVELOPMENTAL ORIGIN

Some primitive autonomic ganglia transform into neurons, some into satellite and neurolemma cells associated with neurons, and others become distinct endocrine elements. The latter stain brown with chrome salts and are thus designated chromaffin cells. This reaction is due to the presence of the hormone epinephrine contained within the cells. The chromaffin system consists of various aggregates of these cells throughout the body. The adrenal medulla is the most prominent member of the group.

Paraganglia, aptly named, consist of chromaffin cells that collect in close approximation to autonomic ganglia and plexuses. They begin to form at about 2 mo of gestation and attain a diameter of about 1 mm by birth.

Chromaffin bodies are chromaffin masses that arise along the course of the aorta. Chromaffin cells are intermingled with strands of connective tissue and are enclosed in a connective-tissue capsule. They develop first at the root of the inferior mesenteric artery at about 2 mo of gestation. At birth they are about 1 cm in diameter. The largest complex in the abdomen, the organ of Zuckerkandl, occurs near the bifurcation of the aorta into the iliac arteries. After birth chromaffin bodies begin to decline in size and nearly disappear by puberty.

Carotid bodies begin as a mesodermal condensation on the wall of each internal carotid in the seventh week. Chromaffin cells and nonchromaffin autonomic ganglion cells invade and branches of the glossopharyngeal nerve innervate the bodies. When mature, the organ functions in the reflex regulation of blood pressure.

The adrenal gland is actually two distinct glands combined in a common capsule. The cortex is derived from mesoderm and secretes steroid hormones. The medulla is derived from ectodermal chromaffin tissue and secretes catecholamines. In lower animals, such as fish, the cortex and medulla present as separate organs. During the seventh week of gestation, chromaffin cells from the celiac plexus collect on the medial side of the already prominent primordial cortex and migrate inward. By the fourth month, the chromaffin tissue occupies a central position in the gland. The tissue becomes organized into cords and masses permeated with a profuse network of sinusoidal capillaries.

The link between the autonomic nervous system and the adrenal medulla is both embryologic and functional. The adrenal medulla functions much like the postganglionic sympathetic neuron, but the neurotransmitter (epinephrine) is released into the blood stream, rather than the synaptic junction. The receptors and effector cells are located throughout the body, rather than just across the synapse. An appreciation of their similarities

From: *Endocrinology: Basic and Clinical Principles, Second Edition*
(S. Melmed and P. M. Conn, eds.) © Humana Press Inc., Totowa, NJ

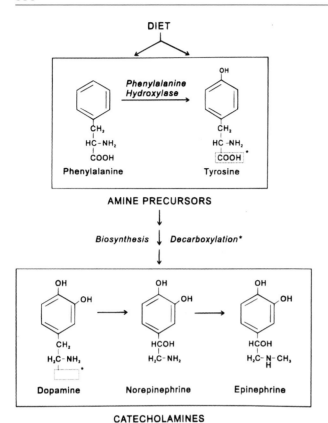

Fig. 1. APUD is a feature characteristic of endocrine and neuroendocrine tissues. The amino acids phenylalanine and tyrosine are the amine precursors that are decarboxylated and subsequently become catecholamines in sympathetic neurons and chromaffin tissue. Both amino acids are derived from the diet, but tyrosine may also be synthesized from phenylalanine in the liver.

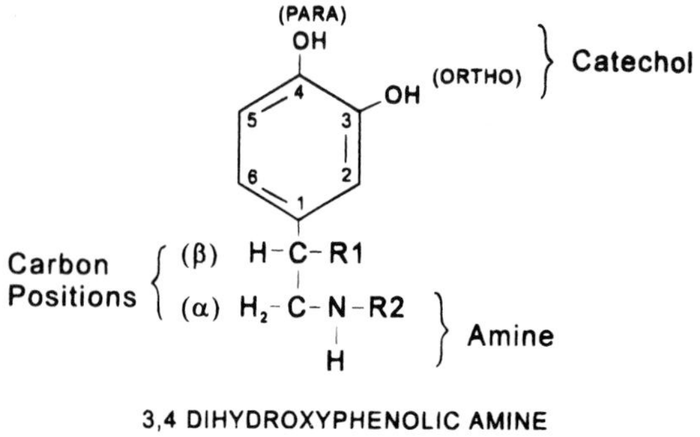

Fig. 2. Structure of catecholamine. The catecholamines are 3,4-dihydroxyphenolic amines. The benzene ring structure numbering is counterclockwise with carbon 1 being bonded to the aliphatic side chain. The catechol group consists of two adjacent hydroxyl groups: one at position 4, or *para* with respect to position 1; and the second at position 3, or *ortho* with respect to the hydroxyl at position 4. The aliphatic side-chain carbon atoms are labeled β and α. As illustrated, the substitutions on these carbons define each of the three most prominent catecholamines.

and differences aids in understanding how one influences the other in both normal and pathophysiologic processes.

2. CATECHOLAMINES

The principal catecholamines found in the body—norepinephrine, epinephrine, and dopamine—are formed by hydroxylation and decarboxylation of the amino acids phenylalanine and tyrosine (Fig. 1). The process of amine precursor uptake and decarboxylation (APUD) is a feature common to a variety of endocrine and neuroendocrine tissues that are embryologically related and secrete polypeptide hormones, hormone precursors, and catecholamines. All three of these catecholamines act as neurotransmitters in the central nervous system (CNS). Norepinephrine also functions as a neurotransmitter in the sympathetic nervous system. Although there are dopamine receptors outside the CNS, the role of dopamine as a hormone or neurotransmitter

peripherally is not fully described. Epinephrine is the circulating hormone secreted by the adrenal medulla and influences processes throughout the body.

2.1. Biosynthesis of Catecholamine

Catecholamines are 3,4-dihydroxylated phenolic amines (Fig. 2). The most prevalent of these are dopamine, norepinephrine and epinephrine. Biosynthesis (Fig. 3) begins with tyrosine, which consists of a benzene ring hydroxylated in the 4 (*para*) position to the two-carbon side chain at the 1 position. The β-carbon, closest to the ring, is saturated with hydrogen and is single bonded to the α-carbon. The α-carbon is bonded to the amino and carboxylic acid groups that define the amino acids. The rate-limiting enzyme, tyrosine hydroxylase, 3-hydroxylates (*ortho* with respect to the 4-position hydroxyl) tyrosine to dihydroxyphenylalanine (DOPA). The α-carbon is decarboxylated by aromatic L-amino acid decarboxylase to form the first catecholamine, dopamine (L-dihydroxy phenylethylamine). Hydroxylation of the β-carbon of dopamine (by dopamine β-hydroxylase) results in the formation of norepinephrine. Dopamine β-hydroxylase requires vita-

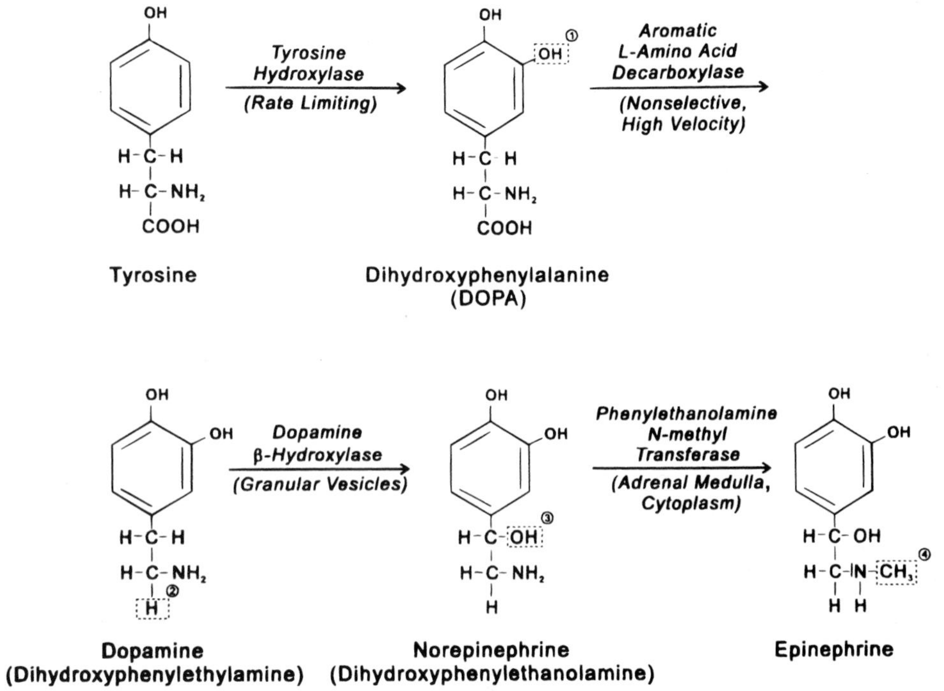

Fig. 3. Biosynthesis of catecholamine. Tyrosine hydroxylase catalyzes the (1) *para*-hydroxylation of tyrosine to form dihydroxy-phenylalanine (DOPA) and is the rate-limiting step in the biosynthesis of catecholamines. The other major steps include (2) decarboxylation of DOPA, (3) β-hydroxylation of dopamine, and (4) *N*-methylation of norepinephrine to form epinephrine.

min C (ascorbic acid) as a cofactor. Norepinephrine can be converted into epinephrine by methylation of the amino group on the α-carbon by phenylethanolamine-*N*-methyltransferase (PNMT).

Tyrosine hydroxylase activity is the rate-limiting step in catecholamine synthesis. Control is achieved through several mechanisms that maintain the synthesis rate of catecholamines proportional to their release. The reaction requires tyrosine (substrate), oxygen, and a reduced pteridine cofactor. Norepinephrine exerts negative feedback with a sensitivity that is inversely proportional to the level of pteridine cofactor. The usual rate of catecholamine production is, therefore, influenced by three factors. First is the intraneuronal (or intracellular) transport of tyrosine, which may be altered by certain drugs that inhibit active transport; other amino acids that compete for the transport system; or other amino acids that act as competitive inhibitors, such as α-methylpara-tyrosine. Second is the activity of dihydropteridine reductase and subsequent concentration of reduced pteridine cofactor. Third is the cytoplasmic concentration of norepinephrine. A high intracellular concentration of norepinephrine is attained by transport of catecholamines out of the cytoplasm, away from tyrosine hydroxylase, and into storage vesicles. In response to a stimulus, catecholamines are released from storage vesicles, not from

activation of tyrosine hydroxylase and *de novo* synthesis. However, as stores are replaced and cytoplasmic norepinephrine is depleted, feedback inhibition of tyrosine hydroxylase is removed. The released norepinephrine binds to a synaptic membrane receptor linked to cyclic adenosine monophasphate (cAMP), which activates a protein kinase that phosphorlyates and activates tyrosine hydroxylase. Gene activation of tyrosine hydroxylase occurs after prolonged stimulation (hours). It has been reported that both cholinergic ganglionic stimulation of sympathetic nerves or the adrenal medulla, and intracellular depletion of catecholamines by reserpine, result in an increase in tyrosine hydroxylase gene transcription rate. Four types of tyrosine hydroxylase mRNAs have been described, produced by a single gene. The multiple forms may provide an additional level of regulation of the enzyme through differential phosphorylation and activation of each subtype. Glucocorticoids and cAMP also stimulate transcription, and cAMP may also stabilize mRNA and prolong its activity.

Aromatic L-amino acid decarboxylase is found in many tissues and defines them as part of the APUD (decarboxylation) system, as above. This enzyme is found in high concentrations and requires a cofactor, pyridoxal 5-phosphate. The affinity for its substrate,

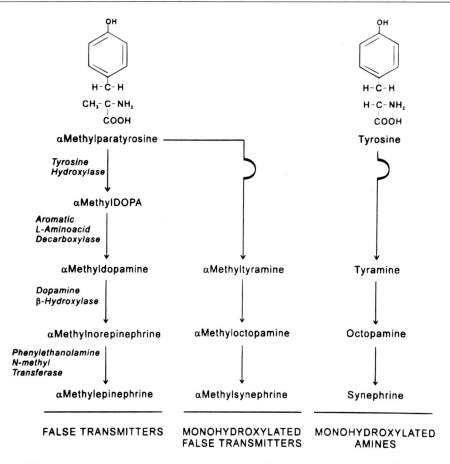

Fig. 4. Synthesis of false transmitters and monohydroxylated amines. Because of the lack of specificity, a host of other compounds can be produced by the enzymes involved in catecholamine synthesis. α-Methylparatyrosine, a competitive inhibitor of tyrosine hydroxylase, may be administered to patients with pheochromocytoma to treat excess secretion of catecholamine. As a result of interaction with tyrosine hydroxylase, the less biologically active α-methyl derivatives or false transmitters are synthesized instead of the normal, active compounds. Both naturally occurring monohydroxylated amines and α-methyl derivatives are produced when the initial reaction with tyrosine hydroxylase is bypassed.

DOPA, is very high, as is its capacity (maximum velocity). It is relatively nonselective but even potent inhibitors (α-methyldopa) have little effect on the synthesis rate of catecholamines.

Dopamine β-hydroxylase is a copper-containing oxidase that requires ascorbic acid and oxygen to hydroxylate dopamine to norepinephrine. The enzyme in both soluble and insoluble forms is found within granular storage vesicles. The granule consists of adenosine triphosphate (ATP), chromogranin A (a macromolecule), dopamine β-hydroxylase, norepinephrine, or epinephrine. Dopamine must be actively transported into the vesicle to be converted into norepinephrine. The transport process requires ATP and is inhibited by reserpine. Stimulation results in fusion of the vesicular membrane with the plasma membrane and release of the entire contents. Thus, dopamine β-hydroxylase, chromogranin A, and catecholamine plasma levels increase with sympathetic stimulation. Exocytosis results from calcium ion (Ca^{2+}) entry at the plasma membrane via nicotinic or voltage-activated channels. The rise in cytosolic Ca^{2+} leads to a reorganization of the cortical actin network and triggers access of the granule to its exocytotic sites. Calpactin, the Ca^{2+}- and phospholipid-dependent annexin protein, has been strongly implicated in the interaction of the granule with the plasma membrane. Calcium channel–blocking agents such as nifedipine and verapamil inhibit catecholamine secretion. Because the enzyme is lost when excreted with the granule, it must be synthesized and replaced in response to the release of catecholamines. There is little substrate specificity despite its name. Many phenylethylamines (Fig. 4) can be hydroxylated, including the monohydroxylated amine tyramine (from the decarboxylation of tyrosine), forming octopamine; α-methylparatyramine (from the decarboxylation of α-methylparatyrosine), forming α-methyloctopamine; and α-methyl dopamine (from the decarboxylation of α-methyl dopa), forming α-methyl norepinephrine. The lack of substrate specificity by aromatic L-amino decarboxylase and dopamine β-hydroxylase can be utilized to ameliorate high catecholamine states by virtue of two effects. One effect involves competitive inhibition decreasing the rate of production of the biologically active catecholamines, and the other involves the storage and release of false neurotransmitters. This latter effect is based on the fact that the α-methyl derivatives just described can displace norepinephrine from sites within the storage vesicles and be released in place of norepinephrine. For the most part, these derivatives have significantly less biologic activity than the catecholamines that they replace.

PNMT is found in the adrenal medulla and chromaffin cells near the adrenal cortex. Although some PNMT activity can be found in a few brain cells, the marked prevalence of enzyme activity in close proximity to the adrenal cortex is owing to the effects of glucocorticoids. It is not clear how glucocorticoids regulate enzyme activity, but it is known that the mechanism does not involve gene activation. It has been speculated that glucocorticoids may regulate a cosubstrate or act to stabilize the enzyme. Whatever the mechanism, it also does not involve the classic (type II) glucocorticoid receptor. Although norepinephrine is the preferred substrate, enzyme is aptly named because it is nonselective and will N-methylate any phenylethanolamine including octopamine, α-methyloctopamine, α-methylnorepinephrine, and structurally related compounds (*see* Fig. 4). PNMT requires *S*-adenosylmethionine for a methyl-group donor, oxygen, and magnesium. Noncompetitive inhibition by its product, epinephrine, is its most potent immediate regulator of activity. Cholinergic stimulation will cause PNMT gene activation in the adrenal medulla. Although angiotensin and imidazolines (clonidine, cimetidine) have been shown to increase PNMT mRNA in adrenal medullary chromaffin cells, the physiologic implications of this effect are unclear at this time.

2.2. Catecholamine Catabolism

There are two primary pathways for the degradation of catecholamines (Fig. 5); one is near the site where catecholamines are synthesized and stored (chromaffin cells and sympathetic neurons), and the second deactivates primarily circulating catecholamines. Monoamine oxidase (MAO) catalyzes the first and catechol-*O*-methyltransferase (COMT), the second. MAO, a mitochrondrial enzyme, cleaves off the terminal aliphatic

amine and oxidizes the α-carbon to carboxylic acid. The product, 3,4-dihydroxymandelic acid, is the same for epinephrine and norepinephrine because the N-methyl group that distinguishes the two is removed. COMT using the methyl-group donor S-adenosylmethionine methylates the 3-hydroxy group, producing metanephrine and normetanephrine, respectively, from epinephrine and norepinephrine. O-Methylation of 3,4-dihydroxymandelic acid by COMT or oxidative deamination of the metanephrines by MAO produces vanillylmandelic acid (VMA). Most of the substrates and products of these reactions may be conjugated to sulfate (primarily) or glucuronide, which reduces further metabolism and enhances excretion.

2.3. Physiology of Adrenal Medullary Catecholamine

2.3.1. Biosynthesis and Release

Most of the catecholamine synthetic steps up to norepinephrine are not significantly different in the adrenal medulla compared to sympathetic nerves (Fig. 6). Biosynthesis begins with tyrosine, which can be obtained from the diet, or synthesized from phenylalanine by phenylalanine hydroxylase, which is found in the liver. Tyrosine is actively transported from the bloodstream into the adrenal. Tyrosine is converted into 3,4-dihydroxyphenylanine (DOPA) by the rate-limiting, mitochrondrial enzyme tyrosine hydroxylase. Feedback inhibition is exerted by norepinephrine. Decarboxylation of DOPA to dopamine is catalyzed by the cytosolic enzyme aromatic L-amino acid decarboxylase. Dopamine must then be actively transported into granulated vesicles that contain dopamine β-hydroxylase to be converted into norepinephrine. For most chromaffin tissue and neurons, the synthesis ends with norepinephrine binding to the granule, which is made up of dopamine β-hydroxylase; a macromolecule; chromogranin A; and ATP. In the noradrenergic neuron, this granule containing norepinephine is secreted into the synapse during depolarization. As with other chromaffin tissue, the adrenal medulla stores and releases norepinephrine in granules; however, the adrenal medulla is the body's primary source of epinephrine and the cytosolic enzyme PNMT, which produces epinephrine from norepinephrine. Because PNMT activity is so dependent on glucocorticoids (cortisol in humans), it is also dependent on pituitary adrenocorticotropic hormone (ACTH) and the rest of the hypothalamic-pituitary-adrenal cortical axis. ACTH also has a tropic effect on adrenal medullary tyrosine hydroxylase activity. For the enzymatic reaction to occur, norepinephrine must be released from its storage granule, combine with PNMT in the cytoplasm to produce epinephrine, and then be transported

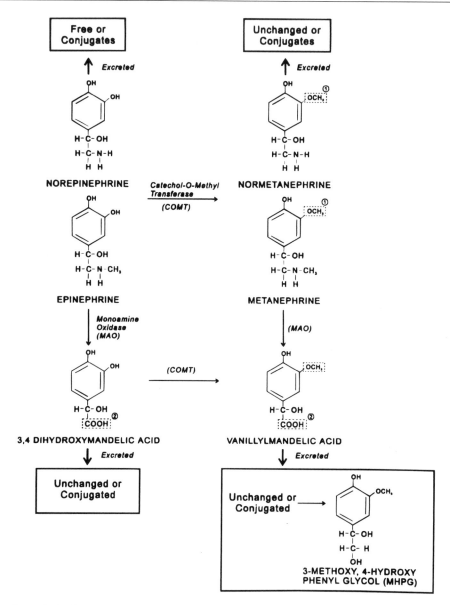

Fig. 5. Catabolism of catecholamines. Regardless of the first step, (1) methylation of the 3-position hydroxyl group, or (2) oxidative deamination, the end product of the sum of the reactions is VMA, which is excreted in the urine or may be further reduced to be excreted as 3-methoxy, 4-hydroxyphenylglycol. Epinephrine and norepinephrine may be excreted in the free form (the source of urinary total catecholamines) or be converted into metanephrine and normetanephrine (the source of urinary metanephrines), respectively, by COMT. Interaction of the catecholamines or metanephrines with (2) MAO results in deamination and, therefore, eliminates any further ability to differentiate the contribution of epinephrine or norepinephrine to the product.

back into another granule. The storage granules in the adrenal medulla contain epinephrine or norepinephrine and the release can be selective. That is, epinephrine can be released independently from norepinephrine, but how this is accomplished is not known. Approximately 80% of the catecholamine output from the adrenal medulla is epinephrine under the usual physiologic circumstances.

2.3.2. Physiologic Function

Although derived from neural tissue, which characteristically induces a discrete sympathetic response in one organ, the adrenal medulla's function is to produce a similar sympathetic response in all organs at approximately the same time. Epinephrine, secreted by the adrenal medulla, is the hormonal equivalent of the sympathetic neuron's neurotransmitter, norepinephrine.

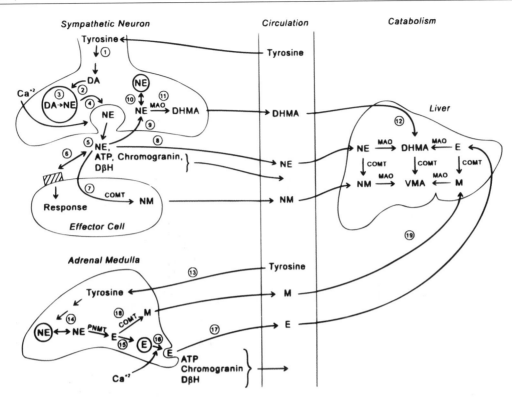

Fig. 6. Comparison of biosynthesis, release, and catabolism of catecholamines in sympathetic neuron and adrenal medulla. (1) Tyrosine is converted into dopamine (DA), which is (2) actively transported into storage granules to be (3) converted into norepinephrine (NE). During depolarization, calcium (Ca^{+2}) moves into the neuron; (4) exocytosis occurs; and (5) NE is released into the synapse along with ATP, chromogranin, and dopamine β-hydroxylase (DβH). NE may then (6) bind to a receptor to produce a response, be internalized (7) and metabolized by COMT to normetanephrine (NM), (8) leak out of the synapse to reach the bloodstream, or (9) be taken up into the neuron to be transported back into (10) a storage granule or metabolized (11) to dihydroxymandelic acid (DHMA). NE, NM, and DHMA can be transported by the circulation to the liver and (12) metabolized to VMA. Tyrosine (13) is taken up by the adrenal medulla and converted into NE, which is then released back into the cytoplasm (14) to be converted into epinephrine (E) by PNMT. E can then be taken up by storage granules (15) and released (16) by exocytosis into the bloodstream (17) along with ATP, chromogranin, and DβH. E can then be transported to distant receptors to produce a hormonal response or be transported (19) to the liver along with M to be metabolized to VMA.

Epinephrine provides a rapid physiologic response to cold, fatigue, shock, hypoglycemia, and other emergencies.

2.4. Mechanism of Action

2.4.1. TYPE AND DISTRIBUTION OF ADRENERGIC RECEPTORS

Catecholamines exert their effects through receptors located on the target organ's cell membrane. Table 1 presents representative listing of the receptors and their responses. There are two main groupings of receptors, α and β. Each of these is divided into two or perhaps three subgroups labeled α_1, α_2, β_1, and so on. Classification of the receptor types is determined by examining the effect of a defined concentration (dose-response) curve of a series of pharmacologic derivatives of the catecholamines (agonists and antagonists) on certain

tissue response systems that act as the standards with which the unclassified drug or tissue response is compared. β_2-Receptors are predominantly found in smooth muscle and glandular cells, and β_1-receptors are most prevalent in the myocardium; however, some tissues possess both types in different proportions. β_1-Receptors or α_1-receptors predominate at postsynaptic sites and convey the primary neuronal signal to the effector cell. α_2-Receptors are located at presynaptic nerve terminal sites and mediate feedback inhibition of neuronally released norepinephrine. Although certain generalizations can be made about the effect and relative potencies of various sympathomimetic amines on certain receptor subtypes, there are usually several exceptions to each generalization. The physiologic state of the tissue, the relative ratio of one receptor type compared with another, aging, temperature, and the pres-

**Table 1
Responses Mediated by α-Adrenergic
and β-Adrenergic Receptor Stimulation**

Tissue or organ response	Type of Receptor
Cardiac	
• Increase in rate (chronotropy)	β
• Increase in contractility (inotropy)	β
• Increase in A-V node conduction	β
Vascular	
• Constriction (arteries and veins)	α
• Dilatation (only arteries)	β
Pulmonary	
• Dilatation of bronchial smooth muscle	β
Liver	
• Gluconeogenesis, glycogenolysis	β
Pancreas	
• Exocrine	
⬧ Decrease in secretion)	α
• Endocrine (insulin, glucagon)	
⬧ Inhibition of secretion	α
⬧ Stimulation of secretion	β
Fat cells	
• Increase in lipolysis (increases free fatty acids)	β
Salivary glands	
• Increase in amylase secretion	β

ence or absence of other seemingly unrelated drugs or hormones can alter adrenergic responses. Many drugs may not even act directly on an adrenergic receptor but cause an increase or decrease in catecholamine levels, or release of endogenous catecholamines that will influence receptor responses. The number of active receptors may decrease during agonist stimulation, resulting in a progressively less maximal response to progressively higher levels of stimulation, termed *downregulation* or *tachyphylaxis*. Exhaustion of a second messenger such as cAMP or its intermediates may result in loss of a response.

2.4.2. Receptor Characteristics: Differential Effects of Epinephrine and Norepinephrine

The physiologic response to epinephrine or norepinephrine is dependent on the relative sensitivity of the receptor to that catecholamine, and the range of physiologic concentrations that can be attained at the receptor site. For example, epinephrine and norepinephrine both stimulate β_1-receptors in the heart and increase heart rate and contractility. Epinephrine can elicit these effects at 1 to 2 nM, which is equivalent to the normal concentration of epinephrine in the blood. By contrast, >20 nM norepinephrine is required to obtain a response from β_1-receptors, which is four- to

fivefold higher than normal plasma levels. Only certain pathologic conditions generate circulating norepinephrine to a level that will stimulate cardiac β_1-receptors. On the other hand, sympathetic noradrenergic neurons innervating the myocardium will readily produce intrasynaptic concentrations exceeding the threshold needed to elicit a β_1-receptor response. Both epinephrine and norepinephrine are secreted by the adrenal medulla, but only epinephrine conveys the biologic response to stimulation. The adrenal medulla produces virtually all of the circulating epinephrine and practically none of the circulating norepinephrine. Plasma norepinephrine is primarily derived from a "leak" of norepinephrine from sympathetic neurons and their synaptic discharges.

The principal effects of epinephrine are to vasodilate arterioles in skeletal muscle and vasoconstrict arterioles in the skin; stimulate the rate and force of myocardial contractions; cause the relaxation of the smooth muscles of the gut, lungs, and urinary bladder, and contraction of the sphincters; stimulate the breakdown of glycogen and inhibit insulin to elevate blood sugar; and stimulate lipolysis to elevate fatty acids and glycerol. The latter two effects provide fuel for muscle action (fatty acids) and glucose for the CNS. Most of these effects are mediated by β-receptors cAMP.

2.5. Pathophysiology

2.5.1. Adrenal Medullary Insufficiency

Adrenal medullary insufficiency is associated with no known diseases. After bilateral adrenalectomy, urinary epinephrine secretion falls, but <10% of norepinephrine and its metabolites is lost and this has no significant physiologic impact. The contribution of the adrenal medulla to circulating norepinephrine is insignificant compared to the sympathetic nervous system because most adrenergic receptors, the mediators of secreted norepinephrine, are associated with synapses. The synaptic concentration of norepinephrine during a stimulus is several orders of magnitude above that in the circulation. It is the leak of norepinephrine from the neurons and synapses that is the major contributor to plasma norepinephrine levels. This source of norepinephrine is the result of adrenergic stimulation and not the cause.

2.5.2. Intra- and Extraadrenal Hyperfunction

Conditions are generally pathologic where circulating levels of norepinephrine are higher than synaptic concentrations. Under these circumstances, circulating levels of norepinephrine are high enough to elicit symptoms of increased sympathetic stimulation. Tumors of chromaffin tissues can produce clinically important syndromes and lead to life-threatening clinical disease.

Pheochromocytoma is the term applied to catecholamine-secreting tumors of the adrenal medulla. *Paraganglioma* is the term that has been used to describe catecholamine-secreting tumors that arise in extra-adrenal chromaffin tissue such as paraganglia, chromaffin bodies, and carotid bodies. It would be preferable to designate all catecholamine-secreting tumors as pheochromocytoma and qualify the description with the anatomic location. There is no advantage to using separate terms because the pathophysiology and treatment of excess catecholamine secretion are changed little by whether the source of the catecholamines is intra- or extraadrenal.

2.5.3. PHEOCHROMOCYTOMA

Catecholamine-secreting tumors of chromaffin tissue, pheochromocytomas, are a rare cause of a common disease, hypertension. Less than 0.1% of the hypertensive population have pheochromocytoma. Finding this "needle in a haystack" has several important clinical aspects. The hypertension caused by pheochromocytoma is usually curable, whereas essential hypertension ordinarily can only be controlled. Administration of the wrong antihypertensive or surgery on a patient with unrecognized pheochromocytoma can be fatal. These tumors may be associated with other potentially fatal but curable diseases. Pheochromocytoma may mimic other diseases such as diabetes mellitus, thyrotoxicosis, severe anxiety, coronary artery disease, or carcinoid syndrome. The high incidence of pheochromocytoma in families as a primary disease in association with multiple endocrine neoplasia (MEN) or in association with other familial diseases indicates the need for genetic counseling in these families. Finally, there is a rational and specific approach to diagnosis and treatment.

2.5.3.1. Pathophysiology. Pheochromocytoma occurs 80% of the time as a benign tumor in one of the adrenal glands. Twenty percent are extraadrenal, with half (10%) below the diaphragm in areas such as along the aorta, near the urinary bladder, and in the organ of Zuckerkandl and the other half above the diaphragm in areas along the aorta, in the lungs or heart, or in the neck or carotid bodies. Ten percent occur in children. In nonfamilial disease, 10% of patients have bilateral adrenal tumors and 10% have multiple extraadrenal tumors, but in familial disease, >80% are bilateral or multiple sites. Malignant pheochromocytoma occurs in 10% of patients and is three times more likely to be malignant. Pheochromocytoma is evenly distributed between the sexes and can occur at any age, although the incidence peaks between the fourth and sixth decades.

Catecholamines are mostly responsible for the signs and symptoms of pheochromocytoma. It is unusual that a tumor will grow large enough or be so invasive as to interfere with the function of surrounding organs such as the liver, kidneys or spinal cord. The manifestations of pheochromocytoma are primarily the result of the excessive secretion of norepinephrine, epinephrine, and dopamine. The most common mix is predominately norepinephrine with epinephrine. Some tumors secrete only norepinephrine, but <10% secrete only epinephrine. Dopamine and its metabolite, HVA, derived from the combined activities of MAO and COMT, have not been measured in the routine laboratory examination of pheochromocytoma. When dopamine levels have been reported, they rarely exceed the concentration of norepinephrine. Dopamine and HVA are more likely to be significantly elevated in children with pheochromocytoma or in malignancy.

The reasons for increased production and secretion of catecholamines are not clear. Abnormally high turnover rates have been noted in small tumors, but the granules and storage mechanisms appeared normal, leading to the logical but as yet unproven conclusion that there is a defect in the systems regulating synthesis and release. Perhaps the negative feedback mechanism of norepinephrine on tyrosine hydroxylase is altered so that sensitivity to feedback is decreased, or metabolism or release is so rapid that feedback does not occur. One animal study has shown that increased cell contact in pheochromocytoma increases tyrosine hydroxylase transcription rate, leading to higher concentrations of the enzyme. Secretion can occur in tumors at a relatively constant high rate, as bursts in between periods of normal secretion, or as a combination of the two. Small tumors tend to secrete high levels of free catecholamines. With more intracellular metabolism occurring in large tumors, high levels of metabolites tend to be released and free catecholamine secretion is reduced.

Some patients are more symptomatic than others. Approximately 50% of patients with pheochromocytoma have sustained hypertension, 45% are normotensive with paroxysms of hypertension, and only 5% are normotensive or even hypotensive. Part of the reason for these differences relates to the patterns of catecholamine secretion. Bursts produce hypertensive episodes. Patients with sustained hypertension and some normotensive patients can have high or normal levels of norepinephrine. How high sustained levels of norepinephrine result in sustained hypertension is not readily understood. However, if an elevated secretion rate persists, α- and β-receptors may become desensitized or downregulated. Hemodynamic mechanisms will no longer respond to the elevated levels of norepinephrine and blood pressure will be normalized. Consequently, for two patients with the same plasma

Table 2
Frequency of Symptoms of Pheochromocytoma

Frequency >50%	*Frequency <50% and >25%*	*Frequency <25% and >10%*
Headache	Pallor	Weakness
Sweating	Nausea	Fatigue
Palpitations	Tremor	Dyspnea
	Anxiety	Weight loss
	Abdominal pain	Flushing
	Chest pain	

concentration of norepinephrine, one could be normotensive and the other hypertensive. Some investigators have reported this finding as indicating that there is no correlation between blood pressure and catecholamine levels. This has been interpreted by some to imply that catecholamines do not affect blood pressure in patients with pheochromocytoma, but this is not the case. The normotensive patient with elevated levels of norepinephrine is capable of responding to an additional burst of catecholamines with a hypertensive episode. Before catecholamines could be measured reliably, this was the observation and rationale for the stimulation tests. Catecholamine levels and blood pressure may not correlate well among patients, but within an individual, a significant change in catecholamine concentration will elicit a blood pressure response. Patients with rare, exclusively epinephrine-secreting tumors can present with normotension or hypotension owing to the predominantly vasodilating effects of epinephrine. Another cause of hypotension is orthostatic hypotension, resulting from the ganglionic blocking activity of excessive amounts of catecholamines that prevent the normal sympathetic response to upright posture.

The pathophysiology of pheochromocytoma has been described primarily in relation to the effects of the catecholamines on blood pressure, because of the ease and accuracy of blood pressure measurements, and the blood pressure's rapid response to changes in catecholamine levels. The excessive secretion of catecholamines has other important pathophysiologic consequences, which are examined in the subsequent sections.

2.5.3.2. Clinical Manifestations. Most symptoms of pheochromocytoma can be readily attributed to the pharmacologic effects of catecholamines. The most frequent symptoms associated with pheochromocytoma are headache, sweating, and palpitations. These symptoms combined with a hypertensive crisis strongly suggest pheochromocytoma and would indicate the need for a careful investigation. A majority of patients do present in this fashion, and these and other symptoms, provided

Table 3
Diseases Mimicked by Pheochromocytoma

- Anxiety states, psychoneuroses, panic attacks
- Carcinoid
- Diabetes mellitus
- Drug abuse (cocaine, amphetamines)
- Essential hypertension
- Hyperthyroidism
- Malignant hypertension
- Megacolon, chronic constipation
- Migraine and other vascular headaches
- Primary cardiac disease
  (coronary insufficiency, congestive cardiomyopathy)
- Toxemia of pregnancy

in Table 2, are usually paroxysmal even if the hypertension is persistent. Paroxysms usually last a few minutes and occur several times a day. However, there is a wide variation up to a duration of 1 wk and a frequency of once every 2 mo. The paroxysms can be precipitated by certain drugs, or by physical activity such as straining, lifting, or even micturition (provoking secretion from a tumor on or near the bladder), or they can be spontaneous.

Many patients present with more subtle signs and symptoms that mimic and can be confused with other diseases (*see* Table 3). Pheochromocytoma and these diseases may need to be differentiated from one another. Essential hypertension and malignant hypertension are obvious conditions that should be considered. Sweating, anxiety, palpitations, tachycardia, weight loss, tremor, and other signs of hypermetabolism can be caused by catecholamines or by hyperthyroidism. Many of these same symptoms also occur in anxiety states, psychoneuroses, and panic attacks, which tend to be the most frequent disorders attributed to pheochromocytoma. Catecholamines are toxic to the myocardium and may cause myocardial necrosis and myocarditis. The toxic effect, vasospasm, or excessive demands on a coronary system compromised by arteriosclerosis can produce a frank myocardial infarct, symptoms of coronary insufficiency, or congestive cardiomyopathy.

Headaches caused by pheochromocytoma are most often associated with rapid changes in catecholamine levels, not persistently elevated blood pressure, and could be confused with migraines or other vascular headaches. Catecholamines cause diabetes mellitus through an α-receptor inhibition of insulin release from the islets, β-receptor-mediated stimulation of gluconeogenesis and glucagon secretion, and insulin resistance. Once the tumor is removed and catecholamine levels fall, the normal regulatory mechanism driven by glucose returns, and carbohydrate intolerance is resolved. Gastrointestinal motility is inhibited by catecholamines and can produce severe constipation and or even mimic megacolon. Abuse of certain drugs, such as cocaine and amphetamines, duplicates all the characteristics of pheochromocytoma including highly elevated catecholamine measurements. No tumor is found, however, and the urinary toxicology screen is positive for the responsible drug. With an unreliable drug history, a drug-screening test should be performed. I am, however, aware of at least one young man who was abusing cocaine and also had a 4-cm adrenal pheochromocytoma.

Pheochromocytoma could be familial or sporadic. As a familial disease, it may be associated with a variety of other familial endocrine tumors, which are mostly all autosomal dominant. Table 4 presents these diseases. Identified families should be screened for pheochromocytoma. MEN type 2 (MEN 2), is characterized by the occurrence of pheochromocytoma, medullary carcinoma of the thyroid, and hyperparathyroidism in some combination in an individual or genetically related family members. MEN 3, includes the type 2 tumors plus mucosal neuromas (lips and tongue) and a marfinoid habitus. All family members should be screened for all three tumors (catecholamine, calcitonin, and calcium measurements). Affected members may have one or two but rarely all three tumors. Because the treatment for medullary carcinoma of the thyroid is surgery—thyroidectomy—all patients should be screened for pheochromocytoma before administering an anesthetic. If present, the pheochromocytoma is removed first. Because medullary carcinoma of the thyroid may be fatal beyond the *in situ* stage, all patients with pheochromocytoma should have at least a screening calcitonin measurement done. The screen for medullary carcinoma in affected families should be more stringent and include pentagastrin- or calcium-stimulated calcitonin tests.

Neurofibromatosis occurs in approx 5% of patients with pheochromocytoma, and pheochromocytoma occurs in approx 1% of patients with neurofibromatosis. Other neuroectodermal syndromes, Sturge-Weber and tuberous sclerosis, occur with increased incidence in

Table 4
Associated Familial Diseases

- MEN 2 and MEN 3
- Neurofibromatosis
- Sturge-Weber
- Tuberous sclerosis
- von Hipple-Lindau

Table 5
Conditions That Increase Catecholamine Secretion

Increase >5-fold	Increase > 2 fold
Acute myocardial infarction	Burns
Congestive heart failure	Depression
and pulmonary edema	Hypoxia
Diabetic ketoacidosis	Mental stress
Hypoglycemia	Shock (hemorrhagic, septic)
Pheochromocytoma	Stroke

Table 6
Drugs Reported to Increase Catecholamine Levels

Increase > 2 fold	Increase < 2 fold
Caffeine	Amphetamine
Clozepine	Hydralazine
Clonidine (abrupt withdrawal >3 fold)	Nitroglycerin
Cocaine	Propranolol
Hydrochlorthiazide	Nicotine
Insulin	
Marihuana	
Nifedipine	
Phenoxybenzamine	
Prazosin	

association with neurofibromatosis and pheochromocytoma.

2.5.3.3. Diagnosis. A careful history is essential to eliminate indiscriminate laboratory testing. Although measurement of catecholamines and their metabolites is very sensitive, it is not very specific. There are many conditions (*see* Table 5) and drugs (*see* Table 6) that can significantly elevate catecholamines. Therefore, unless these conditions are controlled or resolved and interfering drugs eliminated, false positive tests will be obtained, which will require additional expensive and possibly more invasive tests. Catecholamines are not a specific tumor marker, nor is any level of catecholamines diagnostic of pheochromocytoma.

If the conditions in Table 5 have been eliminated or stabilized, the drugs in Table 6 have been discontinued or the dosage minimized, and the history and physical examination are strongly suggestive of pheochromocytoma, then biochemical testing should be done. Hypertension associated with the symptoms and characteristics of pheochromocytoma (*see* Table 2) is the key to selecting the appropriate patients for laboratory testing. This includes hypertension in young adults or teenagers; hypertension unresponsive to three or more antihypertensives; either sustained hypertension or normotension with paroxysms of hypertension accompanied by symptoms; a hypertensive and symptomatic response to exercise, abdominal examination, micturition, or palpation of a neck mass; marked hypertensive response to induction anesthesia; accelerated or malignant hypertension; paradoxical hypertensive response to β-blockers; or markedly labile blood pressure with symptoms. Other conditions for which biochemical testing is appropriate include families with MEN or familial pheochromocytoma, or the other associated diseases provided in Table 4. Finally, incidental adrenal tumors discovered on abdominal computed tomography (CT) or magnetic resonance imaging (MRI) scans require screening tests to eliminate the presence of a hormone-secreting tumor including pheochromocytoma.

The specificity of the most sensitive tests for pheochromocytoma depends, to a large extent, on the proper selection of a symptomatic, hypertensive patient for whom other confounding conditions and drugs have been eliminated. The most sensitive tests for pheochromocytoma are measurement of plasma metanephrines and/or a 24-h urine collection for metanephrines (metanephrine and normetanephrine) and/or total urinary catecholamines by high-performance liquid chromatography (HPLC). Fluorometric methods remain an adequate substitute when HPLC methods are not readily available. If metanephrine or catecholamine levels are greater than threefold above the upper limit of normal in a symptomatic and hypertensive patient, then imaging is indicated. If catecholamine levels are <1.5-fold of the upper limit of normal, then it is unlikely that the patient has pheochromocytoma. If the levels are marginally elevated, between 1.5-fold and 3-fold above the upper limit of normal, then a 12-h, nighttime collection of urine for catecholamines and metanephrines is indicated. Collection at night eliminates the effects of stress and upright posture on the production of catecholamines that occurs during the day in healthy patients and will not affect the secretion of catecholamines in pheochromocytoma. If levels remain marginally elevated or higher, then one should proceed to imaging. If levels are normal, then one should discontinue testing. If the patient has only brief paroxysms that occur only a few times per day or less frequently, then one should obtain the tests as a timed urine collection (2–4 h) during a prominent symptomatic hypertensive episode. If values exceed threefold, then one should proceed to imaging, and if less than threefold, depending on the level of clinical suspicion, one should either discontinue test-

ing or repeat the test during another episode. This combination of urinary catecholamine and metanephrine measurement has been reported by most investigators, for many years, to be a sensitive (98–100%) and specific (96–98%) biochemical test for pheochromocytoma. Plasma metanephrine testing is a recent addition to the diagnostic tools available. Although it has not acquired a fraction of the long experience of urinary studies, it will probably be as reliable (sensitive and specific) as testing for urinary metanephrine. A major advantage of obtaining a sample through venopuncture is that it is far easier than a 24-h urine collection.

A robust biochemical diagnosis is essential before proceeding to imaging tests. Benign, nonfunctioning adrenal masses have a much higher incidence than pheochromocytoma. Performing an unnecessary major surgical procedure to remove a benign, nonfunctioning mass is to be avoided. Alternatively, a mass not found in the initial examination may result in futile, expensive, and more invasive attempts to locate a nonexistent tumor.

The purpose of making a diagnosis of pheochromocytoma is to enable the surgical excision of the source of the excessive secretion of catecholamines causing the patient's hypertension and symptoms. If significantly elevated catecholamines cannot be demonstrated during a hypertensive, symptomatic episode, then catecholamines are not causing the problem and testing should not proceed to imaging. If a high degree of suspicion remains despite the negative biochemical testing, then the patient should be treated medically and reevaluated at a later date. Imaging may be indicated in patients with familial diseases (Table 4) for whom biochemical testing was negative. This has become a more reasonable option as newer imaging techniques have become more sensitive and specific.

Pharmacologic tests developed to elicit or inhibit catecholamine secretion from a pheochromocytoma bear a significant risk and are generally less specific and sensitive than urinary collections. Phentolamine (Regitine), a short-acting α-blocker, administered intravenously will cause a significant fall in blood pressure during a hypertensive episode. It may induce an undesired, profound fall and cause a myocardial or cerebral infarction. Administration of histamine, tyramine, and glucagon all cause release of catecholamines by different mechanisms and have been used to elicit either a blood pressure or catecholamine response from the tumor. An excessive hypertensive response resulting in a stroke or the development of a significant arrhythmia could occur during these stimulation tests. Clonidine is used to exclude false positive plasma catecholamine measurements.

Other biochemical testing offers little or no advantage over measurement of urinary catecholamines and metanephrines. Urinary VMA by colorometric methods is less specific and by HPLC is equivalent to metanephrines but is more costly and less readily available. Measurements of plasma catecholamines produce more false positives and are more expensive to obtain and analyze. Theoretically, measurement of plasma catecholamines would be a more sensitive method of documenting elevated catecholamine secretion during a brief hypertensive, symptomatic episode. The logistics required to obtain such a sample without prolonged hospitalization is problematic. Chromogranin A and dopamine β-hydroxylase are released with catecholamines during exocytosis. Both are frequently elevated in pheochromocytoma but are less specific than measurement of urinary catecholamine.

The diagnosis will have been made prior to imaging based on the history, physical findings, and biochemical measurements. The purpose of localization (imaging) is to find the tumor and plan the approach for surgical removal. Finding a mass with characteristics that are consistent with a pheochromocytoma helps to confirm but does not make the diagnosis. MRI is the preferred method of tumor detection. The sensitivity and specificity of MRI are at least equal to or greater than of CT, and MRI does not expose the patient to ionizing radiation. Pheochromocytoma on T_2-weighted imaging (MRI) presents an especially bright mass in comparison to most other tumors. CT provides no similar distinguishing characteristics of pheochromocytoma compared to other masses. MRI of the abdomen and pelvis is the first examination to be performed, because 90% of tumors are found below the diaphragm. If no tumor is found below the diaphragm, then the chest and neck should be imaged. If no mass is found, then CT imaging with contrast should be performed of the same areas and in the same order. If still no mass is found, then a ^{131}I-metaiodobenzylguanidine (MIBG) scan could be considered. Although this scan is highly specific (100%), it is considerably less sensitive (60–80%) than either the MRI or CT scans (>98%). The isotope is specifically concentrated in intra- and extraadrenal pheochromocytomas. Because it is a ^{131}I-based isotope, it has a short half-life (9 d). The MIBG scan is expensive and not readily available. The ^{123}I-based isotope is more sensitive but even more difficult to obtain. A new imaging technique, 6-[^{18}F]-fluorodopamine ([^{18}F]-DA) by positron emission tomography, is as specific as MIBG, is more sensitive, requires no pretreatment to protect the thyroid, and produces higher resolution images. [^{18}F]-DA plus MRI may be the best combination for the detection of intra-

and extraadrenal tumors, benign or malignant. Unfortunately, [^{18}F]-DA is currently available only at the National Institutes of Health.

There is a high incidence of gallstones in pheochromocytoma, and ultrasound examination of the gallbladder and ducts is warranted prior to surgery.

2.5.3.4. Management. The definitive treatment for pheochromocytoma is surgery. The early, coordinated team effort of the endocrinologist, anesthesiologist, and surgeon helps to ensure a successful outcome. The goals of preoperative medical therapy are to control hypertension; obtain adequate fluid balance; and treat tachyarrythmias, heart failure, and glucose intolerance. The nonselective and long-acting α-adrenergic blocker phenoxybenzamine is the principal drug used to prevent hypertensive episodes. Optimal blockade requires 1 to 2 wk of therapy. Short-acting α_1-blockers such as prazosin could be used as well. The effects of the calcium channel blocker nifedipine on the inhibition of calcium-mediated exocytosis of storage granules are also moderately effective in controlling hypertension. Adequate hydration and volume expansion with saline or plasma is used to reduce the incidence of postoperative hypotension. The addition of α-methyltyrosine (Demser), a competitive inhibitor of tyrosine hydroxylase and catecholamine biosynthesis, to α-adrenergic blockade provides several important advantages. Control of hypertension can be obtained with a lower dose of α-blocker, which minimizes the duration and severity of hypotensive episodes. The side effects of α-methyltyrosine are rarely encountered during the brief 1 to 2-wk preoperative period. β-Adrenergic blockade is usually not required and should not be given unless a patient has persistent tachycardia and some supraventricular arrhythmias. β-Blockade should *never* be instituted prior to α-blockade. The inability to vasodilate (β-receptors blocked) and unopposed α-receptor-stimulated vasoconstriction could precipitate a hypertensive crisis, congestive heart failure, and acute pulmonary edema. If β-blockade is needed, propranolol or a more cardioselective β_1-antagonist, atenolol, can be used. α-Methyltyrosine may reduce the need for β-blockers and is the drug of choice to treat catecholamine-induced toxic cardiomyopathy. Hyperglycemia is best treated with a sliding scale of regular insulin in the immediate preoperative period to maintain blood glucose between 150 and 200 mg%. Glucose intolerance usually ends abruptly after the tumor's blood supply is isolated during surgery. Hypoglycemia during anesthesia is to be avoided.

The advantages of a coordinated team approach are most apparent during surgery. All members of the team will be aware of the patient's complications and relative response to the preoperative preparation. Monitoring of the cardiopulmonary and metabolic status should become more intense and accurate. The selection of premedications, induction anesthesia, muscle relaxant, and general anesthetic to be used in pheochromocytoma is based on those that do not stimulate catecholamine release or sensitize the myocardium to catecholamines. These premedications include diazepam or pentobarbital, meperidine, and scopolamine. Thiopental is the preferred drug for induction and vecuronium for neuromuscular blockade. Isoflurane and enflurane are excellent volatile general anesthetics, but the newest member of this family, desflurane, has the distinct advantage of being very volatile and thus very short acting. Increasing the inhaled concentration of desflurane will rapidly reduce blood pressure (2 min) during a hypertensive episode, and hypotensive effects dissipate just as quickly by reducing the inhaled concentration. The achievement of rapid, stress-free anesthesia reduces the risk of complications during surgery. During surgery, tumor manipulation and isolation of the vessels draining the tumor can result in changes in plasma catecholamine concentrations of 1000-fold within minutes. With modest α-receptor blockade, α-methyltyrosine, and desflurane, the need for urgent application of nitroprusside or phentolamine to control blood pressure during surgery may be eliminated. Pheochromocytomas are very vascular by nature and significant hemorrhage is a potential hazard. Advanced preparation reduces the impact of these complications. Whole blood; plasma expanders; nitroprusside; and esmolol, a short-acting β-blocker, should be immediately available.

When bilateral adrenalectomy is being performed, adrenal cortical insufficiency should be treated with stress doses of hydrocortisone intra- and postoperatively until stable. Mineralocorticoid should be replaced postoperatively.

Hypotension is the most common complication encountered in the recovery room. The loss of the vasoconstrictive and ion tropic effects of catecholamines, persistent α-receptor blockade, downregulated adrenergic receptors, and perioperative blood loss all contribute. The treatment is aggressive volume expansion. Sympathomimetic amines are rarely indicated. Hypoglycemia may result from administered insulin or be reactive. Dextrose should be given during the immediate postoperative period and blood glucose monitored regularly for several hours.

2.5.3.5. Prognosis. Most patients become normotensive within 1 to 2 wk after surgery. Hypertension persists in about one-third of patients either because they have an underlying essential hypertension or because they have residual tumor. Patients with essential hypertension no longer have the symptoms of pheochromocytoma, and their blood pressure is usually easily controlled with conventional therapy. If a patient has a residual tumor, an unidentified second site, or multiple metastases, then the signs and symptoms of pheochromocytoma will gradually or abruptly recur in proportion to the level of catecholamines being secreted.

There are no characteristic histologic changes on which to base the diagnosis of malignancy. The clinical course showing an aggressive, recurrent tumor or finding chromaffin cells in nonendocrine tissue such as lymph nodes, bone, muscle, or liver makes the diagnosis. Factors have been examined to determine their potential role in predicting a malignant course. Extra-adrenal tumors, large size, local tumor invasion, family history of pheochromocytoma, associated endocrine disorders, and young age are significant in predicting a malignant course. DNA flow cytometry has been used retrospectively to determine whether the DNA ploidy pattern could be used in predicting the clinical course of pheochromocytoma. Although no pattern has been diagnostic, abnormal patterns (aneuploid, tetraploid) were best correlated with malignancy, and a diploid pattern has been very strongly correlated with a benign course.

The primary approach to the treatment of malignant pheochromocytoma is surgical debulking with medical management similar to that used for preoperative preparation. All treatment is palliative; there is no cure. Chemotherapy with a combination of cyclophosphamide, vincristine, and dacarbazine produced a 57% response with a median duration of 21 mo. High doses of ^{131}I-MIBG have been used to shrink tumors and decrease catecholamine secretion in some patients who demonstrate high-grade uptake of this compound. Repetitive treatments are needed to obtain a temporary response over 2 to 3-yr, but the therapy is well tolerated. Unlike ^{131}I-MIBG, [^{18}F]-DA used for localization would have no beneficial effect in the treatment of malignant pheochromocytoma.

3. PEPTIDES

3.1. Developmental Origin

The cells of the adrenal medulla have a pluripotential capacity to secrete a variety of other peptide hormones that are usually biologically active. A great deal is known about the development and regulation of the catecholaminergic properties of these cells, but relatively little is known about the developmental control of their peptidergic properties. Evidence suggests that glucocorticoids derived from an intact hypothalamic-pituitary-adrenal cortical axis and splanchnic innervation are essential to the developmental expression of these peptides. Peptide neurotransmitters have been identified in the neurons innervating the adrenal as well as the gland itself. The list of neuropeptides discovered continues to grow and includes Met-enkephalin, Leu-enkephalin, neurotensin, substance P, vasoactive intestinal peptide (VIP), neuropeptide Y (NPY), calcitonin-related peptide, orexin-A, adrenomedullin (AM), and proadrenal medullin N-terminal peptides (PAMPs).

3.2. Potential Physiologic or Pathophysiologic Roles

Some peptide hormone secretion may be only pathophysiologic and derived from a neoplastic process, such as pheochromocytoma. Alternatively, normal physiologic processes can be operative but have yet to be discovered. VIP, ACTH, and a parathyroid hormone–like hormone can be produced by pheochromocytoma and produce symptoms of watery diarrhea, Cushing syndrome, and hypercalcemia, respectively. NPY is secreted in sympathetic storage vesicles along with norepinephrine, chromogranin, dopamine β-hydroxylase, ATP, and AM. Like chromogranin, it is not taken back up into the neuron after release, and measured levels may be used as another marker of sympathetic activity. NPY appears to mediate vasoconstriction through potentiating noradrenergic stimulation of α-receptor responses, and secretion is increased in severe hypertension. VIP and NPY are the most abundant transmitter peptides in the adrenal. Endothelin-1 is another potent vasoconstrictor peptide that has been found along with its mRNA in pheochromocytomas. Both of these peptides could be involved in normal circulatory regulation, contribute to the pathophysiology of sympathetically mediated hypertension, or even be responsible for the unusual hypertensive episodes of pheochromocytoma that do not correlate well with catecholamine levels.

AM testing was proposed as a diagnostic test for pheochromocytoma but has not gained popularity. AM is released by normal adrenals at a low rate and at a higher rate by pheochromocytoma. PAMP regulates intracellular signaling pathways that regulate chromaffin cells in an autocrine manner, and AM acts on the vasculature via paracrine mechanisms.

Two peptides linked to obesity have been identified that affect catecholamine synthesis or release. Orexin-A, a hypothalamic peptide implicated in the regulation of feeding behavior and sleep control, has been reported to stimulate tyrosine hydroxylase activity and catecholamine synthesis in bovine adrenal medullary cells through orexin receptor-1 mRNA. Ghrelin, a peptide that was initially found in the stomach and that regulates appetite and growth hormone secretion, has been shown to inhibit adrenal dopamine release in chromaffin cells. The relationship between the action of these two peptides on the regulation of adrenal catcholamines and weight control has not been explored.

Another role suggested for some of the neuropeptides—Met-enkephalin (also synthesized in chromaffin tissue, stored and released in sympathetic granules) and VIP—is to increase adrenal blood flow in response to cholinergic stimulation and thus enhance the distribution of epinephrine into the bloodstream. By contrast, NPY released by cholinergic stimulation inhibits adrenal blood flow and could, therefore, function to inhibit the distribution of epinephrine.

SELECTED READINGS

Burgoyne RD, Morgan A, Robinson I, Pender N, Cheek TR. Exocytosis in adrenal chromaffin cells. *J Anat* 1993;183:309.

Evans DB, Lee JE, Merrell RC, Hickey RC. Adrenal medullary disease in multiple endocrine neoplasia type 2. Appropriate management. *Endocrinol Metab Clin North Amer* 1994;23:167.

Graham PE, Smythe GA, Lazarus L. Laboratory diagnosis of pheochromocytoma: which analytes should we measure? *Ann Clin Biochem* 1993;30:129.

Ilias I, Yu J, Carrasquillo JA, Chen CC, Eisenhofer G, Whatley M, McElroy B, Pacak K. Superiority of 6-[18F]-fluorodopamine positron emission tomography *versus* [131I]-metaiodobenzylguanidine scintigraphy in the localization of metastatic pheochromocytoma. *J Clin Endocrinol Metab* 2003;88:4083.

Kobayashi H, Yanagita T, Yokoo H, Wada A. Pathophysiological function of adrenomedullin and proadrenomedullin N-terminal peptides in adrenal chromaffin cells. *Hypertens Res* 2003; (Suppl):S71.

Lenders JWM, Pacak K, Walther MM, Linehan WM, Mannelli M, Friberg P, Keiser HR, Goldstein DS, Eisenhofer G. Biochemical diagnosis of pheochromocytoma: which test is best? *JAMA* 2002; 287:1427.

Nagatsu T. Genes for human catecholamine-synthesizing enzymes. *Neurosci Res* 1991;12:315.

Nativ O, Grant CS, Sheps SG, O'Fallon JR, Farrow GM, van Heerden JA, Lieber MM. The clinical significance of nuclear DNA ploidy pattern in 184 patients with pheochromocytoma. *Cancer* 1992; 69:2683.

Raum WJ. Pheochromocytoma. In: Bardin CW, ed. *Current Therapy in Endocrinology and Metabolism*, 5th Ed. St. Louis, MO: Mosby 1994:172.

Whitworth EJ, Kosti O, Renshaw D, Hinson JP. Adrenal neuropeptides: regulation and interaction with ACTH and other adrenal regulators. *Microsc Res Tech* 2003;61:259.

23 Hormones of the Kidney

Masashi Mukoyama, MD, PhD
and Kazuwa Nakao, MD, PhD

1. INTRODUCTION

The kidney plays an essential role in the maintenance of life in higher organisms, not only through regulating the blood pressure and body fluid homeostasis and clearing the wastes, but also by acting as a major endocrine organ. The kidney secretes (1) renin, a key enzyme of the renin-angiotensin system (RAS) that leads to the production of a potent pressor hormone angiotensin, and produces the following hormones and humoral factors: (2) kallikreins, a group of serine proteases that act on blood proteins to produce a vasorelaxing peptide bradykinin; (3) erythropoietin (EPO), a peptide hormone essential for red blood cell (RBC) formation by the bone marrow; and (4) 1,25-$(OH)_2$ vitamin D_3, the active form of vitamin D essential for calcium homeostasis, which is produced by the proximal tubule cells via the enzyme 1α-hydroxylase.

In addition, the kidney serves as an important endocrine target organ for a number of hormones, thereby controlling the extracellular fluid volume, electrolyte balance, acid-base balance, and blood pressure. Among these hormones, angiotensin and aldosterone, both key products in the axis of the RAS, and the natriuretic peptide family, comprising potent diuretic and vasorelaxing hormones secreted from the heart, are regarded as the most important players. Furthermore, the kidney is a major organ for the production and action of various "local hormones," or autocrine/paracrine regulators, such as prostaglandins (PGs), adrenomedullin (AM), and endothelins (ETs). These factors are thought to provide an integrated mechanism for the fine-tuning of microcirculation, solute transport, and various cellular functions in the kidney.

This chapter discusses the roles of the hormones that are produced or have major actions in the kidney, focusing on their functional relationships and implications in physiologic and pathophysiologic conditions. The roles of vitamin D and the kidney in calcium homeostasis as well as the prostanoid system are detailed in other chapters.

2. COMPONENTS OF RAS

The RAS is a proteolytic cascade, composed of a group of proteins and peptides that ultimately produce

From: *Endocrinology: Basic and Clinical Principles, Second Edition*
(S. Melmed and P. M. Conn, eds.) © Humana Press Inc., Totowa, NJ

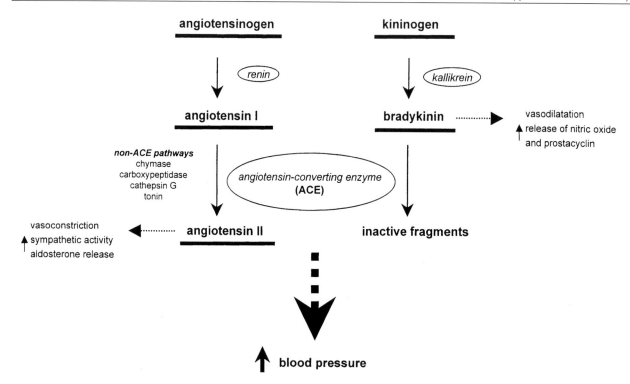

Fig. 1. Biosynthetic cascade of the RAS.

a potent octapeptide, angiotensin II (Ang II) (Fig. 1). Classically, the cascade starts with the proteolytic enzyme renin, released from the juxtaglomerular cells of the kidney (Fig. 2). Renin acts on a liver-derived plasma α_2-globulin, angiotensinogen, to cleave the N-terminal decapeptide sequence and produce Ang I. Subsequently, the C-terminal dipeptide His^9-Leu^{10} is cleaved from Ang I to form Ang II, by angiotensin-converting enzyme (ACE), primarily within the pulmonary circulation. Ang II then acts on various target tissues, resulting in vasoconstriction in the resistance vessels, increased intraglomerular pressure and sodium reabsorption in the kidney, and stimulated biosynthesis and secretion of the mineralocorticoid aldosterone in the adrenal cortex. In addition to such a well-described circulating hormonal RAS, it is now recognized that there are components of the RAS that allow local synthesis of Ang II. Such a system is referred to as the tissue RAS and may serve local actions of Ang II in an autocrine/paracrine manner.

The biologic actions of the RAS are mediated by Ang II via at least two types of the specific membrane receptors: angiotensin type 1 (AT$_1$) and type 2 (AT$_2$) receptors. With the availability of pharmacologic and genetic tools that inhibit ACE and block Ang II receptors, as well as data from a number of clinical studies, it is now revealed that the RAS plays a critical role in

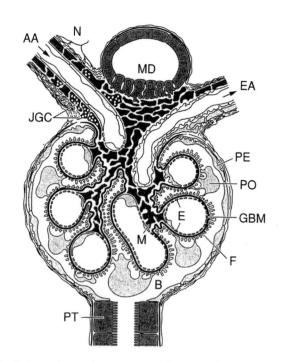

Fig. 2. Juxtaglomerular apparatus. MD = macula densa; JGC = juxtaglomerular cells; AA = afferent arteriole; EA = efferent arteriole; N = sympathetic nerve terminal; M = mesangium; GBM = glomerular basement membrane; E = endothelium; PO = podocyte; F = foot process; PE = parietal epithelium; B = Bowman's space; PT = proximal tubule.

maintaining cardiovascular and renal homeostasis physiologically, and in developing disease states pathologically. Accordingly, interruption of the RAS has become an increasingly important therapeutic strategy for various cardiovascular disorders such as hypertension, heart failure, and renal disease.

2.1. Renin

2.1.1. Synthesis and Biochemistry of Renin

More than a century ago, Tigerstedt and Bergman found a potent pressor activity in rabbit kidney extract. They named a putative substance secreted from the kidney *renin*, after the Latin word *ren* (kidney). Forty years later, Braun-Menéndez et al. and Page et al. showed that this material was of a protease nature, acting on a plasma protein to release another pressor substance, which was later named angiotensin.

Renin (EC 3.4.25.15) is classified as an aspartyl protease and synthesized as a preproprotein. Renin is stored and secreted from the renal juxtaglomerular cells located in the wall of the afferent arteriole, which is contiguous with the macula densa portion of the same nephron (Fig. 2). The human renin gene, spanning 12 kb, is located on chromosome 1 (1q32-1q42) and consists of 10 exons and 9 introns. Hormonal-responsive elements in the 5′-flanking region of the renin gene include consensus elements for cyclic adenosine monophosphate (cAMP) and steroids (glucocorticoid, estrogen, and progesterone). In certain strains of the mouse, there are two renin genes (*Ren-1* and *Ren-2*), both located on chromosome 1, and in the rat, the renin gene is located on chromosome 13. In most mammals, the kidney is the primary source of circulating renin, although renin gene expression is found in a number of extrarenal tissues, including the brain, adrenal, pituitary, submandibular glands, gonads, and heart.

The initial translation product preprorenin, consisting of 406 amino acids, is processed in the endoplasmic reticulum to a 47-kDa prorenin by removal of a 23-amino-acid presegment. Prorenin then enters either a regulated or a constitutive secretory pathway. A substantial portion of prorenin is further processed, when a 43-amino-acid prosegment is removed, to the active 41-kDa mature renin, which is a glycosylated single-chain polypeptide that circulates in human plasma. Prorenin also circulates in the blood at a concentration several times higher than active renin. Active renin can be generated from prorenin by cold storage (cryoactivation); acidification; or a variety of proteolytic enzymes including trypsin, pepsin, and kallikrein. The N- and C-terminal halves of active renin are similar, and each domain contains a single aspartic residue in the active center, which is essential for its catalytic activity.

Angiotensinogen (renin substrate) is the only known substrate for renin. This reaction appears to be highly species specific. Human renin does not cleave mouse or rat angiotensinogen, and human angiotensinogen, in turn, is a poor substrate for rodent renin.

2.1.2. Regulation of Renin Release

Because renin is the rate-limiting enzyme in circulating Ang II production, control of renin release serves as a major regulator of the systemic RAS activity. Restriction of salt intake, acute hemorrhage, administration of diuretics, or acute renal artery clamping results in a marked increase in renin release. The regulation of renin release is controlled by four independent factors: renal baroreceptor, macula densa, renal sympathetic nerves, and various humoral factors:

1. Mechanical signals, via the baroreceptor or vascular stretch receptor, of the juxtaglomerular cells sensing the renal perfusion pressure in the afferent arteriole (Fig. 2): The renal baroreceptor is perhaps the most powerful regulator of renin release, and reduced renal perfusion pressure strongly stimulates renin release.

2. Tubular signals from the macula densa cells in the distal convoluted tubule: The cells function as the chemoreceptor, monitoring the delivery of sodium chloride to the distal nephron by sensing the sodium and/or chloride load through the macula densa cells, and decreased concentrations within the cells stimulate renin release.

3. The sympathetic nervous system in the afferent arteriole: Juxtaglomerular cells are directly innervated by sympathetic nerves (Fig. 2), and β-adrenergic activation stimulates renin release. Renal nerve–mediated renin secretion constitutes an acute pathway by which rapid activation of the RAS is provoked by such stimuli as stress and posture.

4. Circulating humoral factors: Ang II suppresses renin release (as a negative feedback) independent of alteration of renal perfusion pressure or aldosterone secretion. Atrial natriuretic peptide (ANP) and vasopressin inhibit renin release, whereas PGE_2 and prostacyclin (PGI_2) stimulate renin release.

In addition to the major regulators just described, a series of other humoral factors is implicated, considering the finding that the primary stimulatory second messenger for renin release is intracellular cAMP whereas the inhibitory signal is increased intracellular calcium and increased cyclic guanosine monophasphate (cGMP). For example, local paracrine regulators, such as adenosine and nitric oxide (NO), may have significant influences on renin release, perhaps more importantly in certain pathologic conditions.

2.2. Angiotensinogen

Angiotensinogen is the only known substrate for renin capable of producing the family of angiotensin

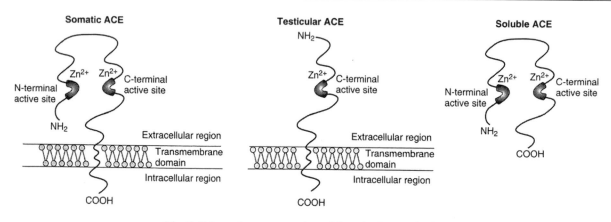

Fig. 3. Schematic representation of three isoforms of ACE.

peptides. In most species, angiotensinogen circulates at a concentration close to the K_m for its cleavage by renin, and, therefore, varying the concentration of plasma angiotensinogen can affect the rate of Ang I production. Because angiotensinogen levels in plasma are relatively constant, plasma concentrations of active renin, not angiotensinogen, would be the limiting factor for the rate of plasma Ang I formation in normal conditions, as determined by the plasma renin activity. However, in certain conditions such as pregnancy and administration of steroids, when angiotensinogen production is enhanced, circulating angiotensinogen would have a major effect on the activity of the systemic RAS. Furthermore, recent studies on the linkage analysis between angiotensinogen gene and human essential hypertension suggest that the alterations in plasma angiotensinogen levels may have a significant impact on the total RAS activity, affecting blood pressure.

Angiotensinogen shares sequence homology with α_1-antitrypsin and belongs to the serpin (for serine protease inhibitor) superfamily of proteins. The human angiotensinogen gene (~12 kb long) is located on chromosome 1 (1q42.3) close to the renin gene locus. The angiotensinogen gene consists of five exons and four introns, and cDNA codes for 485 amino acids, of which 33 appear to be a presegment. The first 10 amino acids of the mature protein correspond to Ang I. The 5′-flanking region of the human angiotensinogen gene contains several consensus sequences for glucocorticoid, estrogen, thyroid hormone, cAMP, and an acute phase–responsive element.

The liver is the primary site of angiotensinogen synthesis and secretion. However, angiotensinogen mRNA is expressed in a variety of other tissues, including brain, large arteries, kidney, adipose tissues, reproductive tissues, and heart, which constitutes an important part of the tissue RAS.

2.3. Angiotensin-Converting Enzyme

ACE, or kininase II (EC 3.4.15.1), is a dipeptidyl carboxypeptidase, which is a membrane-bound ectoenzyme with its catalytic sites exposed to the extracellular surface. It is a zinc metallopeptidase that is required for the final enzymatic step of Ang II production from Ang I (Fig. 1). ACE also plays an important role in the kallikrein-kinin system, by inactivating the vasodilator hormone bradykinin. In vascular beds, ACE is present on the plasma membrane of endothelial cells, where it cleaves circulating peptides; vessels in the lung, as well as in the brain and retina, are especially rich in ACE. ACE is also abundantly present in the proximal tubule brush border of the kidney.

There are primarily two molecular forms of ACE (somatic and testicular) that are derived from a single gene by different utilization of two different promoters. Although the majority of ACE is membrane bound, somatic ACE can be cleaved near the C-terminus, leading to the release of ACE into the circulation. This results in three main isoforms of ACE: somatic ACE, testicular (or germinal) ACE, and soluble (or plasma) ACE (Fig. 3). The human ACE gene consisting of 26 exons and 25 introns, is located on chromosome 17q23. The somatic promoter is located in the 5′-flanking region of the gene upstream of exon 1, whereas the testicular promoter is present within intron 12. Somatic ACE is a 170-kDa protein consisting of 1306 amino acids encoded by a 4.3-kb mRNA, which is transcribed from exons 1 to 26 except exon 13. It is an extensively glycosylated protein, containing two highly homologous domains with an active site in each domain. Testicular ACE is an approx 90-kDa protein consisting of 732 amino acids, harboring only one C-terminal active site. This isoform is found only in the testes. Testicular ACE is encoded by a 3-kb mRNA, transcribed from exons 13 to 26, with exon 13 encoding the unique N-terminus of the testicular isoform.

Somatic ACE is distributed in a wide variety of tissues, including blood vessels, kidney, heart, brain, adrenal, small intestine, and uterus, where it is expressed in the epithelial, neuroepithelial, and nonepithelial cells as well as in endothelial cells. Somatic ACE in these tissues (tissue ACE) is postulated to play a crucial role in the rate-limiting step of the tissue RAS activity. In addition, studies on the human ACE gene revealed the presence of a 287-bp insertion (*I*)/deletion (*D*) polymorphism within intron 16, which may account for the high degree of individual variability of ACE levels. The *D* allele is associated with high plasma and tissue ACE activity and has been linked to cardiovascular diseases such as acute myocardial infarction.

In addition to ACE, it is now known that there are other ACE-independent pathways of Ang II generation from Ang I (Fig. 1). Among them, chymase, which is present abundantly in the human heart, is thought to be most important. The relative importance of such alternative pathways in physiologic and pathophysiologic states, however, is the subject of continuing debate and awaits further clarification.

2.4. Angiotensin Receptors

For many years, it was thought that Ang II exerts its effects via only one receptor subtype that mediates vasoconstriction, aldosterone release, salt-water retention, and tissue remodeling effects such as cell proliferation and hypertrophy. This receptor subtype is now termed the AT_1 receptor. In the late 1980s, it became clear that there was another Ang II–binding site that was not blocked by the AT_1 receptor antagonists. This receptor subtype is now known as the AT_2 receptor. Pharmacologic examinations may suggest the presence of other receptor subtypes, but to date, no other receptors have been isolated or cloned.

Most known biologic effects of Ang II are mediated by the AT_1 receptor. The AT_1 receptor consists of 359 amino acids, with a relative molecular mass of 41 kDa, and belongs to the G protein–coupled, seven-transmembrane receptor superfamily. The principal signaling mechanism of the AT_1 receptor is through a G_q-mediated activation of phospholipase C (PLC) with a release of inositol 1,4,5-trisphosphate and calcium mobilization. Activation of the protein tyrosine kinase pathway may also be involved. In humans, there is a single gene for this receptor, located on chromosome 3. The human AT_1 receptor gene consists of five exons and four introns, with the coding region contained within exon 5. The promoter region contains putative elements for cAMP, glucocorticoid, and activating protein-1 sites for

immediate early gene products. In rodents, there are two isoforms of this receptor, named AT_{1A} and AT_{1B}, encoded by different genes. These isoforms show a very high sequence homology (94%) and AT_{1A} is considered to be a major subtype, although the functional significance of each isoform is not fully clarified. AT_1 receptor mRNA is expressed primarily in the adrenals, vascular smooth muscle, kidney, heart, and specific areas of the brain implicated in dipsogenic and pressor actions of Ang II, and it is also abundantly present in the liver, uterus, ovary, lung, and spleen.

The AT_2 receptor consists of 363 amino acids, with a relative molecular mass of 41 kDa. This receptor also exhibits a seven-transmembrane domain topology but shares only 32% overall sequence identity with the AT_1 receptor. It is likely coupled to a G protein, although it may also be coupled to a phosphotyrosine phosphatase. The AT_2 receptor gene, located on chromosome X, is composed of three exons and two introns, with the entire coding region contained within exon 3. Expression of the AT_2 receptor is developmentally regulated. It is abundantly expressed in various fetal tissues, especially in mesenchyme and connective tissues; it gets down-regulated on birth and is not expressed at significant levels in adult tissues including the cardiovascular system at normal conditions, being limited to adrenal medulla, brain, and reproductive tissues. Interestingly, however, the AT_2 receptor is reexpressed under certain pathologic conditions, such as on tissue injury and remodeling, especially in the cardiovascular system. The signaling mechanism and functional role of the AT_2 receptor have not been fully elucidated, but recent studies have shown that stimulation of the AT_2 receptor induces apoptosis and exerts cardioprotective actions by mediating vasodilatation, probably via activation of NO and cGMP production. Furthermore, the AT_2 receptor exerts an antiproliferative action on vascular smooth muscle cells, fibroblasts, and mesangial cells. Thus, it is now recognized that the AT_2 receptor should act to counterbalance the effects of the AT_1 receptor.

2.5. Angiotensins

A family of angiotensin peptides is derived from Ang I through the action of ACE, chymase, aminopeptidases, and tissue endopeptidases. There are at least four biologically active angiotensin peptides (Table 1). Ang I, decapeptide cleaved from angiotensinogen, is biologically inactive. Ang II acts on AT_1 and AT_2 receptors, with equally high affinities. Ang II can be processed by aminopeptidase A or angiotensinase, to form Ang III. Like Ang II, Ang III circulates in the blood and shows somewhat less vasoconstrictor activity but exerts an almost equipotent activity on aldosterone secretion.

Table 1
Angiotensin Peptides

Peptide	Sequence
Ang I	Asp-Arg-Val-Tyr-Ile-His-Pro-Phe-His-Leu
Ang II	Asp-Arg-Val-Tyr-Ile-His-Pro-Phe
Ang III	Arg-Val-Tyr-Ile-His-Pro-Phe
Ang IV	Val-Tyr-Ile-His-Pro-Phe
Ang 1-7	Asp-Arg-Val-Tyr-Ile-His-Pro

Ang III can be further converted by aminopeptidase B into Ang 3–8, or Ang IV. In addition, Ang 1–7 can be produced from Ang I or Ang II by endopeptidases. It is reported that the fragments Ang IV and Ang 1–7 have pharmacologic and biochemical properties different from those mediated by the AT_1 or AT_2 receptors, perhaps exerting an opposite effect of Ang II such as vasodilatation. The functional significance and receptors of these peptides, however, still remain elusive.

3. PATHOPHYSIOLOGY OF RAS

3.1. Biological Actions of Ang II

Ang II has short-term actions related to maintaining normal extracellular fluid volume and blood pressure homeostasis as well as long-term actions related to cardiovascular remodeling, most of which are mediated via the AT_1 receptor. Six primary short-term actions are as follows:

1. Increasing aldosterone secretion.
2. Constricting vascular smooth muscle, thereby increasing blood pressure and reducing renal blood flow.
3. Increasing the intraglomerular pressure by constriction of the efferent arteriole, contracting the mesangium, and enhancing sodium reabsorption from the proximal tubule.
4. Increasing cardiac contractility.
5. Enhancing the sympathetic nervous activity by increasing central sympathetic outflow, and releasing norepinephrine and epinephrine from the adrenal medulla.
6. Promoting the release of vasopressin.

Long-term actions of Ang II include the following:

1. Increasing vascular smooth muscle hypertrophy and hyperplasia.
2. Promoting cardiac hypertrophy.
3. Enhancing extracellular matrix synthesis, thereby causing tissue fibrosis.
4. Promoting inflammatory reactions by stimulating the migration and adhesion of monocytes to the vessel wall.

These actions are closely associated with the cardiovascular structural manifestations, or cardiovascular remodeling, in both human and experimental hypertension. Ang II also acts on the central nervous system,

increasing thirst and sodium craving. In addition, Ang II may have potential actions in regulating ovarian and placental function.

3.2. Tissue RAS

Many tissues and organs can synthesize Ang II independent of the classic circulating RAS, and locally formed Ang II can exert multiple effects acting as an autocrine and paracrine regulator. Ang II levels may be much higher in tissues than in plasma. A variety of tissues express angiotensinogen, renin, ACE, and other Ang II–generating enzymes, as well as angiotensin receptors. These additional enzyme systems are referred to as the tissue RAS.

The effects of locally generated Ang II are long term, i.e., not just vasoconstriction or salt-water retention, but the induction of tissue remodeling, modulation of cell growth, and inflammation. These effects could be mediated by alternative pathways; thus, these multiple pathways in tissues allow more ways to synthesize Ang II, particularly in the areas of inflammation where mast cells release chymase, monocytes release ACE, and neutrophils secrete cathepsin G. With the presence of such non-ACE pathways of Ang II generation, the inhibition of ACE alone is not theoretically sufficient to completely inhibit Ang II production. Although the importance of the tissue RAS has been suggested and tissue Ang II should be a target for antihypertensive, antihypertrophic, and antiinflammatory effects, it is recognized that many of the data available so far are experimental and there is no definitive proof in humans. The availability of and analysis with several AT_1 receptor blockers in clinical settings should provide an answer to this issue.

3.3. Transgenic and Knockout Approaches

Several types of transgenic and knockout animals have been established to study the functional significance of the RAS in vivo. Transgenic lines of mice and rats harboring both the human renin and angiotensinogen genes develop severe hypertension. Hypertension in the mice likely represents pathologic conditions brought about by the inappropriate secretion of renin from outside the kidneys, including pregnancy-associated hypertension (preeclampsia). Transgenic rats harboring the mouse *Ren-2* gene exhibited fulminant hypertension, which overexpressed the transgene in the adrenal gland. Cardiac-specific overexpression of the AT_1 receptor resulted in hypertrophy and arrhythmia, whereas overexpression of the AT_2 receptor in the heart and vessels showed reduction in hypertrophy and tissue damage. These models may indicate the functional significance of the tissue RAS in cardiovascular control.

Knockout studies of the components of the RAS reveal that each component of the cascade (angiotensinogen, renin, ACE, and AT_{1A} receptor) is indispensible to the maintenance of normal blood pressure. These knockout animal models invariably show low blood pressure by ~30 mmHg. Moreover, mice deficient in any component exhibit severe abnormality in kidney development, characterized by cortical atrophy and hypoplasia. ACE-null male mice show greatly reduced fertility. The AT_2 receptor–knockout mice reveal enhanced pressor response to Ang II and exaggerated cardiovascular remodeling in response to noxious stimuli, again suggesting a potential cardioprotective role of this receptor.

3.4. Genetic Studies and Clinical Implication

Linkage and association studies have been performed using polymorphic markers of ACE, angiotensinogen, renin, and Ang II receptors. In rats, significant linkage has been demonstrated between the ACE locus and blood pressure. In humans, on the other hand, no relation was found between the ACE gene and hypertension. However, affected sib-pair analysis has found a strong linkage between the human angiotensinogen gene and hypertension. Among the polymorphic markers of the angiotensinogen gene, amino acid conversion at codon 235 from methionine to threonine (M235T) was significantly associated with hypertension. 235T subjects also have higher angiotensinogen levels in plasma. In addition, M235T polymorphism was found to be linked with several polymorphisms in the 5´-promoter region of the human angiotensinogen gene, such as A(-20)C, C(-18)T, and A(-6)G.

The human ACE gene contains an *I/D* polymorphism (ACE *I/D*), characterized by the presence/absence of a 287-bp fragment in intron 16. A significant linkage has been shown between a deletion polymorphism of the human ACE gene (ACE *DD*) and myocardial infarction. The deletion allele is associated with significantly increased ACE levels in the tissue and circulation. In addition, several reports have shown an association between the ACE *DD* polymorphism and an increased risk of cardiovascular events such as restenosis after coronary intervention, and progression of renal disease such as IgA nephropathy and diabetic nephropathy. Multiple lines of evidence have shown that ACE inhibitors and AT_1 receptor blockers are particularly effective in reducing morbidity and mortality in heart failure, and in retarding the progression of diabetic and nondiabetic nephropathies. Therefore, the presence of the ACE *DD* polymorphism should provide more compelling indications of these antihypertensive agents.

4. COMPONENTS OF NATRIURETIC PEPTIDE SYSTEM

Following the discovery of atrial natriuretic peptide (ANP) from human and rat atrial tissues, two endogenous congeners, brain natriuretic peptide (BNP) and C-type natriuretic peptide (CNP), were isolated from the porcine brain. These natriuretic peptides share a common ring structure of 17 amino acids formed by a disulfide linkage (Fig. 4), which is the essential part of their biologic actions. The natriuretic peptide system is a potent natriuretic, diuretic, and vasorelaxing hormone system, comprising at least three endogenous ligands and three receptors (natriuretic peptide receptor A [NPR-A], NPR-B, and the clearance receptor) (Fig. 4). The accumulated evidence indicates that this system plays an essential role in the control of blood pressure and body fluid homeostasis by acting on the kidney and vasculature as cardiac hormones, as well as by regulating cardiovascular and renal remodeling, neural control, and bone metabolism as local regulators. Furthermore, the importance of this system in the clinical setting has now been established not only as an excellent diagnostic marker but also as a useful therapeutic agent for cardiovascular diseases.

4.1. Natriuretic Peptide Family

4.1.1. ANP AND BNP AS CARDIAC HORMONES

ANP (28-amino-acid peptide) and BNP (32-amino-acid peptide in humans) act as cardiac hormones. ANP is predominantly synthesized in the cardiac atrium as pro-ANP (also called γ-ANP, with 126 amino acids) in healthy subjects, whereas BNP (from pro-BNP, with 108 amino acids) is mainly produced in the ventricle. Active peptides reside at the C-terminus of the prohormones and are cleaved during storage or in a process of secretion. Plasma ANP levels are well correlated with atrial pressure, thereby providing a good marker of blood volume status. Although BNP was first isolated from the brain, only small amounts of BNP are detected in the brain in humans and rodents.

Synthesis and secretion of ANP and BNP are markedly augmented in animal models of ventricular hypertrophy and in patients with congestive heart failure (CHF) in accordance with the severity, in which ventricular production of ANP as well as BNP is significantly enhanced. In humans, elevation of BNP becomes more prominent than ANP in relation to the severity of heart failure. Therefore, the plasma BNP level is now the most reliable biochemical marker for left ventricular dysfunction. In addition, plasma BNP levels are markedly increased in the early phase of acute myocardial infarction, when plasma ANP is increased only slightly.

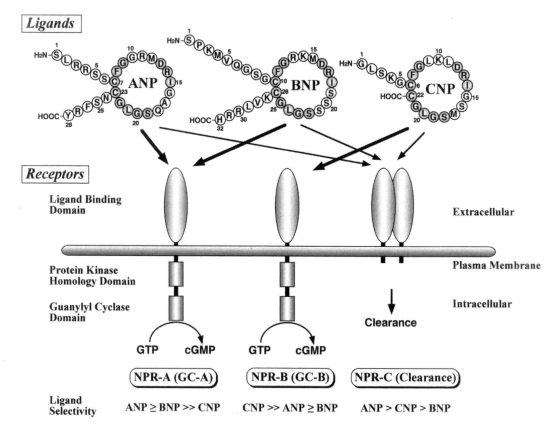

Fig. 4. Natriuretic peptide system.

It is also shown that a sustained increase in plasma BNP is associated with decreased ventricular contractility, increased stiffness, and poor prognosis. These observations suggest that BNP plays an important role in ventricular remodeling.

ANP and BNP activate a common guanylyl cyclase (GC)–coupled receptor subtype, NPR-A or GC-A, that is expressed in a wide variety of tissues. The main distribution of GC-A includes the kidney, blood vessels, heart, lung, adrenal, and brain. Human urine contains another peptide called urodilatin, an N-terminally extended form of ANP by four amino acids, which is synthesized in the kidney and secreted into the tubular lumen. A functional significance of urodilatin is still unclear, but it may act as a local regulator of tubular reabsorption in the distal nephron.

4.1.2. CNP as a Local Hormone

CNP, a 22-amino-acid peptide, is the third member of the natriuretic peptide family with a highly conserved ring structure, but uniquely it lacks the C-terminal extension. The precursor structure of CNP is well preserved among species, and the concentrations of CNP are much higher than those of ANP and BNP in the brain, indicating the significance of CNP as a neuropeptide. CNP is found in the cerebral cortex, brain stem, cerebellum, basal ganglia, and hypothalamus. Furthermore, CNP is expressed in a variety of peripheral tissues, including vascular endothelium, kidney tubules and glomeruli, adrenal gland, thymus, uterus, and macrophages. Endothelial production of CNP represents a potent peptide-type endothelium-derived relaxing factor. Vascular CNP expression may be induced in pathologic states such as septic shock and in injured tissues during vascular remodeling. Notably, CNP and its receptor, NPR-B or GC-B, are abundantly expressed in the chondrocytes in the growth plate of the bone. Transgenic and knockout approaches now reveal that the CNP/GC-B system is an essential regulator of endochondral bone growth.

4.2. Natriuretic Peptide Receptors

The natriuretic peptide family elicits most of its biologic actions by the activation of particulate GC. Three classes of NPRs have been identified (Fig. 4), two of which are the monomeric 130-kDa protein initially designated as the biologically active receptor, containing GC-A and GC-B. The other type of receptor not coupled

tissue kallikrein (24–44 kDa), found principally in the kidney and in the exocrine and endocrine glands such as salivary gland and pancreas, cleaves both low molecular weight and high molecular weight kininogens to release Lys-bradykinin (Fig. 5). The tissue kallikrein gene family comprises a large number of closely related genes. The sizes of this gene family vary among species, up to 20 genes in the rat, 24 in the mouse, and 3 in the human. These members exhibit high sequence homology, suggesting that they share a common ancestral gene.

6.2. Kinin Receptors and Their Function

Kinins act on two receptors, B_1 and B_2 receptors, which differ in tissue distribution, regulation, pharmacologic properties, and biologic activities. The B_2 receptor has a high affinity to bradykinin and Lys-bradykinin, whereas the B_1 receptor is selectively activated by des-Arg^9-bradykinin or des-Arg^{10}-kallidin. These receptors belong to a seven-transmembrane-domain, G protein–coupled receptor superfamily. On stimulation, both B_1 and B_2 receptors lead to activation of PLC with inositol phosphate generation and calcium mobilization. The B_2 receptor gene contains three exons and two introns; the third exon encodes a whole receptor protein of 364 amino acids, which shows 36% amino acid identity with the B_1 receptor. The promoter region of the B_2 receptor gene contains consensus interleukin-6 (IL-6) and cAMP-responsive elements. The B_1 receptor is generally not expressed in normal conditions but appears in pathologic states such as administration of lipopolysaccharide, inflammation, and injury. The B_2 receptor, on the other hand, is widely distributed in many tissues including the kidney, heart, lung, brain, and testis. Therefore, in normal conditions, most of the physiologic effects of kinins are mediated by the B_2 receptor.

Kinins have prominent effects in the cardiovascular, pulmonary, gastrointestinal (GI), and reproductive systems. Kinins, via the B_2 receptor, appear to play an important role in the regulation of local blood flow. In the vasculature, kinins induce vasodilatation with release of various mediators, such as NO, PGs, platelet-activating factor, leukotrienes, and cytokines, and may be involved in vasodilatation and edema formation observed during inflammation. Kinins induce smooth muscle contraction in the GI tract, uterus and bronchioles. The B_2 receptor is also likely to be involved in renal salt handling and in blood pressure regulation in individuals consuming a high-sodium diet. The B_1 receptor may be implicated in the chronic inflammatory and pain-producing responses to kinins, but studies are still needed to clarify their functional significance.

6.3. Renal Kallikrein-Kinin System

Tissue kallikrein is synthesized in the kidney and excreted in urine. Filtered kinins, which are active on the glomerular vasculature, would not be found downstream in the nephron because of the high activity of kininases in the proximal tubule. Renal kallikrein has been localized by immunohistochemical techniques to the distal nephron segments, mostly in the connecting tubule. Kinin receptors are present in the collecting duct. Therefore, a paracrine role for the renal kallikrein-kinin system near the site of action has been proposed to explain the importance of this system. In addition, kinins generated in the cortical distal nephron segments may act on the glomerular vasculature, because the sites are in close association with the glomerular tuft.

Pharmacologic evidence shows that kinins play an important role in the regulation of renal microcirculation and water and sodium excretion. Renal actions of kinins involve glomerular and tubular actions. Bradykinin dilates both afferent and efferent arterioles and can increase renal blood flow without significant changes in glomerular filtration rate, but with a marked increase in fluid delivery to the distal nephron. It appears that natriuresis and diuresis are the result of an effect of kinins on renal papillary blood flow, which inhibits sodium reabsorption. Kinins also inhibit vasopressin-stimulated water permeability and sodium transport in the cortical collecting duct. Because the effect of bradykinin is greatly attenuated by cyclooxygenase inhibition, the natriuretic and diuretic actions of kinins may be mediated mostly, or at least partly, by PGs.

6.4. Pathophysiology of the Kallikrein-Kinin System

Decreased activity of the kallikrein-kinin system may play a role in hypertension. The urinary excretion of kallikrein is significantly reduced in patients with hypertension or in children with a family history of essential hypertension, and the urinary kallikrein levels are inversely correlated with blood pressure. Reduced urinary kallikrein excretion has also been described in various models of genetic hypertension. A restriction fragment length polymorphism for the kallikrein gene family in spontaneously hypertensive rats has been linked to high blood pressure. Collectively, these findings suggest that genetic factors causing a decrease in renal kallikrein activity might contribute to the pathogenesis of hypertension.

Endogenous kinins clearly affect renal hemodynamics and excretory function. This notion is supported by studies using kininogen-deficient Brown Norway rats, which show a brisk hypertensive response to a high-sodium diet. Furthermore, B_2 receptor knockout mice have provided more definitive data supporting the conclusion that kinins can play an important role in preventing salt-sensitive hypertension.

Increased tissue concentrations of kinins and potentiation of their effect may be involved in the therapeutic effects of ACE inhibitors. This hypothesis is supported by the finding that a kinin antagonist partially blocks the acute hypotensive effects of ACE inhibitors. Moreover, beneficial effects on the heart and kidney by ACE inhibition are significantly attenuated or reversed by treating with the kinin antagonist, or in mice lacking the B_2 receptor and kininogen-deficient rats. These data strongly suggest a potential role of kinins in mediating part of the cardioprotective and renoprotective effects exerted by treatment with ACE inhibitors.

7. ADRENOMEDULLIN AND ENDOTHELINS
7.1. Adrenomedullin

AM is a potent vasorelaxing peptide with 52 amino acids that is isolated from the adrenal medulla and shares structural homology with calcitonin gene–related peptide. The preproadrenomedullin gene encodes two active peptides, AM and proadrenomedullin N-terminal 20 peptide (PAMP), which are generated by post-translational processing of the same gene. AM is produced primarily in the vasculature; is released as an endothelium-derived relaxing factor; and is also expressed in the adrenal medulla, brain, heart, and kidney. AM exerts its effects via activation of cAMP production and nitric oxide synthesis. PAMP, on the other hand, does not activate cAMP or NO synthesis and exerts its vasodilatory effects via presynaptic inhibition of sympathetic nerves innervating blood vessels. AM receptors are composed of two components, a seven-transmembrane calcitonin receptor-like receptor and a single-transmembrane receptor–activity-modifying protein, whereas PAMP receptors remain elusive and are yet to be cloned. AM has potent diuretic and natriuretic actions, and AM and PAMP also inhibit aldosterone secretion. Thus, the AM gene encodes two distinct peptides with shared biologic activity, but unique mechanisms of action.

AM increases renal blood flow and has tubular effects to stimulate sodium and water excretion. AM also has a potent inhibitory effect on proliferation of fibroblasts, mesangial cells, and vascular smooth muscle cells. In addition, experiments of AM infusion and AM gene delivery have shown that it has a potent vasodilatory and antifibrotic property, resulting in cardiovascular and renal protective effects. Furthermore, AM exerts a potent angiogenic activity, as demonstrated by AM-deficient mice that exhibit a profound defect in fetal and placental vascular development, leading to embryonic death. In humans, plasma concentrations of AM are elevated in various cardiovascular disorders including CHF, hypertension, and renal failure, which may represent a compensatory role of AM in these disorders. Furthermore, preliminary clinical studies have revealed that the administration of AM causes beneficial effects on CHF and pulmonary hypertension, suggesting the possibility of potential clinical usefulness of AM in such diseases.

7.2. ET Family

The vascular endothelium is able to modulate the vascular tone in response to various mechanical and chemical stimuli, and such modulation is achieved, at least partly, by endothelium-derived humoral factors, relaxing factors and constricting factors. ET was isolated as an endothelium-derived constricting peptide with 21 amino acids that is the most potent endogenous vasoconstrictor yet identified. The first peptide identified is called ET-1, and the ET family now consists of three isoforms, ET-1, ET-2, and ET-3, acting on two receptors, ET_A and ET_B. ET-1 is the primary peptide secreted from the endothelium and detected in plasma, and its mRNA is also expressed in the brain, kidney, lung, uterus, and placenta. Endothelial ET-1 production is stimulated by shear stress, hypoxia, Ang II, vasopressin, thrombin, catecholamines, and growth factors and inhibited by CNP and AM. ET-2 is produced in the kidney and jejunum, and ET-3 is identified in the intestine, adrenal, brain, and kidney. The ET_A receptor is relatively specific to ET-1, whereas the ET_B receptor has an equal affinity to three isoforms. Both receptors are coupled to G proteins, leading to activation of PLC with inositol phosphate generation and calcium mobilization.

Plasma ET-1 concentrations are elevated in renal failure, acute myocardial infarction, atypical angina, essential hypertension, and subarachnoid hemorrhage. ET-1 exerts a positive inotropic action and potent vasoconstriction (coronary, pulmonary, renal, and systemic vasculature) as well as vascular and cardiac hypertrophy. An important synergism exists between ET-1 and Ang II, especially in the heart during cardiac hypertrophy, which is counteracted by ANP and BNP. Pharmacologic blockade of ET receptors has been effective in some forms of experimental hypertension and heart failure, and the nonselective antagonist bosentan has been approved for treatment of primary pulmonary hypertension. In the kidney, the receptors are mainly present in the blood vessels and mesangial cells.

Although these are predominantly the ET_A subtype, the ET_B receptor may have pathophysiologic significance, particularly in the distal tubules, where ET_B receptor activation causes sodium excretion. Involvement of renal ET_B receptor in sodium-sensitive hypertension remains to be clarified. Furthermore, gene knockout approaches have revealed that the ET system plays an essential role during development; the ET-1/ET_A system is crucial in branchial arch development and cardiac septum formation, whose mutation causes mandibulofacial and cardiac abnormalities. By contrast, the ET-3/ET_B system is essential for migration of neural crest cells (melancytes and neurons of the myenteric plexus), whose mutation results in aganglionic megacolon (Hirschsprung disease) and vitiligo.

8. ERYTHROPOIETIN

The kidney is the primary organ responsible for regulating the production of the protein hormone EPO, in response to perceived changes in oxygen pressure. A number of experimental and clinical studies have demonstrated an essential role of the kidney in erythropoiesis, including the development of severe anemia by renal ablation, and in renal failure patients. EPO is a glycosylated protein composed of 165 amino acids with a relative molecular mass of 34 kDa. Plasma concentrations of EPO normally range from 8 to 18 mU/mL and may increase 100- to 1000-fold in anemia. EPO mRNA levels are highly sensitive to changes in tissue oxygenation, and, therefore, its synthesis is regulated primarily at the level of gene transcription.

The site of EPO production in the kidney is now shown to be the interstitial cells of the renal cortex, around the base of the proximal tubule. Oxygen deficiency is sensed effectively by the "oxygen sensor" in these cells. Reduced capillary blood flow may also induce the increased production of EPO. Studies on the EPO gene have shown that its production in response to hypoxia is induced by a transcription factor, hypoxia-inducible factor-1.

Erythropoiesis begins when the pluripotent stem cells in the bone marrow are stimulated by nonspecific cytokines, such as IL-3 and granulocyte-macrophage colony-stimulating factor, to proliferate and transform into the erythroid-committed progenitor cells. EPO then acts on these early progenitor cells bearing its receptor to expand and differentiate into colony-forming unit-erythroid (CFU-E). EPO further continues to stimulate CFU-E to erythroid precursors, which eventually reach the stage of mature RBCs. CFU-E is the key target cell for EPO, which indeed regulates RBC production.

Anemia can develop relatively early in the course of chronic renal failure, which is referred to as renal anemia. The impairment of EPO production appears to parallel the progressive reduction of functional nephron mass, and plasma EPO levels are relatively very low for the degree of severity of anemia in these patients. Recombinant human EPO can potently reverse anemia in such states, and its administration has now widely been performed routinely for correcting anemia in hemodialysis and peritoneal dialysis patients, as well as in patients with moderate renal impairment.

SELECTED READINGS

Cambien F, Poirier O, Lacerf L, et al. Deletion polymorphism in the gene for angiotensin-converting enzyme is a potent risk factor for myocardial infarction. *Nature* 1992;359:641–644.

Candido R, Burrell LM, Jandeleit-Dahm KA, et al.. Vasoactive peptides and the kidney. In: Brenner BM, ed. *The Kidney*, 7th Ed., vol. 1. Philadelphia, PA: W. B. Saunders 2004:663–726.

Chao J, Chao L. New experimental evidence for a role of tissue kallikrein in hypertension. *Nephrol Dial Transplant* 1997;12: 1569– 1574.

Chusho H, Tamura N, Ogawa Y, et al. Dwarfism and early death in mice lacking C-type natriuretic peptide. *Proc Natl Acad Sci USA* 2001;98:4016–4021.

Drewett JG, Garbers DL. The family of guanylyl cyclase receptors and their ligands. *Endocr Rev* 1994;15:135–162.

Dzau VJ. Circulating versus local renin-angiotensin system in cardiovascular homeostasis. *Circulation* 1988;77:I-4–I-13.

Horiuchi M, Akishita M, Dzau VJ. Recent progress in angiotensin II type 2 receptor research in the cardiovascular system. *Hypertension* 1999;33:613–621.

Inagami T. Molecular biology and signaling of angiotensin receptors: an overview. *J Am Soc Nephrol* 1999;10(Suppl 11):S2–S7.

John SW, Krege JH, Oliver PM, et al. Genetic decreases in atrial natriuretic peptide and salt-sensitive hypertension. *Science* 1995; 267:679–681.

Kitamura K, Kangawa K, Kawamoto M, et al. Adrenomedullin: a novel hypotensive peptide isolated from human pheochromocytoma. *Biochem Biophys Res Commun* 1993;192:553–560.

Lifton RP, Gharavi AG, Geller DS. Molecular mechanisms of human hypertension. *Cell* 2001;104:545–556.

Lopez MJ, Wong SKF, Kishimoto I, et al. Salt-resistant hypertension in mice lacking the guanylyl cyclase-A receptor for atrial natriuretic peptide. *Nature* 1995;378:65–68.

Mukoyama M, Nakao K, Hosoda K, et al. Brain natriuretic peptide as a novel cardiac hormone in humans: evidence for an exquisite dual natriuretic peptide system, atrial natriuretic peptide and brain natriuretic peptide. *J Clin Invest* 1991;87:1402–1412.

Nakao K, Ogawa Y, Suga S, Imura H. Molecular biology and biochemistry of the natriuretic peptide system. I: Natriuretic peptides. *J Hypertens* 1992;10:907–912.

Suganami T, Mukoyama M, Sugawara A, et al. Overexpression of brain natriuretic peptide in mice ameliorates immune-mediated renal injury. *J Am Soc Nephrol* 2001;12:2652–2663.

Takahashi N, Smithies O. Gene targeting approaches to analyzing hypertension. *J Am Soc Nephrol* 1999;10:1598–1605.

Tamura N, Ogawa Y, Chusho H, et al. Cardiac fibrosis in mice lacking brain natriuretic peptide. *Proc Natl Acad Sci USA* 2000; 97:4239–4244.

Yanagisawa M, Kurihara H, Kimura S, et al. A novel potent vasoconstrictor peptide produced by vascular endothelial cells. *Nature* 1988;332:411–415.

24 Reproduction and Fertility

Neena B. Schwartz, PhD

1. INTRODUCTION

The crucial participation of hormones in reproduction and fertility is the most complicated story in endocrinology, because it involves several organ systems; gametes as well as hormones; two classes of receptors and intracellular signals; and a myriad of environmental factors such as seasonal signals and, of course, the nearby presence of a conspecific carrier of the opposite gamete type. As complicated as this system is in mammals, being quite different among major classes, it is even more complex when one deals with the vast number of nonmammalian vertebrate species. In a marvelous recent review, Rothchild discussed the evolution of placental mammals from other vertebrates. This chapter is limited to two mammals: the rat, which has been the species of choice for elucidating basic science, and the primate, which is obviously of major interest in dealing with clinical issues. The rat runs a 4- or 5-day estrous cycle, from the onset of follicular growth under the influence of follicle-stimulating hormone (FSH), to ovulation following an luteinizing hormone (LH) surge.

From: *Endocrinology: Basic and Clinical Principles, Second Edition*
(S. Melmed and P. M. Conn, eds.) © Humana Press Inc., Totowa, NJ

If mating does not occur, this cycle is repeated and mature corpora lutea do not form. Primates run a 28-d menstrual cycle, which includes an active progesterone-secreting luteal phase.

Figure 1 is an illustration summarizing the current understanding of the organs and hormones involved in regulating reproduction in male and female mammals. Numbers in the figure are cited in the text in parenthesis. The left side of Fig. 1 represents the components of the system in the female mammal; the right side shows the analogous components in the male.

2. GONADS AND ACCESSORIES

The gonads are characterized by the presence of the germ cells, their accompanying "nurse cells," and cells that secrete sex-specific steroids into the circulation (*see* Table 1). Steroid receptors are intracellular, and when the steroid ligand binds the specific receptor in the target organ, within either the cytosol or nucleus, the combined entity (transcription factor) binds to specific nuclear DNA and causes transcription of target genes. Both the ovaries and testes are totally dependent on two peptide hormones secreted by the gonadotrope cells

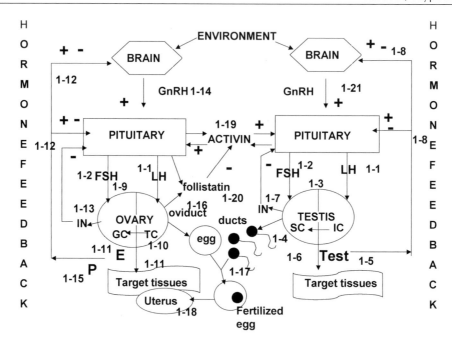

Fig. 1. Illustration summarizing reproductive system in male and female mammals. E = estrogen; P = progesterone; Test = testosterone; LH = luteinizing hormone; FSH = follicle-stimulating hormone; GnRH = gonadotropin-releasing hormone; GC = granulosa cells; TC = thecal cells; SC = Sertoli cells; IC = interstitial cells; In = inhibin.

Table 1
Gonadal Cell Types

	Testis	*Ovary*
Nurse cells	Sertoli cells	Granulosa cells
Gamete	Sperm; renewing	Ova; maximum number fixed at birth
Steroid-secreting cells	Interstitial cells (hormone: testosterone)	Granulosa cells (hormone: estradiol)
	Sertoli cells (hormone: estradiol)	Thecal cells (hormone: testosterone)
		Corpus luteum cells (hormone: progesterone)

within the anterior pituitary gland: LH (1-1) and FSH (1-2). Specific receptors for these hormones are found within gonadal cell membranes; these receptors are of the seven-transmembrane loop variety, requiring intracellular second messengers to transmit signals to the cell nucleus.

2.1. Testis (1-3)

In the adult male, spermatogenesis is continuous, except in seasonal breeders, with a dividing population of spermatogonia. It takes 40 d in the rat and 70 d in humans for a diploid spermatogonium to become four mature haploid spermatozoa, ready to leave the tubule and move into the epididymis, where they are stored and become mature (1-4). Sertoli cells, the "nurse" cells for future sperm, possess FSH receptors and can aromatize testosterone to estradiol. Testosterone is synthesized and

secreted by the interstitial cells of the testis (1-5), which are found outside the spermatic tubules in close proximity to blood vessels, which empty into the spermatic veins, then carrying blood back to the heart. FSH is necessary for the normal functioning of Sertoli cells; in the absence of FSH, even if LH is present, spermatogenesis does not proceed normally. Spermatogenesis also depends on local high levels of testosterone diffusing from the interstitial cells (1-6). Interstitial cells have LH receptors on their cell membranes and secrete testosterone only when LH is present. Sertoli cells also synthesize and secrete a peptide hormone called inhibin (1-7), which can downregulate FSH synthesis and secretion by pituitary gonadotropes. Testosterone (1-8), acting at the hypothalamus and in the gonadotrope, can suppress LH secretion and, in some cases, increase FSH synthesis and secretion.

Table 2
Factors Altering Relative LH and FSH Secretion

Increase FSH/LH	Increase LH/FSH
Low-frequency GnRH	High-frequency GnRH
Low number of GnRH receptors	High number of GnRH receptors
GnRH antagonists	Removal of ovaries
Low inhibin	Removal of testes
High activin	
Low follistatin	
Increased progesterone	
Increased glucocorticoids	
Increased testosterone	

2.2. Ovary (1-9)

Oogenesis stops in mammals before birth, when the oocytes enter the first phase of meiosis. Most oocytes undergo apoptosis ("atresia") and die between the prenatal meiotic event and adulthood. The oocytes are encased within the follicles, where they are surrounded by granulosa cells; the outer layer of the follicle consists of thecal cells (1-10). Granulosa cells initially express only FSH receptors and the thecal cells express LH receptors. Meiosis resumes in surviving mature oocytes only after the LH preovulatory surge occurs during adult cycles.

Within a given cycle in adults, follicular maturation occurs in a stepwise fashion. Once cycles begin at puberty, a surviving follicle (or follicles, in multiovulatory species such as the rat) starts to grow, as the granulosa cells divide under the influence of FSH. The thecal cells, under the influence of LH, start to synthesize and secrete testosterone locally (1-10). The testosterone diffuses into the granulose cell layers and is converted into estradiol by the aromatase enzyme in the granulosa cell. As the granulosa cells continue to divide, estradiol secretion into the bloodstream occurs, and estradiol (1-11) begins to act on target tissues and to exert negative feedback on the pituitary and hypothalamus (1-12). Inhibin secretion from granulosa cells also occurs (1-13), and FSH levels fall. The granulosa cells gradually develop LH receptors. Rising levels of estradiol abruptly initiate a rapid rise in gonadotropin-releasing hormone (GnRH) secretion from the hypothalamus (1-14), which causes the preovulatory surges of LH and FSH. After the preovulatory surge of LH occurs, a series of molecular events ensue in the ovary that lead to suppression of estradiol and inhibin secretion, stimulation of progesterone secretion (1-15), and dispersal of the granulosa cells surrounding the ovum. The ovum then completes the first stage of meiosis, throws off the first polar body, and is extruded from the follicle (1-16) into the oviduct. If sperm are present fertilization may occur (1-17) and the second polar body is cast off, leaving the fertilized diploid egg; if the uterine environment is favorable, owing to proper action of estradiol and progesterone, implantation of the growing blastocyst occurs in the uterine lining (1-18) after about 4 to 5 d in the oviduct.

3. BRAIN AND PITUITARY

The brain and the anterior pituitary gland are linked, with respect to reproduction, by the secretion of a peptide, GnRH, from the hypothalamus (1-14, 1-21) and the presence of GnRH receptors on the cell membranes of the gonadotrope cells. LH and FSH are dimeric proteins, which share a common α-subunit but have different β-subunits, and the entire molecules are recognized by different specific receptors on the cell membranes of the gonads. A pulsatile secretion of GnRH is necessary for continuation of secretion by the gonadotrope cells. Cell lines of GnRH neurons (Gt1 cells) in culture show spontaneous pulses at a frequency of about one per hour. Although GnRH pulses cause secretion of both LH and FSH, differing ratios of the two hormones can be secreted under the influence of alterations in GnRH receptor levels, pulse frequency, and amplitude (Table 2). The GnRH-secreting neurons are found in the arcuate nucleus of the hypothalamus, and GnRH is secreted directly into a portal system that bathes the anterior pituitary cells. LH is more dependent on GnRH than FSH is: increases in GnRH amplitude or frequency enhance LH secretion more than FSH, and GnRH antagonists lower LH more than FSH. The greater the number of GnRH receptors on gonadotropes, the more LH secretion is favored over FSH.

GnRH receptors (two kinds) are of the seven transmembrane domains and are found in the membranes of the gonadotropes. Most gonadotrope cells synthesize and contain both LH and FSH, although the ratio of the hormones within the cells and their distribution across the pituitary varies during the cycle, with maximal levels found just before the LH surge. The second-messenger system transducing the GnRH signal to the gonadotrope is highly complex; it involves the mitogen-activated protein kinase pathway and calcium mobilization. Targets of GnRH activation of its receptor are the genes for the α- and β-subunits of the gonadotropins and the GnRH receptor gene itself.

Progesterone (1-15), testosterone (1-5), and glucocorticoids enhance FSH synthesis when applied directly to pituitaries in culture or in vivo (Table 2). There are also three peptides that are of crucial importance in regulating FSH synthesis and secretion by the pituitary (Table 2). Inhibin is a heterodimer related to the transforming growth factor-β (TGF-β) family and is secreted by the ovarian follicles or Sertoli cells, specifically inhibiting FSH synthesis and secretion directly (1-7, 1-13) in the gonadotrope. Activin is a dimer of the inhibin α-subunit. Activin stimulates FSH synthesis and secretion; activin is made locally in the pituitary gland and is probably as important as GnRH, if not more important, in stimulation of FSH secretion (1-19). The third peptide is follistatin (1-20), which is not homologous to the TGF-β family. It is made in both the ovary and the pituitary gland and acts as an inhibitory binding protein for activin. Follistatin blocks the stimulation of FSH synthesis and secretion from activin, and also from progesterone, testosterone, and glucocorticoids. This suggests that the steroids act on FSH production via stimulation of activin.

Hormonal feedback from gonadal steroids acts at both hypothalamic and pituitary levels (1-8, 1-12) and is primarily negative in nature because removal of the gonads increases GnRH and LH and FSH secretion. The stimulation by estrogen of the preovulatory surges in female mammals is usually labeled "positive" feedback, although if ovulation occurs, ovarian secretion is lowered as the follicle switches to a corpus luteum, thereby dropping estrogen secretion and favoring progesterone secretion.

GnRH secretion (1-14, 1-21) is regulated by many stimulatory and inhibitory neuromodulators released from interneuron synapses acting at the GnRH neurons. Excitatory inputs include norepinephrine and glutamate (L-glutamic acid), which is the major stimulatory agonist in the hypothalamus. Neuropeptide Y stimulates GnRH release, as well as the action of GnRH in releasing LH from the pituitary, in animals previously exposed to estrogen. γ-Amino- butyric acid is probably the major inhibitory input to the GnRH neurons. Opioids are also inhibitors of GnRH release. Because GnRH neurons *in situ* do not contain steroid receptors, steroids probably act on GnRH release frequency and amplitude by acting on interneurons.

4. ONTOGENETIC DEVELOPMENT OF REPRODUCTIVE ABILITY

In the early embryo, a set of primordial germ cells formed in the placental membranes migrates to the urogenital ridge, inducing gonad formation with a somatic contribution from the local epithelium. The Y chromosome contains a gene, *sry* (sex-determining region of the Y chromosome), which codes for a transcription factor that induces formation of Sertoli cells. In the absence of the sry gene, the somatic supporting cell precursors become follicle cells and proceed toward ovarian development. A number of other genes must also be expressed in order for the formation of normal testis and ovary to take place. Müllerian-inhibiting substance (MIS) is secreted by the testis early and diffuses to the locally forming duct systems; MIS kills the cells of the Müllerian duct, which would have formed into oviduct/uterus. In female embryos, this duct system survives but the Wolffian duct system, which is destined to develop into the male accessory ducts, does not survive because it depends on testosterone secretion. Testosterone secretion from the developing testis induces masculinization of the external genitalia. These incipient genitalia cells must convert the testosterone into dihydrotestosterone by means of the enzyme α-5-reductase for this masculinizing of the genitalia to take place. For normal female ovarian, duct, and genitalia differentiation to take place, both X chromosomes must be present, and a number of ovarian genes must be expressed.

Normal anterior pituitary gland and hypothalamic differentiation is also necessary for reproduction to develop normally in both male and female genotypes. The cells that secrete GnRH in the mature individual actually are derived embryologically from cells in the olfactory region and migrate during brain development to the hypothalamus. Two "orphan" nuclear receptors (SF1 and DAX1) that appear throughout the hypothalamus, gonadotropes, gonads, and adrenals are heavily involved with normal gonadal differentiation and function in both sexes.

Newborn animals are sexually immature. Puberty occurs when the central drive for GnRH secretion kicks in, and the threshold for negative feedback of gonadal hormones increases. Premature puberty in human males is usually associated with central nervous system malfunction. Reproductive menopause occurs in females when the supply of oocytes remaining in the ovaries becomes inadequate to secrete sufficient estrogen to trigger LH surges. In males, testosterone levels drop with aging, but generally reproduction is attenuated later than in females.

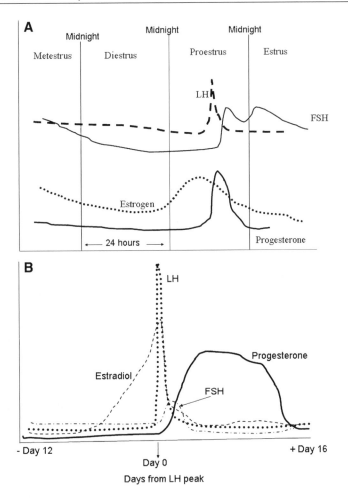

Fig. 2. Time course of changes in estrogen, progesterone, LH, and FSH during rat and primate nonpregnant cycle: (**A**) rat estrous cycle. (**B**) Primate menstrual cycle.

5. ENVIRONMENT

The connection of the reproductive system to the brain via GnRH provides the conduit whereby the environment provides input to the system. For mammals, there is a value for birth to occur in the spring, when food supplies are most plentiful. Sheep ovulate and mate in the fall, as the ratio of dark to light increases, and with the long gestation period give birth in the spring. Small rodents, by contrast, with a 20-d gestation period, mate and ovulate in the spring, when the light/dark ratio is increasing. For some species near the equator, because the hours of light and dark remain equal throughout the year, rainfall rather than light may serve as a seasonal signal.

Other species, such as the domestic cat, the rabbit, and the camel, are coitus-induced ovulators. In these species, estradiol stimulates mating behavior, and the cervical stimulus received during coitus triggers a neural reflex that causes a large release of GnRH. This triggers a preovulatory surge of LH that causes ovulation.

6. CYCLICITY: WHAT MAKES THE SYSTEM CYCLE IN FEMALES?

Figure 2 illustrates the changes in the pituitary and ovarian hormones during the nonpregnant rat and primate cycles. The female rat (Fig. 2A) and primate (Fig. 2B) manifest repetitive cycles because the rising levels of estrogen stimulated by background levels of LH and FSH cause the release of a burst of GnRH, which causes the abrupt increase in LH (and FSH) release. These preovulatory surges of LH and of FSH not only cause resumption of meiosis in the most mature follicle(s), but also a cascade of enzymatic changes within the granulosa cells, which terminate estradiol secretion. The resultant corpus luteum begins secreting progesterone. (By contrast, in the male mammal, testosterone and LH levels are maintained at steady levels from day to day, except for the oscillations in both that track GnRH pulses.)

There are two principal operational differences between the rodent and primate cycles. The first is that the rodent cycle is tightly tied to the daily light-dark timing. Not only is the rising estrogen level in the blood a necessary signal for the GnRH release that precedes the LH surge, but there is also a daily circadian signal that occurs between 2:00 PM and 4:00 PM in rats kept in a room lighted from 5:00 AM to 7:00 PM. This neural signal acts in conjunction with the estrogen to closely time the LH/FSH release (Fig. 2A). There is no evidence that such a circadian signal operates with estrogen in the primate. The second difference between the rodent and the primate has to do with the luteal phase. In the rat, mouse, and hamster, there is no spontaneous luteal phase analogous to that in the primate following ovulation. In the primate, the LH surge that triggers ovulation is also adequate to maintain progesterone secretion from the corpus luteum, until placental secretion takes over. In the rat, if pregnancy does not occur, blood levels of both estradiol and progesterone remain low; the resulting absence of steroidal negative feedback (1-12) permits FSH and LH to rise. The prolonged FSH secretion in the rodent cycle ("secondary FSH surge") (Fig. 2A) occurs because inhibin secretion by the ovary is terminated by the LH surge; this elevated FSH initiates the growth of the next crop of follicles. However, in the presence of a male, the precedent estrogen secretion followed by the brief proestrous progesterone surge induces sexual receptivity in the female late in the afternoon and mating occurs. The stimulation of the cervix by mating turns on twice daily surges of prolactin in the female, which maintain the progesterone secretion for 12 d or so, permitting implantation. Pregnancy occurs when a developing embryo implants into the lining of the uterus, prepared by the preceding estrogen and progesterone secretion. In the primate, the corpus luteum formed after the LH surge secretes progesterone spontaneously for about 12 d. For pregnancy to continue, the corpus luteum needs to continue secreting progesterone for about 14 d in the rat and 2 mo in the primate. This steroid is critical for suppressing uterine contractions. Once the embryo is securely implanted in the uterine lining (1-18), the placenta (part maternal, part embryonic) secretes the chorionic gonadotropin necessary to maintain the corpus luteum and eventually also secretes the steroids necessary for maintenance of the pregnancy and the onset of lactation.

7. CONTRACEPTION

The population of our planet continues to grow exponentially, threatening the environment and outpacing food and water supplies. An understanding of the linkages in Fig. 1 is crucial to the design of contraceptives. The oral contraceptive pill, used by vast numbers of females worldwide, is predominantly progesterone-like, and suppresses GnRH, FSH, and LH secretion (1-8), so that ovulation does not occur (1-12). Depoprovera is a progestin implant that frees females from having to ingest pills on a daily basis. Testosterone implants have been tested in males as a contraceptive; the high levels of testosterone suppress GnRH, LH, and FSH secretion, thus suppressing spermatogenesis, without depriving the recipient of testosterone necessary for libido and potency (1-8). Condoms block the gametes from meeting and have the advantage of detering the spread of sexually transmitted diseases. In the age of acquired immunodeficiency syndrome and relative sexual freedom, this advantage is extremely important. Tying of the oviducts (1-16) in females or of the vas deferens (1-4) in males, obviously, prevents the gametes from meeting. These simple methods have the advantage of a brief surgery and no drugs with possibly harmful side effects. They are popular in older, stable couples who have completed their families. However, they must be regarded as irreversible, at present. The intrauterine device is a loop that is inserted into the uterus. It alters the uterine luminal environment (1-18) such that implantation cannot take place normally. Antisera to LH or FSH (1-1, 1-2) have been tested in animals and in some human studies; questions of reversibility, side effects, and efficacy are still unsettled. GnRH antagonists have been tested in men as a contraceptive. Because they reduce LH and FSH (1-21), they also reduce testosterone secretion so potency falls; if they are to be useful they must be accompanied by testosterone.

In females, the "morning after pill," an estrogen analog, diethylstilbestrol, can prevent pregnancy from occurring after unprotected sex, apparently by rendering the oviductal environment unsuitable for fertilization or survival of the fertilized egg. RU486, an antagonist of the progesterone receptor, can be ingested within a couple of weeks of the onset of pregnancy to cause loosening of the implanted embryo. Following RU486, a prostaglandin-like drug is taken, which initiates uterine contraction, thus expelling the embryo.

8. INFERTILITY

If differentiation of the gonads or the tracts does not occur normally, as in the absence of the sry gene responsible for testicular development, or any of the cascade of genes responsible for steroid synthesis, irreversible infertility results. If chromosomal abnormalities such as XO or XXY occur, the resultant inadequate ovary (XO: Turner syndrome) or inadequate testis (XXY: Klinefelter syndrome) will result in infertility. Mutation of steroid receptors or of peptide receptors in target tissue can cause infertility, by preventing gamete maturation, fertilization, or implantation. If the cells that secrete GnRH do not reach the hypothalamus during development, infertility occurs because of "hypogonadotropic hypogonadism" and is detected when puberty does not occur. Fertility can be induced in such patients by implantation of a pump that injects pulses of GnRH into the bloodstream.

Most frequently, infertility occurs in the presence of normal sexual differentiation, because of failure of the female to ovulate or of the male to have viable sperm. The complexity of the system seen in Fig. 1 sometimes makes it difficult to diagnose the specific site of the problem. In females with normal duct morphology, but no spontaneous ovulation, ovulation can be induced by injection of LH or of GnRH. Eggs can be harvested and fertilized in vitro and implanted back into a suitably prepared uterus, or cryopreserved for future use. Artificial insemination by donor sperm can be used by couples when sperm are inadequate in the male. Intracellular sperm injection has also been used when the male partner has inadequate numbers of sperm; a sperm is directly injected into the egg to be fertilized.

9. NEW FRONTIERS IN REPRODUCTION

New technologies have had an impact on reproductive science and practice, just as they have in other areas of biomedical research. However, some of them have been particularly controversial. Molecular biology techniques have enabled the detection of genetic aberrations that cause some infertility. In vitro fertilization has permitted many couples to bear children, but overproduction of ova with induced ovulation can yield multiple fetuses with resultant health problems. Direct fertilization by means of injection of a single sperm into a harvested ovum has been criticized because of developmental abnormalities detected in some fetuses. Genetic testing of embryos *in utero* in order to detect abnormalities has protected some parents from bearing children with extreme abnormalities such as Tay-Sachs disease, but some religious groups oppose the testing. The sex of a child can now be determined noninvasively using ultrasound; in some countries such as India, this technique has permitted abortion of "less desirable" female fetuses, resulting in badly skewed sex proportions, which may have social and political implications as the generation of children matures. Stem cell research offers possible tissue harvesting for treatment of disease, such as of insulin-producing cells, but may be employed to create new individuals by reproductive cloning, opening a Pandora's box of ethical and moral issues. Hormone replacement therapy in postmenopausal women has been seen as a boon for women suffering extreme hot flashes and has been proven to help prevent osteoporosis. However, there may be risk of breast cancer with the treatment. The subject of reproduction and sex is not a neutral subject sociologically or politically, and knowledge of endocrinology *per se* is not the last word on how the science can be applied acceptably to these important areas.

SUGGESTED READINGS

Achermann JC, Ozisik G, Meeks JJ, Jameson LJ. Perspective—genetic causes of human reproductive disease. *J Clin Endocrinol Metab* 2002;87:2447–2454.

Bohnsack BL, Kilen SM, Nho J, Schwartz, NB Follistatin suppresses steroid-enhancing follicle-stimulating hormone release in vitro. *Biol Reprod* 2000;62:636–641.

Clarke AE. *Disciplining Reproduction: Modernity, American Life Sciences and the Problems of Sex.* Berkeley, CA: University of California Press 1998.

Herbison AE. Multimodal influence of estrogen upon gonadotropin-releasing hormone neurons. *Endocr Rev* 1998;19:302–330.

Millar RP. GnRH II and type II GnRH receptors. *Trends Endocrinol Metab* 2002;14:35–43.

Rothchild I. Perspective: the yolkless egg and the evolution of eutherian viviparity. *Biol Reprod* 2003;68:337–357.

Schwartz, NB. Gonadotropins. *Encyclopedia of Neuroscience,* 3rd Ed., CD-Rom version. Adelman, G, Smith BH, eds. Elsevier 2004.

Schwartz NB. Perspective: reproductive endocrinology and human health in the 20th century—a personal retrospective. *Endocrinology* 2001;142:2163–2166.

Tilmann C, Capel B. Cellular and molecular pathways regulating mammalian sex determination. *Recent Prog Horm Res* 2002;57:1–18.

Tsai, MJ, O'Malley BW. Molecular mechanisms of action of steroid/thyroid receptor superfamily members. *Annu Rev Biochem* 1994;63:451–486.

25 Endocrinology of Fat, Metabolism, and Appetite

Rachel L. Batterham, MBBS, PhD
and Michael A. Cowley, PhD

CONTENTS

1. HOMEOSTASIS

An organism's ability to interact with a changing external environment while preserving its own integrity is a critical requirement for life. French scientist Claude Bernard first suggested this concept of homeostasis in the nineteenth century in his studies on the maintenance of stability in the *milieu intérieur*. American physiologist Walter Cannon first coined the term *homeostasis* (derived from the Greek words for "same" and "steady") in the 1930s. He used it to describe "the coordinated physiological processes which maintain most of the steady-states in the organism" and realized that such processes "are so complex and so peculiar to living beings—involving, as they may, the brain and nerves, the heart, lungs, kidneys and spleen, all working coop-

From: *Endocrinology: Basic and Clinical Principles, Second Edition*
(S. Melmed and P. M. Conn, eds.) © Humana Press Inc., Totowa, NJ

eratively —that I have suggested a special designation of these states, homeostasis."

1.1. Regulation of Energy Balance: A Homeostatic Process

The preservation of the internal constancy of the cellular environment needs to be coupled with the dependence of living organisms on external energy sources and the dynamic nature of their life processes. Maintaining an appropriate balance between energy intake and energy expenditure is critical for survival. For example, a sustained negative imbalance between energy intake and expenditure is potentially life-threatening within a relatively short period of time.

There is substantial evidence in mammalian systems that the level of whole-body energy stores is tightly regulated by homeostatic mechanisms. For example, over the course of a decade, an average human consumes approx 10 million kcal but generally this is accompanied by a weight change of only a few kilograms. To accomplish this tight regulation of energy balance, it has been calculated that energy intake must match energy expenditure to within 0.17% over a decade. Much human obesity involves an increase in weight of less than 1 lb of body fat/yr. This corresponds to an energy surplus, or dysregulation, of about 11 calories/d. Randy Seeley has elegantly restated this as a surplus intake of "a potato chip a day" (personal communication, October 24, 2003).

Significant negative energy balance is highly detrimental for an organism, and many pathways and mechanisms have evolved to prevent this from occurring. However, it has become clear that excess energy storage in the form of increased adiposity also has significant adverse effects on mammalian well-being. The current epidemic of obesity in human populations is associated with significant increases in morbidity and mortality. Understanding the mechanisms that regulate energy homeostasis and the nature of any defects in these systems in obese subjects will therefore have significant implications for health care.

The regulation of body weight is a highly complex process with multiple interrelated systems controlling caloric intake, energy expenditure, and fuel metabolism. To maintain energy balance, the organism must assess energy stores within the body; assess the nutrient content of the diet; determine whether the body is in negative energy balance; and adjust hormone levels, energy expenditure, nutrient movement, and feeding behavior in response to these assessments. For example, over the course of a single day the amount of energy ingested can be influenced by a wide range of variables such as food availability and choice as well as by physical, social, economic, and emotional factors. However, despite the short-term variability in energy intake, body fuel stored in the form of adipose tissue remains relatively constant over time, suggesting the existence of precise control mechanisms. Experimental evidence for the existence of adipostatic mechanisms includes observations that manipulations in body fat content induced by such diverse interventions as dieting, behavior modification, surgical removal of fat or experimental overfeeding induce compensatory responses that gradually restore adiposity to baseline levels.

Fifty years ago, Kennedy hypothesized that the biologic system that regulates body adiposity involves humoral signals generated in proportion to body fat stores that act in the brain to alter food intake and energy expenditure. The understanding of the anatomic, neu-

ronal, and molecular components of the central nervous system (CNS) element of this system has progressed rapidly in recent years. Likewise the understanding of the identity and mechanisms of action of humoral signals that act as adiposity signals has increased. These studies have complemented each other and often been interrelated, but for clarity, in this chapter we first will review the anatomic, neuronal, and molecular components of the CNS system focusing on the role of the hypothalamus. Subsequently, we review the role of peripheral humoral factors such as leptin, insulin, and gut peptides in the regulation of energy homeostasis.

2. HYPOTHALAMIC PATHWAYS REGULATING ENERGY HOMEOSTASIS

2.1. Historical Perspective

Brain lesioning and electrical stimulation studies performed more than six decades ago first implicated the hypothalamus as a major center controlling food intake and body weight. Hetherington and Ranson observed that medial hypothalamic lesions within the arcuate hypothalamic (ARH), ventromedial hypothalamic (VMH), paraventricular hypothalamic (PVH), and dorsomedial hypothalamic (DMH) nuclei resulted in uncontrolled hyperphagia and obesity. By contrast, destruction of the lateral hypothalamus resulted in decreased food intake and starvation. From these observations, a model emerged in which the lateral and ventromedial hypothalamic areas were believed to be the brain centers that controlled hunger and satiety, respectively, working in a reciprocal fashion to maintain energy homeostasis. It must be recognized that these were gross manipulations of the central homeostatic circuitry and left many questions unanswered. As researchers have developed tools that enable finer analysis, they have developed models that are more detailed than the "two-center" view of system.

Although this review focuses on the role of the hypothalamus in energy homeostasis, there is a developing body of work that highlights similar effects, at least in the control of short-term energy homeostasis, for the brain stem. One of the evolving challenges in the field will be understanding the contributions of these two sites of signal processing, and how they interact with each other.

2.2. Arcuate Nucleus

The ARH nucleus in the mediobasal hypothalamus, adjacent to the base of the third ventricle, consists of an elongated collection of neuronal cell bodies occupying nearly one-half of the length of the hypothalamus. The ARH nucleus has been implicated in the control of feeding behavior by a number of different approaches. First,

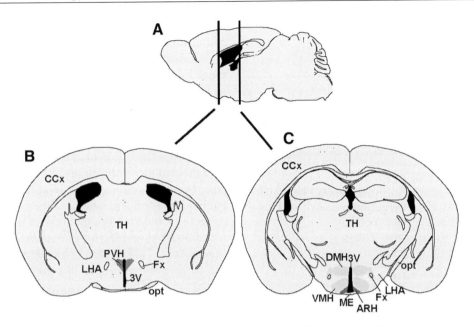

Fig. 1. Main hypothalamic regions involved in the regulation of food intake. (**A**) Longitudinal view of mouse brain, anterior end on left and caudal hindbrain on right. (**B,C**) Cross-sections of brain at two levels (indicated by vertical lines in [A]). One population of first-order neurons is found in the arcuate nucleus (ARH) and project anteriorly to the paraventricular nucleus (PVH), fornix (Fx), and lateral hypothalamic area (LHA). Several other regions are strongly implicated in regulating food intake, including the ventromedial nucleus (VMH) and the dorsomedial nucleus (DMH). 3V = third ventricle; CCx = cerebral cortex; opt = optic tract; TH = thalamus.

the studies on discrete CNS lesions, either experimentally induced in animals or as part of clinical observations in humans, demonstrate that damage to this region results in hyperphagia and obesity. Second, capillaries in the median eminence, which lies below the ARH nucleus, lack tight junctions. Therefore, this region effectively lies outside the blood-brain barrier, and, thus neurons of the ARH nucleus are accessible to circulating hormones and nutrients. Furthermore, nutrients and hormones may also gain access to the ARH nucleus by diffusion across the ependyma from the cerebrospinal fluid (CSF) in the third ventricle. The ARH nucleus is therefore positioned to act as a site of metabolic sensing and to receive and integrate endocrine information about the energy status of the body. Neurons within the ARH nucleus are thought to act as sensors of whole-body energy status and to initiate downstream responses designed to maintain fuel stores at a constant level. It must be acknowledged that there is still some debate about the degree to which neurons in the ARH can sample plasma. The ARH nucleus also has extensive reciprocal connections with other hypothalamic regions, including the PVH nucleus, DMH nucleus, VMH nucleus, and lateral hypothalamus (Fig. 1). However, reciprocal connections with the hindbrain appear to be limited, at least in rodents.

2.3. Paraventricular Hypothalamic Nucleus, Ventromedial Hypothalamus, and Dorsomedial Hypothalamus

The PVH constitutes a dense cluster of heterogeneous neurons, which form a distinct pattern on both sides of the roof of the third ventricle in the anterior hypothalamus (Fig. 1B). The PVH is regarded as a key integrating center; whereby many of the neural pathways that influence energy homeostasis converge onto this nucleus. The PVH controls the secretion of peptides from both the posterior and the anterior pituitary and projects to nuclei with sympathetic or parasympathetic afferents. The VMH is one of the largest nuclei of the hypothalamus and was long considered to be a "satiety center." Stimulation of the VMH has been shown to inhibit feeding, whereas lesions in this region cause overeating and weight gain. The main output of the VMH is to areas that control sympathetic tone. The DMH is located immediately dorsal to the VMH and has extensive connections with other hypothalamic nuclei such as the PVH and the lateral hypothalamus. The DMH also connects to the brain stem and has inputs to the parasympathetic nervous system and the cortico/limbic system, which does not have a direct projection to PVH. The VMH and the lateral hypothalamus have no direct connections but connect indirectly through the DMH and the PVH.

Table 1
**Selection of Hormones, Neurotransmitters,
and Peptides Implicated in Stimulation
or Inhibition of Feeding Behavior** [a]

Increase food intake	Decrease food intake
AgRP	α-MSH
β-endorphin	Amylin
Dynorphin	Bombesin
Galanin	Calcitonin gene–related peptide
Ghrelin	CART
GHRH	CCK
MCH	Ciliary neurotrophic factor
Noradrenaline	Corticotropin-releasing hormone
NPY	GLP-1 (7–36)
Opioids	Glucagon
Orexin-A and –B	Leptin
PYY	Noradrenaline
	Oxyntomodulin
	PP
	PYY$_{3-36}$
	Serotonin
	Somatostatin
	TRH

[a]AgRP = agouti-related peptide; GHRH = growth hormone–releasing hormone; MCH = melanin-concentrating hormone; NPY = neuropeptide Y; PYY = peptide YY; α-MSH = α-melanocyte-stimulating hormone; CCK = cholecystokinin; CART = cocaine- and amphetamine-regulated transcript; GLP-1 (7–36) = glucagon-like peptid-2 (7-36); PP = pancreatic polypeptide; TRH = thyrotropin-releasing hormone.

2.4. Lateral Hypothalamic Area

The lateral hypothalamic area (LHA) is vaguely defined and comprises a large, diffuse population of neurons. The LHA was classically viewed as the "feeding center." Stimulation of this nucleus increases food intake, and destruction of it attenuates feeding and causes weight loss. The LHA has projections both within and outside the hypothalamus and is known to modulate the activity of the parasympathetic nervous system. The lateral hypothalamus also has extensive connections to the higher cortex and to limbic areas and is thus well connected to mediate some of the rewarding and cognitive aspects of energy regulation.

3. NEUROTRANSMITTERS AND NEUROPEPTIDES SYSTEMS

As knowledge of the neuronal networks that regulate energy balance has expanded, the view of functional anatomic centers has been replaced by the concept that discrete neuronal populations underlie such control mechanisms. These neurons express neurotransmitters that mediate particular effects on energy homeostasis and are in turn regulated by specific signals of nutri-

tional state. In the next section, we discuss the neurotransmitter and neuropeptide systems.

Information about nutrient stores, satiety, hunger, and palatability of food is communicated from the periphery to the brain, where it is integrated and translated into appropriate changes in energy balance. These responses are mediated via activation or inhibition of discrete neurotransmitter and neuropeptide signaling pathways expressed in the hypothalamus and other brain regions. A number of these neurotransmitters and neuropeptides have been shown to increase food intake when administered into the CNS, whereas others have been shown to decrease food intake, and some of these peptides and transmitters have differing effects depending on the site of exposure. Table 1 details the peptides implicated in the pathways controlling this complex neuronal circuitry.

Many of these neurotransmitters have been found within discrete neuronal populations within the hypothalamic nuclei described above. For example, neuropeptide Y (NPY) and agouti-related peptide (AgRP), both potent stimulators of food intake, are colocalized in a population of neurons in the ARH (although NPY is expressed in many other sites as well), and α-melanocyte-stimulating hormone (α-MSH) and cocaine- and amphetamine-regulated transcript (CART), which induce an anorectic response, are colocalized in an adjacent set of ARH neurons. The PVH is rich in terminals containing numerous appetite-modifying neurotransmitters, including NPY, α-MSH, serotonin, galanin, noradrenaline, and the opioid peptides. Within the LHA there is a defined subpopulation of neurons that express orexins and melanocortin-concentrating hormone (MCH), peptides that stimulate food intake. NPY nerve terminals are abundant in the LHA, in contact with orexin and MCH-expressing cells.

4. OVERVIEW OF HYPOTHALAMIC REGULATORY CIRCUITS

Over the last two decades, a large body of work has defined the basic model for the function of the hypothalamic circuits that regulate energy homeostasis. This model, which we describe next, is outlined in Fig. 2. We then describe in more detail some of the molecular and cellular components of this system. In particular, we focus on NPY, the melanocortin circuitry, and the peripheral factors that are known to act on these pathways.

4.1. ARH as a Primary Sensor of Peripheral Signals

Two adjacent groups of cells in the ARH, the AgRP/NPY neurons (orexigenic) and the POMC/CART neurons (anorectic), act as the primary site in the brain for receiving the humoral signals that reflect body energy status. Projections between ARH AgRP/NPY and POMC/CART allow cross talk and, hence, a coordinated response.

4.2. Second-Order Neuronal Pathways in Hypothalamus

Projections from the ARH to the PVH and LHA, which contain second-order neurons, allow transduction of peripheral signals into behavioral and metabolic responses that attempt to maintain body fat stores at a constant level. For example, ARH AgRP/NPY and POMC/CART project to TRH neurons in PVH, resulting in changes in energy expenditure.

5. NEUROPEPTIDE Y

NPY is a member of the peptide family that includes pancreatic polypeptide (PP), peptide YY (PYY), and NPY. PP was the first member discovered in 1968, as a contaminant of insulin extracted from chicken pancreas. The second member, PYY, was discovered from porcine intestine extracts. Subsequently, NPY was discovered from extracts of porcine brain. All members of the family consist of 36 amino acids with a C-terminal amide group and display a characteristic hairpin tertiary structure. NPY and PYY show >70% identity in amino acid sequence and both share >50% identity with PP. NPY shows remarkable evolutionary conservation, which implies an important functional role. In all species so far investigated, from lamprey to human, of the 36 amino acids in the sequence, 22 are identical in the mature peptide.

5.1. Central Distribution of NPY

In mammals, NPY is found in cells derived from the neural crest and is widely distributed within the central and peripheral nervous systems. Within the brain, NPY-containing cell bodies have a broad distribution with prominent levels in neocortex, hippocampus, and thalamus; in brain-stem nuclei, particularly within the A1 nucleus, the locus coeruleus, and the nucleus of the solitary tract (NTS); and in the hypothalamus. Within the hypothalamus, the arcuate nucleus (ARH) is the major site of NPY expression, where 90% of the NPY neurons also contain another orexigenic peptide, AgRP. These ARH NPY/AgRP neurons project dorsally and anteriorly into the perifornical LHA, PVH, DMH, and medial preoptic area and ventrally into the median eminence; the ARH-PVH projection is particularly dense. In addition, NPY expression is seen in the DMH of many obese animals.

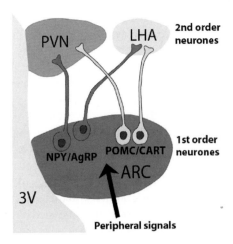

Fig. 2. ARH first- and second-order neurons. The NPY/AgRP and proopiomelanocortin (POMC)/CART neurons in the ARH, adjacent to the median eminence, are the best-characterized first-order neurons in the hypothalamic response to circulating peripheral signals. NPY/AgRP and POMC neurons project to the PVH and to the LHA, where some of the second-order neurons involved in the regulation of appetite and energy expenditure are located. 3V = third ventricle; ARC = arcuate; LHA = lateral hypothalamic area, PVN = paraventricular nucleus.

5.2. Orexigenic Effects of NPY

NPY has been attributed a formidable list of effects, ranging from memory processing and retention, to the control of blood pressure and circadian body temperature. Here, we focus on the effects of NPY on energy homeostasis.

A physiologic role for the hypothalamic NPY system in energy homeostasis is suggested because its production and release are affected by changes in energy balance. For example, hypothalamic NPY concentrations increase during fasting and return to normal with refeeding. Conversely, inhibition of NPY biosynthesis in the ARH, by direct application of antisense oligonucleotides, causes reduced food intake and a blunted hyperphagic response to fasting in rats.

NPY strongly stimulates feeding when injected into the cerebral ventricles or various hypothalamic areas, notably the PVH and perifornical LHA. NPY increases food intake primarily by increasing meal size, and by reducing the latency to feeding initiation, without substantially increasing meal frequency. Repeated doses of NPY cause a consistent increase in feeding without evidence of tolerance. Thus, repeated injection into the PVH over a period of several days results in sustained hyperphagia, body weight gain, and a marked increase in body fat accumulation. In addition to the feeding effects, chronic administration of central NPY also exerts effects in peripheral tissues that promote fat accumulation. These include increased acetyl coenzyme A carboxylase activity with increased *de novo* fatty acid and triglyceride synthesis in both white adipose tissue and the liver. NPY is also reported to increase circulating insulin levels, thus favoring deposition of triglycerides. However, increased food intake alone cannot fully account for the range of metabolic and hormonal effects elicited by the administration of NPY. This conclusion is supported by studies in which NPY-induced hyperphagia is prevented by pair feeding animals to the food intake of vehicle-treated animals. In this paradigm, the metabolic and hormonal responses induced by NPY are only partially attenuated. However, the mechanisms underlying these metabolic effects are not fully known but are thought to involve decreased expression of uncoupling proteins in brown adipose tissue, decreased activity of the sympathetic nervous system, and altered glucocorticoid release.

5.3. Physiologic Role of ARH-NPY Neurons: First-Order Neurons

One of the primary physiologic roles of the ARH-NPY/AgRP neurons may be to sense and respond to states of negative energy balance. These neurons become more active following a critical fall in the body's energy stores. Once activated these neurons initiate appropriate behavioral and metabolic responses to restore energy balance. Such states of negative energy balance include starvation, untreated insulin-dependent diabetes mellitus, and lactation. All of these states are characterized by increased hunger, active food-seeking behavior, reduced thermogenesis, and increased ARH-NPY/AgRP neuronal activity. In vivo stereotaxic sampling from the brain during starvation and in insulin-deficient diabetes has confirmed that NPY release is elevated. Furthermore, peripheral injection of ghrelin (*see* below) stimulates feeding and activates NPY neurons in vivo (as seen by increased c-fos expression in NPY neurons) in the ARH. The suggestion that NPY drives the hyperphagia in these conditions is supported by the observation that NPY gene expression and peptide levels increase in the hypothalamus of streptozotocin-diabetic rats before any increase in food intake occurs. Overall, these data indicate that the ARH-NPY/AgRP neurons act homeostatically to restore normal energy balance and body fat stores under conditions of energy deficit.

5.4. Role of NPY in Obesity

Several genetic rodent models of obesity (*ob/ob* mouse, *db/db* mouse, and *fa/fa* fatty rats) exhibit elevated NPY mRNA levels together with raised NPY peptide levels in specific hypothalamic nuclei, including the ARH, PVH, and DMH. These findings suggest that overactivity of the ARH-PVH projection plays a role in the hyperphagia and reduced energy expenditure that contributes to obesity in these models. Chronic activation of NPY neurons by daily ghrelin treatments increases body weight in rats.

5.5. NPY Knockout Mice

The premise that NPY plays a key role in the normal control of food intake is challenged by the phenotype of the NPY-null mice. Initial reports suggested that NPY-deficient mice have normal body weight and food intake under basal conditions. Refeeding in response to a fast was also initially reported to be normal in these mice. However, a more recent report demonstrated that when NPY-null mice were backcrossed onto a congenic C57 background, they showed decreased refeeding in response to 24- and 48-h fasting. In addition NPY-null mice fail to develop hyperphagia in response to uncontrolled diabetes. Moreover, when NPY-null mice are crossed with obese leptin-deficient *ob/ob* mice, the offspring have reduced food intake, reduced body weight, and increased fertility. These findings suggest a role for NPY in the regulation of food intake. The comparatively mild phenotype of this knockout mouse may be owing to developmental compensatory mechanisms.

6. NPY RECEPTORS

The members of the PP family act on the same family of receptors called the NPY receptors. Because the members of the PP family contain many tyrosine residues, the NPY receptors are designated by a *Y*, the single-letter amino acid code for tyrosine. Currently, six different NPY receptors have been characterized. All belong to the G protein–coupled receptor (GPCR) superfamily and share the common feature of seven-transmembrane-spanning regions but differ in their ligand affinity profiles. All the NPY receptors seem to inhibit cyclic adenosine monophosphate (cAMP) production.

6.1. Historical Aspects of Subdivision of NPY Receptors

Historically, the subdivision of NPY receptors comes from the observation that C-terminal fragments of NPY or PYY, e.g., NPY$_{13-36}$, can mimic some of the responses elicited by full-length NPY. Receptors activated by only holopeptides were designated Y1, and those activated by holopeptides and C-terminal fragments were designated Y2. This initial subdivision of NPY receptors into Y1R and Y2R subtypes has stood the test of time and is supported by additional data. First, analogs of NPY and

PYY synthesized with a proline residue at position 34 are far more potent at Y1R than Y2R. Second, nonpeptide antagonists have been synthesized that competitively block Y1R but not Y2R. Third, cDNAs and genes have been cloned that encode Y1R and Y2R from several species.

6.2. Present Definition of NPY Receptors

Five distinct NPY receptors have been cloned. Sequence comparisons show that receptors Y1, Y4, and y6 are more closely related to each other than to the receptors Y2 and Y5. Y2R and Y5R are equally distantly related to one another as to the Y1/Y4/y6 group. In fact, the Y1/Y4/y6 group and Y2R and Y5R are more divergent than any other GPCRs that bind the same endogenous ligand.

6.3. Y1R

Y1 receptor cDNA was first cloned from rats in 1990. An order of potency of NPY $\geq$ PYY $\geq$ [Pro^{34}] substituted analog >> C-terminal fragments > PP is characteristic for the Y1R. Y1R mRNA has been detected in a variety of tissues, including brain, heart, kidney, and gastrointestinal (GI) tract. In the brain, nutritional status has been demonstrated to regulate Y1R mRNA expression, with levels decreasing with fasting. Initial evidence suggested that Y1R mediated the hyperphagic effects of NPY. For example, ^{34}[Pro]NPY, a full Y1R agonist, was found to stimulate food intake, and the potent selective Y1R antagonist BIBO3304 significantly reduced the hyperphagia induced by NPY or 24-h fasting. Surprisingly, Y1R-null mice have increased body weight and white adipose tissue, despite a small decrease in daily food intake and markedly reduced fast-induced refeeding. However, Y1R-null mice have decreased locomotor activity, and this may cause decreased energy expenditure and, hence, explain the increased fat deposition observed.

6.4. Y2R

A cDNA for Y2R was first cloned from human SMS-KAN cells and subsequently from human brain cDNA libraries. The prototypical response for the Y2R is presynaptic inhibition of neurotransmitter release. Y2R mRNA has been detected in various parts of the CNS. Mice with germ-line deletion of Y2R develop hyperphagia and reduced energy expenditure resulting in mild obesity with increased fat deposition. These Y2R-null mice showed a normal response to fasting and administration of NPY but an attenuated response to leptin. Furthermore, we have shown that Y2R-null mice are resistant to the anorexic effects of PYY$_{3-36}$, and we have shown that PYY$_{3-36}$ is a physiologic regulator of feeding in rodents and humans. These findings suggest that Y2R may be involved in the basal control of food intake and body weight.

6.5. Putative Y3R

The existence of Y3R was suggested on the basis that PYY was considerably less active than NPY in several animal models including the rat CNS, rat colon, and rat lung. However, such a receptor has not been cloned and no specific agonist or antagonists have been described.

6.6. Y4R

The gene for Y4R was initially cloned from a human genomic library and called PP1. The principal feature of Y4R is high affinity for PP of the same species, suggesting that PP is the primary endogenous ligand. Human Y4R mRNA is expressed in the colon, small intestine, prostate gland, and various CNS regions. Recently, Y4R has been deleted and the Y4R-null mice crossed with *ob/ob* mice. Y4R deficiency was found to have no beneficial effects on the body weight of the *ob/ob* mice. However, fertility in the *ob/ob* mice was greatly improved by Y4R deletion.

Y4R is expressed at many sites in the brain. Within the hypothalamus, Y4R is highly expressed on neurons in the LHA that also express orexin, a peptide that is involved in both CNS arousal and energy balance.

6.7. Y5R

Y5R cDNA was cloned in 1996 and its pharmacologic profile demonstrated to be NPY $\geq$ PYY ~ [Pro^{34}] substituted analog ~ NPY$_{2-36}$ ~ PYY$_{3-36}$ >> NPY$_{13-36}$. Y5R was proposed as the "feeding" receptor on the basis that CGP71683A, a Y5 antagonist, inhibited NPY-induced hyperphagia. Furthermore, administration of an antisense oligonucleotide directed against Y5R inhibited NPY-induced feeding and the hyperphagia of Zucker rats and *ob/ob* mice. However, there are conflicting reports on the role of Y5R from different groups. Flynn et al. found that antisense oligonucleotides targeting Y5R had no effect on NPY-induced 2-h food intake and only caused a reduction in food intake after 10 h. These results suggest that Y5R may act to maintain feeding but is not involved in the initial feeding response elicited by NPY. Y5R has been deleted and young Y5R-null mice have normal food intake and body weight. Paradoxically, older animals have increased body weight and fat pads, further complicating the understanding of the role of this receptor in energy homeostasis. Deletion of either the Y1 or the Y5 receptor causes late-onset mild obesity, and it appears that there may be redundancy of NPY receptors at the neurons that respond to NPY. NPY appears to stimulate feeding via both Y1R and Y5R. Interestingly, the genes encoding these two receptors are very close together .

6.8. y6

An additional receptor subtype has been cloned from mouse genomic DNA; the intronless gene encodes a 371-amino-acid protein that was originally designated Y5R. Homologs were cloned from monkey, rabbit, and human and designated Y2B. However, in primates the y6 gene appears to have become nonfunctional because a frameshift mutation results in a truncated nonfunctional protein product.

7. MELANOCORTIN SYSTEM AND AGRP

The melanocortin system is defined as the hypothalamic and brain-stem neurons expressing POMC, the hypothalamic neurons coexpressing NPY/AgRP, and the neurons downstream of these systems. In addition, two ancillary proteins, mahogany and syndecan-3, have been found to modulate the activity of the melanocortin system.

7.1. Proopiomelanocortin

The POMC gene encodes a 31- to 36-kDa preprohormone, from which seven mature peptide hormones (adrenocorticotropic hormone, α-MSH, β-MSH, γ-MSH, corticotropin-like intermediate lobe peptide, β-lipotrophin, and β-endorphin) are derived via posttranslational cleavage by prohormone convertases. Posttranslational processing of the POMC prohormone is tissue specific, resulting in the production of different POMC peptides by different cell types. The POMC gene is expressed primarily in the CNS, where it is expressed in the ARH, NTS of the caudal brain stem, and pituitary. POMC neurons project broadly to many brain regions including hypothalamic nuclei (PVH, DMH, VMH). The POMC gene is also expressed by cutaneous keratinocytes and melanocytes. In addition, POMC mRNA and immunoreactivity have been reported in a number of peripheral human tissues, including the genitourinary tract, GI tract, adrenal gland, spleen, lung, and thyroid and in cells of the immune system. Within the hypothalamus, POMC neurons are found only within the ARH, where they are colocalized with CART, a neuropeptide with anorectic effects.

7.2. Melanocortin Receptors

Five melanocortin receptors (MCRs) have been cloned, all having differing affinity for POMC products and with varied levels of expression in different tissues. These G_s protein–coupled receptors function through adenylyl cyclase to increase intracellular cAMP. Three melanocortin receptors (MC3R, MC4R, and MC5R)

have been identified within the brain, and both MC3R and MC4R are expressed in hypothalamic nuclei implicated in energy homeostasis, including the VMH, DMH, PVH, and ARH.

The initial function ascribed to the melanocortin system was the regulation of pigmentation via changes of melanin production in the skin and hair. Its importance in the control of body weight was first highlighted by the agouti (A^y/a) mouse. The *Agouti* gene was cloned in 1992 and found to encode a 131-amino-acid protein. In mammals, agouti is primarily expressed in the skin, where it acts in a paracrine manner to regulate pigmentation by antagonism of MC1R. In the absence of agouti protein, α-MSH binds to MC1R on the surface of melanocytes, leading to the production of brown-black pigment (eumelanin). The agouti protein antagonizes MC1R and induces a switch from eumelanin to yellow-red (phaeomelanin) pigment.

In the A^y/a mouse, a dominant mutation in the mouse *Agouti* gene results in ectopic expression of the protein. This ubiquitous expression gives rise to a pleiotropic obesity syndrome referred to as the obese yellow syndrome. The A^y/a mice develop a yellow coat color, hyperphagia, hyperinsulinaemia, hyperglycemia, obesity, and increased body length. In 1994, it was postulated that the phenotype of the A^y/a mouse resulted from antagonism of other MCRs. Murine agouti protein was found to be a high-affinity antagonist of α-MSH binding to both MC1R and MC4R but appeared to have no effect on binding to MC3R or MC5R. These findings suggested that antagonism of MC4R at the hypothalamic level by agouti protein abolished neural melanocortin signaling, thereby altering appetite circuits and resulting in obesity.

The human *Agouti* gene was cloned in 1994 and found to encode a 131-amino-acid protein termed *agouti-signaling protein* (ASP). The mouse and human *agouti* products were found to exhibit 80% homology, suggesting that agouti may be functionally similar in both species. In contrast to the mouse, human *Agouti* gene is expressed in high levels in adipose tissue, heart, testis, and ovary, but with no expression observed in the CNS. In vitro studies found ASP to be a potent antagonist on human MC1R, MC2R, and MC4R, and a relatively weak antagonist at human MC3R and MC5R. The differing properties of human and murine agouti protein regarding both tissue expression and MCR affinity suggested that agouti may be regulating additional or distinct physiologic processes in humans.

Additional studies with synthetic MC3R and MC4R ligands confirmed the importance of the central melanocortin system in the regulation of appetite. The synthetic MC3/4R-specific agonist melanotan II was found to inhibit feeding following icv administration into four different rodent models of hyperphagia: fasted mice, A^y/a mice, *ob/ob* mice, and mice injected with NPY. These findings suggested that the melanocortin system serves not only to regulate pigmentation but also to play an important role in hypothalamic appetite control circuits.

7.3. AgRP

The fact that agouti is a highly specific MC4R antagonist, even though it is normally expressed only in hair follicles, suggested the existence in the brain of an "agouti-like" protein. The *Agouti-related transcript* (*AgRT*) gene was isolated in 1997. *AgRT* is normally expressed at high levels in the hypothalamus and adrenal gland. AgRP, the 132-amino-acid peptide product of *AgRT*, acts as a competitive antagonist at both MC3R and MC4R. Within the ARH, AgRP mRNA and peptide are found in virtually all NPY-expressing, first-order neurons.

Several lines of evidence suggest that AgRP plays a key role in the regulation of body weight. *AgRT* mRNA levels in the ARH are altered by nutritional state. An 18-fold increase was observed after a 48-h fast, whereas levels are reduced by diet-induced obesity. Injections of AgRP and synthetic AgRP analogs stimulate food intake and body weight gain. The importance of AgRP in the regulation of appetite was confirmed by the development of transgenic mice overexpressing *AgRT*. These transgenic mice, although retaining their wild-type coat color, were found to resemble phenotypically the A^y/a mice. However, AgRP knockout mice have no major phenotype and display normal feeding behavior.

7.4. MC3R and MC4R

The highest concentration of MC3R expression levels are found in the medial habenula, hypothalamic regions, and limbic system, including the VMH, ARH, preoptic nucleus, LHA, and posterior hypothalamic area. MC3R mRNA is also found in the septum, hippocampus, thalamus, amygdala, and brain stem.

POMC and AgRP neurons in the ARH selectively express MC3R but not MC4R, suggesting a role for this receptor in feedback regulation of the melanocortin circuitry. Recently, we have demonstrated in electrophysiologic studies that data from labeled POMC neurons in the ARH show an autoreceptor role for MC3R. The altered body composition of MC3R knockout mice confirms a role for MC3R in regulating energy homeostasis. Young MC3R mice are not hyperphagic or significantly overweight, but they have increased adiposity and an increased feeding efficiency.

In the rodent brain, MC4R mRNA appears to be less abundant though more widely expressed than MC3R and is seen in virtually all brain regions including the cerebral cortex, hypothalamus, thalamus, brain stem, and spinal cord. MC4R is highly expressed in the PVH, DMH, and dorsal motor nucleus of the vagus in the caudal brain stem. Targeted deletion of MC4R results in mice with an obesity syndrome virtually identical to the obese yellow syndrome, characterized by hyperphagia, hyperinsulinemia, hyperglycemia, reduced oxygen consumption, and increased linear growth with no abnormalities of reproductive or adrenal axes. Heterozygous mice display a phenotype intermediate between that of wild-type and homozygous littermates.

An important consequence of AgRP-expressing neurons and α-MSH-expressing neurons both projecting to MC4R is that the ratio of activation of the two neuronal pathways will determine the final activity at MC4R. Thus, to understand the activity of MC4R it is necessary to understand the activity of both populations of neurons. Currently, it appears that most peripheral signals act in a reciprocal manner on the two populations; for example, leptin inhibits AgRP neurons and activates POMC neurons. Ghrelin acts in the opposite manner; it activates NPY neurons and inhibits POMC neurons.

8. OTHER CNS REGIONS INVOLVED IN REGULATION OF ENERGY BALANCE

8.1. Brain Stem

The hypothalamus is not solely responsible for the control of feeding behavior. This has been underscored by studies of chronic decerebrate rats. In this model, the forebrain has been experimentally disconnected by a mesencephalic knife cut so that the animal relies solely on neural components caudal to the lesion to regulate its food intake. The feeding response to manipulations of GI content is not affected by decerebration, but if the total caloric availability is decreased, the animal becomes anorectic. These studies suggest that while forebrain structures add information on the metabolic state of the animal, nuclei in the brain stem are capable of integrating and responding appropriately to feedback signals from the digestive tract. Such signals include both positive orosensory and negative viscerosensory information provided by cranial nerves. The major input of viscerosensory transmission comes through the afferent portion of the vagus nerve, which terminates in the NTS and the area postrema. The peripheral branches of the vagus nerve, whose cell bodies are located in the nodose ganglion, supply sensory terminals to several internal organs, including the GI tract. The NTS is an important brain-stem area that processes satiety-related information. Neurohumoral signals arising in the GI tract comprise the first step in a series of events mediating postprandial satiety. These signals are conveyed to the NTS via blood-brain barrier–free area postrema and gastric vagal afferents.

The NTS contains POMC neurons and MC4R. Local administration of MC4R agonists or antagonists into the fourth ventricle elicits feeding responses that are indistinguishable from those induced by injecting these compounds into the lateral ventricles. Moreover, leptin receptors are present with the NTS, and recent evidence indicates that leptin can act directly in the NTS to reduce food intake and body weight. Thus, the NTS contains neurons that not only respond to satiety signals, but also might act as first-order neurons that respond directly to peripheral signals of energy balance. The NTS neurons have extensive reciprocal connections with forebrain areas such as the PVH, suggesting that the integration of satiety and energy homeostasis information probably involves multiple brain areas.

8.2. Higher Centers

Energy homeostasis requires the ability to sense changes in energy balance, to initiate appropriate compensatory signals, and to translate those signals into a motivated behavior. The motivation to eat, the sensation of eating, and the pleasure associated with consumption of a palatable meal all depend on higher brain functions that must be integrated within the hypothalamus. Some of this integration is thought to occur in the striatum, the portion of the basal ganglia that includes the caudate nucleus, putamen, and nucleus accumbens.

It is worth remembering that few people overeat because of chronic hunger; rather, it is the rewarding or comforting aspects of food that many overeaters crave. Thus, it is likely that clues to the etiology of, and potential treatments for, human obesity will be discovered as researchers further understand how reward signals are integrated with signals of energy state.

9. PERIPHERAL SIGNALS OF ENERGY STATUS

The neuronal and molecular hypothalamic circuits described above are now known to represent a major component of the brain centers that Kennedy proposed as responding to humoral adiposity signals. However, in contrast to the complexity and significant numbers of factors involved in hypothalamic function, the search for peripherally produced adiposity signals has, to date, revealed only a few key molecules. The pancreatic hormone insulin, which enters the brain from the circulation and acts there to reduce energy intake, was the first hormonal signal implicated in the control of body weight by the CNS. However, it was the subsequent identification of the adipocyte hormone leptin

and the delineation of its role in the CNS regulation of energy homeostasis that provided the impetus for many of the recent advances in the understanding of these pathways and mechanisms. More recently, factors such as resistin and adiponectin have received considerable attention.

9.1. Leptin

Body fat stores remain very constant over time, in spite of large changes in energy intake and energy expenditure. This constancy led Kennedy to propose that body fat generates a signal proportional to adipose stores, and that this signal exerted feedback control over brain function. Twenty years later, in parabiosis experiments, Coleman surgically coupled normal mice with two spontaneously occurring murine models of genetic obesity (*ob/ob* or *db/db* mice), creating a cross-circulation between two animals: one normal and one obese. Coleman showed that the parabiotic partner could exert remarkable changes in food intake and body weight of the coupled animal. Furthermore, he showed that the *ob* locus was responsible for the production of a circulating factor that limited food intake, and that the *db* locus was necessary for the response to the circulating satiety signal. The positional cloning of the gene implicated in the obese phenotype of the *ob/ob* mouse in 1994 has led to a new era of obesity research. The *ob* gene encodes a hormone, leptin (from the Greek word *leptos*, meaning thin), that is expressed in adipose tissue and at lower levels in gastric epithelium and the placenta. The plasma level of leptin is highly correlated with adipose tissue mass and decreases in both humans and mice after weight loss. The levels of protein are increased in several genetic and environmentally induced forms of rodent obesity and in obese humans. Administration of recombinant leptin either by injection or as a constant sc infusion to wild-type mice results in a dose-dependent decrease in body weight at increments of plasma leptin levels within the physiologic range.

ob/ob mice show many of the abnormalities seen in starved animals, including decreased body temperature, hyperphagia, decreased energy expenditure, decreased immune function, and infertility. Leptin replacement corrects all of these abnormalities, implying that *ob/ob* mice exist in a state of "perceived starvation" and that the resulting biologic response in the presence of food leads to obesity. The possibility that falling plasma leptin levels signal nutrient deprivation is further suggested by the observation that exogenous leptin attenuates the neuroendocrine responses to food restriction. Fasted wild-type mice treated with leptin continue to ovulate, whereas fasted controls given saline experience an ovulatory delay of several days. Leptin treatment blunts the changes in circulating thyroid hormone and corticosterone levels that are normally associated with food deprivation. Starvation is associated with decreased immune function, and leptin also corrects these abnormalities. In *ob/ob* mice, leptin stimulates proliferation of CD4[+] T-cells and increases production of cytokines by T-helper-1 cells. These results indicate that leptin may also be a key link between nutritional state and the immune system. Leptin is also important in regulating the onset of puberty.

The identification of leptin led rapidly to the cloning of its cognate receptor. The leptin receptor is a member of the cytokine family of receptors that have a single transmembrane domain and are generally expressed as monomers or dimers on the cell surface. Ligand binding induces dimerization, activation of the receptor, and signal transduction. Ob-R is predicted to have two separate leptin-binding regions and binds leptin with low nanomolar affinity. Five splice forms of the leptin receptor that differ at the carboxyl terminus have been identified. Four of these receptor forms are membrane bound, whereas Ob-Re encodes a secreted form of the receptor that circulates in plasma. Mutations that disrupt the leptin receptor have been identified in each of the available strains of diabetic (*db/db*) mice. *db/db* mice are also genetically obese and manifest a phenotype that is nearly identical to that evident in leptin-deficient *ob/ob* mice. DNA sequence analyses of the available *db* strains have implicated the Ob-Rb form of the receptor as mediating many, if not all, of leptin's weight-reducing effects. The Ob-Rb form is expressed in the POMC and NPY neurons of the ARH, and in other brain regions involved in the regulation of energy homeostasis, suggesting that the brain is an important target of leptin action. This is further supported by the high potency of leptin to reduce food intake when delivered directly into the CNS. Neuron-specific deletion of Ob-Rb using Cre/loxP-mediated recombination techniques in mice recapitulates the phenotype of the *ob/ob* mice. In addition, we have shown that leptin directly modulates the electrical activity of NPY and POMC neurons in brain slice preparations.

In human subjects, a highly significant correlation between body fat content and plasma leptin concentration has been observed, and obese humans generally have high leptin levels. These data suggest that in most cases human obesity is likely to be associated with reduced sensitivity to leptin. The basis for leptin resistance in the overwhelming majority of obese hyperleptinemic humans is unknown. Data from animal studies indicate that this condition is likely to be very heterogeneous and that many factors are likely to influence the activity of the neural circuits that regulate feeding

behavior and body weight. It has also been shown that entry of leptin into the CSF is limiting in some obese subjects thus contributing to leptin resistance by decreasing the concentration of leptin that is available to stimulate leptin receptors at sites that are protected by the blood-brain barrier.

Overall, leptin appears to function largely as a "long-term" signal of energy balance—influencing the quantity of food consumed and the amount of energy that is expended. Leptin levels do not increase significantly after a meal, and administration of leptin does not acutely lead to termination of a meal. Thus, leptin is an adiposity signal rather than a classic satiety factor. However, leptin and other components of the long-term system interact extensively with the components of the short-term system.

9.2. Insulin

In addition to its central role in the control of blood glucose levels, Woods and Porte proposed some 25 yr ago that the pancreatic hormone insulin is an afferent signal to the brain that couples changes in body adiposity to compensatory changes in food intake. The role of insulin as a signal of adiposity has not been irrefutably established, but the insulin hypothesis is supported by the facts that insulin circulates in proportion to body fat, that insulin receptors are present in the brain, and that icv infusion of insulin decreases food intake and reduces body weight. Insulin receptor expression has been shown to be high in the ARH. Intracerebroventricular administration of insulin has also been shown to decrease fasting-induced increases in AgRP/NPY mRNA and to reverse the hyperphagia associated with insulin deficiency. Furthermore, many neurons in the ARH that are electrophysiologically inhibited by leptin are also inhibited by insulin. Thus, it has been suggested that insulin provides an inhibitory input to the ARH neurons. More recently, it has been shown that deleting insulin receptor specifically in neurons results in moderate weight gain in mice. Similarly, studies using antisense oligonucleotides to attenuate insulin receptor expression in the hypothalamus, or direct administration of insulin mimetics into the ARH, have implied a role for insulin in the central regulation of energy homeostasis.

10. SIGNALS FROM GI TRACT

Leptin, and perhaps insulin, represent long-term adiposity signals. However, in response to a meal, hunger is reduced for several hours. Intravenous infusion of nutrients does not have this long-lasting effect, suggesting that gut-derived factors and neural signals are important. Such factors may act as satiety factors or regulate meal initiation or termination. However, it is only recently that multiple gut-derived factors have been demonstrated to regulate feeding, and their role in the hypothalamic circuits regulating energy homeostasis is still not yet well defined.

10.1. Cholecystokinin

In the early 1970s, based on a series of experiments, Gibbs and colleagues first proposed a role for the brain/gut peptide cholecystokinin (CCK) in the control of food intake. They demonstrated that peripherally administered CCK caused immediate and short-lasting inhibition of food intake. These studies were among the first to provide a chemical identity to the gut signals involved in producing postingestive satiety and meal termination. The mechanism by which CCK promotes satiety is hypothesized to involve both inhibition of gastric emptying, which stimulates vagal afferents sensitive to gastric distension, and direct activation of vagal afferent fibers that terminate in the brain stem. Evidence to support the latter mechanism includes the finding that CCK receptors are present on afferent vagus nerve fibers. Moreover, the satiety effects of peripherally-administered CCK are abolished by vagal deafferentation but remain intact in the chronic decerebrate rat, demonstrating that they are mediated by the vagus-nerve brain-stem complex. Several aspects of CCK action exemplify the distinction between long- and short-term hormonal signals that regulate appetite. When CCK is administered prior to each meal in rats, a consistent reduction in meal size is observed (~50%). However, rather than losing weight, the rats responded by eating these smaller meals twice as frequently.

10.2. Glucagon-Like Peptide-1

Glucagon-like peptide-1 (GLP-1) is synthesized and released from intestinal endocrine cells (L-cells). GLP-1 is also produced by neurons in the NTS. Initial studies of biologic activity of GLP-1 in the mid-1980s utilized the full-length N-terminal extended forms of GLP-1 (1–37 and 1–36 amide). These larger GLP-1 molecules were generally devoid of biologic activity. In 1987, three independent research groups demonstrated that removal of the first six amino acids resulted in a shorter version of the GLP-1 molecule with substantially enhanced biologic activity. The majority of circulating biologically active GLP-1 is found as the GLP-1(7–36) amide form, with lesser amounts of the bioactive GLP-1(7–37) form also detectable. Both peptides appear equipotent in all biologic paradigms studied to date. GLP-1 is a potent stimulator of insulin release and has been shown to be a physiologic incretin in humans. GLP-1 also inhibits glucagon release. The insulinotropic and glucagon-inhibiting effects of GLP-1 are glucose dependent, thus preventing GLP-1 from inducing hypoglycemia. In view of this effect of incretin, GLP-1R agonists are currently being evaluated as a potential treatment for type 2 diabetes.

A large body of evidence demonstrates that icv GLP-1 can reduce food intake in both acute and chronic studies. Conversely, icv administration of the GLP-1 antagonist exendin (9-39) can acutely increase food intake and promote weight gain in chronic rodent studies. More than a dozen human studies in both healthy subjects and patients with obesity or type 2 diabetes have examined the relationship between GLP-1 infusion and food intake. The majority of studies have shown a small but significant inhibition of short-term food intake with concurrent GLP-1 infusion. A metaanalysis of these studies has concluded that there is a dose-dependent reduction in food intake associated with a reduction in gastric emptying in human subjects.

Paradoxically, despite the effects of GLP-1 on food intake in rodents, GLP-1 receptor–/– CD1 mice are lean and do not exhibit disturbances of food intake or body weight regulation. Furthermore, GLP-1R–/– mice do not develop obesity with age, or following several months of high-fat feeding.

10.3. Ghrelin

Studies on the stimulation of growth hormone (GH) secretion led to the discovery of ghrelin. Synthetic compounds called GH secretagogues were found to increase the release of GH acting via a novel GPCR named the GH secretagogue receptor found in the pituitary and hypothalamus.

In 1999, an endogenous ligand for this orphan receptor was discovered and purified from the stomach. The ligand, a 28-amino-acid peptide, was named ghrelin from the Indo-European root *ghre*, meaning to grow. Ghrelin has a unique octanoyl fatty acyl side chain essential for biologic activity. Ghrelin is primarily secreted from X/A-like endocrine cells in the stomach. Its immunoreactivity has been increased under conditions of negative energy balance such as starvation, cachexia, and anorexia nervosa, whereas it is decreased under conditions of positive energy balance such as feeding, hyperglycemia, and obesity. Circulating ghrelin levels are suppressed by meal ingestion or intragastric glucose, but not by gastric distension, and have been shown to rise during fasting. Administration of ghrelin increases food intake, decreases fat oxidation, increases adiposity in rodents, and triggers hunger and increased food intake in humans.

Several lines of evidence suggest that peripheral ghrelin stimulates food intake by altering the activity of neurons within the ARH. First, after microinjection into defined hypothalamic sites, ghrelin was found to stimulate feeding most markedly when administered in the ARH. Second, peripheral injection of ghrelin causes an increase in expression of c-fos in ARH-NPY neurons. Third, molecular genetic studies have shown that deletion of the genes for AGRP and NPY prevents ghrelin from stimulating food intake in mice. Finally, electrophysiologic studies have demonstrated that ghrelin activates NPY neurons and indirectly inhibits POMC neurons. However, more recently, a series of studies by Date et al. has shown that ghrelin receptors are present on vagal afferents and that ghrelin suppresses firing of these afferents.

In collaboration with Tamas Horvath, we have recently described ghrelin production in the hypothalamus of mouse and rat, and others have shown that ghrelin is produced in the hypothalamus of monkeys. We have also shown that these ghrelin neurons project to many of the hypothalamic nuclei that we know regulate energy homeostasis. However, the relative contribution of central vs peripheral ghrelin to the regulation of hunger and food intake is not yet clear.

10.4. Peptide YY$_{3-36}$

PYY is a 36-amino-acid GI hormone first isolated from porcine small intestine by Tatemoto in 1980 and named PYY owing to the presence of an amino acid–terminal (Y) tyrosine and a carboxyl-terminal tyrosine amide (Y). The enteroendocrine L-cells of the GI tract are the major source of PYY. In addition to producing and secreting PYY, the L-cells cosecrete three additional hormones that have been shown to reduce food intake in rodents and man: GLP-1, CCK; and, more recently, oxyntomodulin.

There are two main endogenous forms of PYY: PYY$_{1-36}$ and PYY$_{3-36}$. PYY$_{1-36}$ binds to and activates at least three Y receptor subtypes in rats and humans (Y1, Y2, and Y5), while removing the first two amino acids at the N-terminal changes the receptor selectivity such that PYY$_{3-36}$ is more selective for Y2 receptor. The percentage of these two forms in human blood has been reported to differ according to the feeding status. In the fasted state, the concentration of PYY$_{1-36}$ predominates over that of PYY$_{3-36}$. By contrast, after a meal, PYY$_{3-36}$ is the major circulating form. Following ingestion of food, plasma levels increase within 15 min, reach a peak at approx 90 min and then remain elevated for up to 6 h.

PYY has been shown to have several biologic actions, including vasoconstriction, inhibition of gastric acid secretion, reduction of pancreatic and intestinal secretion, and inhibition of GI motility. When injected into the cerebral ventricles, the PVH or hippocampus PYY increases food intake. Indeed, among all the orexigenic peptides and neurotransmitters described to date, PYY is the most potent stimulant of food intake; this effect is thought to be mediated by Y1R and Y5R. However, many of the sites that express Y1R and Y5R are protected behind the blood-brain barrier, and, thus, circulating PYY$_{3-36}$ (or NPY for that matter) is not able to bind to them. Circulating PYY$_{3-36}$ therefore binds to receptors around circumventricular organs. Within the ARH, PYY$_{3-36}$ binds to NPY Y2R, which is highly expressed on NPY neurons and inhibits these neurons. As we have shown, this leads to activation of POMC neurons in vivo and in vitro, because PYY$_{3-36}$ decreases the tonic inhibitory activity of NPY neurons onto POMC neurons; PYY$_{3-36}$ disinhibits POMC neurons. Of course, the inhibition of NPY/AgRP neurons by PYY$_{3-36}$ means that in addition to reduced NPY release, AgRP secretion will be decreased.

We have demonstrated that the anorectic effects of PYY$_{3-36}$ require the NPY Y2R, and that PYY$_{3-36}$ inhibits fasting-induced refeeding and nighttime free feeding and decreases body weight gain in mice and rats. We have also shown that peripherally-administered PYY$_{3-36}$ inhibits food intake in human volunteers. More recently, our studies in obese humans have demonstrated that PYY levels are low in obesity, implicating a role for PYY in the pathogenesis of obesity. Moreover, administration of PYY reduces appetite and food intake in obese subjects, suggesting that PYY$_{3-36}$ analogs, and NPY Y2R agonists, may be good therapies for obesity. In pursuit of this goal, we are conducting studies to determine the effect of chronic PYY$_{3-36}$ treatment on body weight in rhesus macaques.

10.5. Pancreatic Polypeptide

In response to ingestion of food, PP is released from the pancreatic islets in proportion to the calories ingested, suggesting that PP may act as a signal from the gut to the brain as to how much food has been ingested. More than 30 yr ago, PP was first shown to reduce food intake in *ob/ob* mice. The role of PP as a satiety signal is further supported by studies performed in wild-type mice showing that peripheral injection of PP reduces food intake. Moreover, transgenic mice overexpressing PP have reduced body weight and decreased adiposity. Further evidence for PP as a satiety factor comes from the findings that plasma levels of PP are low in obesity but elevated in patients with anorexia. Recently, we have shown that peripheral infusion of human PP in normal weight volunteers reduces appetite and food intake. Indeed, of all the gut hormones so far investigated, administration of PP results in the most prolonged reduction in food intake.

PP is thought to affect appetite by altering the levels of neuropeptides that regulate energy homeostasis within the brain. Indeed, PP has been shown to reduce the release of NPY in vitro and to reduce NPY synthesis, suggesting that PP mediates its effects via NPY. PP likely mediates its effects via Y4R, which was originally named the PP receptor because of its high affinity for PP. Y4R expressed within the brain stem and hypothalamus, key brain areas involved in the regulation of appetite and accessible to the peripheral circulation. Establishing the receptor and underlying mechanisms by which PP mediates its effects will enable more accurate prediction of the other biologic systems that PP treatment may have an impact on, and it may enable the future development of drugs that treat obesity by acting on the PP/Y4R system.

Like ghrelin and GLP-1, PYY and PP are expressed in the periphery and in neurons in the brain. Peripheral administration of PYY or PP inhibits food intake, but central administration stimulates food intake. Unraveling the complex interaction between central and peripheral contributions to energy homeostasis will require considerable effort.

11. RELEVANCE OF ENERGY REGULATORY PATHWAYS TO HUMAN DISEASE

The large body of evidence described above (which has exploited a wide range of experimental paradigms from neuroanatomy, neuropeptide identification, neuronal mapping studies, and electrophysiology through to murine gene targeting and positional cloning approaches and in vivo analysis of rodents and humans) has recently been informed by studies on rare human cases of obesity with a monogenic basis. These cases have provided evidence that many elements of the regulatory pathways are highly evolutionarily conserved and have given new insights into the mechanisms of energy homeostasis in humans.

11.1. Mutations in Leptin Pathway and Human Obesity

In 1997, Montague and colleagues provided the first description of human congenital leptin deficiency. They described two cousins of Pakistani origin homozygous for a frameshift mutation in the leptin gene that resulted in the loss of the last 34 amino acids of leptin including the C-terminal cysteine, which is essential for biologic activity and secretion. The children with this mutation had no detectable circulating leptin and had a clinical phenotype characterized by profound early onset obe-

sity, hyperphagia, and endocrine abnormalities. Subsequently, two more children with an identical mutation, again of Pakistani origin, have been identified. Treatment of these four children with leptin has resulted in a remarkable reversal of their massive obesity. A distinct homozygous missense mutation in the leptin gene that resulted in extreme obesity has been found in three members of a Turkish family. Two of these individuals were studied in detail and were found to have hypogonadism and delayed puberty. These studies provided evidence that leptin also plays a role in the onset of puberty in humans.

The phenotype of leptin-deficient humans parallels that seen in *ob/ob* mice in terms of food intake, adiposity, and gonadal function. However, there are phenotypic differences. For example, *ob/ob* mice display low body temperature and decreased energy expenditure, which is less evident in humans, and *ob/ob* mice are short whereas leptin-deficient humans are of normal height. *ob/ob* mice have marked activation of the hypothalamic-pituitary axis, which is not observed in leptin-deficient humans, suggesting that this may underlie some of the phenotypic differences. As well as finding the human equivalent of the *ob/ob* mouse, rare defects in the ObR resulting in obesity have been found. Clement and coworkers identified three French family members with mutations of leptin receptor resulting in reproductive abnormalities and obesity. In addition, these siblings had central hypothyroidism requiring treatment for dwarfism. These rare mutations in the leptin signaling pathway have provided new insights into the role of leptin in human energy balance and neuroendocrine function.

11.2. Mutations in Melanocortin System and Human Obesity

In addition to finding mutations in the peripheral signaling elements of the energy homeostatic pathway, defects in the CNS pathways and, in particular, in the melanocortin system have recently been described. Approximately 5% of children with severe early onset obesity have a mutation in the coding region of MC4R, and these mutations greatly reduce the activity or expression of MC4R. In these cases, the obesity is inherited in a dominant (heterozygous) fashion, producing a phenotype analogous to that demonstrated by disruption of the murine MC4R gene and suggesting haploinsufficiency at this locus. Interestingly, these mutations not only result in an increase in fat mass but also in lean mass with accelerated linear growth. Individuals who are homozygous for MC4R loss-of-function mutations are very hyperinsulinemic, analogous with the phenotype of MC4R-null mice.

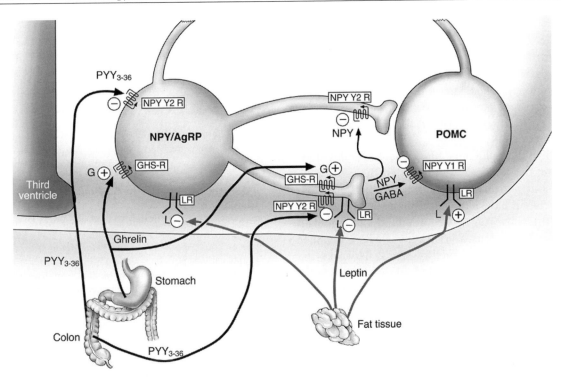

Fig. 3. Convergence of multiple signals upon ARH melanocortin neurons. NPY/AgRP neurons are inhibited by leptin via actions on the leptin receptor (LR), and by PYY$_{3-36}$ via actions on the neuropeptide Y2R (NPY Y2R). NPY/AgRP neurons are activated by ghrelin acting via the GH secretagogue receptor (GHS-R). NPY/AgRP neurons tonically inhibit POMC neurons, so changes in NPY/AgRP neuron activity are reciprocated by opposite changes in POMC neuron activity. POMC neurons are directly activated by leptin. NPY and γ-aminobutyric acid (GABA) inhibit POMC neurons. This melanocortin neuronal circuit is simultaneously sensitive to multiple peripheral signals of energy state. (Reproduced with permission from Cowley et al., 2003.)

It might be expected that researchers will discover that many more obese individuals have mutations in the promoter/enhancer region of MC4R that lead to decreased expression of MC4R. The high levels of mutations in MC4R observed in many human populations suggest that these mutations may provide an evolutionary advantage in some environments.

The importance of α-MSH signaling is further confirmed by the development of obesity in two individuals with mutations in the POMC gene. Two children with bright red hair, pale skin, and adrenal failure at birth subsequently developed severe hyperphagia and obesity. They essentially had no function related to their POMC gene. More recently, a heterozygous POMC mutation, Arg3267Gly, has been described, and this appears to be more common among obese than lean subjects. This mutation disrupts a dibasic cleavage site in POMC and leads to the production of a fusion protein comprising β-MSH and β-endorphin. Obesity has also been observed in a woman with a mutation in the prohormone convertase-1 gene, a protease known to cleave neuropeptide precursors including POMC.

12. A HIERARCHY OF SIGNALS: SHORT- AND LONG-TERM REGULATORS OF INGESTIVE BEHAVIOR

Feeding behavior lies at the interface of free will and physiology and is influenced by many factors. In addition to food availability, feeding is affected by metabolic, neural, and endocrine factors, and it is modified by powerful visual, olfactory, emotional, and cognitive inputs. Ultimately, all of these factors must be integrated to make decisions to begin and end periods of feeding. Implicit in this model of energy homeostasis is a mechanism for integrating short-term, meal-related signals into the long-term control of energy balance. It has been suggested that the response of the brain to short-term signals is influenced by the prevailing concentration of circulating adiposity signals. This hypothesis is supported by the findings that neural signals of gastric distension in vivo are potentiated by systemic leptin treatment and that satiety induced by administration of CCK is potentiated by icv infusion of insulin or systemic injection of leptin. Thus, long-term controllers of energy balance may regulate adipose stores in part by modulating the sensitivity of short-term signals such as gastric distension or CCK.

It is difficult to imagine that we will ever develop a complete, formal hierarchy of signals that inform the brain about body energy state, partly because these signals can all have a range of intensities, which will change the "importance" accorded to those signals in energy balance calculations. Rather, we hope to understand the complex, interacting neural networks that inform the brain about whole-body energy balance. We have already shown that the melanocortin circuits in the hypothalamus are a common target of many short-, medium-, and long-term signals of energy state. We have also shown that the anorexigenic and orexigenic arms of the melanocortin circuitry are reciprocally regulated by most signals (Fig. 3). A detailed understanding of this circuitry has enabled us to propose several new targets for therapies to alter energy homeostasis. In the future, we hope to define how this circuit integrates several separate inputs at the same time, e.g., determining whether the melanocortin circuits respond to leptin and PYY additively. Further challenges are to define how other neural inputs to the melanocortin circuits carry information from brain-stem sites, how the information from melanocortin circuits influences the autonomic nervous system to regulate energy expenditure, and how the melanocortin circuitry influences higher cortical centers where decisions to eat are made.

ACKNOWLEDGMENT

This work was supported by grants DK 62202 and RR 0163 from the National Institute of Health.

REFERENCE

Cowley MA, Cone RD, Enriori P, Louiselle I, Williams SM, Evans AE. Electrophysiological actions of peripheral hormones on melanocortin neurons. *Ann NY Acad Sci* 2003;994:175–186.

SUGGESTED READING

Barsh GS, Schwartz MW. Genetic approaches to studying energy balance: perception and integration. *Nat Rev Genet* 2002;3: 589–600.

Batterham RL, Cowley MA, Small CJ, et al. Gut hormone PYY(3-36) physiologically inhibits food intake. *Nature* 2002;418: 650–654.

Cone RD, Cowley MA, Butler AA, Fan W, Marks DL, Low MJ. The arcuate nucleus as a conduit for diverse signals relevant to energy homeostasis. *Int J Obes Relat Metab Disord* 2001;25 (Suppl 5):S63–S67.

Cowley MA, Smart JL, Rubinstein M, et al. Leptin activates anorexigenic POMC neurons through a neural network in the arcuate nucleus. *Nature* 2001;411:480–484.

Cowley MA. Hypothalamic melanocortin neurons integrate signals of energy state. *Eur J Pharmacol* 2003;480:3–11.

Crowley VE, Yeo GS, O'Rahilly S. Obesity therapy: altering the energy intake-and-expenditure balance sheet. *Nat Rev Drug Discov* 2002;1:276–286.

Farooqi IS, Jebb SA, Langmack G, et al. Effects of recombinant leptin therapy in a child with congenital leptin deficiency. *N Engl J Med* 1999;341:879–884.

Farooqi IS, Keogh JM, Yeo GS, Lank EJ, Cheetham T, O'Rahilly S. Clinical spectrum of obesity and mutations in the melanocortin 4 receptor gene. *N Engl J Med* 2003;348:1085–1095.

Grill HJ, Kaplan JM. The neuroanatomical axis for control of energy balance. *Front Neuroendocrinol* 2002;23:2–40.

Michel MC, Beck-Sickinger A, Cox H, et al. XVI. International Union of Pharmacology recommendations for the nomenclature of neuropeptide Y, peptide YY, and pancreatic polypeptide receptors. *Pharmacol Rev* 1998;50:143–150.

Saper CB, Chou TC, Elmquist JK. The need to feed: homeostatic and hedonic control of eating. *Neuron* 2002;36:199–211.

Yeo GS, Farooqi IS, Aminian S, Halsall DJ, Stanhope RG, O'Rahilly S. A frameshift mutation in MC4R associated with dominantly inherited human obesity. *Nat Genet* 1998;20:111–112.

Zhang Y, Proenca R, Maffei M, Barone M, Leopold L, Friedman JM. Positional cloning of the mouse obese gene and its human homologue. *Nature* 1994;372:425–432.

26 Endocrinology of the Ovary

Denis Magoffin, PhD, Ashim Kumar, MD,
Bulent Yildiz, MD, and Ricardo Azziz, MD, MPH, MBA

Contents

1. STRUCTURE AND ULTRASTRUCTURE OF OVARY

1.1. Structure of Ovary

The ovary is a complex endocrine organ with both a cortex and a medulla. The medulla contains primarily loose connective tissue, blood vessels, and nerves, but few follicles. The ovarian cortex is composed of primordial and developing follicles, corpora lutea, and corpora albicantia distributed in loose connective tissue known as the interfollicular stroma (Fig. 1).

1.2. Ovarian Follicle

The functional unit of the ovary is the follicle. Within the ovary are follicles at various stages of development, from resting primordial follicles through large Graafian follicles ready to ovulate. Developing follicles are classified according to their morphology (Fig. 2), which, as discussed below, is correlated with their function.

The primordial follicle consists of a meiotically arrested oocyte surrounded by a zona pellucida, a single

From: *Endocrinology: Basic and Clinical Principles, Second Edition*
(S. Melmed and P. M. Conn, eds.) © Humana Press Inc., Totowa, NJ

layer of flattened granulosa cells, and a basal lamina. Preantral follicles are characterized by a growing or fully grown oocyte surrounded by a zona pellucida; one to approximately five layers of cuboidal granulosa cells; a basal lamina; and once the follicle attains approximately two layers of granulosa cells, one or more layers of theca interna cells and the theca externa. Antral follicles develop from preantral follicles with the formation of the fluid-filled antrum and the separation of the corona radiata from the mural granulosa cells (Fig. 2).

1.3. Ultrastructure of Endocrine Cells in Ovary

Both theca and granulosa cells are capable of secreting steroid hormones. Theca cells are steroidogenic cells throughout their life-span; however, granulosa cells become active steroidogenically in the antral stage of development. Steroidogenic cells are characterized by a specialized ultrastructure (Fig. 3). They have mito-

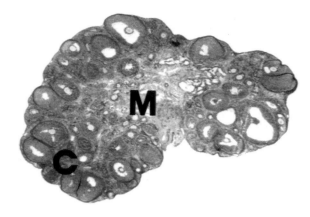

Fig. 1. Morphology of ovary. A cross-section of a rat ovary showing the cortex (C) containing numerous developing follicles and the medulla (M) containing mainly connective tissue, nerves, and blood vessels is shown (magnification: ×18).

chondria with vesicular cristae, an abundant agranular endoplasmic reticulum (ER), and lipid vesicles. These morphologic adaptations are related to the steroidogenic function of the cells. The vesicular cristae are likely related to the expression of the cholesterol side-chain cytochrome P450 (CYP11A) and the abundance of cholesterol in the inner mitochondrial membrane as opposed to the lamellar cristae of nonsteroidogenic cells. The agranular ER reflects the expression of steroidogenic enzymes. In nonsteroidogenic cells, the ER appears "granular" owing to the abundance of ribosomes involved in protein synthesis. The lipid vesicles are a storage site for the cholesteryl esters that can serve as precursor for steroid hormone biosynthesis. Because high concentrations of cholesterol are toxic to cells, they are isolated from the cytosol by encapsulation in membrane-bound vesicles.

2. NORMAL FOLLICLE DEVELOPMENT

Under normal conditions, women produce a single dominant follicle that ovulates a single oocyte each menstrual cycle. The process begins when a cohort of primordial follicles is recruited to initiate growth. Once a primordial follicle initiates growth, the theca and granulosa cells and the oocyte begin to express a developmental program in which a precise sequence and temporal pattern of gene activity occurs. If the entire developmental program is carried out, the follicle ovulates and luteinizes; if there are alterations or errors in this program, the follicle is destroyed by atresia.

In women, the dominant follicle in each cycle originates from a primordial follicle that was recruited to grow about 1 yr earlier. It takes approx 300 d for a primordial follicle to progress through the preantral stages

of development. Preantral follicle development can occur in the absence of gonadotropin stimulation and is therefore referred to as the gonadotropin-independent phase of development. There is recent evidence, however, indicating that the rate of follicle growth can be somewhat accelerated in the presence of high concentrations of follicle-stimulating hormone (FSH).

The rate of follicle growth accelerates markedly when the follicle enters the antral stages of development at approx 2 to 3 mm in diameter. From this point onward, follicle development is highly dependent on FSH stimulation. At the end of the luteal phase of the menstrual cycle, there is a small increase in circulating FSH concentrations that is believed to stimulate the development of the cohort of small antral follicles from which one follicle will be selected to ovulate during the next menstrual cycle. Withdrawal of FSH support is sufficient to cause the follicle to die by the process of atresia that is mediated by apoptosis. Although there is a rapid rate of proliferation of granulosa cells during antral follicle growth, the principal factor causing the tremendous expansion of the follicular diameter is the production of follicular fluid. A 4-mm follicle contains approx 30 µL of fluid, whereas a preovulatory follicle contains up to 6.5 mL of antral fluid. Progression through the antral stages of development occurs in 40–50 d, equivalent to just over two menstrual cycles.

2.1. Initiation of Follicle Growth

Recruitment of nongrowing primordial follicles into the developing pool of follicles begins during embryonic life shortly after the primordial follicles have formed in the ovary and continues until the population of primordial follicles is exhausted. In excess of 6 million primordial follicles are formed in a woman's ovaries between 6 and 9 mo of gestation. At birth, the number of primordial follicles in each ovary is approx 400,000. If the rate of disappearance of primordial follicles were constant throughout a woman's lifetime, it is estimated that the primordial follicles would not be exhausted until the age of 74; however, there is an approximately threefold increase in the rate of disappearance of primordial follicles after the age of 35 that is paralleled by an increase in circulating FSH concentrations, perhaps owing to a decline in negative feedback signals from the ovary.

Primordial follicles consist of a small primary oocyte arrested in prophase of meiosis I surrounded by a single layer of flattened granulosa cells and a basal lamina. When a primordial follicle is recruited into the pool of developing follicles, the granulosa cells transform into cuboidal cells and begin to divide. Although the oocyte does not yet resume meiosis, there is an increase in

Primordial   Primary   Secondary   Small Antral

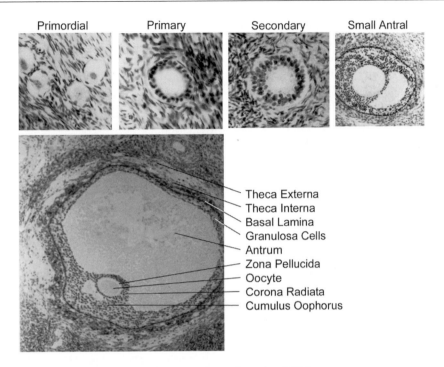

Theca Externa
Theca Interna
Basal Lamina
Granulosa Cells
Antrum
Zona Pellucida
Oocyte
Corona Radiata
Cumulus Oophorus

Fig. 2. Morphology of ovarian follicle.

mRNA and protein synthesis in the oocyte, and it begins to increase in size.

The signal for follicle recruitment is unknown. It is known that recruitment can occur in hypophysectomized animals, indicating that recruitment is not dependent on luteinizing hormone (LH) or FSH. There is evidence that the rate of recruitment can be modulated by intraovarian and environmental factors. The rate of recruitment is related to the total number of primordial follicles in the ovaries, indicating that intraovarian mechanisms are important for regulating recruitment. Evidence from experiments in rodents indicates that recruitment can be attenuated by neonatal thymectomy, starvation, or administration of exogenous opioid peptides, suggesting that there may be endocrine signals capable of modulating the rate of recruitment.

2.2. Selection of Dominant Follicle

The selection of the dominant follicle is one of the final steps in the year-long program of follicle development. In women, the follicle that will ovulate is selected in the early follicular phase of the menstrual cycle. At that time, each ovary contains a cohort of rapidly growing follicles 2–5 mm in diameter. These small antral follicles contain a fully grown oocyte, approx 1 million granulosa cells, and several layers of theca cells. From this cohort, the follicle most advanced in the developmental program is selected to become dominant. Once

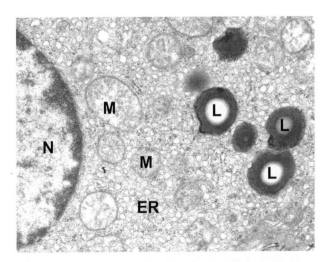

Fig. 3. Ultrastructure of ovarian steroid-secreting cells. The specialized ultrastructure of steroid-producing cells includes mitochondria (M) with vesicular cristae, abundant agranular ER, and numerous lipid vesicles (L) containing cholesteryl esters. N = nucleus (magnification: ×21,000)

it reaches a size of 6–8 mm in the early follicular phase, changes occur, possibly in the structure of the basal lamina, that permit FSH to enter the follicle and begin to stimulate the granulosa cells. The granulosa cells and theca cells of the selected follicle show a high rate of cell proliferation, whereas mitosis stops in the cells of other cohort follicles. The ability to sustain a high capacity for rapid cell division is a characteristic feature seen only in dominant follicles. The smaller follicles in the cohort with slower growth inevitably undergo atresia.

When biologically active FSH first enters the follicle at about 6 to 7 mm, the granulosa cells begin to express the aromatase enzyme and to secrete estradiol. In addition, the granulosa cells begin to secrete increasing amounts of inhibin B. Together, these hormones cause a small but significant and progressive decrement in the circulating FSH concentration owing to their inhibitory effects on pituitary secretion. The lack of FSH support to the cohort follicles causes developmental failure and certain atresia. Counteracting the FSH withdrawal by administration of exogenous FSH is the basis for ovulation induction protocols that are used clinically to develop multiple preovulatory follicles for assisted reproduction techniques.

In contrast to the cohort follicles, the dominant follicle preferentially sequesters FSH in the follicular fluid, thus enabling it to maintain adequate FSH support even though circulating FSH concentrations decline. Another important mechanism that confers a developmental advantage to the dominant follicle is sensitization of the follicle cells to FSH. The granulosa cells of the dominant follicle produce growth and differentiation factors, such as insulin-like growth factors (IGFs) and inhibin, that augment the stimulatory effects of FSH. By virtue of these mechanisms, the dominant follicle can continue to grow and thrive while the cohort follicles die. By simply changing the concentration of FSH during the follicular phase of the cycle, the number of preovulatory follicles can be determined.

The theca cells do not respond to FSH but are regulated by LH. The mean circulating concentrations of LH do not change appreciably during the follicular phase of the menstrual cycle. At the time theca cells first appear in secondary follicles, they have steroidogenic capacity, but the stimulatory effects of LH are attenuated by granulosa cell–secreted factors. Because estradiol is a key mediator of follicle selection and theca cell steroidogenesis is essential for the follicle to secrete estradiol, it is important for thecal steroidogenesis to increase in dominant follicles. It is likely that the same factors that sensitize the granulosa cells to FSH also augment the stimulatory effects of LH on theca cell steroidogenesis. Thus, theca cell steroidogenesis is enhanced only when the granulosa cells have expressed the aromatase enzyme. In women, the capacity to secrete large amounts of estrogen is the exclusive property of dominant follicles.

2.3. Atresia

Greater than 99% of the follicles present in the ovaries die by atresia. Atresia occurs in both preantral and antral follicles and is not exclusively related to the failure of a follicle to become dominant. Indeed, approx 95% of the follicles become atretic prior to the first ovulation.

The process of follicle atresia occurs by apoptosis. The granulosa cells undergo nuclear and cytoplasmic condensation, plasma membrane blebbing, and the release of apoptotic bodies containing cellular organelles. The nuclear DNA undergoes internucleosomal cleavage, and the cellular fragments are removed from the ovary by phagocytosis. It is clear that removal of FSH support from follicles in the gonadotropin-dependent stages of follicle development will trigger atresia, but the causes of apoptosis in preantral follicles are less certain.

3. STEROID HORMONE PRODUCTION

3.1. Two-Cell, Two-Gonadotropin Concept of Follicle Estrogen Production

The production of large quantities of estradiol is one of the most important endocrine functions of the dominant follicle. It is through estradiol concentrations that the state of follicle development is communicated to the hypothalamus and pituitary such that the midcycle ovulatory surge of LH is timed appropriately. Another key function of estradiol is to prepare the endometrium for implantation of the embryo.

Experiments conducted during the 1950s demonstrated that both the theca interna and the granulosa compartments of the ovarian follicle are required for estradiol production. In addition, both LH and FSH stimulation are required for estradiol production to occur. These observations have been confirmed many times in a variety of mammalian species, and the molecular basis for the two-cell, two-gonadotropin concept for follicle estrogen biosynthesis has been established (Fig. 4).

From the time the theca cells first differentiate into endocrine cells, they contain LH receptors and the key steroidogenic enzymes required for androgen biosynthesis from cholesterol: cholesterol side-chain cleavage cytochrome P450 (CYP11A), 3β-hydroxysteroid dehydrogenase (3β-HSD), and 17α-hydroxylase/C_{17-20} lyase cytochrome P450 (CYP17). Thus, the theca cells are endowed with the capacity to synthesize androgens from cholesterol *de novo* under the control of LH. Although the principal androgen secreted by the theca cells is androstenedione, the human CYP17 enzyme is extremely inefficient at converting 17β-

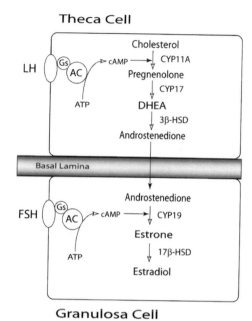

Theca Cell

Granulosa Cell

Fig. 4. Two-cell, two-gonadotropin concept of follicle estrogen production. LH stimulates the theca cells to differentiate and produce androstenedione from cholesterol. FSH stimulates the differentiation of the granulosa cells. The androstenedione diffuses across the basal lamina and is metabolized to estradiol in the granulosa cells. Gs = stimulatory G-protein; AC = adenylate cyclase, ATP = adenosine triphosphate; cAMP = cyclic adenosine monophosphate.

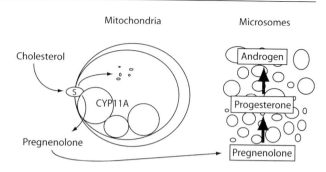

Fig. 5. Compartmentalization of steroidogenic enzymes. Diffusion of cholesterol across the mitochondrial membranes is facilitated by StAR (S). The function of StAR is terminated by proteolysis. Cholesterol in the mitochondria is converted into pregnenolone by CYP11A. Pregnenolone diffuses out of the mitochondria and is metabolized to other steroids in the microsomes. In the ovary, depending on the cell type, the final product may be progesterone or androgen.

hydroxyprogesterone to androstenedione. Consequently, steroidogenesis proceeds via the delta 5 pathway, where 17β-hydroxypregnenolone is metabolized into dehydroepiandrosterone (DHEA) by the CYP17 enzyme, and then DHEA is converted into androstenedione by the 3β-HSD. The theca cells in women do not express aromatase CYP19 and, hence, cannot produce estradiol. In certain species, notably the horse and pig, theca cells do express low levels of CYP19 and can produce small amounts of estrogen; however, cooperation with the granulosa cells is still required to secrete high concentrations of estradiol.

In contrast to the theca cells, the granulosa cells are incapable of *de novo* steroidogenesis in the follicular phase of the menstrual cycle. It is not until the periovulatory period that the granulosa cells express LH receptors and CYP11A as they begin to luteinize. Therefore, in the follicular phase of the cycle, the granulosa cells cannot produce the androgen substrate required by the CYP19 enzyme. When a follicle is selected to become dominant, the granulosa cells express high levels of CYP19 and 17β-hydroxysteroid dehydrogenase (17β-HSD) under the control of FSH. This enables the granulosa cells to metabolize the androstenedione pro-

duced by the theca cells to estradiol. Thus, it takes two cells, theca and granulosa, and two gonadotropins, LH and FSH, for the ovarian follicle to produce estradiol.

3.2. Intracellular Compartmentalization of Steroidogenic Enzymes

The regulation of steroid hormone production occurs in two ways. Acute regulation of the rate of steroidogenesis takes place by controlling the rate of cholesterol access to the CYP11A enzyme. This is possible because the CYP11A is localized in the inner leaflet of the inner mitochondrial membrane (Fig. 5). Because cholesterol is sparingly soluble in water, diffusion from the outer to the inner mitochondrial membrane is very slow. Acute stimulation with LH causes production of the steroidogenesis acute regulatory protein (StAR) that facilitates the transport of cholesterol across the mitochondrial membranes. StAR is thought to function by bringing the outer and inner mitochondrial membranes into contact at focal points, thus facilitating the movement of cholesterol from the outer to the inner membrane. The activity of the StAR protein is rapidly terminated by proteolytic cleavage. When cholesterol is present in the inner mitochondrial membrane, the CYP11A enzyme readily metabolizes it to pregnenolone. Pregnenolone is able to diffuse out of the mitochondria, where it is metabolized to other steroids that, in the ovary, are localized in the microsomes.

3.3. Hormonal Regulation of Cellular Differentiation

The second means for regulating steroid hormone biosynthesis is to control cellular differentiation by

Table 1
Autocrine/Paracrine Factors Regulating Ovarian Steroid Hormone Production

Factor [a]		Cellular origin	Effect on LH-dependent androgen production in vitro [b]	Effect on FSH-dependent estrogen production in vitro [b]
Growth factors	• IGF-I	GC	+	+
	• Activin	GC	–	+
	• Inhibin	GC	+	–
	• TGF-β	GC/TC	–	+
	• TGF-α	TC	–	–
	• bFGF	GC	–	–
	• NGF	TC	+	?
	• GDF-9	Oocyte	+	–
	• HGF	TC	–	–
	• KGF	TC	–	?
Cytokines	• TNF-α	Oocyte/GC/resident ovarian macrophages	–	–
	• IL-1β	GC/resident ovarian macrophages	–	–

[a] IGF-1 = insulin-like growth factor-1; TGF-β = transforming growth factor-β; bFGF = basic fibroblast growth factor; NGF = nerve growth factor; GDF-4 = growth differentiation factor-9; HGF = hepatocyte growth factor; KGF = keratinocyte growth factor; TNF-α = tumor necrosis factor-α; IL-1β = interleukin-1β.

[b] +, augments; –, inhibits; ?, unknown.

altering the concentrations of the various steroidogenic enzymes expressed in the cells. Changes in the concentrations of steroidogenic enzymes occur over more prolonged and developmentally regulated time frames on the order of days or longer, whereas the acute regulation of steroidogenesis occurs on the order of minutes.

The signal initiating granulosa cell growth and differentiation has not been fully defined. It is clear that gonadotropins are not involved because the granulosa cells in primordial follicles do not express FSH or LH receptors. Evidence is beginning to emerge indicating that proteins secreted by the oocyte such as growth differentiation factor-9, a member of the transforming growth factor-β (TGF-β) superfamily, play an essential role in initiating follicle development. Prior to the selection of the dominant follicle, the granulosa cells do not express CYP19 and therefore do not contribute to estradiol production.

When preantral follicles contain approximately two layers of granulosa cells, the granulosa cells secrete proteins into the stroma that cause undifferentiated mesenchymal cells to differentiate into theca cells. The signals have not been fully defined, but it appears that several small molecular weight proteins potentially including IGF-1 and stem cell factor or kit ligand may be components of the differentiation signal. When the theca cells first differentiate, they contain LH receptors, StAR, CYP11A, 3β-HSD, and CYP17. Thus, they are capable of producing androstenedione at the preantral stage of follicle development.

Excessive androgens can have detrimental effects on ovarian function; therefore, it is beneficial to ensure that androgens do not accumulate before CYP19 is expressed in the granulosa cells. The granulosa cells secrete several factors that inhibit the stimulatory actions of LH on theca cell steroidogenic enzyme gene expression and androgen production including activin and TGF-β (Table 1).

If a follicle becomes selected, the inhibitory signal from the granulosa cells changes to one in which the stimulatory effects of LH are enhanced. Many of the same molecules both enhance the effects of LH on theca cell differentiation and sensitize the granulosa cells to the stimulatory effects of FSH. It is through the enhancement of LH and FSH action by factors such as IGF-1 and inhibin family members (Table 1) that expression of steroidogenic enzymes in the theca cells and CYP19 in the granulosa cells is increased even though the concentrations of LH and FSH do not increase in the circulation. Although the nature of the signals is not fully understood, it is clear that there is a detailed system of communication among the oocyte, granulosa cells, and theca cells that ensures that the differentiation and function of the follicle cells are coordinated. Successful completion of this developmental program results in a preovulatory follicle ready to ovulate.

4. OVULATION

Ovulation is the end process of a series of events initiated by the gonadotropin surge and resulting in the release of a mature fertilizable oocyte from a Graafian follicle. During the second half of the follicular phase and as follicles grow, plasma estradiol concentrations begin to rise. About 24–48 h after plasma estradiol levels reach a peak, the midcycle LH surge takes place. This preovulatory LH surge occurs at around d 14 of a 28-d cycle, with a total duration of approx 48 h. Ovulation occurs 36 h after the onset of the LH surge. Progesterone and FSH levels remain low in the follicular phase until just before ovulation. At this time, a small FSH surge accompanies the greater LH surge, and progesterone levels rise slightly just before ovulation.

The precise hormonal regulation mechanisms operating during ovulation are not fully elucidated. However, it is well known that the gonadotropin surge at the end of the follicular phase is essential for ovulation. The midcycle LH surge results from activation of positive estradiol feedback at the level of both the pituitary and hypothalamus. The increasing amounts of estradiol secreted by the dominant follicle trigger the hypothalamic gonadotropin-releasing hormone (GnRH) surge. The administration of a GnRH antagonist in women prevents the surge or interrupts it if it has already started. This suggests that GnRH is necessary not only for the surge to occur but also for the maintenance of the surge. Additionally, the pituitary LH surge is facilitated by an increased responsiveness of gonadotrope cells to GnRH observed following exposure to rising estradiol and by an increase in GnRH receptor number. The feedback signal to terminate the LH surge is unknown. The decline in LH may be owing to the loss of the positive feedback effect of estrogen, resulting from the increasing inhibitory feedback effect of progesterone, or owing to a depletion of LH content of the pituitary from downregulation of GnRH receptors. The rise in progesterone concentrations may lead to a negative feedback loop and inhibit pituitary LH secretion by decreasing GnRH pulse frequency. Moreover, LH downregulates its own receptors just before ovulation, resulting in decreased estrogen production.

The LH surge stimulates resumption of meiosis I in the oocyte with release of the first polar body. The oocyte nucleus or germinal vesicle undergoes a series of changes that involve germinal vesicle breakdown and the progression of meiosis to the second meiotic metaphase or first polar body stage. It has been suggested that the LH surge overcomes the arrest of meiosis by inhibiting the oocyte maturation inhibitor (OMI) secretion. This inhibitor is produced by granulosa cells and leads to the arrest of meiosis during folliculogenesis. It appears that OMI exerts its inhibitory action on meiosis, not directly on the oocyte, but acts to increase the concentrations of cAMP in the cumulus cells, which

then passes via gap junctions into oocyte and halts meiotic maturation. The LH surge, by inhibiting OMI secretion and thereby decreasing cAMP, allows the resumption of meiosis. The second meiotic division is completed at the time of fertilization, if it occurs, yielding the ovum with the haploid number of chromosomes and the second polar body that is released.

With the LH surge, the production of antral fluid in the dominant follicle increases, and the follicle enlarges markedly. This results in a relatively thin peripheral rim of granulosa cells and regressing thecal cells to which the oocyte, with its associated cumulus cells, is attached only by a tenuous and thinning stalk of granulosa cells. The increasing size of the follicle and its position in the cortex of the ovarian stroma cause it to bulge out from the ovarian surface, leaving only a thin layer of epithelial cells between the follicular wall and the peritoneal cavity. At one site on its surface, the follicle wall becomes even thinner and avascular; the cells in this area dissociate and then appear to degenerate and the wall balloons outward. The follicle then ruptures at this site, the stigma, causing the fluid to flow out on the surface of the ovary, carrying with it the oocyte and its surrounding mass of cumulus cells. Follicle rupture and oocyte extrusion are evoked by LH and progesterone-induced expression of proteolytic enzymes such as collagenases. Enzymatic degradation of the follicle wall is a primary hypothesis to explain the rupture. Increased prostaglandin (PG) synthesis also appears to play a role in the extrusion of the oocyte. PGs probably contribute to the process of ovulation through various pathways, such as affecting the contractility of the smooth muscle cells on the ovary and activating proteolytic enzymes, especially those associated with collagen degradation.

5. LUTEINIZATION

Luteinization is the process that transforms the granulosa and theca cells into luteal cells. This process is triggered by the surge of LH at midcycle, once the granulosa cells have acquired receptors for LH, and does not necessarily signify that ovulation has occurred. The LH surge causes profound morphologic changes in the follicle that becomes corpus luteum. These include acquisition by the granulosa cells of the capacity of *de novo* synthesis of steroids (mainly progesterone and estrogen) and invasion of the previously avascular granulosa cell layer by a vascular supply.

After ovulation and expulsion of the unfertilized egg, the granulosa cells continue to enlarge, become vacuolated in appearance, and begin to accumulate a yellow pigment called lutein, and they are now called as granulosa lutein cells. Luteinization of granulosa cell involves the appearance of lipid droplets in the cytoplasm, development by the mitochondria of a dense matrix with tubular cristae, hypertrophy of the ER and enlargement of the granulosa cell into the "large luteal cell." Thecal cells are also luteinized (theca-lutein cells) and make up the outer portion of the corpus luteum. These "small luteal cells" are much less active in steroidogenesis and have no secretory granules. The basal lamina of the follicle dissolves, and capillaries invade into the granulosa layer of cells in response to secretion of angiogenic factors such as vascular endothelial growth factor by the granulosa and thecal cells.

The corpus luteum is a transient endocrine organ that predominately secretes progesterone, and its primary function is to prepare the estrogen-primed endometrium for implantation of the fertilized ovum. The granulosa-lutein cells express cholesterol side-chain cleavage enzyme and 3β-HSD, and, accordingly, they have a high capacity to produce progesterone and estradiol. Blood vessels penetrating the follicle basal lamina provide these cells with low-density lipoproteins, the main source of cholesterol as a substrate for progesterone and estradiol synthesis in luteal cells. Seven days after ovulation, approximately around the time of expected implantation, peak vascularization is achieved. This time also corresponds to peak serum levels of progesterone and estradiol. The secretion of progesterone and estradiol is episodic and correlates with the LH pulses. During the process of luteinization, LH is required to maintain steroidogenesis by granulosa-lutein cells. The role of other luteotropic factors such as prolactin (PRL), oxytocin, inhibin, and relaxin remains unclear. Theca-lutein cells that express the enzymes in the androgen biosynthetic pathway and produce androstenedione are also involved in steroid biosynthesis.

The life-span of the corpus luteum is 14 days after ovulation and depends on continued LH support. The mechanism involved in maintaining the function of the corpus luteum for 14 d and in precipitating the process of luteolysis (programmed cell death) at the end of this period is incompletely understood. It is clear, however, that LH maintains the functional and morphologic integrity of the corpus luteum, yet it is insufficient to prevent luteolysis. Corpus luteum function declines by the end of the luteal phase unless human chorionic gonadotropin (hCG) is produced by a pregnancy. Luteolysis can be viewed as a default response to lack of stimulation by hCG. If pregnancy does not occur, the corpus luteum undergoes luteolysis under the influence of luteolytic factors. These factors include estradiol, oxytocin, and PGs. The luteolytic effect of both estrogen and oxytocin appears to be mediated, at least in part, by local formation of PGF_{2a}. PGF_{2a} exerts its effects via

the synthesis of endothelin-1 (ET-1), which inhibits steroidogenesis and stimulates the release of a cytokine, tumor necrosis factor-α (TNF-α), which induces cell apoptosis.

Corpus luteum starts to undergo luteolysis approx 8 d after ovulation. Luteolysis involves fibrosis of the luteinized cells, a dramatic decrease in the number of secretory granules with a parallel increase in lipid droplets and cytoplasmic vacuoles, and a decrease in vascularization. The luteal cells become necrotic, progesterone secretion ceases, and the corpus luteum is invaded by macrophages and then by fibroblasts. Endocrine function is rapidly lost, and the corpus luteum is replaced by a scarlike tissue, the corpus albicans.

6. DEFECTS IN OVULATORY FUNCTION

Ovulatory defects can be classified into three groups based on the World Health Organization (WHO) definition. These classes suggest different etiologies and, consequently, different optimal treatment approaches.

1. Group I: hypogonadotropic hypogonadism: Patients with hypogonadotropic hypogonadism comprise 5–10% of anovulatory women. These patients have low serum FSH and estradiol levels. This category includes women with hypothalamic amenorrhea (HA), stress-related amenorrhea, anorexia nervosa, and Kallman syndrome. These women will respond to gonadotropin therapy for ovulation induction.
2. Group II: eugonadotropic hypogonadism: Patients are eugonadotropic, normoestrogenic, but anovulatory and constitute the majority of anovulatory women evaluated (60–85%). They exhibit normal FSH and estradiol levels. This category includes women with polycystic ovary syndrome (PCOS), among other disorders. These women respond to most ovulatory agents.
3. Group III: hypergonadotropic hypogonadism: Patients with hypergonadotropic hypogonadism account for 10–30% of women evaluated for anovulation. These patients tend to be amenorrheic and hypoestrogenic, a category that includes all variants of premature ovarian failure (POF) and ovarian resistance syndromes. These patients will not respond to ovulation induction but are candidates for oocyte donation.

Hyperprolactinemia accounts for 5–10% of women with anovulation, and these patients respond well to medications that lower PRL secretion. Although many of these women have normal estrogen levels (i.e., are euestrogenic) and therefore can be categorized as having a WHO Group II ovulatory defect, some of these women may be hypoestrogenic and be more similar to Group I patients. Consequently, these patients are often considered separately from those women meeting the standard WHO classification of ovulatory disorders.

Table 2
Etiologies of POF

Decrease in initial pool of oocytes	Increase rate of loss of oocytes
Gonadal dysgenesis	X-chromosome defects
Thymic aplasia	Autoimmune
	Iatrogenic (surgical/chemotherapy)
	Enzymatic abnormalities
	Infection/toxins

Following we discuss in some detail the pathophysiology and clinical presentation of patients with HA (WHO Group I), PCOS (WHO Group II), and POF (WHO Group III).

6.1. Hypothalamic Amenorrhea

Amenorrhea with signs or symptoms of hypoestrogenism and low gonadotropin levels with exclusion of related disorders confirms a diagnosis of HA. WHO classifies HA as Group I anovulation. Hypothalamic or pituitary dysfunction may involve the amount of products (e.g., GnRH, FSH) secreted or the pulse frequency of the products.

A thorough history and physical examination can help elucidate potential etiologies. Hyperprolactinemia and hypo/hyperthyroidism should be ruled out in all women with amenorrhea. An imaging study of the hypothalamus and pituitary is imperative to evaluate for tumors. The accuracy of the assays used for FSH and LH is poor in the lower ranges. Therefore, the "lab results" for FSH and LH in patients with HA may be "low" or "low normal."

Anatomic or developmental lesions of the hypothalamus or pituitary gland can lead to hypothalamic amenorrhea. Patients with Kallman syndrome have a failure of migration of the GnRH neurons from the nasal placode to the hypothalamus. They present with amenorrhea and anosmia. Patients with idiopathic hypogonadotropic hypogonadism present similar to those with Kallman syndrome, but without anosmia. Treatment options include the GnRH pump or gonadotropin ovulation for infertility, and HRT for osteoporosis prevention and estrogen replacement.

Hypothalamic lesions, tumors, or space-occupying lesions (e.g., sarcoidosis) can lead to HA. Craniopharyngiomas are the most common tumor affecting the reproductive function of the hypothalamus. They are treated surgically in combination with radiotherapy. Iatrogenic HA may result from damage during surgery or irradiation of the hypothalamus. These patients should be tested for insufficiency of all pituitary secretagogues and replaced as indicated.

HA from pituitary lesions can be the result of tumors (micro/macroadenomas), infarction (e.g., Sheehan syndrome), empty sella syndrome, trauma (with transection of the pituitary stalk), space-occupying lesions (e.g., sarcoidosis), and lymphocytic hypophysitis.

Prolactinomas are the most common type of adenomas found in the pituitary. Initial treatment of PRL-secreting micro- or macroadenomas is with dopamine agonists, e.g., bromocriptine or cabergoline. The effects of dopamine analogs on PRL levels can be detected within weeks. Surgery is reserved for refractory cases. Other secretory products of adenomas include GH, adrenocorticotropic hormone, and FSH.

Patients with empty sella syndrome may present with normal, low, or elevated levels of pituitary hormones. Those with trauma or infarction may have aberrations of various pituitary hormones, and assessment of patients should include the adrenal, thyroid, ovary, and GH. These women need to be treated on an individualized basis as indicated.

Nonanatomic defects of the pituitary are indistinguishable from hypothalamic lesions. A GnRH stimulation test is not routinely used in clinical practice to differentiate between pituitary and hypothalamic dysfunction because of difficulties in interpretation of test results and little effect on patient management.

Functional lesions disrupting the hypothalamic pituitary axis can result from a variety of stressors. Physical stressors such as anorexia nervosa or excessive exercise lead to HA. Diagnosis is based on history or findings of severe weight loss or cachexia with laboratory findings consistent with HA. Treatment includes resolution of the stressor and HRT to prevent osteoporosis.

6.2 Polycystic Ovary Syndrome

Androgens are C19 steroids secreted by the zona reticularis of the adrenal cortex and the theca and stroma of the ovaries, produced through *de novo* synthesis from cholesterol. The ovarian theca is responsible for secreting approx 25% of circulating testosterone, and for 50% of all androstenedione, the most important precursor of dihydrotestosterone and testosterone. Androgen excess

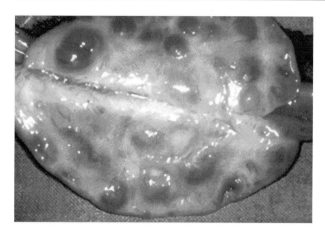

Fig. 6. Polycystic ovary bivalved during ovarian wedge resection. Note the multiple follicular cysts measuring 2–6 mm in diameter, and the increased stromal volume.

or hyperandrogenism affects 5–10% of reproductive-age women.

A common feature of androgen excess disorders is ovulatory dysfunction, which may arise from a disruption of gonadotropin secretion or from direct ovarian effects. Androgens may directly alter the secretion of gonadotropins in women. However, the effect of androgens on the hypothalamic-pituitary-ovarian axis appears to be primarily dependent on their aromatization to estrogens. Excessive androgen levels may also directly inhibit follicle development at the ovarian level, which may result in the accumulation of multiple small cysts within the ovarian cortex, the so-called polycystic ovary (Fig. 6).

By far the most common cause of androgen excess is the PCOS, accounting for approx 80–85% of patients with androgen excess, and 4–6% of reproductive-age women. Although there is continuing debate regarding the definition of PCOS, useful diagnostic criteria arose from a 1990 National Institutes of Health (NIH) conference on the subject. These criteria note that PCOS should include, in order of importance, (1) clinical and/or biochemical evidence of hyperandrogenism; (2) ovulatory dysfunction; and (3) the exclusion of other causes of androgen excess or ovulatory dysfunction, including adrenal hyperplasia, hyperprolactinemia, thyroid dysfunction, and androgen-secreting neoplasms (ASNs).

The presence of polycystic ovaries on ultrasound was not included as part of the definition arising from the 1990 NIH conference. However, in approx 70% of patients with PCOS, the ovaries contain intermediate and atretic follicles measuring 2–5 mm in diameter, resulting in a "polycystic" appearance at sonography (Fig. 7). Diagnostic criteria for PCOS using ovarian morphologic

features have been suggested. However, note that "polycystic ovaries" on sonography or at pathology might simply be a sign of dysfunctional folliclar development. For example, this ovarian morphology is frequently seen in patients with other androgen excess disorders, including nonclassic and classic adrenal hyperplasia. It is also frequently observed in patients with hyperprolactinemia, type 2 diabetes mellitus, and bulimia nervosa, independent of the presence of hyperandrogenism. Up to 25% of unselected women have polycystic ovaries on ultrasound, many of whom are normoandrogenic regularly cycling. Hence, we consider the presence of polycystic ovaries to be only a sign, albeit nondiagnostic, of androgen excess or PCOS. A recent expert conference has suggested including the presence of polycystic ovaries as part of the diagnostic scheme for PCOS (Rotterdam, 2004)

Classically, pathologic features of the ovaries in PCOS includes thickening and collagenization of the tunica albuginea, a paucity of corpus luteum, basal membrane thickening, an increased number of follicles in various stages of development and atresia, and stromal/thecal hyperplasia (hyperthecosis) (Fig. 8A). Although the number of cysts measuring 4–6 mm is greater than normal, the fact that most of these are in various stages of atresia leads to a relative deficiency in granulosa cells and/or predominance of theca/stromal cells. Although we and others have reported that the theca/stromal cells in PCOS frequently demonstrate "luteinization" (Fig. 8B), Green and Goldzieher (1965) did not observe any abnormality of the follicular or theca cells on light or electron microscopy.

The presence of multiple follicular cysts typically results in "polycystic"-appearing ovaries, which give the syndrome its name. However, note that patients with PCOS demonstrate a spectrum of histologic findings. Givens (1984) has described ovaries with an increased number of follicular cysts and minimal stromal hyperplasia, classified as type I. Alternatively, type IV ovaries demonstrated a small number of follicular cysts, with marked stromal hyperplasia and "hyperthecosis." Types I and IV ovaries appear to represent the two extremes of a continuum. Kim et al. (1979) studied nine patients with clinical evidence of androgen excess. Four of these patients demonstrated "polycystic" ovaries, and the remaining five had histologically normal ovaries. In these patients, adrenocortical suppression with dexamethasone (2 mg daily for 3 d) minimally suppressed androgen levels in all patients, whereas an oral contraceptive administered for 21 d normalized androgens in both groups of patients with androgen excess. Thus, ovarian hyperandrogenism was present in patients with and without polycystic-appearing ovaries.

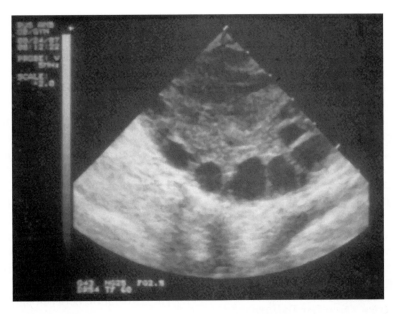

Fig. 7. Transvaginal ultrasound visualization of a polycystic ovary. Note the string of subcapsular follicles measuring 3–6 mm in diameter, with increased central stroma mass.

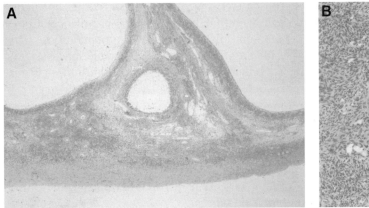
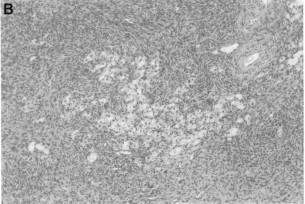

Fig. 8. Section of polycystic ovary. Note (**A**) the markedly thickened ovarian capsule with multiple subcapsular Graafian follicles (hematoxylin adn eosin [H&E] stain, ×2.5) and (**B**) the islands of luteinized stromal cells, characteristic of hyperthecosis (H&E stain, ×10).

In addition to the direct effects of androgens on ovarian function, hyperinsulinism and excess LH levels appear to contribute to the ovarian androgen excess present in PCOS. Many women with PCOS appear to be uniquely insulin resistant, with compensatory hyperinsulinemia, independent of body weight. The compensatory hyperinsulinemia, resulting from the underlying insulin resistance, augments the stimulatory action of LH on the growth and androgen secretion of ovarian thecal cells, while inhibiting the hepatic production of sex hormone–binding globulin. Overall, insulin resistance and secondary hyperinsulinemia affect a large fraction of patients with PCOS and may cause or augment ovarian androgen excess in these patients.

The LH/FSH ratio is also elevated in 35–95% of patients with PCOS, although recent ovulation appears to be associated with a transient normalization in the ratio. The use of insulin sensitizers to treat patients with PCOS may result in lower circulating levels of LH, suggesting that insulin resistance or, more likely, hyperinsulinemia is in part responsible for the gonadotropic abnormalities observed in many women with PCOS although not all researchers agree. The excess LH present contributes to the stimulation of theca cell biosynthesis, further leading to the excess ovarian secretion of androgens.

Ovulatory dysfunction in PCOS frequently results in oligoovulatory infertility. As a general rule, women with PCOS require ovulation induction with either clomiphene citrate or gonadotropins. In this context, women with PCOS are at especially increased risk of developing the hyperstimulation syndrome, a syndrome of massive enlargement of the ovaries; development of rapid and symptomatic ascites, intravascular contraction, hypercoagulability, and systemic organ dysfunction; and multiple gestations. These complications occur generally following treatment with gonadotropins, although ovarian hyperstimulation has even been reported in women with PCOS conceiving a singleton pregnancy spontaneously or after the use of clomiphene or pulsatile GnRH.

6.3. Premature Ovarian Failure

Menopause occurring prior to 40 yr of age is termed POF. The diagnosis is based on findings of amenorrhea, hypoestrogenism, and elevated gonadotropins. In a study of 15,253 women attending menopause clinics in Italy, the Progetto Menopausa Italia Study Group found that 1.8% of the women reported POF. Coulam et al. (1986) reported a 1% risk incidence of POF in a group of 1858 women in Rochester, Minnesota. The prevalence of POF in women with primary amenorrhea is estimated at 10–28%. Women with secondary amenorrhea have a lower prevalence, at approx 4–18%. Risk factors for POF include nulliparity and lifelong irregular menses; however, age at menarche, oral contraceptive use, and smoking were not associated with the condition.

These findings may not imply irrevocable quiescence of follicular activity, because there are numerous reports of reinitiation of menses in women previously diagnosed with POF. Because of the multiple possible etiologies and the unresolved nature of the damage, there are no predictors of remission. Little is known about these periods other than that they do occur spontaneously and can result in viable pregnancy. Failure of oocytes secondary to depletion or inhibition of their function results in POF. Histologic examination of the ovaries reveals minimal follicular activity; dense connective tissue and/or lymphocytic infiltrates may be seen. Nelson et al. (1994) reported on follicular activity in women with POF with normal karyotypes. They found that although almost half of the patients had estradiol levels consistent with follicular activity, the follicles were not functioning normally.

Approximately 50% of POF is of an idiopathic etiology. Other causes include chromosomal anomalies leading to gonadal dysgenesis, autoimmunity, chemotherapeutics, ovarian surgery, inherited enzymatic defects, and infections. In these settings, POF may result from a reduction in the initial pool of follicles, or an accelerated loss of oocytes (Table 2). Pure gonadal dysgenesis (46, XX) results in women born with ovaries lacking oocytes. More common is the increased destruction of oocytes. Women with X-chromosome defects (Turner syndrome, Turner mosaic, translocations, deletions, and heterozygote fragile X) show accelerated loss of oocytes, which is clearly associated with POF. Specifically, a critical region on Xq appears to play a key role in ovarian function, and a disruption of this region leads to premature activation of follicular apoptosis. The thymus is essential to ensure appropriate number of oocytes at birth; therefore, thymic aplasia can also lead to POF.

The association between autoimmunity and POF is clear. POF was associated with other endocrine autoimmune conditions including those of the adrenal (Addison disease: 2.5%) and thyroid glands (hypothyroidism: 27%), as well as diabetes mellitus, in a prospective analysis of 120 women with POF and normal karyotype. Women with POF have increased prevalence of other autoimmune diseases such as hypoparathyroidism, myasthenia gravis, pernicious anemia, and systemic lupus erythematosus. Antibodies against various ovarian antigens have been isolated in higher frequency in women with POF. Antiovarian antibodies have been targeted against oocytes, theca, granulosa, and gonadotropin receptors. Several investigators have found antibodies against steroid-producing antibodies and antibodies toward steroidogenic enzymes (CYP21, CYP17, CYP19, and 3β-HSD) in women with Addison disease and POF.

Surgical and chemotherapeutic treatments can lead to POF. Women undergo oophorectomy and ovarian cystectomy for a variety of reasons including dermoids, endometriosis, persistent cysts, and cancer. Women with multiple ovarian surgeries are at increased risk of POF. Alkylating agents used in chemotherapy are associated with oocyte damage and POF. The use of GnRH analogs and ovarian autografts may prevent oocyte damage.

Several enzymatic defects have been implicated as the etiology for POF. Women with defects in galactose-1-phosphate uridyl-transferase have a high prevalence of POF. Women with this disorder appear to have an adequate number of follicles but show evidence of accelerated loss prior to menarche. 17α-Hydroxylase deficiency has also been associated with POF.

Infections with varicella, shigella, or malaria were found in 3.5% of women with POF. Exposure to environmental toxins has been associated with POF. Polcyclic aromatic hydrocarbons, from combustion of fossil fuels or in cigarette smoke, can stimulate apoptosis in oocytes leading to POF. POF was found to be secondary to exposure to 2-bromopropane in a study of 16 women exposed to the cleaning solvent.

The patient's history and physical examination should include assessment for the possible etiologies just discussed. Laboratory evaluation should include levels of FSH, LH, estradiol, thyroid-stimulating hormone, prolactin, fasting glucose, calcium, phosphate, and electrolytes. A chromosomal analysis should be done on those under 35 yr of age.

Treatment for POF should focus on supporting and educating the patient, treating symptoms of hypoestrogenemia, and preventing osteoporosis. Infertility should be addressed by educating the patient regarding possible remission with resumption of menses and fertility, ovum donation, and adoption. The patient may be started on any regimen of hormone replacement therapy (HRT) with estrogen and progesterone as indicated, with appropriate counseling regarding the risks of thrombosis and breast cancer. Patients with POF should be followed closely and evaluated for other endocrinopathies, especially adrenal insufficiency, on an annual basis. There is little prospective evidence to support the use of glucocorticoids in the treatment of POF, and this management has significant risks such as avascular necrosis of the femoral head, and knee, as well as iatrogenic Cushing syndrome. Numerous case reports offer the promise of potential therapies for POF to restore ovarian function, but these should be avoided until proven with appropriate studies.

REFERENCES

Coulam CB, Adamson SC, Annegers JF. Incidence of premature ovarian failure. *Obstet Gynecol* 1986;67:604–606.
Givens JR. Polycystic ovaries—a sign, not a diagnosis. *Semin Reprod Endocrinol* 1984;2:271–280.
Green JA, Goldzieher JW. The polycystic ovary. IV. Light and electron microscope studies. *Am J Obstet Gynecol* 1965;91:173–181.
Kim MH, Rosenfield RL, Hosseinian AH, Schneir HG. Ovarian hyperandrogenism with normal and abnormal histologic findings of the ovaries. *Am J Obstet Gynecol* 1979;134:445–452.

Nelson LM, Anasti JN, Kimzey LM, et al. Development of luteinized graafian follicles in patients with karyotypically normal spontaneous premature ovarian failure. *J Clin Endocrinol Metab* 1994;79:1470–1475.
The Rotterdam ESHRE/ASRM-Sponsored PCOS Consensus Workshop Group. Revised 2003 consensus on diagnostic criteria and long-term health risks related to polycystic ovary syndrome. *Fertil Steril* 2004;81:19–25.

SUGGESTED READINGS

Chabbert-Buffet N, Bouchard P. The normal human menstrual cycle. *Rev Endocr Metab Disord* 2002;3:173–183.
Clayton RN, Ogden V, Hodgkinson J, Worswick L, Rodin DA, Dyer S, Meade TW. How common are polycystic ovaries in normal women and what is their significance for the fertility of the population. *Clin Endocrinol* 1992;37:127–134.
Goldzieher JW, Green JA. The polycystic ovary. I. Clinical and histologic features. *J Clin Endocrinol Metab* 1962;22:325–338.
Hillier SG. Gonadotropic control of ovarian follicular growth and development. *Mol Cell Endocrinol* 2001;179:39–46.
Knochenhauer ES, Key TJ, Kahsar-Miller M, Waggoner W, Boots LR, Azziz R. Prevalence of the polycystic ovarian syndrome in unselected Black and White women of the Southeastern United States: A prospective study. *J Clin Endocrinol Metab* 1998;83:3078–3082.
LaBarbera AR, Miller MM, Ober C, Rebar RW. Autoimmune etiology in premature ovarian failure. *Am J Reprod Immunol Microbiol* 1988;16:115–122.
Laml T, Preyer O, Umek W, Hengstschlager M, Hanzal H. Genetic disorders in premature ovarian failure. *Hum Reprod Update* 2002;8:483–491.
Marshall JC, Eagleson CA, McCartney CR. Hypothalamic dysfunction. *Mol Cell Endocrinol* 2001;183:29–32.
Polson DW, Wadsworth J, Adams J, Franks S. Polycystic ovaries—a common finding in normal women. *Lancet* 1988;1:870–872.
Progetto Menopausa Italia Study Group. Premature ovarian failure: frequency and risk factors among women attending a network of menopause clinics in Italy. *Br J Obstet Gynaecol* 2003;110:59–63.
Rebar RW, Connoly HV. Clinical features of young women with hypergoandotropic amenorrhea. *Fertil Steril* 1990:53:804–810.
Richards JS, Russell DL, Robker RL, Dajee M, Alliston TN. Molecular mechanisms of ovulation and luteinization. *Mol Cell Endocrinol* 1998;145:47–54.
Yen SS, Rebar R, Vandenberg G, Judd H. Hypothalamic amenorrhea and hypogonadotropinism: responses to synthetic LRF. *J Clin Endocrinol Metab* 1973;36:811–816.
Zawadzki JK, Dunaif A. Diagnostic criteria for polycystic ovary syndrome: towards a rational approach. In: Dunaif A, Givens JR, Haseltine F, Merriam GR, eds. *Polycystic Ovary Syndrome*. Boston, MA: Blackwell Scientific 1992;377–384.

27 The Testis

Amiya Sinha Hikim, PhD, Ronald S. Swerdloff, MD, and Christina Wang, MD

1. INTRODUCTION

The mammalian testis has two basic compartments: the interstitial (intertubular) compartment and the seminiferous tubule compartment (Fig. 1A). The interstitial compartment is highly vascularized and contains Leydig cells clustered near or around the vessels. These cells are responsive to luteinizing hormone (LH) and secrete testosterone, which subsequently accumulates in the interstitium and the seminiferous tubules at relatively high concentrations. The Leydig cell possesses abundant smooth endoplasmic reticulum (SER) and mitochondria, both of which contain the enzymes associated with steroid biosynthesis (Fig. 1B). The seminiferous tubule compartment contains Sertoli cells and developing and mature germ cells. The formation of spermatozoa from stem spermatogonia (spermatogenesis) includes mitotic and meiotic division, followed by cellular differentiation (spermiogenesis). Thus, the two major areas of activity within the testis center on steroidogenesis and spermatogenesis. A large body of literature provides evidence that LH (via stimulation of testosterone) and follicle-stimulating hormone (FSH) are the key regulators of spermatogenesis.

2. LEYDIG CELLS AND STEROIDOGENESIS

In this section, we briefly review the endocrine and paracrine regulation of Leydig cell function and testicu-

From: *Endocrinology: Basic and Clinical Principles, Second Edition*
(S. Melmed and P. M. Conn, eds.) © Humana Press Inc., Totowa, NJ

lar steroidogenesis. The detailed description of steroid hormone action is discussed in another chapter.

2.1. Regulation of Leydig Cell Function

2.1.1. GONADOTROPIN-RELEASING HORMONE

The regulation of testicular function depends on gonadstropin-releasing hormone (GnRH) secretion by the small numbers of GnRH neurons scattered in the anterior hypothalamus (Fig. 2). GnRH is then transported through axons to the median eminence, where it enters the capillaries of the hypothalamic portal blood to the anterior pituitary. GnRH secretion is affected by many neurotransmitters including glutamate acting via nitric oxide, dopamine, γ-aminobutyric acid, neuropeptide Y, opiates, galanin, and galanin-like peptide. GnRH is released into the portal blood in pulses, and the pulse frequency is regulated by a pulse generator in the mediobasal hypothalamus. Changes in cell membrane potential may predispose the GnRH neurons to bursts of GnRH release that are in synchrony with LH secretory bursts.

GnRH binds and activates a G protein cell membrane receptor on the gonadotropes in the anterior pituitary. Binding of GnRH to its receptor activates the membrane-associated phospholipase C and increases intracellular inositol phosphate. Inositol triphosphate mobilizes intracellular calcium and opens the voltage-gated calcium channels, resulting in increases in intra-

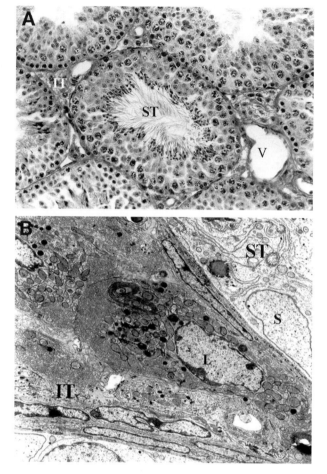

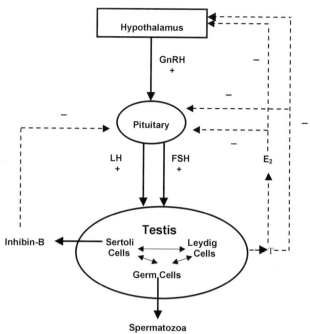

Fig. 2. Regulation of hypothalamic-pituitary-testis. The solid lines represent stimulating effects and the dashed lines negative feedback actions.

Fig. 1 (A) Light micrograph showing interstitial (intertubular) and seminiferous tubular (ST) compartments of mouse testis. The interstitial compartment contains Leydig cells (L) clustered around the blood vessels (V). **(B)** Electron micrograph showing interstitial (IT) and seminiferous tubular (ST) compartments of mouse testis. Leydig cells (L) are seen in the IT compartment. A portion of a Sertoli cell (S) with distinct nucleus is seen in the seminiferous tubular compartment.

cellular calcium. Rises in intracellular calcium result in the release of both LH and FSH. GnRH also increases the transcription of genes for the gonadotropins via diacylglycerol, phosphokinase C, and mitogen-activated protein kinase/JNK pathways. GnRH receptors are upregulated by pulsatile GnRH. On the other hand, continuous GnRH results in desensitization of the GnRH receptors followed by suppression of LH and FSH and disturbance of gonadal function.

2.1.2. Gonadotropins

Both LH and FSH production are dependent on GnRH. Both gonadotropins are glycoproteins consisting of a common α-subunit and a hormone-specific β-

subunit. GnRH increases gene transcription of both the LH and FSH β-subunit gene via specific transcription factors (e.g., LH via SF-1, EGR-1, and SP1 and FSH via *fos* and *jun* as well as androgen response elements). The α-subunit is less rigorously regulated and both pulsatile and continuous GnRH increase gene expression. Studies in monkeys and humans have shown that bursts of GnRH secretion are necessary for the pulsatile release of LH. In the human, LH pulses occur every 60–120 min. In pubertal boys, there is increased LH pulsatile secretion during sleep. With aging there are decreases in the pulse amplitude of LH secretion. The synthesis of testosterone by the testis is under the regulation of LH through a G protein–associated transmembrane receptor. LH binds to the receptors to initiate signaling through activation of G_s protein, adenylate cyclase, cycxlic adenosine monophosphate (cAMP), and protein kinase A (PKA), stimulating testicular steroidogenesis.

GnRH and LH/FSH secretion is regulated by negative feedback mechanisms. In primates including humans, testosterone suppresses LH synthesis and secretion primarily through its action on the GnRH neurons and pulse generator. FSH secretion is also under the negative feedback of testosterone. In humans, it has been shown that the nonaromatizable androgen 5α-dihydrotestosterone decreases LH pulse frequency, suggesting that androgens act via the androgen receptor

(AR) to regulate GnRH secretion. Testosterone also decreases LH secretion by gonadotropes in rodent pituitary, but its role in the negative feedback of human pituitary is less clear. Estradiol (E_2), acting predominantly through the estrogen receptor α (ERα), also plays a role in the negative feedback of GnRH and gonadotropin secretion. When administered to men estrogen antagonists (clomiphene) and aromatase inhibitors (testolactone) result in elevation of both LH and FSH. Men with ERα gene mutation and aromatase deficiency also have elevated FSH and LH. These pharmacologic manipulations and models in nature indicate that E_2 plays a role in the negative regulation of GnRH and gonadotropin secretion.

2.1.3. ACTIVINS, INHIBINS, AND FOLLISTATIN

Although FSH secretion is primarily regulated by GnRH and gonadal steroids, there are other paracrine and endocrine factors such as pituitary activin and follistatin and testicular inhibin β that only regulate FSH without affecting LH secretion and synthesis. Activin stimulates FSH β gene transcription through activation of the Smad family of proteins. Follistatin binds to activin and inhibits its biologic activity. The testicular protein inhibin β, secreted by Sertoli cells, competes with activin for binding to the activin receptor, preventing the initiation of signaling of Smads and thus decreasing FSH gene transcription.

2.1.4. CLINICAL IMPLICATIONS

Serum FSH, LH, and inhibin β levels are useful in the diagnosis of hypogonadism and infertility. In men with hypothalamic-pituitary dysfunction, serum LH and FSH levels are low (hypogonadotropic hypogonadism), whereas in men with primary testicular dysfunction, serum LH levels are elevated if Leydig cell function is compromised, and serum FSH is also elevated if Sertoli cell function or seminiferous tubule damage occurs (hypergonadotropic hypogonadism). Because inhibin selectively suppresses FSH secretion, circulating inhibin β and FSH are inversely related in healthy men and men with primary or testicular disease. Circulating inhibin β reflects Sertoli cell function and is decreased in men with seminiferous tubule dysfunction.

2.2. Leydig Cell Function

2.2.1. LEYDIG CELLS

The structure of the adult Leydig cell is shown in Fig. 1B. The predominant cytoplasmic organelle is the SER, which is characteristically more abundant in steroidogenic cells. Mitochondria and lipid droplets are also numerous in Leydig cells, playing important roles in steroidogenesis. Leydig cells are believed to be mesenchymal in origin though recent evidence suggests that there may be a neural crest component. In the human, fetal Leydig cells become apparent at 8 wk and multiply to reach a maximum at 15 wk of gestation, coinciding with a rise in androgen concentration in testis and blood, and then remain inactive for the rest of gestation. The number of Leydig cells increases at 2 to 3 mo after birth, which is associated with the surge of serum testosterone at this early age. Leydig cells then enter into a period of quiescence until puberty. During puberty the number of adult Leydig cells increases further and reaches a maximum of 500 million at about the age of 20 yr. The increased number of cells and their stimulation by increasing LH levels results in a peak of serum testosterone in early adulthood. The number of Leydig cells remains stable between age 20 and 60, and then gradually decreases after the age of 60. The decrease in the number of Leydig cells and function may be responsible for the androgen deficiency associated with aging in men.

2.2.2. TESTICULAR STEROIDOGENESIS (FIG. 3)

The biosynthetic pathway of testosterone production is shown schematically in Fig. 3. The conversion of cholesterol into pregnenolone occurs within the mitochondria via the enzyme cytochrome P450 side-chain cleavage ($P450_{scc}$). Pregnenolone then diffuses into the cytoplasm and can be converted via the Δ5 (Fig. 3, right) or Δ4 pathway (Fig. 3, left) into the end product, testosterone. In the Δ5 pathway, pregnenolone is converted by $P450_{c17}$/C17 hydroxylase into 17α-pregnenolone and then into dehydroepiandrosterone (DHEA) by $P450_{C17}$/C17, 20 lyase/desmolase. This Δ5 pregnenolone pathway is predominant over the Δ4 progesterone pathway in the human testis. Although DHEA can then be converted by the 17β-hydroxysteroid dehydrogenase (17β-HSD) via androstenediol into testosterone, the dominant pathway in the human testis is for DHEA to be converted into androstenedione by 3β-hydroxysteroid dehydrogenase (3β–HSD) and then into testosterone. In the Δ4 pathway, predominant in rodents, pregnenolone is converted into progesterone by 3β–HSD. Progesterone is then converted into 17α-hydroxyprogesterone and androstenedione via $P450_{C17}$. Androstenedione is converted into testosterone by 17β-HSD.

2.2.3. MECHANISMS OF TESTOSTERONE ACTIONS

Testosterone can act on the androgen receptor (AR) directly or as a prohormone. (Discussion of the binding of testosterone to the AR and the complexity of regulation of the AR action is beyond the scope of this chapter.) Mutations of AR transcription events result

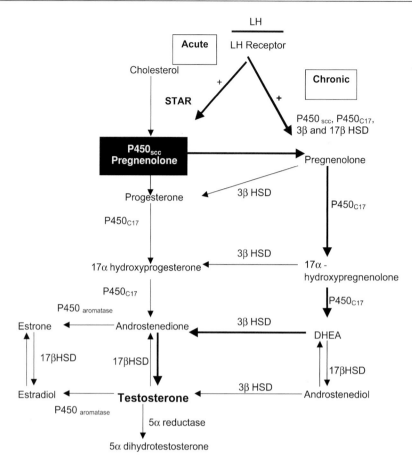

Fig. 3. Regulation of testicular steroidogenesis by LH. The black box represents the mitochondria and the heavy solid lines the predominant steroidogenic pathway in humans. STAR = steriodogenic acute regulatory protein.

in the syndrome of androgen insensitivity that spans the clinical manifestations from male infertility to a female phenotype. The 5α-reductase enzyme converts testosterone into 5α-dihydrotestosterone (5α-DHT), an irreversible reaction. 5α-DHT is then metabolized to 5α-androstane-3α (and -3β), 17β-diols, and the triols. 5α-DHT binds to the AR to exert its action. There are two 5α-reductase enzymes: 1 and 2. 5α-Reductase 2 enzyme is expressed in male reproductive tissues (prostate, testis, epididymis, seminal vesicles) from the embryogenesis to adulthood, genital skin, hair follicles, and liver. 5α-Reductase 1 enzyme is present in nongenital skin, sebaceous gland, and liver, and more recently, it was found to be expressed in bone and brain. Genetic mutations of 5α-reductase enzyme 2 result in males with ambiguous genitalia, small hypospadiac phallus, and blind vagina. These males may achieve partial virilization at puberty owing to the surge of serum testosterone allowing some conversion to 5α-DHT. Males with 5α-reductase 2 deficiency have small

prostates, decreased facial and body hair and relatively normal bone mineral density (BMD).

Testosterone is also converted by the aromatase enzyme into E_2. This conversion occurs in the Leydig cells and accounts for <10% of E_2 produced in the adult male. The majority of E_2 in males is derived from the peripheral conversion of testosterone into E_2 or androstenedione into estrone and then into E_2. E_2 acts via ERα and ER-β. The action of E_2 in various tissues depends on the balance of expression and transcription between ERα and ERβ. In the human, aromatization of testosterone to E_2 appears to be important for achieving and maintaining bone mass and BMD. In rodents, conversion of androgens into estrogens is important for male aggressive and sexual behavior. In primates and in humans, the requirement of conversion of testosterone into estrogens for brain functions is much less clear. Recent development of knockout mouse models for ERα and ERβ and reports of aromatase and ERα gene mutations in human males allows better understanding of the functions of these receptor subtypes. There is also recent evidence in mice suggesting that in the prostate, 5αDHT is converted into 5α-androstane 3β, 17β-diol. This steroid binds and exerts its effect via ERβ rather than through the AR crosslinking the androgens and estrogen actions in the male.

2.2.4. REGULATION OF LEYDIG CELL STEROIDOGENESIS

LH is the major regulator of Leydig cell function; however, in the fetus, recent evidence suggests that factors such as pituitary adenylate cyclase–activating polypeptide (PACAP) may regulate Leydig cell function. LH elicits two types of responses in the Leydig cells: acute or chronic. LH binds to the transmembrane G protein receptor and signals through the PKA-cAMP pathway. The acute response results in a rapid production of testosterone within minutes and does not require new transcription of mRNA. In the acute response, carrier proteins deliver the substrate cholesterol for P450$_{scc}$ enzyme complex in the mitochondria. This mitochondrial transport of cholesterol is regulated by the steroidogenic acute regulatory (StAR) protein. Mutations of the StAR gene result in lipoid congenital adrenal hyperplasia in which steroidogenesis is absent in both the adrenals and gonads owing to absence of shuttling of cholesterol to P450$_{scc}$ complex within the mitochondria. Although StAR is important for cholesterol shuttling to the mitochondrial, other proteins such as PBR may also be important for this trafficking.

Chronic stimulation by LH has tropic effects on the Leydig cells requiring both transcription and increased translation of the proteins. There is increased expression of the steroidogenic enzymes P450$_{scc}$, P450$_{c17}$, 3β-HSD and 17β-HSD. The steroidogenic organelle including the mitochondrial membrane potential and SER volume are both supported by LH.

In addition to LH, local cell-to-cell interactions and paracrine factors produced by Sertoli cells, germ cells, peritubular cells, and macrophages may affect Leydig cell function. FSH receptors are located only in Sertoli cells. FSH can act via Sertoli cell secretory proteins to regulate Leydig cells. Using FSH β and FSH receptor knockouts, recent studies showed that LH alone is sufficient for normal postnatal development of Leydig cells only when FSH receptors are present. In the absence of LH, FSH stimulates Leydig cell steroidogenesis. Sertoli cell factors such as insulin-like growth factor-1 increase whereas transforming growth factor-β (TGF-β) and interleukin-1 (IL-1) inhibit Leydig cell steroidogenesis. Other peptide hormones including PACAP, vasoactive intestinal peptide, and arginine vasopressin have been shown to regulate Leydig cell steroidogenesis in vitro, but the significance of these findings is not clear.

2.2.5. CLINICAL IMPLICATIONS

Decreased Leydig cell function is associated with decreased production of testosterone and may manifest clinically with symptoms and signs of male hypogonadism. Men with low serum testosterone levels may complain of decreased libido and erectile dysfunction, lack of energy, tiredness, mood changes, decreased muscle mass, and bone pain and fractures. Physical examination and tests may show loss of body hair and regression of secondary sex characters, low lean body mass and low BMD. When intratesticular testosterone decreases to a low level, spermatogenesis will be impaired, resulting in infertility. Except for the infertility, these clinical features ameliorate with testosterone treatment. Leydig cell numbers and volume decrease with aging. In addition the steroidogenic machinery appears to be impaired with aging. Leydig cell dysfunction associated with aging may result in declining serum testosterone levels in older men. Androgen deficiency is treated by testosterone replacement therapy. However, the benefits and risks must be considered especially in the treatment of older males with low serum testosterone levels.

3. SPERMATOGENESIS AND SERTOLI CELL FUNCTION

Spermatogenesis is an elaborate process of cell differentiation in which stem spermatogonia, through a series of events, become mature spermatozoa and occurs continuously during the reproductive lifetime of the individual. Stem spermatogonia undergo mitosis to produce two types of cells: regenerating stem cells and differentiating spermatogonia, which undergo rapid and successive mitotic divisions to form primary spermatocytes. The spermatocytes then enter a lengthy meiotic phase as preleptotene spermatocytes and proceed through two cell divisions (meiosis I and II) to give rise to haploid spermatids. These in turn undergo a complex process of morphologic and functional differentiation resulting in the production of mature spermatozoa. The formation of spermatozoa takes place within the seminiferous epithelium, consisting of germ cells at various phases of development and supporting Sertoli cells. The different generations of germ cells form associations with fixed composition or stages, which constitute the cycle of seminiferous epithelium (12 in mouse, 14 in the rat). When germ cell development is complete, the mature spermatids are released from the Sertoli cells into the tubular lumen and proceed through the testicular excurrent duct system, known as the rete testis, until they enter the epididymis via ductus efferens. During passage through the epididymis, the spermatids undergo a series of biochemical changes to become the motile spermatozoa capable of fertilization.

This review highlights the hormonal and genetic control of spermatogenesis. A brief overview of testicular organization, germ cell development, and cascade of cell–cell interactions in the testis is also presented.

3.1. Organization of Spermatogenesis

The general organization of spermatogenesis is essentially the same in all animals and can be divided into three main phases, each involving a class of germ cells.

3.1.1. Spermatogonial Phase

The initial phase (also known as spermatocytogenesis) is the proliferative or spermatogonial phase, during which stem spermatogonia undergo mitosis to produce two types of cells: additional stem cells and differentiating spermatogonia, which undergo rapid and successive divisions to form preleptotene spermatocytes. In both rat and mouse, there are three types of spermatogonia: stem cell (A_{is}, or $A_{isolated}$), proliferative (A_{pr}, or A_{paired} and A_{al}, or $A_{alinged}$), and differentiating [A_1, A_2, A_3, A_4, In (intermediate), and B] spermatogonia. The stem cells, A_{is}, divide sporadically to replicate themselves as isolated entities and to produce pairs of A_{pr} spermatogonia. The latter engage in a series of synchronous divisions leading to the formation of chains of A_{al} spermatogonia connected to each other by the intracellular bridges. The A_{al} spermatogonia do not divide but, rather, differentiate into A_1 spermatogonia. The type A1 cells, however, divide to give rise to more differentiating (A_2, A_3, A_4, In, and B) cells. In men, mostly three different types of spermatogonia (the dark type A [Ad], pale type A [Ap], and B type) have been identified. The Ap cells have the capacity to give rise to new Ap cells as well as to the more differentiated B spermatogonia and are considered to be the renewing stem cells. The Ad spermatogonia are reserve stem cells, which normally divide only rarely. The precise mechanism by which stem spermatogonia transform into differentiating spermatogonia and simultaneously renew their own population is not known.

3.1.2. Meiotic or Spermatocyte Phase

The meiotic or spermatocyte phase leads to the formation of haploid spermatids from young primary spermatocytes and is traditionally divided into five sequential stages: leptotene, zygotene, pachytene, diplotene, and diakinesis. The meiotic phase involves DNA synthesis in the youngest primary spermatocytes (preleptotene) entering into the long meiotic prophase and RNA synthesis in the diplotene stage. Elaborate morphologic changes occur in the chromosomes as they pair (synapse) and then begin to unpair (desynapse)

during the first meiotic prophase. These changes include (1) initiation of intimate chromosome synapsis at the zygotene stage, when the synaptonemal complex begins to develop between the two sets of sister chromatids in each bivalent; (2) completion of synapsis with fully formed synaptonemal complex and occurrence of crossing over at the pachytene stage; and (3) dissipation of the synaptonemal complex and desynapsing (allowing the chromosomal pairs to separate except at regions known as chiasmata) at the diplotene stage. Following the long meiotic prophase, the primary spermatocytes rapidly complete their first meiotic division to form two secondary spermatocytes, each containing duplicated autosomal chromosomes and either a duplicated X or a duplicated Y chromosome. These cells undergo a second maturation division, after a short interphase with no DNA synthesis, to produce four spermatids, each with a haploid number of single chromosomes.

Responding to unknown signals, type B spermatogonia divide to form young primary spermatocytes, the preleptotene cells. These cells are the last cells of the spermatogenic sequence to go through the S-phase of the cell cycle. The morphology of preleptotene cells is very similar to that of B cells except that the preleptotene cells are slightly smaller and have less chromatin along the nuclear envelope (Fig. 4). The presence of leptotene cells signals the initiation of the meiotic prophase. During the leptotene phase, the chromosome appears as single, randomly coiled threads, which thicken and commence pairing during the zygotene phase through the formation of synaptonemal complex. The long pachytene phase that occupies over a week in the mouse commences with the completion of synapses and is associated with further thickening and shortening of the chromosome. During this phase, exchange of chromosomal material between maternal and paternal homologous chromosomes occurs by a "crossing over," with the chromosomes linked at such sites by chiasmata. The pachytene phase is further characterized by nuclear and cytoplasmic growth, during which the cell and its nucleus progressively increase in volume. As desynapsis occurs during the next phase, known as the diplotene phase, the paired chromosomes partially separate but remain joined at their chiasmata. The diplotene cells are the largest primary spermatocytes and also the largest of any of the germ cell types. Subsequently, in the diakinetic phase, further shortening of the chromosomes occurs, as they detach from the nuclear membrane. Soon after this phase, the primary spermatocytes rapidly complete their first meiotic division, or meiosis I, going through metaphase, anaphase, and telophase, during which the homologous chromosomes separate and migrate to the poles of the cell, which then splits to

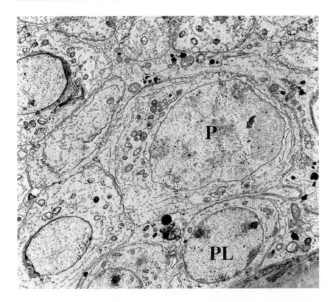

Fig. 4. A portion of the mouse stage VII tubule shows preleptotene (PL) and pachytene (P) spermatocytes and step 7 (7) spermatids. Two of the PL spermatocytes are connected by intercellular bridges.

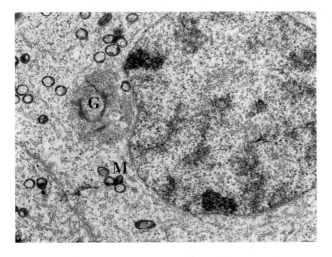

Fig. 5. Mouse secondary spermatocyte. The mitochondria (M) are round dispersed within the cytoplasm and often aggregated into small groups. The Golgi apparatus (G) is extensive, but no proacrosomal granules characteristic of step 1 spermatids are seen.

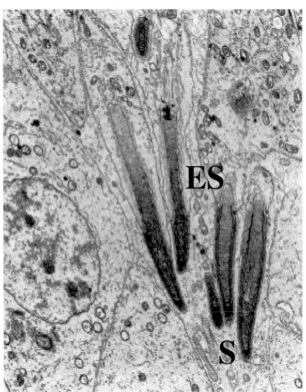

Fig. 6. Portion of mouse stage XI tubule showing elongated spermatids (ES) embedded deeply in the Sertoli cell (S) cytoplasm.

form two daughter cells called secondary spermatocytes.

Thus, at the end of meiosis I, the chromosomal complement has been reduced from tetraploid to diploid and two secondary spermatocytes have formed from one primary spermatocyte. An electron micrograph of a secondary spermatocyte is shown in Fig. 5. The mitochondria are round dispersed within the cytoplasm and often aggregated in small groups. The Golgi apparatus is extensive, but no proacrosomal granules

characteristic of step 1 spermatids are seen. The second meiotic division, or meiosis II, quickly follows, consisting of a transient interphase II with no chromosome replication, followed by prophase II, metaphase II, anaphase II, and telophase II. Thus, at the end of meiosis II, each secondary spermatocyte gives rise to two spermatids so that there are a total of four spermatids derived from the individual primary spermatocyte.

3.1.3. Spermiogenesis

The spermiogenic phase (spermiogenesis) involves morphologic and functional differentiation of newly formed spermatids into mature spermatozoa. Early in this transformation, the Golgi apparatus packages material that initiates acrosome formation. A flagellum forms from the centrioles and becomes associated with the nucleus. The nucleus progressively elongates as its chromatin condenses. These elongated spermatids are deeply embedded in the Sertoli cell cytoplasm (Fig. 6). During spermiogenesis the genome is repackaged with protamins rather than histones, which is necessary to reduce the volume of the genetic payload from the relatively bulky round spermatids to the streamlined spermatozoa (compare the size of the elongated spermatids

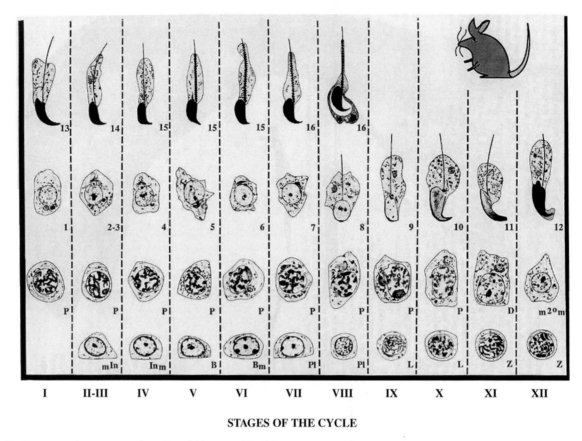

STAGES OF THE CYCLE

Fig. 7. Diagrammatic representation of seminiferous epithelial cycle in mouse. The columns numbered with Roman numerals show the various types of cells present at each cellular association, which are encountered in the various cross-sections of the seminiferous tubule. Different types of A spermatogonia are not indicated in the cycle map. mIn = dividing intermediate spermatogonium; B = B spermatogonium; Pl = preleptotene; L = leptotene; Z = zygotene; P = pachytene; Di = diakinesis; m2^{0}m, dividing spermatocytes; 1–16 = 16 steps of spermiogenesis. (Reproduced from Russell et al., 1990.)

shown in Fig. 6 with that of the round spermatids in Fig. 4). Late spermatids are released (spermiation) almost simultaneously through the activity of the Sertoli cell. The release of spermatids is associated with the loss of the residual cytoplasm. The process of spermiogenesis occurs without cell divisions, is one of the most phenomenal cell transformations in the body, and can be subdivided into many characteristic steps. For example, this process can be divided into 16 steps in the mouse and 6 steps in the human.

3.1.4. STAGES OF THE SEMINIFEROUS EPITHELIUM

An intriguing feature of spermatogenesis is that the developing germ cells form associations with fixed composition or stages (Fig. 7), which constitute the cycle of the seminiferous epithelium (12 in the mouse and 14 in the rat). Each stage lasts for a fixed period of time at the end of which each germ cell type within that stage will progress into the next stage. For example, in the Sprague-Dawley rat, the progression of stage VII to

stage VIII will take little more than 2 d. The time interval between the successive appearances of the same cell association at a given area of the tubule is known as the cycle of the seminiferous epithelium (which is about 8.8 d in mice and 12.9 d in Sprague-Dawley rats). The duration of the seminiferous epithelial cycle in the human is about 16.0 d. However in humans, unlike rodents, individual tubular profile almost always contains more than one cell association or stage. Stages in human tubules may be mapped by drawing stage boundary lines among individual cell associations in a cross-sectioned tubule.

3.1.5. SERTOLI CELLS

The Sertoli cells provide the fundamental organization and integrity of the seminiferous epithelium. These tall, irregularly columnar cells span the distance from the base of the tubule into the tubular lumen and are elaborately equipped to support spermatogenesis. The Sertoli cell nucleus is large, with its characteristic tripartite nucleolus (Fig. 8), and located within the basal aspect of the cell, which rests on the basement membrane. Adjacent Sertoli cells form contacts (tight junctions) with each other at their lateral surfaces and near their base to effectively compartmentalize and separate the two populations of germ cells. Thus, at each stage of the seminiferous epithelial cycle, the germ cells are in intimate association with Sertoli cells in a predictable fashion, with the more immature cells (spermatogonia and young spermatocytes) located near the basal compartment and the advanced (most spermatocytes and spermatids) germ cells in the adluminal compartment.

The elaborate configuration and numerous processes to encompass developing germ cells result in a much greater surface of these cells. In comparison to the rat hepatocyte, e.g., the surface-to-volume ratio of the Sertoli cell is about 11 times greater than that of hepatocytes. This high surface-to-volume ratio is reflective of the extremely irregular shape and extensive surface process of these cells. Perhaps the most notable feature of the Sertoli cell of many species is the compartmentalization of organelles within its cytoplasm. This is reflective of regional functioning of the Sertoli cell in relationship to the physiologic needs of various germ cell types as well as polarized function/secretion of the cell. The SER is the most abundant organelle during active spermatogenesis. The rough endoplasmic reticulum is relatively sparse in the Sertoli cell. The mitochondria occupy about 6% of the Sertoli cell cytoplasmic volume. Compared with normal rats with active spermatogenesis, Sertoli cells from the regressed testes of hypophysectomized rats show a significant reduction in the cell volume and surface area and absolute volumes and surface areas of nearly all of their organelles.

3.2. Hormonal Regulation of Spermatogenesis

The hormonal control of spermatogenesis has been studied for several decades since its dependence on pituitary gonadotropins was first described. This process is thought to be primarily under the control of pituitary gonadotropins, FSH, and LH (via the stimulation of testosterone), and on the interplay between Sertoli and germ cells. Sertoli cells possess receptors for both FSH and androgen, and it is likely that these hormones exert their stimulatory effects on Sertoli cells, which, in turn, results in stimulation of intratubular factors for the survival of germ cells through a paracrine mechanism. However, despite the considerable attention that hormonal control of spermatogenesis has received to date, the specific role and relative contribution of FSH and

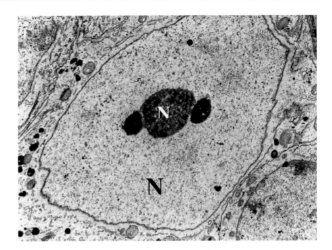

Fig. 8. Electron micrograph showing typical mouse Sertoli cell nucleus (N) with its characteristic tripartite nucleolus (white N).

testosterone on the regulation of spermatogenesis are still debatable.

3.2.1. GONADOTROPINS AND ANDROGEN REGULATION OF SPERMATOGENESIS

The hormonal control of spermatogenesis has been the subject of numerous studies over many years. Previous studies have shown that quantitatively normal spermatogenesis (assessed by measurements of homogenization-resistant advanced [steps 17–19] spermatids) can be restored by exogenous administration of testosterone alone in adult rats made azoospermic by treating them with implants of testosterone and estradiol or by active immunization against either GnRH or LH. A separate study reported that testosterone alone is capable of maintaining advanced spermatid numbers in adult rats actively immunized against GnRH. These results of quantitative maintenance or restoration of spermatogenesis by testosterone alone in rats in the absence of both radioimmunoassayable LH and FSH suggest that FSH has no effect on the regulation of spermatogenesis in the adult rat. Quantitative maintenance of spermatogenesis has also been achieved in adult rats in which LH and FSH had been suppressed pharmacologically by a GnRH antagonist (GnRH-A) with testosterone alone, when the testosterone was administered at higher doses. However, because testosterone supplementation increases both the serum concentrations and pituitary content of FSH in GnRH-A-treated rats, the observed quantitative maintenance of spermatogenesis in these rats cannot be attributed with certainty to testosterone. Others have further shown that spermatogenesis is not quantitatively restored in GnRH-immunized rats that received even the same larger amount of testosterone as used in the earlier studies and further emphasized the need for both FSH and testosterone in the restoration of spermatogenesis. In additional studies, it was shown that cotreatment of testosterone with an FSH antiserum to prevent T-induced restoration of serum FSH levels in these GnRH-A-immunized rats is not effective in restoring spermatogenesis. This implies the need of FSH for restoration of spermatogenesis in adult rats after chronic gonadotropic suppression. Supportive of this implication is the demonstration of the failure of quantitative restoration of spermatogenesis in gonadotropin-deficient (hpg) mice by androgens alone. Similarly, in most studies of hypophysectomized rats, spermatogenesis was not quantitatively maintained or restored by exogenous administration of testosterone, suggesting that FSH and/ or other pituitary hormones might be required for complete regulation of spermatogenesis in this species. Clinical studies in men also suggest that both LH and FSH are required to maintain quantitatively normal spermatogenesis.

A number of investigators have previously suggested a definitive role of FSH on the regulation of spermatogenesis in the adult rats under various experimental situations. These studies were, however, of limited duration (1 to 2 wk). Thus, stimulatory effects of FSH on spermatogenesis that are obvious after 1 or 2 wk of gonadotropin and/or testosterone deprivation might not become so obvious after long-term treatment. The most definitive evidence, however, comes from an earlier study that showed that replacement of recombinant human FSH GnRH-A-treated rats fully attenuated the early (1 wk) GnRH-A-induced reduction in germ cell numbers at stage VII as well as the number of advanced (steps 17–19) spermatids and effectively prevented the GnRH-A-induced reduction in the number of pachytene and step 7 spermatids for 2 wk. In addition, replacement of FSH in GnRH-A-treated rats was able to increase the number of B spermatogonia available for entry into meiosis and maintain the number of preleptotene spermatocytes throughout the treatment period. The observed beneficial effects of recombinant human FSH in spermatogenesis in GnRH-A-treated rats are most likely not owing to the stimulation of Leydig cell function (via paracrine interaction between Sertoli and Leydig cells), because the addition of FSH to GnRH-A had no discernible effect on intratesticular or plasma testosterone levels, accessory sex organ weight, and total volume of the Leydig cells when compared with GnRH-A alone. Mice deficient in FSH β-subunit exhibited a striking decrease in testis weight, seminiferous tubule volume, and epididymal sperm number (up to 75%) compared with littermate controls. This 75% reduction in epididymal sperm

number is identical to the reported 76% decrease in the transformation of round to elongated spermatids following immunoneutralization of FSH in the adult rat. Thus, the reduction in epididymal sperm number in FSH-deficient mice is most likely attributed to a decrease in the number of elongated spermatids during spermiogenesis. However, the absence of any apparent fertility defect, despite a 75% reduction in the epididymal sperm number, in these mice suggest that there is far more sperm produced in the adult mice than is required to achieve fertility. Moreover, in the FSH receptor knockout mice, the testes volume may be smaller but the mice may still be fertile.

The role of FSH in the regulation of spermatogenesis in primates and humans has been documented. For example, administration of exogenous testosterone implants in adult macaque monkeys for 20 wk induced azoospermia in some animals and variable degrees of spermatogenic suppression in others. Interestingly, such variability in testosterone-induced spermatogenic suppression was not associated with differences in residual intratesticular androgens, LH, or inhibin B levels but, rather, was associated with differences in the degree of FSH suppression between azoo- and nonazoospermic animals. These results suggest that FSH is a key factor in the maintenance of spermatogenesis in monkeys. Testosterone treatment of healthy men suppressed gonadotropins, and intratesticular testosterone also induced azoospermia in some individuals and variable degrees of suppression in others. When these testosterone-treated men were supplemented with LH or human chorionic gonadotropin (hCG), their spermatogenesis recovered qualitatively; the sperm count remained suppressed (25–50 million/mL) from the pretreatment concentrations (75–100 million/mL). FSH supplementation also stimulated spermatogenesis, though not quantitatively, in these men. Spermatogenesis of these men, however, was restored by the simultaneous administration of both LH and FSH. Data from men with a mutation in the gene encoding either the FSH-R or the FSH β-subunit further provided an opportunity to evaluate the role of FSH in human spermatogenesis. Men homozygous for an inactivating mutation of FSH receptor gene experienced variable suppression of both spermatogenesis and fertility. Men with markedly impaired secretion of FSH caused by a homozygous mutation in the gene for FSH β-subunit had azoospermia and severely reduced testis size. From these experiments of nature, it appears that FSH may not be an absolute requirement for spermatogenesis in men but may be necessary for quantitatively normal spermatogenesis. Some other conditions/factors in addition to FSH deficiency may cause the azoospermia, since one of the men was resistant to FSH therapy, and the other also had low testosterone and high LH, indicating primary Leydig cell failure. Whatever the final role of FSH in spermatogenesis, its effects seem to be mediated through action on the Sertoli cells, given that the receptors for FSH are limited to these cells.

3.3. Sertoli Cell Regulation of Spermatogenesis

While circulating hormones clearly play an important role in initiating and regulating the process of spermatogenesis, the Sertoli cell barrier prevents most substances from entering the seminiferous tubule compartment and directly influencing germ cell development. Therefore, the tubules must independently produce their own regulatory substances. Sertoli cells, the somatic cells of the seminiferous tubules, play an especially prominent role in the cell-to-cell interactions necessary for germ cell development by their physical association with and the transfer of molecules to the developing germ cells. Sertoli cells also establish an important physiologic separation between basal (consisting of primarily spermatogonia) and adluminal (consisting of meiotic and postmeiotic) compartments of germ cells by the formation of a Sertoli–Sertoli cell barrier. This compartmentalized organization of the seminiferous epithelium allows bidirectional movement of Sertoli cell products to different populations of developing germ cells. Sertoli cells secrete many products, including activin, inhibin, Müllerian-inhibiting substance, stem cell factor (SCF) (c-kit ligand), IL-1, IL-6, transferrin, ceruloplasmin, cathepsin L, α_2 macroglobulin, TGF-α, TGF-β, androgen-binding protein, retinol-binding protein, sulfated glycoproteins 1 and 2, and testibumin. All of these products have been proposed to have putative actions on germ cells. Evidence is now beginning to indicate that some of these Sertoli cell products are also regulated by specific hormones. For example, SCF gene expression (at both transcriptional and posttranscriptional levels) in the rat seminiferous tubule was upregulated by FSH in a stage-specific manner. By contrast, testosterone, estradiol, TGF-α, TGF-β, and activin had no effect on SCF gene expression. A paracrine role of glial-derived neurotropic factor (GDNF), secreted by the Sertoli cells, in modulating the cell fate of undifferentiated spermatogonia has also been shown. Gene-targeted mice with one GDNF-null allele show depletion of stem cell reserves, whereas mice overexpressing GDNF show accumulation of undifferentiated spermatogonia. Sertoli cells also have typical ARs that mediate the effects of testosterone on spermatogenesis. The fact that testosterone exerts its effects on somatic cells rather than germ cells was highlighted by recent germ cell transplantation studies, in which spermatogonia from AR-deficient mice developed into spermatozoa in wild-type recipient mice. Likewise, a Sertoli cell–selective knockout of the AR caused spermatogenic arrest in meiosis and complete absence of elongated spermatids. In summary, Sertoli cells thus appear to mediate the biologic actions of both circulating hormones and the paracrine regulatory factors.

3.4. Genes Regulating Spermatogenesis

An exciting advance in the understanding of the genetic regulation of spermatogenesis is the use of genetically altered mice either overexpressing or harboring null mutation of specific genes. Studies using these mice are making an increasing contribution to the understanding of the roles of various genes in regulating spermatogenesis (Table 1).

There is clear evidence that homozygous disruption of a number of genes results in spermatogenic disruption and, in turn, infertility. These findings give a first glimpse of the mechanisms involved in the regulation of spermatogenesis. In adult mammals, including human, germ cell death is conspicuous during normal spermatogenesis and plays a pivotal role in sperm output. A growing body of evidence now demonstrates that both spontaneous (during normal spermatogenesis) germ cell death and that triggered by various regulatory stimuli occur via apoptosis. Recent studies in humans have further demonstrated that both spontaneous and increased germ cell death in conditions of abnormal spermatogenesis involve apoptosis and implicate a prominent role of programmed germ cell death in male fertility. Thus, it is not surprising that genes, which regulate cell death, are also required for normal spermatogenesis. For example, the ablation of the Bax gene (proapoptotic) by homologous recombination also results in male sterility owing to accumulation of atypical premeiotic germ cells but with accelerated apoptosis of mature germ cells leading to complete cessation of sperm production. Expression of high levels of Bcl-2 or Bcl-x_L proteins (antiapoptotic) in the germ cells results in hyperplasia within the spermatogonial compartment with subsequent disruption of spermatogenesis due to accelerated apoptosis of the mature germ cells. These results also suggest that a proper balance between germ cell proliferation and death is critical for normal spermatogenesis. A deficiency of Bcl-w, another antiapoptotic member of the Bcl-2 family, has also been reported to cause male sterility. Mutant animals have a block in the later phases of spermatogenesis and exhibit progressive depletion of germ cells through accelerated apoptosis to a Sertoli-cell-only phenotype by approx 6 mo of age followed by loss of Sertoli cells. It is pertinent to note here that Bcl-

Table 1
Some Genes Involved in Regulation of Spermatogenesis in Mice

Gene deleted	Phenotype
A-myb	Arrest at pachytene spermatocyte stage, complete absence of post-meiotic cells such as spermatids or spermatozoa, infertile
Apaf-1	Spermatogenic disruption and infertility
Atm	Complete arrest at pachytene spermatocyte phase, increased germ cell apoptosis, infertile
Bax	Accumulation of atypical premeiotic germ cells but no mature spermatozoa, marked increase in germ cell apoptosis, infertile
Bclw	Progressive depletion of germ cells through accelerated apoptosis to a Sertoli-cell-only phenotype by approx 6 mo followed by a loss of Sertoli cells
BMP 8A	Progressive infertility, spermatogenic impairment and epididymal defects
BMP 8B	Variable degrees of germ cell deficiency and infertility
Camk4	Infertile with impairment of spermatogenesis involving elongated spermatids
CREM	Complete absence of late spermatids and a significant increase in germ cell apoptosis
Cyp 19 (ArKO)	Progressive disruption of spermatogenesis
Dazla	Complete absence of meiotic and postmeiotic germ cells, infertile
Desert hedgehog	Infertile, defects in germ cell development
Egr4	Premature germ cell death with severely impaired spermatogenesis and oligozoospermia
ERKO	Disrupted spermatogenesis and infertility
H2AX	Male infertility with spermatogenic arrest at pachytene phase, increased apoptosis.
HR6B	Severely impaired spermatogenesis with a few predominantly abnormal sperm, increased germ cell apoptosis
Hsp70-2	Failure of meiosis with a marked increase in spermatocyte apoptosis, infertile
iNOS	Increased testis size and sperm numbers owing to less spontaneous germ cell apoptosis, no change in the rate of germ cell proliferation
MLH-1	Spermatogenic arrest at pachytene phase, accelerated germ cell apoptosis, infertile
Man2a2	Failure of germ cells to adhere to Sertoli cells and prematurely released, infertile
Mili	Complete absence of postmeiotic germ cell, infertile
RARα	Infertile secondary to severe loss of germ cells
RARβ	Male infertility owing to failure of sperm release and oligoasthenoteratozoospermia
SCARKO	Spermatogenic arrest in meiosis
Trf2	Sterile owing to severe spermatogenic defects

w is expressed in the elongated spermatids and in Sertoli cells. It is likely that the death of late spermatids is owing to the absence of Bcl-w function in those germ cells, whereas depletion of the entire germ line in adults reflects the loss of Bcl-w function in the Sertoli cell.

Other regulators of germ cell apoptosis have also been identified. For example, the ubiquitin system is also required for spermatogenesis, because inactivation of the HR6B ubiquitin-conjugating DNA repair enzyme in mice results in male infertility associated with disturbance in chromatin remodeling and accelerated germ cell apoptosis. Another protein that has recently been implicated in the regulation of meiosis is the mouse DMC1, an *Escherichia coli* RecA homolog that is specifically expressed in leptotene and zygotene spermatocytes. Targeted gene disruption of DMC1 (disrupted meiotic cDNA) results in failed meiosis, accelerated spermatocyte apoptosis, and male infertility. Surprisingly, null mutation of some genes, which are merely overexpressed in the testis, and are also expressed elsewhere, can accelerate germ cell apoptosis and cause specific defects in spermatogenesis. Examples of these mutations that affect germ cell apoptosis are knockouts of the Hsp (heat shock protein) 70-2, CREM (cAMP-responsive element modulator) gene, and Atm (ataxia telangiectasia mutated) gene.

Consequently, future studies with these and other genetically manipulated mice will continue to have an impact on our understanding of how various extrinsic factors (such as survival factor deprivation, chemotherapeutic drugs and testicular toxins, DNA damage, heat stress) through life and death signals in germ cells may affect spermatogenesis. How precisely these mouse mutations model human fertility will only become clear as the molecular basis of human fertility is elucidated. Nonetheless, these observations in mice clearly define important genetic principles that may apply to genes important for human fertility.

3.5. Summary of Regulation of Spermatogenesis

Spermatogenesis is an elaborate process of cell differentiation in which stem spermatogonia, through a series of events, become mature spermatozoa. The process can be divided into three main phases—mitotic, meiotic, and postmeiotic—each involving a class of germ cells. The process is primarily under the control of pituitary gonadotropins, FSH, and LH (via the stimulation of testosterone) and on interplay between Sertoli and germ cells. Sertoli cells are crucial for providing essential supports for germ cell proliferation and progression for various phases of development. The functions of Sertoli cells are also modulated directly and indirectly by various hormones, particularly FSH and LH. The striking changes in Sertoli cell morphology between active and inactive states of spermatogenesis are structural manifestations of alterations of these cells in response to concomitant endocrine changes in the testis. Studies using genetically altered mice either overexpressing or harboring a null mutation of specific genes further suggest that the process of spermatogenesis is regulated by multiple genes that control spermatogonial proliferation, meiosis, and spermiogenesis. Future efforts toward improved fertility control and clinical management of infertility associated with reduced sperm production in men are hampered by an incomplete understanding of the processes responsible for the regulation of normal spermatogenesis. Elucidation of the mechanisms by which these genes control the process of germ cell development will fill a major gap in the knowledge of this fundamental biologic process.

3.6. Clinical Implications

The understanding of the process and regulation of spermatogenesis has important implications in male infertility, male contraception and reproductive toxicology.

3.6.1. MALE INFERTILITY

Male factor accounts for at least 20% of infertility and may contribute to another 25% of infertility when causal factors are identified in both partners. Disorders of the hypothalamic pituitary account for a small proportion of male infertility. These patients usually have decreased secretion of both gonadotropins, resulting in cessation of spermatogenesis. Return of fertility is possible with treatment by exogenous hCG (or recombinant hLH) and recombinant hFSH. Primary testicular failure including congenital abnormalities such as Klinefelter syndrome, cryptorchidism, androgen insensitivity syndrome, and 5α-reductase deficiency and acquired disorders such as orchitis, trauma, torsion, and chemotherapeutic agents and, in some cases, severe damage of the seminiferous tubule epithelium resulting in Sertoli-cell-only syndrome and hyalinization of tubules (as commonly seen in patients with Klinefelter syndrome) may be associated with varying degrees of hypospermatogenesis. In many patients with primary testicular failure, there is depletion of germ cells in the testes and the infertility cannot be treated.

Recent studies have shown that up to 20% of men with azoospermia (no spermatozoa in the ejaculate) or severe oligozoospermia (<1 or 3 million/mL of sperm cells in the ejaculate) may have microdeletions in the long arm of the Y chromosome. Many of these mapped to the Yq6 region known as the AZF (azoospermia factor) region. Deletions can occur at the AZFa, AZFb, and AZFc regions, and larger deletions can occur in two to three regions. Studies of the phenotype-genotype relationship suggest that when the entire AZF region is deleted, the patient is azoospermic. Deletions in the AZFa and AZFb regions are also frequently associated with azoospermia rather than oligozoospermia. However, there is no apparent relationship that exists between the microdeletion region and the testicular phenotype. Because of the common occurrence of these Y chromosome abnormalities, patients with severe oligozoospermia or azoospermia are advised to be tested in Y chromosome microdeletions.

Obstructive azoospermia may be associated with obstruction at the epididymis and vas deferens, which might be associated with past genital tract infections. Congenital bilateral absence of the vas deferens occurs in about 30–50% of patients with obstructive azoospermia. These patients are usually heterozygous for a severe mutation in one allele in combination with another mild irritation of the cystic fibrosis transmembrane conductance regulator gene. Examination of the testes shows normal spermatogenesis.

Despite recent advances, there remains a substantial proportion of infertile men for whom the etiologic cause cannot be found. Treatment of male infertility owing to testicular defects has been significantly changed with the utilization of assisted reproductive technology and intracytoplasmic injection of spermatozoa into the eggs of the female partner.

3.6.2. MALE CONTRACEPTION

Currently, there are two male methods of contraception: condom and vas occlusion. Although the use of condoms can prevent both sexually transmitted infection and pregnancy, this method has a high user failure rate of 12–14% and may not be acceptable by many couples with stable relationships. Vas occlusion is considered irreversible, involves a minor surgery, and is not useful for couples desiring to have a family in the future. The hormonal methods of male contraception are based on the suppression of both FSH and LH by exogenous androgens or androgens in combination with a progestin or GnRH antagonist. Note that because LH and endogenous testosterone are suppressed by the exogenous hormone, an androgen is always required in hormonal male contraceptive methods to prevent the occurrence of hypogonadism. As indicated in the review above, exogenous hormones suppressed FSH action on the Sertoli cells and intratesticular testosterone to very low levels resulting in accelerated apoptosis, inhibition of spermation, and perhaps decreased proliferation of germ cells. As the spermatogonia are spared, after withdrawal of the exogenous hormones, full return of spermatogenesis to normal occurs. Currently, a large phase III clinical study is under way in China using an injectable testosterone ester alone as the male contraceptive, and a multicenter trial utilizing an injectable testosterone ester and a progestin implant is undergoing phase II studies in Europe. It is anticipated that a hormonal male contraceptive will be available for use in 7–10 yr.

3.6.3. MALE REPRODUCTIVE TOXICOLOGY

In recent years, several studies have implicated that semen quality is declining in men. Although this issue remains controversial, there is agreement that there are significant differences among sperm concentration in different regions in Europe and the United States. These differences in semen quality have been primarily ascribed to the differences in environmental pollutants. The most studied of these include the "endocrine disrupters" found in pesticides and herbicides. These endocrine disrupters are chemicals that bind and act via the ER as weak estrogen agonists, act via the AR as antiandrogens, or are coactivators or corepressors of these sex hormone receptors. The influence of such endocrine disrupters on male reproductive tract development is supported by some epidemiologic studies demonstrating increases in the incidence of hypospadias and cryptorchidism in boys in some countries. The issue of environmental pollutants of reproductive health is under intense study.

REFERENCE

Russell LD, Etllin RA, Sinha Hikim AP, Clegg ED. *Histological and Histopathological Evaluation of the Testis*. Clearwater, FL: Cache River Press, 1990:1–286.

SUGGESTED FURTHER READING

De Kretser DM, Kerr JB. The cytology of the testis. In: Knobil E, Neil JD, eds. The *Physiology of Reproduction*, 2nd Ed., New York, NY: Raven Press 1994:1177–1290.

De Kretser DM, Loveland KL, Meehan T, O'Bryan MK, Phillips DJ, Wreford NG. Inhibins, activins, and follistatin: actions on the testis. *Mol Cell Endocrinol* 2001;180:87–92.

McLachlan RI, O'Donnell L, Meachem SJ, Stanton PG, de Kretser DM, Pratis K, Robertson DM. Identification of specific sites of hormonal regulation in spermatogenesis in rats, monkeys, and man. *Recent Prog Horm Res* 2002;57:149–179.

Payne AH, Hardy MP, Russell LD, eds. *The Leydig Cell*. New York, NY: Cache River Press 1996.

Plant TM, Marshall GR. The functional significance of FSH in spermatogenesis and the control of its secretion in male primates. *Endocr Rev* 2001;22:764–786.

Sealfon SC, Weinstein H, Millar RP. Molecular mechanisms of ligand interaction with the gonadotropin-releasing hormone receptor. *Endocr Rev* 1997;18:180–205.

Sharpe RM. Regulation of spermatogenesis. In: Knobil E, Neil JD, eds. *The Physiology of Reproduction*, 2nd Ed., New York, NY: Raven 1994:1363–1434.

Stocco DM, Clark BJ. Regulation of the acute production of steroids in steroidogenic cells. *Endocr Rev* 1996;17:221–244.

Themmen APN, Huhtaniemi IT. Mutations of gonadotropins and gonadotropin receptors: elucidating the physiology and pathophysiology of pituitary-gonadal function. *Endocr Rev* 2000;21: 551–583.

28 Endocrinology of Aging

Steven W. J. Lamberts, MD, PhD

Contents

1. INTRODUCTION

Throughout adult life, all physiologic functions gradually decline. There is a diminished capacity for cellular protein synthesis, a decline in immune function, an increase in fat mass, a loss of muscle mass and strength, and a decrease in bone mineral density (BMD). Most elderly individuals die from the complications of atherosclerosis, cancer, or dementia. However, in an increasing number of the healthy elderly, loss of muscle strength is the limiting factor that determines their chances of living an independent life until death. Muscle weakness can be caused by aging of muscle fibers and their innervation, pain related to osteoarthritis, and chronic debilitating diseases. In addition, a sedentary lifestyle and decreased physical activity and disuse seem, to be very important determinants in this decline in muscle strength, because exercise training even at a very old age has been demonstrated to reverse significantly the decline in physical capacity. In other words, "use it or lose it;" activity is an extremely important treatment for aging.

As the average length of life in Western societies increases further, so does the interest in understanding the considerable variations that have been observed in the course and speed of the aging process within groups

From: *Endocrinology: Basic and Clinical Principles, Second Edition*
(S. Melmed and P. M. Conn, eds.) © Humana Press Inc., Totowa, NJ

of otherwise healthy individuals, with some people exhibiting extensive decline in physiologic functions with age and others little or none. Genetic factors, lifestyle, and societal investments in a safe and healthy environment are considered to be important determinants of successful aging. As life expectancy increases further in the coming years, it becomes more and more important to find interventions that might compress morbidity during the last part of life, with the goal to increase the number of years of healthy life with a full range of functional and mental capacity, without necessarily prolonging life.

Traditionally, the endocrine system in humans has been implicated as a driving part of the aging process. The availability of hormone replacement of all known hormones that might play a role in the aging process has supported this idea. Many signs and symptoms observed in young individuals with selected hormone deficiencies are similar to changes observed during the aging process, and hormone replacement in young individuals reverses virtually all these problems. Apart from these considerations concerning the role of hormones in the physiology of the aging process, the two clinically most prevalent and important changes in endocrine activity during aging that represent pathology (i.e., diseases) are in glucose tolerance and thyroid function.

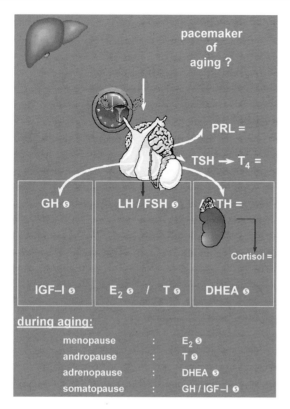

Fig. 1. During aging, declines in the activities of a number of hormonal systems occur. Prolactin (PRL), TSH (thyrotropin), and T$_4$ (thyroxin) levels in general remain unchanged. (Left) A decrease in growth hormone (GH) release by the pituitary gland causes a decrease in the production of insulin-like growth factor-1 (IGF-1) by the liver and other organs (somatopause). (Middle) A decrease in the release of luteinizing hormone (LH) and follicle-stimulating hormone (FSH) and decreased secretion at the gonadal level (from the ovaries, decreased E$_2$ causes menopause, and from the testicles, decreased testosterone [T] causes andropause, respectively). Immediately after the initiation of menopause, serum LH and FSH levels sharply increase. (Right) The adrenocortical cells responsible for the production of dehydroepiandrosterone (DHEA) decrease in activity (adrenopause), without clinically evident changes in adrenocorticotropic hormone and cortisol secretion. A central pacemaker in the hypothalamus or higher brain centers (or both) is hypothesized, which together with changes in the peripheral organs (the ovaries, testicles, and adrenal cortex) regulates the aging process of these endocrine axes. (Reproduced with permission from Lamberts et al., 1997.)

1.1. Glucose Tolerance and Diabetes Mellitus

Approximately 40% of individuals 65–74 yr old and >50% of individuals over 80 have impaired glucose tolerance or diabetes mellitus, and nearly half of these elderly diabetics are undiagnosed. These persons are at risk of developing secondary, mainly macrovascular complications at an accelerated rate. Pancreatic insulin receptor and postreceptor changes associated with aging are critical components of the endocrinology of aging; apart from relative decreased insulin secretion by β-cells, peripheral insulin resistance related to poor diet, physical inactivity, increased abdominal fat mass, and decreased lean body mass contribute to the deterioration of glucose metabolism. Dietary management, exercise, oral hypoglycemic agents, and insulin are the four components of treatment of these patients, whose medical care is costly and intensive.

1.2. Changes in Thyroid Function

Age-related thyroid dysfunction is common in the elderly. Lowered concentrations of plasma levorotators thyroxine (T$_4$) and increased thyrotropin-stimulating hormone (TSH) occur in 5–10% of elderly women. These abnormalities seem to be mainly caused by autoimmunity and may therefore be an expression of age-associated disease, rather than a consequence of the aging process.

It is well recognized that the general symptoms of aging can be easily confused with hypothyroidism, and in the past, decreased thyroid function was believed to be one of the hallmarks of the aging process. During aging a complex number of changes occur in thyroid hormone concentrations. Reduced outer-ring deiodination mediated by type I deiodinase results in a decline in T$_4$ degradation, with a reduced generation of triiodothyronine (T$_3$) and a decreased clearance of reverse T3. In addition, TSH secretion appears to be slightly decreased in healthy elderly humans when subjects with subclinical hypothyroidism are carefully excluded. The reason for such age-dependent reduction of TSH is uncertain. However, in spite of these complex changes in biochemical parameters, recent studies suggest that normal aging is associated with essentially normal thyroid function. The slight decrease in plasma T$_3$ concentration occurs largely within the broad normal range of the healthy elderly population, and this decrease has not been convincingly causally related to functional changes during the aging process. Evaluation of thyroid function in the elderly is necessary on a regular basis because of the increased prevalence of autoimmune subclinical hypothyroidism and nonthyroidal illness.

2. CHANGES IN HORMONE ACTIVITY DURING AGING

During aging three other hormonal systems show decreasing circulating hormone concentrations (Figs. 1 and 2), and these decreases have been considered mainly physiologic. In recent years, hormone replacement strat-

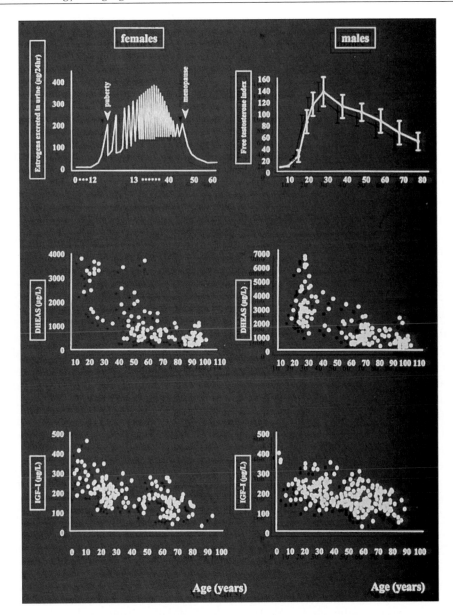

Fig. 2. Changes in hormone levels of healthy women (left) and men (right) during aging process. **(A,B)** Estrogen secretion throughout an individual healthy woman's life (expressed as urinary estrogen excretion) (A) and mean free testosterone index (ratio of serum total testosterone to sex hormone–binding globulin levels) during the life of healthy men (B). **(C,D)** Serum DHEAS and E and F serum IGF-1 levels in healthy women and men during aging process. Note the difference in the distribution of ages in different panels. (Reproduced with permission from Lamberts et al., 1997.)

egies have been developed in each case, but many of their aspects remain controversial, and increasing hormone blood levels to those found in 30- to 50-yr-old individuals has not been universally proven to be safe and of benefit.

3. MENOPAUSE

The most dramatic and rapidly occurring change in women around the age of 50 is menopause. Cycling

estradiol (E_2) production from the ovarian follicles is suddenly exhausted, reproduction stops, and (very) low, constant E_2 levels remain, mainly produced by aromatization of adrenal androgens in nonendocrine tissues, such as adipose tissue.

This acute drop in circulating estrogen levels and the permanent cessation of menstruation around age 50 yr is often accompanied by vasomotor reactions, sleep disturbances, changes in skin and body composition, and a depressed mood. The use of hormone replacement therapy ([HRT], estrogens or estrogen plus progestogen) rapidly alleviates these symptoms of menopause. In women with these symptoms, HRT also improves verbal memory, vigilance, reasoning, and motor speed, but there is no enhancement of other cognitive functions. Generally, no benefits of HRT are observed in asymptomatic women.

Currently, the long-term use (5–10 yr or more) of HRT after menopause is surrounded by controversy; many studies in the past indicated advantages regarding prevention of the three chronic disorders most common in elderly women: cardiovascular diseases, osteoporosis, and dementia. However, these beneficial effects are a double-edged sword because long-term HRT is accompanied by a significant increase in the incidence of breast cancer, thrombosis, and stroke. The controversy has arisen partly because of differences in the selection of participating menopausal women in the large prospective trials with HRT. For example, the inclusion of nurses, who are probably more aware of the advantages of healthy lifestyle than the "normal" population of menopausal women, might have introduced a "healthy user bias" in several of the best prospective clinical trials, which were, however, mostly observational and not randomized controlled.

In 2002, the interim results of the Women's Health Initiative Trial were published. This is a randomized controlled trial to assess the risks and benefits of intervention strategies in the postmenopausal population in t he United States. The trial has in fact shown that HRT increases the risk of developing cardiovascular disease, including coronary heart disease (the primary outcome) and stroke, although it showed benefits for preventing hip fractures and bowel cancer. The relative risks of developing invasive breast cancer, coronary heart disease, and stroke were increased, although the absolute risks remained very small. One treatment arm of the trial included more than 16,000 postmenopausal women who were taking continuous combined estrogen-progestagen HRT, using conjugated equine estrogens (0.625 mg) plus medroxyprogesterone acetate (2.5 mg daily), tested against placebo. This primary prevention study was due to run for 8.5 yr, but was halted at just over 5 yr because the number of cases of breast cancer had reached a prespecified safety limit. For 10,000 women taking HRT each year, compared with those not taking it, there would be an additional eight cases of invasive breast cancers, seven heart attacks, eight strokes, and eight pulmonary embolisms. However, there would also be six fewer bowel cancers and five fewer hip fractures. Overall mortality was not increased with therapy.

The decision to stop the trial and to change US recommendations for the use of postmenopausal HRT for primary prevention of chronic conditions might not be automatically applicable. First, one should realize that the weight and BMI of the US female population were, in general, high, and these factors alone make the participants more prone to breast cancer, stroke, thrombosis, and cardiovascular disease while in their excess adipose tissue enough estrogens might have been produced by aromatization of adrenal androgens, making the intake of additional HRT a pharmacologic rather than a replacement therapy. Second, more and more evidence is provided that genetic testing, such as for estrogen receptor (ER) polymorphisms and factor V Leiden, will not only better predict a positive outcome of HRT on cardiovascular disease, but the chances of developing thrombosis as well. Third, HRT's potential impact on the incidence of dementia needs to be considered.

Women seem to be at higher risk of developing Alzheimer disease, and this is in part owing to their increased longevity. It has been suggested that the abrupt decline of estrogen production at menopause may be associated with a vulnerability of the female brain. Elderly men have an intrinsic supply of estrogen because they aromatize testosterone into estradiol within the brain. There is strong experimental evidence that in the intact brain estradiol might play a key neuroprotective role by delaying the initiation phase of onset of neurodegenerative disease. It was demonstrated that in mice lacking the ERα, estrogen protects the brain from injury by accelerating and amplifying the activity of this receptor. As a consequence, genes that help the brain cells survive are activated, or genes that harm the brain cells are suppressed.

Postmenopausal HRT was considered to prevent or delay cognitive decline and dementia in postmenopausal women. In a systematic review and metaanalysis of all observational studies conducted thus far, it was concluded that HRT started at age 50, at the start of menopause, is associated with a decreased risk of dementia (summary odds ratio: 0.66; 95% confidence interval: 0.53–0.82). However, many of these studies also have important methodologic limitations, with the healthy user bias mentioned earlier an important one. In the Women's Health Initiative Trial, a randomized controlled trial, in which HRT was started at age 65, no improvement of cognitive function was observed.

HRT administered for 1 yr in women with mild to moderate Alzheimer disease did not slow disease progression, nor did it improve global, cognitive, or functional outcome. However, the use of high-dose estrogens to improve cognition in women with dementia was reported in a small study. In a prospective study of incident dementia among 1357 men (mean age: 73.2 yr) and 1889 women (mean age: 74.5 yr) residing in a single county in Utah, it was again demonstrated that prior HRT use is very closely associated with reduced risk of dementia. There was a highly statistical HRT duration-dependent decrease in incident dementia in women after the age of 80, with a decrease in incident dementia in women who had used HRT more than 10 yr in the past compared with that found in men. There was no apparent benefit of current HRT in the older group of women.

These considerations on the advantages and risks of HRT in healthy postmenopausal women are very sobering. There is no doubt that early HRT, taken immediately at menopause, alleviates most symptomatology and is, in principle, safe in the shortterm. In women in whomcardiovascular disease is symptomatic, other (preventive) medications including β-blockers, ACE-inhibitors, aspirin, and/or statins have been proven to be effective. In addition, in symptomatic osteoporosis, bisphosphonates have preventive efficacy similar to or even better than HRT.

Recent studies demonstrated that a higher than usual dietary intake of phytoestrogens (isoflavones and lignans) is associated with a lower aortic stiffness in postmenopausal women, suggesting that phytoestrogens have a protective effect on the risk of atherosclerosis and arterial degeneration through an effect on arterial walls, especially among older women. Interestingly, alcohol consumption was also inversely associated with aortic stiffness, supporting the concept that moderate alcohol consumption decreases the risk of cardiovascular disease in postmenopausal women.

In summary, the verdict on the use of HRT in health-conscious women is, in general, negative at present. With the further development of genetic testing to identify those women who might benefit most, and/or are most at risk for thrombotic events and/or breast cancer, the decision to prescribe HRT early after menopause in order to obtain the early beneficial effects on subjective well-being, as well as possible late delaying effects on dementia, might remain an option.

3.1. Selective ER Modulators

A new development in the preventive treatment of the consequences of long-term estrogen deficiency in menopause is the availability of targeted estrogen replacement therapy using selective estrogen receptor modulators (SERMs). Early studies using tamoxifen in the treatment of breast cancer indicated variable estrogenic and antiestrogenic actions of the compound in different organs. Tamoxifen suppresses the growth of ER-positive breast cancer cells; in addition, long-term tamoxifen treatment of patients surviving breast cancer indicated a partial protection against age-related decrease in BMD. These observations were explained by the fact that tamoxifen, and other compounds such as raloxifene, have antiestrogenic actions on normal and cancerous breast tissue, but agonistic actions on bone, lipids, and blood vessel walls. The differential effects of these SERMs in different organs may be explained by the activation of different forms of ER, in which the form is the "classic" estrogen, whereas the β form mediates the vascular and bone effects of estrogens. Raloxifene, in contrast to tamoxifen and estradiol, does not stimulate endometrial thickness and vaginal bleeding. It has protective effects for vertebral fractures in menopausal women with osteoporosis. A very promising effect of raloxifene is its reported chemoprotective action on breast cancer.

4. ANDROPAUSE

Age-associated hypogonadism develops not as clearly in men as in women. The key difference from menopause is the gradual, often subtle change in androgen levels in men compared with the precipitate fall of estrogen production in women (Fig. 2). There is general agreement that as men age, there is a decline in the concentration of serum total testosterone that begins after age 40. In cross-sectional studies, the annual decline in total and "free" testosterone is 0.4 and 1.2%, respectively. The higher decline in free testosterone levels is related to the increase in levels of SHBG with aging. "Andropause" is characterized by a decrease in testicular Leydig cell numbers and in their secretory capacity, as well as by an age-related decrease in episode and stimulated gonadotropin secretion.

It remains unclear whether the well-known biologic changes during aging in men, such as reduction in sexual activity, in muscle mass and strength, and in skeletal mineralization, are causally related to these changes in testosterone bioactivity ("andropause").

In a group of more than 400 independently living elderly men ages 73–94 (mean age: 78 yr), a positive association was observed between serum total and free testosterone concentrations and muscle strength as well as an inverse relationship with fat mass. In addition, low bioavailable testosterone was associated with a depressed mood in a population-based study in 856 men (age: 50–89).

Many persuasive reports in the literature demonstrate that treatment of men of all ages (young, adult, and old) with clear clinical and biochemical hypogonadism with testosterone replacement instantly reverses vasomotor activity (flushes and sweats): improves libido, sexual activity, and mood; increases muscle mass, strength, and bone mineralization; prevents fractures; decreases fat mass; and decreases fatigue and poor concentration. Additionally, the treatment of adult healthy men with supraphysiologic doses of testosterone, especially when combined with resistance exercise training, increases fat-free mass and muscle size and strength.

A search for studies reporting the results of androgen therapy in older men demonstrates that most studies were small, short-term, noncontrolled, and without uniform endpoints.

Numerous studies of large populations of healthy men have shown a marked rise in the incidence of impotence to >50% in men ages 60–70. Although this increase in impotence occurs in the same age group that shows a clear decline in serum (free) testosterone levels, no causal relationships have been demonstrated. Testosterone replacement therapy in elderly men is in most instances not effective for the treatment of loss of libido or impotence in individuals with serum testosterone concentrations within the normal age-matched range; other factors such as atherosclerosis, alcohol consumption, smoking, and the quality of personal relationships seem to be more important denominators. Only in the case of clear hypogonadism are the decrease in libido and potency restored by testosterone therapy. This suggests that there is a theshold level of testosterone in the low normal range, below which libido and sexual function are impaired and above which there is no further enhancement of response.

Summarizing the literature available on the preventive treatment of healthy elderly men with testosterone at a dose that increases serum testosterone concentrations to those observed in 20-to 30-yr-olds demonstrates limited anabolic effects on body composition (a slight decrease in fat mass, and a slight increase in muscle mass). In addition, minor beneficial effects on muscle strength or physical performance have been observed in a minority of studies.

Detailed analysis of a number of studies in which elderly men selected on the basis of the presence of "low" pretreatment serum testosterone concentrations suggests a beneficial effect of testosterone replacement therapy on muscle strength, BMD, mood, as well as (subjective) aspects of the quality of life.

In conclusion, testosterone at supraphysiologic doses when administered to eugonadal men increases muscle mass and strength. "Replacement" therapy directed at restoring serum testosterone therapy in healthy elderly males to levels observed between the age of 30 and 50 lowers fat mass and increases lean mass to a limited extent without a clear beneficial effect on muscle strength and physical performance. At present, it remains uncertain whether testosterone replacement produces clinically meaningful improvements in muscle function without significant adverse effects in frail older men or in elderly men with serum testosterone concentrations between 7.0 and 11.4 nmol/L.

If one decides to start testosterone replacement the major goal of therapy is to replace testosterone levels to as close to "physiologic" age-matched levels as possible. The dose should thus be titrated according to serum levels. At present, the duration of administration of testosterone is uncertain. Control of prostate size, prostate-specific antigen levels, and hematocrit levels is mandatory. The identification of elderly men who might benefit most from testosterone treatment remains uncertain, and the risks to the prostate and possible effects on the process of atherosclerosis remain subjects for study. The concept of developing androgenic compounds with variable biologic action in different organs (selective androgen receptor modulation) is currently being pursued.

5. ANDRENOPAUSE
5.1. Dehydroepiandrosterone

Humans are unique among primates and rodents because the human adrenal cortex secretes large amounts of the steroid precursors DHEA and its sulfate derivative DHEAS. Serum DHEAS concentrations in adult men and women are more than 100 times higher than those of testosterone and more than 1000 times higher than those of estradiol. In healthy subjects, serum concentrations of DHEAS and its sulfate are highest in the third decade of life, after which the concentrations of both gradually decrease, so that by the age of 70–80 yr, the values are about 20% of peak values in men and 30% of peak values in women (Fig. 2).

Both DHEA and DHEAS seem to be inactive precursors, which, via a number of enzymes, are transformed within human tissues by a complicated network of enzymes into androgens and/or estrogens. The key enzymes are aromatase, steroid sulfatase, 3β-hydroxysteroid-dehydrogenases, and at least seven organ-specific 17β-hydroxysteroid dehydrogenases. Labrie introduced the name "intracrinology" to describe this synthesis of active steroids in peripheral target tissues, where the action is exerted in the same cells in which synthesis takes place, without release in the extracellular space and general circulation. In postmenopausal women, nearly 100% of sex steroids are synthesized in peripheral tissues from precursors of adrenal origin except for a small contribution from ovarian and/or adrenal testosterone and androstenedione. Thus, in postmenopausal women, virtually all active sex steroids are made in target tissues by an intracrine mechanism. Also in elderly males the intracrine production of androgens is important: less than 50% of androgens is derived from testicular production.

As already stated, the situation of a high secretion rate of adrenal precursor sex steroids in men and women is completely different from animal models used in the laboratory, in which the secretion of sex steroids takes place exclusively in the gonads. In many experiments, it has been demonstrated that (long-term) administration of DHEA to rats and mice prevents obesity, diabetes mellitus, cancer, and heart disease, while it enhances immune function.

These experimental animal data have been used as an argument that administration of DHEA in adult/elderly individuals prolongs life-span and might be an "elixir of youth." Supportive data in humans are few, however, and highly controversial.

Several randomized placebo-controlled studies demonstrated that oral administration of DHEA might have beneficial effects on perceived physical and psychologic well-being in both sexes without an effect on libido. A number of other, well-controlled trials with DHEA subsequently did not demonstrate a clinically significant effect.

A physiologic functional role of DHEA in women has been demonstrated. However, in a careful double-blind study in women with adrenal insufficiency, administration of DHEA (50 mg/d) normalized serum concentrations of DHEA, DHEAS, androstenedione and testosterone. DHEA significantly improved overall well-being, as demonstrated by scores for depression and anxiety, the frequency of sexual thoughts, sexual interest, as well as satisfaction with both mental and physical aspects of sexuality.

In conclusion, DHEA(S) is a universal precursor to the peripheral local production and action of estrogens and androgens in the elderly. The addition of DHEA (50 mg) to the existing big pool of DHEA(S) in unselected elderly individuals has no or only limited clinical effects, especially in elderly women. It is unknown whether the increase in sex steroid levels induced by long-term administration of DHEA is safe regarding the development of ovarian, prostate, or other types of steroid-dependent cancers. DHEA is currently widely used within the United States as a "treatment against aging." With the scientific verdict still out, without further confirmation of DHEA's reported beneficial actions in humans, and without a better understanding of its potential risks, it is premature to recommend the routine use of DHEA for delaying or preventing the physiologic consequences of aging.

5.2. Cortisol

Cortisol production by the adrenals seems to have a major impact on memory and cognition. In cross-sectional as well as longitudinal studies, it was demonstrated that higher cortisol levels are associated with poorer memory performance and a higher likelihood of memory decline, especially in women. The detrimental effects of cortisol seem to be directed at the hippocampus. An iv bolus of 35 mg of hydrocortisone reduces hippocampal glucose metabolism, as measured by positron emission tomography scan, in elderly individuals by 12–16%, and the hippocampal volume, measured by magnetyic resonance imaging, is smaller in patients with Cushing's syndrome.

In a small prospective study in healthy elderly individuals, an association between adrenal steroid hormones and cognitive function was confirmed. Free cortisol levels appeared to be associated with cognitive impairment, and a lower degree of cortisol suppression after administration of dexamethasone was associated with an increased risk of cognitive decline. These findings support the concept that stress and anxiety have important consequences regarding to the degree and speed of the decline in memory and other cognitive abilities in the elderly. Clear clinical developments regarding to medical intervention in this process remain elusive, however.

6. SOMATOPAUSE

The third endocrine system that gradually declines in activity during aging is the GH/IGF-1 axis. Mean pulse amplitude, duration and fraction of GH secreted, but not pulse frequency, gradually decrease during aging. In parallel, there is a progressive fall in circulating IGF-1 levels in both sexes. There is no evidence for a "peripheral" factor in this process of somatopause, and its triggering pacemaker seems mainly localized in the hypothalamus, because pituitary somatotropes, even in very old individuals, can be restored to their youthful secretory capacity during treatment with GH-releasing peptides.

The expectation that this decline in GH and IGF-1 secretion contributes to the decline in functional capacity in the elderly ("somatopause") is mainly derived from studies in which GH replacement therapy of GH-deficient adults was shown to increase muscle mass, muscle strength, bone mass, and the quality of life. A beneficial effect on the lipid profile and an important decrease in fat mass were also observed in such patients. As in hypogonadal individuals, adult GH deficiency can thus be considered a model of normal aging, because a number of catabolic processes that are central in the

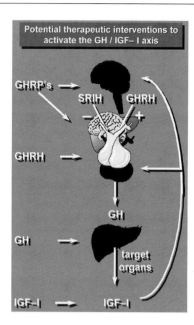

Fig. 3. Schematic representation of the regulation of GH/IGF-1 axis, as well as potential hormonal intervention of different compounds to activate this axis on different levels (left).

biology of aging can be reversed by administration of GH.

In 1990, Rudman published the findings of a trial that provoked headlines in the popular press. In this trial, healthy older men were administered recombinant human GH, heralded as a treatment for aging. The initial optimism prompted many investigators to start clinical trials to investigate the possible benefits of GH in older people. However, today it seems fair to state that GH remains a promising treatment still looking for a proven indication.

Rudman's study concerned men with IGF-1 levels that were deficient by young adult standards. In the 12 men receiving active treatment for 6 mo, fat mass fell, lean body mass rose by 8.8% ($p < 0.05$), and lumbar vertebral density (but not other bone sites) rose by 1.6% ($p < 0.05$). Compared with age-related differences observed in cross-sectional studies, these were massive effects. However, the trial should only be regarded as a pilot study because the treatment groups were not randomized and the subjects were not blinded. In a subsequent similar study, only 18 of 62 subjects completed 12 mo of treatment without experiencing one or more of the three common side effects: carpal tunnel syndrome, gynecomastia, and hyperglycemia. Patients who produced higher IGF-1 levels experienced more side effects. Subsequent trials have generally confirmed the changes in fat and lean tissue but shown inconsistent effects on bone density.

Furthermore, in contrast to the findings in younger GH-deficient adults with pituitary disease, the potentially beneficial changes in muscle and other lean body tissue obtainable in older people have not translated into improved functional abilities. Exercise programs have proven ability to enhance muscle mass and strength, even in very frail elderly people. Adding GH treatment to an exercise intervention produced no additional benefit for healthy males. Although the exercise-related GH responses of older people are attenuated, it has not been shown that a youthful GH response is necessary for older people to benefit maximally from exercise.

Other components of the GH/IGF-1 axis are effective in activating GH and IGF-1 secretion (Fig. 3). Long-acting derivatives of the hypothalamic peptide GH-releasing hormone (GHRH) given twice daily subcutaneously for 14 d to healthy men 70 yr old increased GH and IGF-1 levels to those encountered in 35-yr-olds. This finding supports the concept that somatopause is primarily hypothalamically driven, and that pituitary somatotropes retain their capacity to synthesize and secrete high levels of GH. GH-releasing peptides (GHRPs) are oligopeptides with even more powerful GH-releasing effects. Originally developed by design, it has recently been demonstrated that GHRPs mediate their GH-secretory effects through endogenous specific receptors. Nonpeptide analogs such as MK-677 and L692,429 have powerful GH-releasing effects, restoring IGF-1 secretion in the elderly to levels encountered in young adults. Long-term oral administration of MK-677 to healthy elderly individuals increased lean body mass, but not muscle strength. If proven to be GH specific, these orally active GHRP derivatives might be important alternatives to subcutaneously administered GH for studies in the reversal of somatopause, in the prevention of frailty, and in the reversal of acute catabolism.

Recombinant IGF-1 produces less fluid retention and lower blood glucose than GH. Four weeks of treatment of healthy older women (mean age: 71 yr) with either GH or recombinant human IGF-1 (rhIGF-1) produced potentially beneficial and adverse effects similar to those seen in men, although rhIGF-1 was better tolerated. In combination with a reducing diet and a program of exercise, these treatments produced weight loss in healthy but obese older women without compromising lean body mass or gains in muscle strength, but side effects were a problem, causing 5 of 33 subjects to drop out.

In a 26-wk randomized, double-blind, placebo-controlled parallel-group trial in healthy elderly men and women, the effects of GH and/or sex steroids (testosterone in men, estrogens and progesterone in women) on body composition, strength, and endurance, as well as adverse effects were studied. GH with or without sex steroids induced in these healthy aged women and men the well-known increase in lean body mass and decrease in fat mass. The combination of GH and testosterone caused a marginal increase in muscle strength and maximum oxygen uptake in men, but women had no significant change in strength or cardiovascular endurance. Formation of edema, carpal tunnel syndrome, arthralgias, and deterioration of glucose tolerance or even development of diabetes frequently occurred, limiting the use of GH in aging.

Another still unsolved issue is the safety of long-term administration of GH. Epidemiologic studies, together with many experimental data, suggest that the IGF-1 system is involved in tumor development and progression. It remains uncertain at present whether long-term GH treatment in the elderly thereby might contribute to the risk of prostate, breast, and/or colon cancer.

In conclusion, the use of GH and/or other compounds that activate IGF-1 bioactivity in the treatment of the elderly, either as a preventive intervention delaying the aging process or as a treatment to counteract frailty and/or catabolism, has not been proven to be safe and successful. At present, the use of GH therefore cannot be advised in elderly individuals.

REFERENCE

Lamberts SW, van den Beld AW, van der Lely AJ. The endocrinology of aging. *Science* 1997;278:419–424.

SUGGESTED READINGS

Blackman MR, Sorkin JD, Münzer T, et al. Growth hormone and sex steroid administration in healthy aged women and men. *JAMA* 2002;288:2282–2292.

Grady D. Postmenopausal hormones: therapy for symptoms only. *N Engl J Med* 2003;348:1835–1854.

Labrie F, Luu-The V, Lin SX. Intracrinology: role of the family of 17 beta-hydroxysteroid dehydrogenases in human physiology and disease. *J Mol Endocrinol* 2000;25:1–6.

Lamberts SW. The endocrinology of aging and the brain. *Arch Neurol* 2002;59:1709–1711.

Li CI, Malone KE, Porter PL, Weiss NS, Tang MC, Cushing-Haugen KL, Daling JR. Relationship between long durations and different regimens of hormone therapy and risk of breast cancer. *JAMA* 2003;289:3254–3263.

Riggs BL, Hartmann LC. Selective estrogen-receptor modulators: mechanisms of action and application to clinical practice. *N Engl J Med* 2003;348:618–629.

Rowe JW, Kahn RL. Human aging: usual and successful. *Science* 1987;237:143-149.

Rudman D, Feller AG, Nagraj HS. Effect of human growth hormone in men over 60 years old. *N Engl J Med* 1990;323:1–6.

Vermeulen A. Androgen replacement therapy in the aging male: a critical evaluation. *J Clin Endocrinol Metab* 2001;86:2380–2390.

INDEX